**Cardiac Pacing
and ICDs**

To my parents, Roslyn and Leon Ellenbogen, who inspired a lifelong thirst for learning. To my wife, Phyllis, and children, Michael, Amy and Bethany, whose patience and love made this project successful.

Kenneth A Ellenbogen, MD, FACC

To my parents William B. Wood, PhD and Donna S. Wood, EdD, for their enduring examples of scholarship; to my wife Helen E. Wood, PhD for her love and support, and to Grand Master Seung Gyoo Dong for his guidance – "thinking before acting".

Mark A Wood, MD, FACC

Cardiac Pacing and ICDs

FIFTH EDITION

Kenneth A Ellenbogen, MD, FACC
Kontos Professor of Medicine
Director, Electrophysiology and Pacing Laboratory
Virginia Commonwealth University Medical Center
Richmond, VA, USA

Mark A Wood, MD, FACC
Professor of Medicine
Assistant Director, Electrophysiology and Pacing Laboratory
Virginia Commonwealth University Medical Center
Richmond, VA, USA

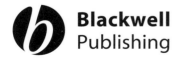

Blackwell
Publishing

Library of Congress Cataloging-in-Publication Data
Cardiac pacing and ICDs / edited by Kenneth A. Ellenbogen, Mark A. Wood. -- 5th ed.
    p. ; cm.
  Includes bibliographical references and index.
  ISBN 978-1-4051-6350-7 (alk. paper)
  1. Cardiac pacing. 2. Implantable cardioverter-defibrillators. I. Ellenbogen, Kenneth A. II. Wood, Mark A.
  [DNLM: 1. Cardiac Pacing, Artificial. 2. Defibrillators, Implantable. 3. Pacemaker, Artificial. WG 168 C26333 2008]
  RC684.P3C29 2008
  617.4'120645--dc22

                                                                                              2008008379

ISBN: 978-1-4051-6350-7

A catalogue record for this book is available from the British Library.

Set in 9.5/12 pt Palatino by Sparks, Oxford – www.sparkspublishing.com
Printed and bound in Singapore by Markono Print Media Pte Ltd

1   2008

Contents

A PDA version of this book by Skyscape is available from:
www.blackwellpublishing.com/9781405163507

Contributors

Amin Al-Ahmad, MD
Associate Director, Cardiac Arrhythmia Service
Assistant Professor of Cardiovascular Medicine
Stanford University School of Medicine
Stanford, California

Mark L Blitzer, MD
Clinical Instructor in Medicine
Yale University School of Medicine
Hospital of Saint Raphael
New Haven, Connecticut

Jeffrey A Brinker, MD
Professor of Medicine and Radiology
Johns Hopkins University School of Medicine
Baltimore, Maryland

Sumeet S Chugh, MD, FACC
Section Head, Clinical Electrophysiology
Director, Cardiac Arrhythmia Prevention Center
Oregon Health and Science University
Portland, Oregon

Joshua M Cooper, MD
Assistant Professor of Medicine
University of Pennsylvania Health System
Philadelphia, Pennsylvania

Frank Cuoco, MD
Senior Electrophysiology Fellow
Medical University of South Carolina
Charleston, South Carolina

Michael R Gold, MD, PhD
Michael E Assey Professor of Medicine
Chief of Cardiology
Associate Dean, Interdisciplinary Clinical
Programs
Medical University of South Carolina
Charleston, South Carolina

David L Hayes, MD
Chair, Division of Cardiovascular Diseases and
Internal Medicine, Mayo Clinic
Professor of Medicine, Mayo College of Medicine
Rochester, Minnesota

G Neal Kay, MD
Director, Clinical Electrophysiology Section
Professor of Medicine
Division of Cardiovascular Disease
The University of Alabama at Birmingham
Birmingham, Alabama

Joseph E Marine, MD
Director of Electrophysiology
Johns Hopkins Bayview Medical Center
Assistant Professor of Medicine
Johns Hopkins University School of Medicine
Baltimore, Maryland

Suneet Mittal, MD
Director, Electrophysiology Laboratory
The St. Luke's-Roosevelt Hospital Center
Columbia University College of Physicians and
Surgeons
New York City, New York

Robert W Peters, MD
Chief of Cardiology
Baltimore VA Medical Center
Professor of Medicine
The University of Maryland School of Medicine
Baltimore, Maryland

Dwight W Reynolds, MD
Chief, Cardiovascular Section
Professor of Medicine
The University of Oklahoma Health Sciences
Center
Oklahoma City, Oklahoma

Mark H Schoenfeld, MD
Clinical Professor of Medicine
Yale University School of Medicine
Director Cardiac Electrophysiology and
Pacemaker Laboratory
Hospital of Saint Raphael
New Haven, Connecticut

Bruce S Stambler, MD
Professor of Medicine
University Hospitals Case Medical Center
Case Western Reserve University
Cleveland, Ohio

Michael O Sweeney, MD
Cardiac Arrhythmia Service
Brigham and Women's Hospital
Associate Professor of Medicine
Harvard Medical School
Boston, Massachusetts

Pugazhendhi Vijayaraman, MD
Fellowship Director
Geisinger Medical Center
Danville, Pennsylvania

Paul J Wang, MD
Professor of Medicine
Director Cardiac Arrhythmia Services and Cardiac
Electrophysiology Laboratory
Stanford University School of Medicine
Stanford, California

Preface

The world of device therapy continues to be full of exciting new technological developments and important clinical trials since the last edition. We have worked hard to further integrate new developments in the fields of pacing, defibrillation and cardiac resynchronization into this edition. We continue to strive to make the material accessible to beginning and intermediate students of cardiology and electrophysiology, regardless of whether they are residents or fellows in training, physicians in private practice, physicians at academic medical institutions, nurses in clinics or hospitals, engineers from industry or other allied healthcare professionals.

We have thoroughly revised this book with a number of new authors and several completely rewritten new chapters. We have worked vigorously to delete old figures and difficult to read figures, and at the same time have added many new and revised figures, as well as many new tables and flowcharts throughout.

This revision is made possible by the scholarship of our contributors, who have worked assiduously to help us turn out a first-rate book. For our contributors and ourselves, we are indebted to the inspiration and dedication of our fellows, faculty and colleagues. We learn from their questions, and their inquisitiveness helps make us better teachers and doctors. We are also indebted to our family and friends, who encouraged us through this project. We thank Dr George Vetrovec for his support of our scholarly activities and Gina Almond and Beckie Brand for their encouragement during this project.

Kenneth A Ellenbogen, MD, FACC
Mark A Wood, MD, FACC

A PDA version of this book by Skyscape is available from:
www.blackwellpublishing.com/9781405163507

CHAPTER 1

Indications for permanent and temporary cardiac pacing

Robert W Peters, Pugazhendhi Vijayaraman, Kenneth A Ellenbogen

Anatomy

To understand the principles and concepts involved in cardiac pacing more completely, a brief review of the anatomy and physiology of the specialized conduction system is warranted (Fig. 1.1, Table 1.1).

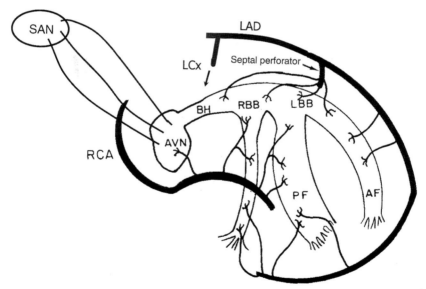

Fig. 1.1 A schematic diagram of the conduction system (SAN, sinus node; AVN, AV node; BH, bundle of His; LBB, left bundle branch; RBB, right bundle branch; AF, left anterior superior fascicle; PF, posterior inferior fascicle of the left bundle branch). The arterial supply is shown (RCA, right coronary artery; LAD, left anterior descending coronary artery; LCx, left circumflex coronary artery). For further description, see text.

Cardiac Pacing and ICDs, 5th edition. Edited by Kenneth A. Ellenbogen and Mark A. Wood.
© 2008 Blackwell Publishing, ISBN: 978-1-4051-6350-7

Table 1.1 The specialized conduction system

Structure	Location	Histology	Arterial blood supply	Autonomic innervation	Physiology
SA node	Subepicardial; junction of SVC and HRA	Abundant P cells	SA nodal artery from RCA 55% or LCx 45%	Abundant	Normal impulse generator
AV node	Subendocardial; interatrial septum	Fewer P cells, Purkinje cells, "working" myocardial cells	AV nodal artery from RCA 90%, LCx 10%	Abundant	Delays impulse, subsidiary pacemaker
His bundle	Membranous septum	Narrow tubular structure of Purkinje fibers in longitudinal compartments; few P cells	AV nodal artery, branches of LAD	Sparse	Conducts impulses from AV node to bundle branches
Bundle branches	Starts in muscular septum and branches out into ventricles	Purkinje fibers; highly variable anatomy	Branches of LAD, RCA	Sparse	Activates ventricles

AV, atrioventricular; HRA, high right atrium; LAD, left anterior descending coronary artery; LCx, left circumflex coronary artery; RCA, right coronary artery; SA, sinoatrial; SVC, superior vena cava.

Sinoatrial node

The sinoatrial (SA) node is a subepicardial structure located at the junction of the right atrium and superior vena cava. It has abundant autonomic innervation and a copious blood supply; it is often located within the adventitia of the large SA nodal artery, a proximal branch of the right coronary artery (55%), or the left circumflex coronary artery. Histologically, the SA node consists of a dense framework of collagen that contains a variety of cells, among them the large, centrally located P cells, which are thought to contain the principal pacemaker cells which initiate impulses and spontaneous electrical activity; transitional cells, intermediate in structure between P cells and regular atrial myocardial cells; and Purkinje-like fiber tracts, extending through the perinodal area and into the atrium. Once the impulse exits the sinus node and the perinodal tissue it traverses the atrium to the atrioventricular (AV) node.

Atrioventricular node

The AV node is a small subendocardial structure within the interatrial septum located at the convergence of the specialized conduction tracts that course through the atria. Like the SA node, the AV node has extensive autonomic innervation and an abundant blood supply from the large AV nodal artery, a branch of the right coronary artery, in 90% of patients, and from the left curcumflex artery in 10%. Histological examination of the AV node reveals a variety of cells embedded in a loose collagenous network including P cells (although not nearly as many as in the SA node), atrial transitional cells, ordinary myocardial cells and Purkinje cells.

His bundle

Purkinje fibers emerging from the area of the distal AV node converge gradually to form the His bundle, a narrow tubular structure that runs through the membranous septum to the crest of the muscular septum, where it divides into the bundle branches. The His bundle has relatively sparse autonomic innervation, although its blood supply is quite ample, emanating from both the AV nodal artery and septal branches of the left anterior descending artery. Longitudinal strands of Purkinje fibers, divided into separate parallel compartments by a collagenous skeleton, can be discerned by histological examination of the His bundle. Relatively sparse P cells can also be identified, embedded within the collagen. The rapid conduction of electrical impulses across the His–Purkinje system is responsible for the almost simultaneous activation of the right and left ventricles.

Bundle branches

The bundle branch system is an enormously complex network of interlacing Purkinje fibers that varies greatly among individuals. It generally starts as one or more large fiber bands that split and fan out across the ventricles until they finally terminate in a Purkinje network that interfaces with the myocardium. In some cases, the bundle branches clearly conform to a trifascicular or quadrifascicular system. In other cases, however, detailed dissection of the conduction system has failed to delineate separate fascicles. The right bundle is usually a single, discrete structure that extends down the right side of the interventricular septum to the base of the anterior papillary muscle, where it divides into three or more branches. The left bundle more commonly originates as a very broad band of interlacing fibers that spread out over the left ventricle, sometimes in two or three distinct fiber tracts. There is relatively little autonomic innervation of the bundle branch system, but the blood supply is extensive, with most areas receiving branches from both the right and left coronary systems.

Physiology

The SA node has the highest rate of spontaneous depolarization (automaticity) in the specialized conduction system and, under ordinary circumstances, it is the major generator of cardiac impulses. Its unique location astride the large SA nodal artery provides an ideal milieu for continuous monitoring and instantaneous adjustment of heart rate to meet the body's changing metabolic needs. The SA node is connected to the AV node by several specialized fiber tracts, the function of which has not been fully elucidated. The AV node appears to have three major functions: it delays the passing impulse for approximately 0.04s under normal circumstances, permitting complete atrial emptying with appropriate loading of the ventricles; it serves as a subsidiary impulse generator, as its concentration of P cells is second only to that of the SA node; and it acts as a type of filter, limiting ventricular rates in the event of an atrial tachyarrhythmia.

The His bundle arises from the convergence of Purkinje fibers from the AV node, although the exact point at which the AV node ends and the His bundle begins has not been delineated either anatomically or electrically. The separation of the His bundle into longitudinally distinct compartments by the collagenous framework allows for longitudinal dissociation of electrical impulses. Thus, a localized lesion below the bifurcation of the His bundle (into the bundle branches) may cause a specific conduction defect (e.g. left anterior fascicular block). The bundle branches arise as a direct continuation of the His bundle fibers. Disease within any aspect of the His bundle branch system may cause conduction defects that can affect AV synchrony or prevent synchronous right and left ventricular (LV) activation. The accompanying hemodynamic consequences have considerable clinical relevance. These consequences have provided the impetus for some of the advances in pacemaker technology that will be addressed in later chapters.

Although a detailed discussion of the histopathology of the conduction system is beyond the scope of the present chapter, it is worth noting that conduction system disease is often diffuse. For example, normal AV conduction cannot necessarily be assumed when a pacemaker is implanted for a disorder seemingly localized to the sinus node. Similarly, normal sinus node function cannot be assumed when a pacemaker is implanted in a patient with AV block.

Indications for permanent pacemakers

The decision to implant a permanent pacemaker is an important one and should be based on solid clinical evidence. A joint committee of the American College of Cardiology (ACC) and the American Heart Association (AHA) was formed in the 1980s to provide uniform criteria for pacemaker implantation. These guidelines were first published in 1984 and most recently revised in 2002.[1] It must be realized, however, that medicine is a constantly changing science, and absolute and relative indications for permanent pacing may change as a result of advances in the diagnosis and treatment of arrhythmias. Accordingly, it should be noted that the joint committee is again revising its recommendations for pacemaker implantation and the new guidelines should be available in the near future. It is useful to keep the ACC/AHA guidelines in mind when evaluating a patient for pacemaker implantation. When approaching a patient with a documented or suspected bradyarrhythmia, it is important to take the clinical setting into account. Thus, the patient's overall general medical condition must be considered as well as their occupation or desire to operate a motor vehicle or equipment, where the safety of other individuals may be at risk.

In the ACC/AHA classification, there are three classes of indications for permanent pacemaker implantation, defined as follows:

Class I
Conditions for which there is evidence and/or general agreement that a pacemaker implantation is beneficial, useful, and effective.

Class II
Conditions for which there is conflicting evidence and/or a divergence of opinion about the usefulness/efficacy of pacemaker implantation.

Class IIa
Weight of evidence/opinion in favor of efficacy.

Class IIb
Usefulness/efficacy less well established by evidence/opinion.

Class III
Conditions for which there is evidence and/or general agreement that a pacemaker is not useful/effective and in some cases may be harmful.

Level of evidence

Additionally, the ACC/AHA Committee ranked evidence supporting their recommendations by the following criteria.

- Level A: Data derived from multiple randomized trials involving a large number of patients.
- Level B: Data derived from a limited number of trials involving a relatively small number of patients or from well-designed analyses of non-randomized studies or data registries.
- Level C: Recommendations derived from the consensus of experts.

Acquired atrioventricular block

Acquired AV block with syncope (e.g. Stokes–Adams attacks) was historically the first indication for cardiac pacing. The site of AV block (e.g. AV node, His bundle, or distal conduction system) will to a great extent determine the adequacy and reliability of the underlying escape rhythm (Figs 1.2–1.4). It is worth noting that, in the presence of symptoms documented to be due to AV block, permanent pacing is indicated, regardless of the site of the block (e.g. above the His bundle as well as below the His bundle). Because of different indications for permanent pacing of heart block due to acute myocardial infarction (MI), congenital AV block and increased vagal tone, these indications are discussed in other sections.

The indications for permanent pacing with AV block follow.

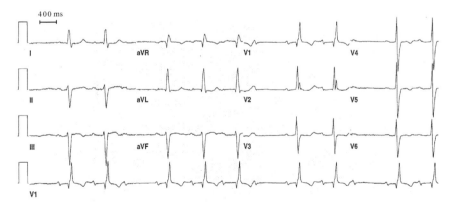

Fig. 1.2 A 70-year-old man with known right bundle branch block, left anterior fascicular block and first-degree atrioventricular (AV) block was seen in the emergency department with a complaint of recurrent syncope. Electrocardiogram revealed type I second-degree AV block. On electrophysiological study, the site of block was found to be infranodal and he was referred for a permanent pacemaker. It should be noted that approximately 65% of patients who develop complete heart block with a wide QRS escape complex have antecedent right bundle branch block with left anterior fascicular block. In this situation, even type I second-degree AV block is frequently infranodal and warrants permanent pacemaker implantation, especially when there is a history of syncope, since idioventricular escape rhythms are notoriously unreliable.

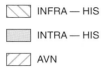

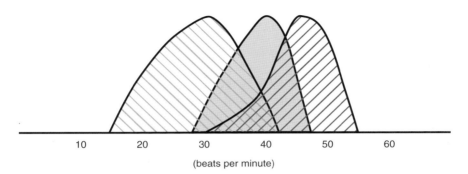

(beats per minute)

Fig. 1.3 A diagram outlining the rate of the escape rhythm in patients with high-grade atrioventricular (AV) block. As can be seen, the escape rate in a patient with block at the AV node (AVN) is usually considerably faster than in individuals with intra-Hisian or infra-Hisian block, although there is considerable overlap between groups.

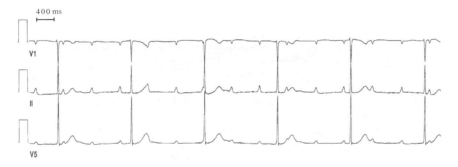

Fig. 1.4 A 70-year-old man was admitted to the hospital complaining of weakness and presyncopal episodes. Rhythm strips revealed complete atrioventricular block and a slow junctional escape rhythm with narrow QRS complexes. He received a permanent dual-chamber pacemaker, which completely relieved his symptoms.

Class I
1 Third-degree and advanced second-degree AV block at any anatomical level, associated with any one of the following conditions:
    a Bradycardia with symptoms (including heart failure) presumed to be due to AV block. (Level of evidence: C.)

b Arrhythmias and other medical conditions requiring drugs that result in symptomatic bradycardia. (Level of evidence: C.)

c Documented periods of asystole ≥3.0 s or any escape rate <40 bpm in awake, symptom-free patients. (Levels of evidence: B, C.)

d After catheter ablation of the AV junction. (Levels of evidence: B, C.) There are no trials to assess outcome without pacing, and pacing is virtually always planned in this situation unless the operative procedure is AV junction modification.

e Postoperative AV block that is not expected to resolve after cardiac surgery. (Level of evidence: C.)

f Neuromuscular diseases with AV block, such as myotonic muscular dystrophy, Kearns–Sayre syndrome, Erb's dystrophy and peroneal muscular atrophy, with or without symptoms, because there may be unpredictable progression of AV conduction disease. (Level of evidence: B.)

2 Second-degree AV block regardless of type or site of block, with associated symptomatic bradycardia. (Level of evidence: B.)

Class IIa

1 Asymptomatic third-degree AV block at any anatomical site with average awake ventricular rates of ≥40 bpm, especially if cardiomegaly, ventricular arrhythmias or LV dysfunction are present. (Levels of evidence: B, C.)

2 Asymptomatic type II second-degree AV block with a narrow QRS. When type II second-degree AV block occurs with a wide QRS, pacing becomes a class I recommendation. (Level of evidence: B.)

3 Asymptomatic type I second-degree AV block at intra- or infra-His levels found at electrophysiology study performed for other indications. (Level of evidence: B.)

4 First- or second-degree AV block with symptoms similar to those of pacemaker syndrome. (Level of evidence: B.)

Class IIb

1 Marked first-degree AV block (>0.30 s) in patients with LV dysfunction and symptoms of congestive heart failure in whom a shorter AV interval results in hemodynamic improvement, presumably by decreasing left atrial filling pressure. (Level of evidence: C.)

2 Neuromuscular diseases such as myotonic muscular dystrophy, Kearns–Sayre syndrome, Erb's dystrophy, and peroneal muscular atrophy with any degree of AV block (including first-degree AV block), with or without symptoms, because there may be unpredictable progression of AV conduction disease. (Level of evidence: B.)

Class III

1 Asymptomatic first-degree AV block. (Level of evidence: B.)

2 Asymptomatic type I second-degree AV block at the AV nodal level or not known to be intra- or infra-Hisian. (Levels of evidence: B, C.)

3 AV block expected to resolve and/or unlikely to recur (e.g. drug toxicity, Lyme disease, or during hypoxia in sleep apnea syndrome in the absence of symptoms). (Level of evidence: B.)

The majority of these diagnoses can be made from the surface electrocardiogram (ECG). Invasive electrophysiology studies are only rarely necessary, but may be helpful or of interest in elucidating the site of AV block (Figs 1.5–1.7). Regarding the first two items in class II, it is likely that permanent pacemakers are more frequently implanted in patients with wide QRS complexes and/or documented infranodal block than in patients with narrow QRS complex escape rhythms.

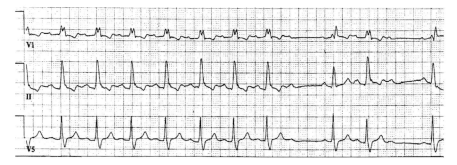

Fig. 1.5 A rhythm strip recorded from a patient with recurrent syncope showing right bundle branch block, left posterior fascicular block and type II second-degree atrioventricular (AV) block. Type II second-degree AV block is almost always infranodal (this was documented by intracardiac recordings). Symptomatic second-degree AV block is a class I indication for permanent pacing.

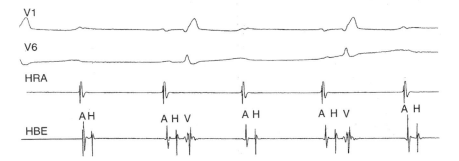

Fig. 1.6 An example of 2:1 atrioventricular (AV) block with the level of block occurring within the His–Purkinje system. In the presence of a narrow QRS complex, 2:1 AV block is usually situated at the AV node, whereas a wide QRS complex in the conducted beats often indicates infranodal block. Note that every other P wave is blocked below the His bundle. The paper speed is 100 mm s^{-1}. From top to bottom: V$_1$ and V$_6$ are standard ECG leads; HRA is the high right atrial recording and HBE is the intracardiac recording of the His bundle electrogram. A, atrial electrogram; H, His bundle electrogram; V, ventricular electrogram.

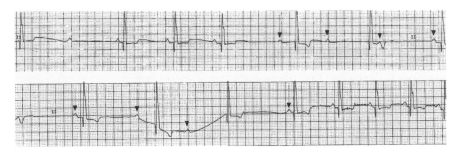

Fig. 1.7 An example of "vagotonic" block. P waves are indicated by the arrows. The simultaneous occurrence of atrioventricular (AV) block and slowing of the sinus rate is diagnostic of hypervagotonia. This type of block is located at the level of the AV node. It is generally considered benign and does not warrant a permanent pacemaker unless the patient is very symptomatic with medically refractory recurrences.

It is worth emphasizing that 2 : 1 AV block may be either type I or type II, but this cannot always be discerned from the surface ECG (Table 1.2). As a rough approximation, if the QRS complex is narrow, the block is probably localized to the AV node and considered type I. If the QRS complex is wide, the level of block may be in the AV node or His bundle, and the site of the block can best be determined from an invasive electrophysiological study (His bundle recording). The causes of acquired high-grade AV block are listed in Table 1.3.

Table 1.2 Differential diagnosis of 2 : 1 atrioventricular (AV) block

Condition	Block above AV node	Block below AV node
Exercise	+	+/− or −
Atropine	+	+/− or −
Carotid sinus massage	−	+ or +/−
Isoprenaline	−	+ or +/−

+ Represents improved AV conduction, − represents worsened AV conduction.

Table 1.3 Causes of acquired high-grade atrioventricular (AV) block

Ischemic
    Acute myocardial infarction
    Chronic ischemic heart disease
    Prinzmetal's angina

Non-ischemic cardiomyopathy
    Hypertensive
    Idiopathic dilated

Fibrodegenerative
    Lev's disease
    Lenègre's disease

Table 1.3 (*Continued.*)

After cardiac surgery/cardiac catheterization laboratory
    Coronary artery bypass grafting
    Aortic valve replacement or aortic root replacement
    Ventricular septal defect repair
    Septal myomectomy or ethanol ablation of the interventricular septum

Other iatrogenic
    After His bundle (AV junction) ablation
    After ablation of septal accessory pathways, AV nodal re-entry
    After radiation therapy (e.g. lung cancer, Hodgkin's lymphoma)

Infectious disease
    Bacterial endocarditis
    Chagas' disease
    Lyme disease
    Syphilis
    Myocarditis
    Rheumatic fever
    Other (viral, rickettsial, fungal, etc.)

Neuromuscular disease
    Myotonic dystrophy
    Muscular dystrophies (fascioscapulohumeral)
    Kearns–Sayre syndrome
    Friedreich's ataxia

Infiltrative disease
    Amyloid
    Sarcoid
    Hemochromatosis
    Carcinoid
    Malignant tumors

Connective tissue disease
    Rheumatoid arthritis
    Systemic lupus erythematosus
    Systemic scleroderma
    Ankylosing spondylitis

Cardiac tumors

Drug induced
    Digitalis
    β-Blockers
    Calcium channel blockers
    Lithium
    Class I or III antiarrhythmic drugs

Congenital
    Congenital heart disease
    Maternal systemic lupus erythematosus

Chronic bifascicular or trifascicular block

Patients with chronic bifascicular block [right bundle branch block (RBBB) and left anterior hemiblock, RBBB and left posterior hemiblock, or complete left bundle branch block (LBBB)] and patients with trifascicular block (any of the above and first-degree AV block) are at an increased risk of progression to complete AV block.

In the 1980s, the results of several large prospective studies of the role of His bundle recordings in asymptomatic patients with chronic bifascicular block were published. In the combined analysis of these studies, more than 750 patients were observed for 3–5 years. The incidence of progression from bifascicular to complete heart block was low, varying from 2% to 5% per year. Most important, the total cardiovascular mortality was 19–25%, and the mortality from sudden cardiac death was 10–20%. In these patients, the presence of bifascicular block on the ECG can be taken as a sign that there is a high likelihood of coexisting structural heart disease. We can conclude from these studies that patients with chronic asymptomatic bifascicular block and a prolonged HV interval (HV interval represents the shortest conduction time from the His bundle to the ventricular endocardium over the specialized conduction system) have more extensive organic heart disease and an increased risk of sudden cardiac death. The risk of spontaneous progression to complete heart block is small, although it is probably slightly greater in patients who have a prolonged HV interval. Permanent pacing appears to prevent recurrent syncope in these patients, but does not reduce the incidence of sudden death, which may often be due to heart failure or ventricular arrhythmias. Routine His bundle recordings are therefore of little value in evaluating patients with chronic bifascicular block and no associated symptoms (e.g. no syncope or presyncope) (Fig. 1.8).

In patients with bifascicular or trifascicular block and associated symptoms of syncope or presyncope, electrophysiological testing is useful. A high incidence of sudden cardiac death and inducible ventricular arrhythmias is noted in this patient group. Electrophysiological testing may be helpful for identifying the disorder responsible for syncope and potentially avoiding implantation of a pacemaker (Fig. 1.9). In patients who have a markedly prolonged HV interval (> 100 ms) and syncope not attributable to other causes, there is a high incidence of subsequent development of complete heart block, and permanent pacing is warranted. However, these patients comprise a relatively small percentage of patients undergoing electrophysiological testing with cardiac symptoms and bifascicular block. In the majority of patients, the HV interval is normal (HV 35–60 ms) or only mildly prolonged, and His bundle recording does not effectively separate out high-risk and low-risk subpopulations with bifascicular block who are likely to progress to complete heart block. Electrophysiological testing will often provoke sustained ventricular arrhythmias, which are the cause of syncope in many of these patients. In patients with LV systolic dysfunction, advanced heart failure and bundle branch block, espe-

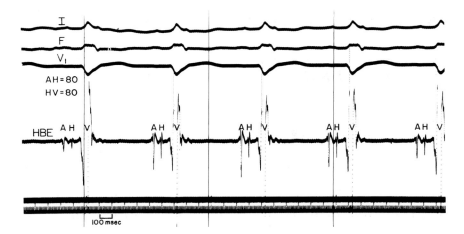

Fig. 1.8 An intracardiac recording in a patient with left bundle branch block. The prolonged HV interval (80 ms) is indicative of infranodal conduction disease, but in the absence of transient neurological symptoms (syncope, dizzy spells, etc.), no specific therapy is indicated. From top to bottom: I, F and V₁ are standard ECG leads; HBE is the intracardiac recording of the His bundle electrogram. A, atrial depolarization; H, His bundle depolarization; V, ventricular electrogram. Paper speed is 100 mm s⁻¹.

cially LBBB, and a QRS interval > 120–130 ms, defibrillators with biventricular pacing have been shown to improve symptoms from heart failure and reduce mortality.[2]

Barold has pointed out that the standard definition of trifascicular block is often too loosely applied.[3] Thus, in patients with RBBB and either left anterior or left posterior fascicular block or in patients with LBBB and first-degree AV block, the site of block could be located either in the His–Purkinje system or in the AV node. The term "trifascicular block" should be reserved for alternating RBBB and LBBB or for block of either bundle in the setting of a prolonged HV interval.

The indications for pacing in the setting of chronic bifascicular/trifascicular block are listed below.

Class I
1 Intermittent third-degree AV block. (Level of evidence: B.)
2 Type II second-degree AV block. (Level of evidence: B.)
3 Alternating bundle branch block. (Level of evidence: C.)

Class IIa
1 Syncope not demonstrated to be due to AV block when other likely causes have been excluded, specifically ventricular tachycardia (VT). (Level of evidence: B.)

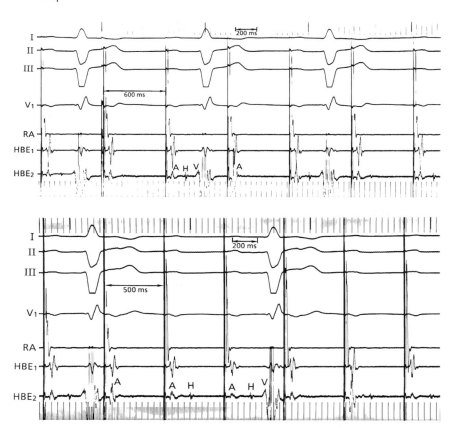

Fig. 1.9 A 68-year-old man was admitted complaining of recurrent dizziness and syncope. His baseline 12-lead ECG showed a PR interval of 0.20s and a right bundle block QRS morphology. During the electrophysiological study, the patient's baseline HV interval was 90ms. Top: During atrial pacing at a cycle length of 600ms (100ppm), there is block in the atrioventricular node. Bottom: During pacing at 500ms (120ppm), there is block below the His bundle. These findings are indicative of severe diffuse conduction system disease. A permanent dual-chamber pacemaker was implanted, and the patient's symptoms resolved. From top to bottom: I, II, III and V₁ are standard ECG leads; intracardiac recording from the right atrial appendage (RA) and His bundle (HBE₁ for the proximal His bundle and HBE₂ for the distal His bundle). A, atrial depolarization; H, His bundle depolarization; V, ventricular depolarization.

2 Incidental finding at electrophysiology study of markedly prolonged HV interval (≥100ms) in asymptomatic patients. (Level of evidence: B.)

3 Incidental finding at electrophysiology study of pacing-induced infra-His block that is not physiological. (Level of evidence: B.)

Class IIb

1 Neuromuscular diseases such as myotonic muscular dystrophy, Kearns–Sayre syndrome, Erb's dystrophy and peroneal muscular atrophy with any degree of fascicular block with or without symptoms, because there may be unpredictable progression of AV conduction disease. (Level of evidence: C.) Class IIa indication in European guidelines.

Class III
1 Fascicular block without AV block or symptoms. (Level of evidence: B.)
2 Fascicular block with first-degree AV block without symptoms.

Permanent pacing for chronic neuromuscular disorders
The frequent involvement of the cardiac conduction system in chronic neuromuscular disorders should not be surprising, considering the many similarities between cardiac and skeletal muscle. In some of these conditions, cardiac disease may be responsible for greater morbidity and mortality than the neuromuscular manifestations, highlighting the importance of evaluating the extent of cardiac involvement. Most often, bradyarrhythmias in neuromuscular disorders are due to direct involvement of the specialized AV conduction system, with symptomatic sinus node dysfunction being unusual. The relatively small numbers of patients involved and the absence of randomized, placebo-controlled clinical trials make it difficult to provide definitive guidelines for pacemaker implantation. In general, the recommendations for permanent pacing in these patients are similar to those in other groups with conduction system disease. However, since mortality and the incidence of sudden cardiac death are high in this group of disorders, and because conduction system disease tends to be unpredictable, the development of second- or third-degree AV block, even in the absence of symptoms, is considered a class I indication for permanent pacing. In addition, suggestive symptoms such as syncope should be promptly and aggressively investigated. Some authorities recommend yearly ECGs and 24-h ambulatory recordings for patients with one of these disorders to facilitate early recognition of AV block. It should also be realized, however, that life-threatening ventricular arrhythmias are also fairly common in this population, especially when LV function is impaired or complicated by hypertrophic cardiomyopathy, so use of a permanent pacemaker will not necessarily prevent sudden cardiac death. There is almost no definitive information available on determining whether pacemakers or defibrillators should be implanted in this population. The neuromuscular disorders most frequently associated with symptomatic conduction system disease are as follows:
1 Duchenne's muscular dystrophy—A progressive X-linked disease that usually becomes clinically apparent in the mid-teens and is fatal by the end of the third decade. The ECG typically shows prominent R waves in V_1 with deep narrow Q waves in the lateral precordial leads. Although cardiac involvement is almost universal, the incidence of arrhythmias is variable, with many patients dying from heart failure. In the absence of definitive data, it seems prudent to recommend permanent pacemaker implantation in patients who

develop second-degree or higher degrees of AV block, especially in the setting of a wide QRS complex.

2 Becker muscular dystrophy—An X-linked condition closely related to Duchenne's muscular dystrophy. It has similar electrocardiographic abnormalities, but progresses more slowly. The severity of cardiac involvement does not parallel the severity of neuromuscular disease. Although there is less experience with this disorder, the indications for permanent pacing appear similar to Duchenne's muscular dystrophy.

3 Myotonic muscular dystrophy—An autosomal dominant disorder that usually becomes clinically manifest in the third decade. Cardiac involvement is common and is mostly confined to the conduction system. Most adults have electrocardiographic abnormalities. Both bradyarrhythmias and tachycardias are common, and suggestive symptoms should be promptly evaluated. Permanent pacemakers are warranted for second- or third-degree AV block, even in the absence of symptoms. A recent large prospective study has suggested that HV ≥ 70 ms identifies a subgroup likely to benefit from prophylactic (no documented high-degree block) permanent pacing.[4]

4 Emery–Dreyfuss muscular dystrophy—A slowly progressive X-linked muscular dystrophy with a high incidence of conduction system disease and arrhythmias. Sudden cardiac death due to bradyarrhythmias has been well documented, and permanent pacemakers are often necessary.

5 Limb girdle muscular dystrophy—A heterogeneous group of disorders that usually begin with weakness in the upper legs and pelvic musculature. Cardiac involvement is variable, although there is a familial form with a high incidence of conduction disease. Patients with a family history of heart block or sudden death should be considered for permanent pacing relatively early in the course of their disease.

6 Kearns–Sayre syndrome—A multisystem mitochondrial disorder characterized by progressive external ophthalmoplegia, pigmentary retinal degeneration and AV block. Involvement of the distal conduction system is the rule and high-degree AV block is common. Although definitive data are lacking, it seems prudent to implant a permanent pacemaker prophylactically when marked first-degree AV block is appreciated.

Infiltrative disorders

The infiltrative disorders are a diverse group of conditions characterized by infiltration of the myocardium by a tissue or substance. These include hematological malignancies (leukemia, lymphoma, myeloma), primary tumors of the heart (primarily sarcomas), "solid" tumors that reach the heart by local extension (breast, lung) or metastases, and non-malignant conditions such as amyloidosis, sarcoidosis, and some of the collagen vascular diseases. The prognosis of these disorders is usually more closely related to the underlying disease, although the actual cause of death may be cardiac. For example, malignancies involving the heart, especially "solid" tumors, tend to have a uniformly poor prognosis. Nonetheless, infiltrative disorders may directly affect the conduction system and cause life-threatening bradyarrhythmias and tachyarrhythmias. In these situations, permanent pacemakers or defibrillators can be life saving.

1 Amyloidosis—A group of disorders in which deposition of an insoluble protein within the myocardium can produce a restrictive cardiomyopathy, resulting in congestive heart failure and arrhythmias.[5] This protein can infiltrate the intramural vasculature, causing microvascular ischemia. The resulting perivascular fibrosis can affect the specialized conduction system, causing sinus node disease, intraventricular conduction defects or AV block. Permanent pacemakers may be helpful in alleviating symptoms, but have not been demonstrated to provide a survival benefit.

2 Sarcoidosis—A relatively common disorder of unknown etiology. Cardiac involvement, with the characteristic non-caseating granulomas, is frequent and, when extensive, portends a poor prognosis. The conduction system is often involved, and permanent pacemakers are often required for symptomatic sinus node disease or AV block. Implantable defibrillators are most often necessary because of recurrent malignant ventricular tachyarrhythmias. Unfortunately, death from progressive heart failure is not uncommon.

3 Collagen vascular diseases—Cardiac involvement is relatively frequent in individuals with a collagen vascular disease, especially polymyositis. Arrhythmias are not common, but fibrosis of the conduction system can cause AV block, necessitating a permanent pacemaker.

Sinus node dysfunction

Sinus node dysfunction, or sick sinus syndrome and its variants, is a heterogeneous clinical syndrome of diverse etiologies. This disorder includes sinus bradycardia, sinus arrest, SA block, chronotropic incompetence, and various supraventricular tachycardias (atrial or junctional) alternating with periods of bradycardia or asystole (Table 1.4). Sinus node dysfunction is quite common, and its incidence increases with advancing age. In patients with sinus node dysfunction, the correlation of symptoms with bradyarrhythmias is critically important. This is because there is a great deal of disagreement about the absolute heart rate or length of pause required before pacing is indicated. If the symptoms of sinus node disease are dramatic (e.g. syncope, recurrent dizzy spells, seizures, or severe heart failure), then the diagnosis may be relatively easy. However, the symptoms are often extremely non-specific (e.g. easy fatigability, depression, listlessness, early signs of dementia) and in the elderly may be easily misinterpreted. Instead, many of these patients have symptoms as a result of an abrupt change in heart rate (e.g. termination of tachycardia with a sinus pause or sinus bradycardia) (Fig. 1.10). It is important to realize that the degree of bradycardia that may produce symptoms will vary depending on the patient's physiological status, age, and activity at the time of bradycardia (e.g. eating, sleeping or walking) (Fig. 1.11). In patients with sinus node dysfunction whose symptoms have not been shown to cor-

Table 1.4 Diagnosis of sinus node dysfunction

Sinus bradycardia—Sinus rates persistently < 60 bpm and associated with symptoms. Prolonged sinus node recovery time (atrial pacing) may help in the diagnosis.

Chronotropic incompetence—Sinus rate does not increase with exertion. Diagnosis made with exercise test or continuous electrocardiographic monitoring.

Sinoatrial (SA) block—Sinus beats are "dropped" in a regular pattern (e.g. 2:1 SA block, 3:2 SA Wenckebach, etc.) due to blocking of impulses in the perinodal area between the sinus node and atrial muscle (by disease, medications, etc.). Diagnosis is made by continuous electrocardiographic monitoring. It may be facilitated by sinus node potential recordings.

Sinoatrial pause—Failure of impulse formation in the sinus node due to pathology, medications, etc. The diagnosis is made electrocardiographically by an absence of sinus P waves that occurs without any discernible pattern.

Bradycardia–tachycardia syndrome—The diagnosis is made electrocardiographically by alternating periods of sinus bradycardia and tachycardia (most commonly atrial fibrillation or flutter). The bradycardia is often manifested by periods of sinus node arrest which often occur when the tachycardia terminates.

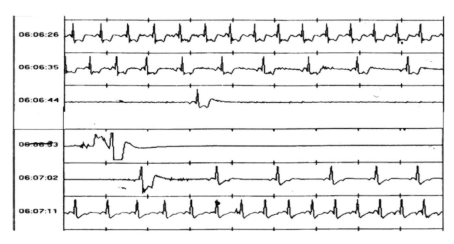

Fig. 1.10 A dramatic example of sinus node dysfunction manifested by 7 and 10 s of asystole as documented by an implantable loop monitor in a patient with recurrent undiagnosed syncope. He underwent permanent pacemaker implantation.

relate with electrocardiographic abnormalities, a simple exercise test may be helpful (to assess the degree of chronotropic incompetence, especially in the individual with vague symptoms) or an electrophysiological study may be considered.

More permanent pacemakers are implanted for sinus node disease than for any other indication in the USA. Patients with alternating periods of brady-

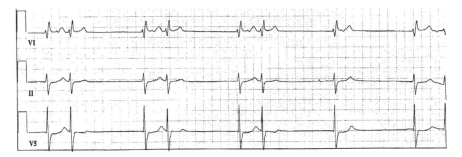

Fig. 1.11 A 69-year-old man had been started on atenolol 75 mg/day for treatment of hypertension approximately 2 weeks earlier. He was seen in the emergency room complaining of feeling weak and lightheaded. The ECG shows a slow junctional escape rhythm followed by a sinus beat in a pattern termed "escape capture bigeminy." Discontinuation of atenolol resulted in return of normal sinus rhythm within 36 h. Patients with sinus node dysfunction may be dependent upon sympathetic stimulation, and β-blockers, even in low doses, may result in profound bradycardia.

cardia and tachycardia (i.e. tachy–brady syndrome) are especially likely to require permanent pacing because medical treatment of the tachycardia often worsens the bradycardia and vice versa (Fig. 1.12). Up to 30% of patients with sinus node disease will also have AV nodal or distal His–Purkinje conduction system disease. Thus, atrial fibrillation, which is a common expression of sinus node disease, may be accompanied by a slow ventricular response, even in the absence of medications that depress AV conduction. Other important complications of sinus node disease include systemic emboli, especially in the setting of alternating periods of bradycardia and tachycardia, and congestive heart failure, usually related to the slow heart rate. In addition, many commonly used medications may exacerbate sinus node dysfunction (Table 1.5). For many patients, an acceptable alternative cannot be found, and pacing is necessary so that they can continue their medications. In some patients, the AV nodal conduction disturbance may not resolve even after discontinuation of drugs that may cause conduction system disturbance.

A group of patients has been identified who have a relatively fixed heart rate during exercise; this condition is referred to as chronotropic incompetence. These patients frequently have other symptoms of sinus node dysfunction. Some may have symptoms at rest (generally non-specific), but most of these patients will note symptoms such as fatigue or shortness of breath with exercise. In some cases, the diagnosis is straightforward; there is no or only a very slight increase in heart rate with exercise. In other cases, the diagnosis is difficult and will require comparison of the patient's exercise response with that of age-matched, gender-matched patients using specific exercise protocols.

Although the indications for permanent pacing for sinus node dysfunction are fairly well delineated, there is considerable debate as to which pacing mode is most appropriate. Because of the high incidence of chronotropic in-

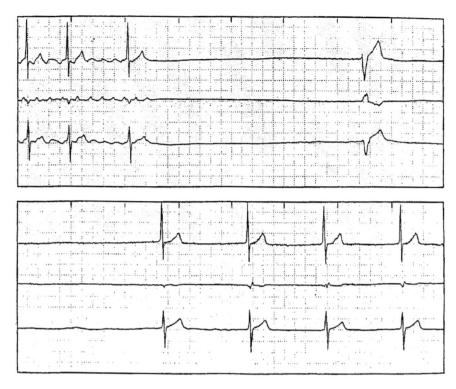

Fig. 1.12 A 53-year-old man with a history of atrial flutter complained of syncope preceded by palpitations. Twenty-four-hour ambulatory recordings (Holter) revealed prolonged periods of asystole following spontaneous termination of atrial flutter. Alternating periods of tachycardia and bradycardia ("bradycardia–tachycardia syndrome") are notoriously difficult to manage without a permanent pacemaker.

Table 1.5 Commonly used medications that may cause sinus node dysfunction or atrioventricular block

---

- Digitalis (especially in the setting of hypokalemia)
- Antihypertensive agents (clonidine, methyldopa, guanethidine)
- Beta-adrenergic blockers (inderal, metoprolol, nadolol, atenolol), and administration as eyedrops
- Calcium channel blockers (verapamil, diltiazem)
- Type 1A antiarrhythmic drugs (quinidine, procainamide, disopyramide)
- Type 1C antiarrhythmic drugs (flecainide, propafenone)
- Type III antiarrhythmic drugs (amiodarone, sotalol)
- Psychotropic medications
  Tricyclics
  Phenothiazines
  Lithium
  Phenytoin
  Cholinesterase inhibitors

---

competence, the need for rate-responsive pacing is generally accepted. However, whether dual-chamber (DDD/DDDR) pacing confers any advantage over the VVIR mode is less well established.[6] Pacing to maintain AV synchrony (AAI/DDD) has been shown to reduce the incidence of atrial fibrillation, but does not prevent strokes or prolong survival.[7] Similarly, there is debate about whether patients with intact AV conduction might benefit more from AAI/AAIR than from DDD/DDDR pacing. Single-chamber devices are less complicated and cheaper and allow for normal ventricular activation. These issues are discussed in a separate chapter.

The indications for pacemaker implantation in patients with sinus node dysfunction are listed below.

Class I
1 Sinus node dysfunction with documented symptomatic bradycardia or sinus pauses. Sinus node dysfunction as a result of essential long-term drug therapy of a type and dose for which there are no acceptable alternatives. (Level of evidence: C.)
2 Symptomatic chronotropic incompetence. (Level of evidence: C.)

Class IIa
1 Sinus node dysfunction occurring spontaneously or as a result of necessary drug therapy, with heart rates < 40 bpm, when a clear association between significant symptoms consistent with bradycardia and the actual presence of bradycardia has not been documented. (Level of evidence: C.)
2 Syncope of unexplained origin when major abnormalities of sinus node function are discovered or provoked in electrophysiological studies. (Level of evidence: C.)

Class IIb
1 In minimally symptomatic patients, chronic heart rates < 40 bpm while awake. (Level of evidence: C.)

Class III
1 Sinus node dysfunction in asymptomatic patients, including those in whom substantial sinus bradycardia (heart rate < 40 bpm) is a consequence of long-term drug treatment.
2 Sinus node dysfunction in patients with symptoms suggestive of bradycardia that are clearly documented as not associated with a slow heart rate.
3 Sinus node dysfunction with symptomatic bradycardia due to non-essential drug therapy.

Neurocardiogenic syncope/hypersensitive carotid sinus syndrome
Neurally mediated syncope is a form of abnormal autonomic control of the circulation. It may take one of three forms:

1 The cardioinhibitory type is characterized by ventricular asystole of ≥3s due to sinus arrest or (occasionally) complete heart block.

2 The pure vasodepressor response is marked by a decrease in arterial pressure of at least 20–30 mmHg, but little or no change in heart rhythm.

3 The mixed type has features of both the cardioinhibitory and vasodepressor types.

Syncope is a common disorder that is estimated to account for up to 6% of all hospital admissions in the USA annually. Despite extensive evaluation, the cause of syncope may not be found in up to 50% of cases. It is believed that a substantial proportion of these cases may be due to neurally mediated syncope. The exact mechanism of neurally mediated syncope has not been fully elucidated, but appears to be initiated by an exaggerated response of the autonomic nervous system to a variety of stimuli. Although the syncope is sometimes an isolated event with an obvious precipitating cause such as severe fright or emotional upset, in many individuals these episodes are recurrent and without apparent triggers. A variety of other stimuli may give rise to cardioinhibitory or mixed cardioinhibitory responses. These conditions, when recurrent and refractory, may also be treated with permanent pacemakers. The conditions include pain, coughing, micturition, swallowing, defecation, and the relatively common vasovagal syndrome. In general, pacemakers may be considered in these patients only when symptoms are recurrent, severe, and cannot be controlled by more conservative measures [e.g. avoidance of stimuli, β-blockers, midodrine hydrochloride (ProAmatine), and/or fludrocortisone acetate (Florinef)]. Pacemaker therapy is thought more likely to be successful in patients who predominantly experience the cardioinhibitory type of response. The advent of head-upright tilt testing has had a major impact on the area of neurocardiogenic syncope. Vasodepressor and/or cardioinhibitory responses may be elicited, which appear to correlate only modestly with the clinical symptoms (Figs. 1.13–1.15). In some studies, the response to tilt table testing has been found to be different from that recorded with an implantable recorder during a spontaneous syncopal episode. The development of permanent pacemakers with the "rate-drop response," which initiates an interval of relatively rapid pacing when the heart rate suddenly drops below a pre-set limit, has stimulated renewed interest in the use of pacing for neurocardiogenic syncope and related disorders. Initial randomized but uncontrolled clinical trials had documented the ability of pacemakers with this feature to reduce syncopal recurrences compared with patients without pacemakers.[8] One double-blind, randomized controlled clinical trial (control group received pacemakers, but programmed to the ODO mode) has shown only a trend toward a reduction in frequency of syncope with active pacing without reaching statistical significance.[9] The final role of pacing in prevention of neurocardiogenic syncope is uncertain; at present, pacing is used only in truly refractory cases in which a significant bradycardic component has been well demonstrated.

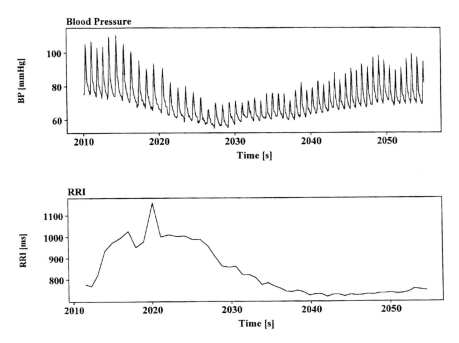

Fig. 1.13 An example of a pure vasodepressor response to tilt testing. The upper panel shows blood pressure and the lower panel shows heart rate (R–R intervals, expressed in milliseconds). Note the marked decrease in blood pressure at a time when the heart rate is actually increasing (the R–R interval is shortening). This type of individual is less likely to respond to permanent pacing.

One variant of neurally mediated syncope is the hypersensitive carotid sinus syndrome. A mildly abnormal response to vigorous carotid sinus massage may occur in up to 25% of patients, especially if coexisting vascular disease is present. Some patients with an abnormal response to carotid sinus massage may have no symptoms suggestive of carotid sinus syncope. On the other hand, the typical history of syncope—blurred vision and lightheadedness or confusion in the standing or sitting position, especially during movement of the head or neck—should be suggestive of this entity. Classic triggers of carotid sinus syncope are head turning, tight neckwear, shaving, and neck hyperextension. Syncopal episodes usually last only several minutes and are generally reproducible in a given patient. Symptoms associated with this syndrome may wax or wane over several years. Carotid sinus hypersensitivity is most often predominantly cardioinhibitory in nature, so that permanent pacing may be very helpful (Fig. 1.16). In contrast, other forms of neurocardiogenic syncope often have a significant vasodepressor component, so that permanent pacing has a more limited role.

The indications for pacemaker implantation in patients with neurally mediated syncope and hypersensitive carotid sinus syndrome are listed below.

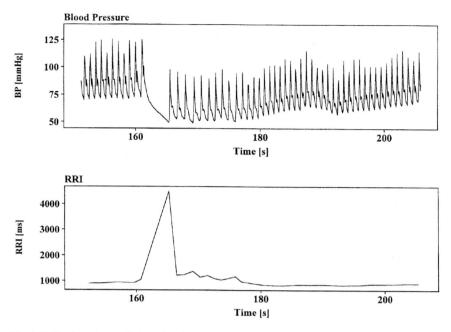

Fig. 1.14 Tracings from a tilt test showing a pure cardioinhibitory response. Note the abrupt increase in cardiac cycle length (R–R interval) reflecting marked bradycardia.

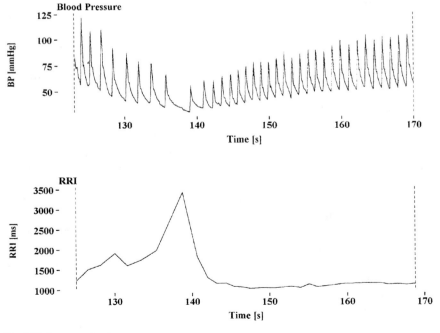

Fig. 1.15 An example of a "mixed" cardioinhibitory and vasodepressor response to tilt testing. An initial decrease in blood pressure is followed by a marked increase in cardiac cycle length.

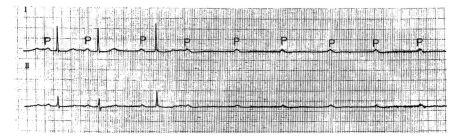

Fig. 1.16 A 49-year-old man complained of near-syncope, which typically occurred while shaving or turning his neck. Carotid sinus massage was performed shortly before the second QRS complex. Note that the sinus rate slows prior to the third QRS complex, followed by complete heart block with ventricular asystole.

Class I

1 Recurrent syncope caused by carotid sinus stimulation; minimal carotid sinus pressure induces ventricular asystole of >3s duration in the absence of any medication that depresses the sinus node or AV conduction. (Level of evidence: C.)

Class IIa

1 Recurrent syncope without clear, provocative events and with a hypersensitive cardioinhibitory response. (Level of evidence: C.)
2 Significantly symptomatic and recurrent neurocardiogenic syncope associated with bradycardia documented spontaneously or at the time of tilt table testing. (Level of evidence: C.)

The new European guidelines state that recurrent severe vasovagal syncope with prolonged asystole during ECG recording or tilt table testing, after failure of medical therapy and informing patients of the conflicting results of clinical trials, is a class IIa indication in patients >40 years old and a class IIb indication in patients <40 years old.

Class III

1 A hyperactive cardioinhibitory response to carotid sinus stimulation in the absence of symptoms or in the presence of vague symptoms such as dizziness, lightheadedness, or both.
2 Recurrent syncope, lightheadedness or dizziness in the absence of a hyperactive cardioinhibitory response.
3 Situational vasovagal syncope in which avoidance behavior is effective.

Idiopathic orthostatic hypotension is a related neurocirculatory disorder that may respond to permanent pacing. Several reports have documented a beneficial response to atrial or AV sequential pacing in a small number of patients with idiopathic orthostatic hypotension refractory to salt and steroid therapy.[10] The rationale for pacing in this condition is that by increasing the paced rate (the lower rate in these series varies from 80 to 100 bpm), the cardiac output increases and potentially leads to more vasoconstriction. This therapy usually results in some clinical improvement, but it varies considerably from patient to patient. There are currently no class I or class II indications for permanent pacing for idiopathic orthostatic hypotension.

Hypertrophic cardiomyopathy

Hypertrophic cardiomyopathy is a disorder of the myocardium characterized by excessive myocardial hypertrophy, with a predilection for the interventricular septum. Although there may be obstructive (i.e. a demonstrable gradient across the LV outflow tract) and non-obstructive forms, there might be little difference between them because the gradient is dynamic and affected by preload, afterload, and other factors. Difficulty with diastolic relaxation (and ventricular filling) of the thickened and non-compliant ventricular musculature is present in both forms of this disorder and may be an important determinant of the clinical presentation. Pacing is thought to exert a beneficial effect by inducing paradoxical septal motion and ventricular dyssynchrony and dilation, thereby improving ventricular filling and reducing the outflow tract gradient. This is generally achieved with dual-chamber pacing with a short PR interval (i.e. usually 50–125 ms) to produce maximal ventricular preexcitation. The acute hemodynamic effects of dual-chamber pacing may be quite dramatic, with a major reduction in LV cavity obliteration and a concomitant decrease in LV outflow tract gradient (Fig. 1.17). More intriguing is the suggestion that the beneficial effects of dual-chamber pacing in this condition do not dissipate immediately once the pacing has been terminated.[11]

The mechanism of the beneficial effects of pacing is incompletely understood and the population who would most reliably benefit has not been fully elucidated. In a multicenter trial (the M-PATHY study) using a randomized, double-blind crossover design, Maron and colleagues have found that symptomatic improvement (quality of life and functional class) was not necessarily accompanied by improvement in objective indices such as treadmill exercise time and peak oxygen consumption.[12] Similarly, in the Pacing in Cardiomyopathy (PIC) study, Linde and colleagues have found significant improvement in both the active pacing and inactive pacing (placebo) group, although the improvement was greater in those assigned to active pacing.[13] These two studies suggest that some of the improvement seen in earlier studies may be partly due to placebo effect or the known variability in clinical course of the disorder. These studies, together, suggest a benefit from DDD pacing with a short AV delay in some patients with hypertrophic cardiomyopathy, but there is no way to predict which patients will respond to this therapy. Because prolongation of life has not been documented with this therapy, the current role of permanent pacemakers in hypertrophic cardiomyopathy is unclear. Accordingly, it should be remembered that surgical myotomy–myectomy is still considered the gold standard for treatment of this condition. Septal ethanol ablation is an emerging therapy also. The clinician managing these patients must determine

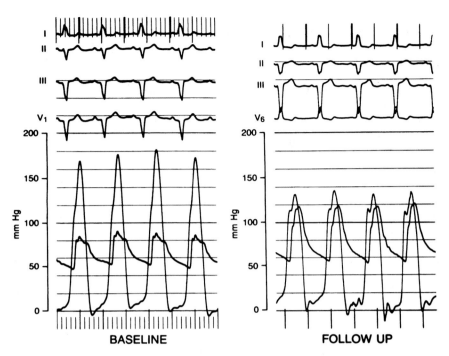

Fig.1.17 Tracings show reduction of left ventricular outflow tract obstruction after chronic dual-chamber pacing. Left panel: At baseline, the left ventricular systolic pressure and left ventricular outflow gradient were 180 mmHg and 90 mmHg, respectively. Right panel: On follow-up assessment, the left ventricular systolic pressure and left ventricular outflow tract gradient, also measured in sinus rhythm, were reduced to 135 mmHg and 15 mmHg, respectively, despite the temporary inhibition of ventricular pacing. This finding suggests remodeling of ventricular function or anatomy by chronic pacing. From top to bottom: I, II, III, V_1 and V_6 are standard ECG leads.

if the device to be implanted will be a dual-chamber pacemaker or a dual-chamber defibrillator. Defibrillators are generally implanted when patients have one risk factor for sudden cardiac death (see Chapter 8).

The indications for permanent pacing for hypertrophic cardiomyopathy are as follows.

Class I
1 Class I indications for sinus node dysfunction or AV block as previously described. (Level of evidence: C.)

Class IIb
1 Medically refractory, symptomatic hypertrophic cardiomyopathy with significant resting or provoked LV outflow tract obstruction. (Level of evidence: A.)

Class III

1 Patients who are asymptomatic or medically controlled.

2 Symptomatic patients without evidence of LV outflow tract obstruction.

Dilated cardiomyopathy (left ventricular systolic dysfunction)

A related area in which permanent pacing may be of benefit is dilated cardio-myopathy. Early studies have suggested that dual-chamber pacing, especially with a short AV delay, may have important hemodynamic benefit in patients with severe congestive heart failure. Although the exact mechanism has not been determined, it was postulated that the improvement in hemodynamics may be related to optimization of ventricular filling or reduction of diastolic mitral regurgitation. However, controlled studies from several groups have failed to confirm these beneficial effects.[14] Studies of right ventricular (RV) out-flow tract pacing for LV systolic dysfunction have been negative or mixed.[15]

In contrast, there is considerable evidence that the use of LV or biventricular permanent pacing improves hemodynamics in some patients with congestive heart failure. Because LV contraction is a key determinant of cardiac output, in theory the properly synchronized contraction of the left ventricle or both ventricles should enhance cardiac performance in patients with prolongation of the QRS duration. Randomized, double-blind, controlled clinical trials have clearly established the beneficial role of biventricular pacing therapy in ad-vanced heart failure patients with prolonged QRS duration.[16]

The indications for pacing in patients with heart failure and impaired LV systolic function are:

Class I

1 Class I indications for sinus node dysfunction or AV block as previously described. (Level of evidence: C.)

2 Biventricular pacing in medically refractory, symptomatic New York Heart Association (NYHA) class III or IV patients with idiopathic dilated or ischemic cardiomyopathy, prolonged QRS interval ($\geq 120\,ms$), LV end-diastolic diam-eter $\geq 55\,mm$ and ejection fraction $\leq 35\%$. (Level of evidence: A.) Most of these patients will qualify for implantable cardioverter defibrillator (ICD) therapy, as listed in Chapter 8. The choice between a biventricular pacemaker and a biventricular ICD should be made based upon the patient's age and a variety of other clinical factors.

Class IIa

1 Biventricular pacing for heart failure patients with NYHA class III or IV symptoms, left ventricular ejection fraction (LVEF) $\leq 35\%$, LV dilation and a concomitant indication for permanent pacing (first implant or upgrading of conventional pacemaker). (Level of evidence: C.)

2 Biventricular pacing for patients with permanent atrial fibrillation and NYHA class III–IV heart failure on optimal medical therapy with an LVEF

≤35%, LV dilation, and indication for AV junction ablation. (Level of evidence: C.)

Class III
1 Asymptomatic dilated cardiomyopathy.
2 Symptomatic dilated cardiomyopathy when patients are rendered asymptomatic by drug therapy.
3 Symptomatic ischemic cardiomyopathy when the ischemia is amenable to intervention.

Prevention and termination of tachyarrhythmias including the prolonged QT syndrome

Permanent pacing can be used in some situations to prevent or terminate supraventricular [supraventricular tachycardia (SVT)] and ventricular arrhythmias. Individuals with prolongation of the QT or QT–U interval may be prone to a type of polymorphic ventricular tachycardia known as torsades de pointes (Fig. 1.18). Tachycardia is often preceded by a short–long–short series of changes in cycle length. Episodes tend to be paroxysmal, recurrent, and may become life-threatening. Therefore, it is critical that the clinical syndrome be recognized, any offending drugs be stopped, and any electrolyte deficiencies be corrected. A summary of the various conditions associated with torsades de pointes is provided in Table 1.6.

Permanent pacing may also be of help in patients with the long QT syndrome, especially for bradycardic patients who have a history of ventricular arrhythmias or syncope. It provides more uniform repolarization and an increased heart rate, which will shorten the QT interval. Permanent pacing may also permit the use of β-blockers, known to be of benefit in this syndrome, without worsening the resting bradycardia. Currently, many of these patients undergo implantation of defibrillators instead of pacemakers, depending mostly on whether the episode was caused solely by bradycardia or whether underlying structural or repolarization abnormalities are present.

Because radiofrequency ablation successfully treats most types of SVT, antitachycardia pacing is now rarely used for the treatment of these arrhythmias.

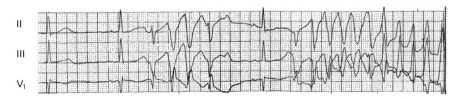

Fig. 1.18 A rhythm strip of ECG leads II, III and V₁ shows paroxysms of polymorphic ventricular tachycardia in an individual with QT interval prolongation and recurrent syncope. Note the short–long–short cycle length sequence that initiates the arrhythmia. In the absence of an identifiable cause, the patient received an implantable cardioverter defibrillator.

Table 1.6 Causes of torsades de pointes

Electrolyte abnormalities
  Hypokalemia
  Hypomagnesemia
  Hypocalcemia

Antiarrhythmic agents
  Quinidine
  Procainamide
  Disopyramide
  Amiodarone
  Sotalol
  Dofetilide
  Ibutilide

Hereditary long QT syndrome(s)

Bradyarrhythmias

Liquid protein diets

Myocardial ischemia/infarction

Neurological events
  Subarachnoid hemorrhage
  Head trauma

Non-cardiac drugs
  Antihistamines (astemizole, terfenadine)
  Tricyclic and tetracyclic antidepressants
  Phenothiazines
  Cisapride
  Erythromycin
  Trimethoprim sulfamethoxazole
  Chloroquine
  Amantadine
  Pentamidine

Toxins
  Organophosphates
  Arsenic

See www.torsades.org or www.longqt.org/medications for updated list.

There is, however, growing interest in permanent pacing therapies for atrial fibrillation. In patients with concomitant sinus bradycardia, dual-site atrial pacing combined with drug therapy may reduce the recurrence rates of atrial fibrillation. In addition, preliminary data suggest that antitachycardia pacing may terminate atrial flutter and other atrial tachycardias that frequently coexist in some patients with atrial fibrillation. Specialized algorithms have been developed that increase the frequency of atrial pacing based on the hypothesis that suppression of premature atrial contractions and decreasing atrial heterogeneity may reduce the frequency and duration of episodes of atrial fibrillation. Ventricular antitachycardia pacing without back-up defibrillation is contraindicated due to the risk of tachycardia acceleration.

The indications for permanent pacing to prevent or terminate tachycardias are:

Class I
1 Sustained pause-dependent VT, with or without prolonged QT, in which the efficacy of pacing is thoroughly documented. (Level of evidence: C.)

Class IIa
1 High-risk patients with congenital long-QT syndrome. (Level of evidence: C.)
2 Symptomatic recurrent SVT that is reproducibly terminated by pacing in the unlikely event that catheter ablation and/or drugs fail to control the arrhythmia or produce intolerable side effects. (Level of evidence: C.)

Class IIb
1 Recurrent SVT or atrial flutter that is reproducibly terminated by pacing as an alternative to drug therapy or ablation. (Level of evidence: C.)
2 AV re-entrant or AV node re-entrant SVT not responsive to medical or ablative therapy. (Level of evidence: C.)
3 Prevention of symptomatic, drug-refractory recurrent atrial fibrillation in patients with coexisting sinus node dysfunction. (Level of evidence: B.)

Class III
1 Tachycardias frequently accelerated or converted to fibrillation by pacing.
2 The presence of accessory pathways with the capacity for rapid anterograde conduction whether or not the pathway(s) participate in the mechanism of the tachycardia.
3 Frequent or complex ventricular ectopic activity without sustained VT in the absence of the long-QT syndrome.
4 Torsades de pointes VT due to reversible causes.

Pacing for children and adolescents, including congenital heart block

The general indications for pacing in children and adolescents are similar to those for adults with several additional considerations. The diagnosis of significant bradycardia in children depends on age, presence and type of congenital heart disease, and cardiac physiology. Following surgery for congenital heart disease, patients may have postoperative AV block that, if untreated by pacing, will worsen their prognosis.[17] Congenital heart disease patients may also have tachycardia–bradycardia syndrome, but the benefits of pacing for this indication are less clear. Congenital heart diseases such as corrected transposition of great arteries, ostium primum atrial septal defects and ventricular septal defects may be associated with complete heart block.

Congenital complete AV block is a rare anomaly that results from abnormal embryonic development of the AV node and is not associated with structural heart disease in 50% of cases. Congenital complete heart block is also associated with maternal lupus erythematosus. Most children with isolated congenital complete AV block have a stable escape rhythm with a narrow complex. Pacing is generally indicated in children with complete heart block if the heart rate in the awake child is < 50 bpm or if associated with LV systolic dysfunction or ventricular arrhythmias. The indications for pacing in congenital complete AV block have been clarified by a prospective study demonstrating improved survival and reduced syncope, myocardial dysfunction and mitral regurgitation even among asymptomatic patients.[18] Exercise testing does not predict future cardiac events in this population.

The indications for permanent pacing in children and adolescents are:

Class I
1 Advanced second- or third-degree AV block associated with symptomatic bradycardia, ventricular dysfunction, or low cardiac output. (Level of evidence: C.)
2 Sinus node dysfunction with correlation of symptoms during age-inappropriate bradycardia. The definition of bradycardia varies with the patient's age and expected heart rate. (Level of evidence: B.)
3 Postoperative advanced second- or third-degree AV block that is not expected to resolve or persists at least 7 days after cardiac surgery. (Levels of evidence: B, C.)
4 Congenital third-degree AV block with a wide QRS escape rhythm, complex ventricular ectopy, or ventricular dysfunction. (Level of evidence: B.)
5 Congenital third-degree AV block in the infant with ventricular rate < 50–55 bpm or with congenital heart disease and a ventricular rate < 70 bpm. (Levels of evidence: B, C.)
6 Sustained pause-dependent VT, with or without prolonged QT, in which the efficacy of pacing is thoroughly documented. (Level of evidence: B.)

Class IIa
1 Bradycardia–tachycardia syndrome with the need for long-term antiarrhythmic treatment other than digitalis. (Level of evidence: C.)
2 Congenital third-degree AV block beyond the first year of life with an average heart rate < 50 bpm, abrupt pauses in ventricular rate that are two or three times the basic cycle length, or associated with symptoms due to chronotropic incompetence. (Level of evidence: B.)
3 Long-QT syndrome with 2:1 AV or third-degree AV block. (Level of evidence: B.)

4 Asymptomatic sinus bradycardia in the child with complex congenital heart disease with resting heart rate <40 bpm or pauses in ventricular rate >3 s. (Level of evidence: C.)

5 Patients with congenital heart disease and impaired hemodynamics due to sinus bradycardia or loss of AV synchrony. (Level of evidence: C.)

Class IIb

1 Transient postoperative third-degree AV block that reverts to sinus rhythm with residual bifascicular block. (Level of evidence: C.)

2 Congenital third-degree AV block in the asymptomatic infant, child, adolescent or young adult with an acceptable rate, narrow QRS complex, and normal ventricular function. (Level of evidence: B.)

3 Asymptomatic sinus bradycardia in the adolescent with congenital heart disease with resting heart rate <40 bpm or pauses in ventricular rate >3 s. (Level of evidence: C.)

4 Neuromuscular diseases with any degree of AV block (including first-degree AV block), with or without symptoms, because there may be unpredictable progression of AV conduction disease.

Class III

1 Transient postoperative AV block with return of normal AV conduction. (Level of evidence: B.)

2 Asymptomatic postoperative bifascicular block with or without first-degree AV block. (Level of evidence: C.)

3 Asymptomatic type I second-degree AV block. (Level of evidence: C.)

4 Asymptomatic sinus bradycardia in the adolescent with longest RR interval <3 s and minimum heart rate >40 bpm. (Level of evidence: C.)

Permanent pacing after the acute phase of acute myocardial infarction

Bradyarrhythmias and conduction defects are relatively common after acute MI. In patients who have these problems, a decision about permanent pacing must be made prior to the patient's discharge from the hospital. It is important to realize that the indications for temporary pacing in the setting of acute MI are different from those for permanent pacing following infarction. Unfortunately, there is some uncertainty regarding permanent pacing for these patients, because large prospective controlled trials have not been performed. In addition, the criteria for permanent pacing in patients after an MI do not necessarily require the presence of symptoms, and the need for temporary pacing in the acute stages of infarction is not by itself an indication for permanent pacing.

The prognosis for these patients is strongly influenced by the amount of underlying myocardial damage.[19] In general, sinus node dysfunction tends to be benign and reversible, and permanent pacemakers are rarely required. Similarly, second-degree and even third-degree AV block after inferior wall

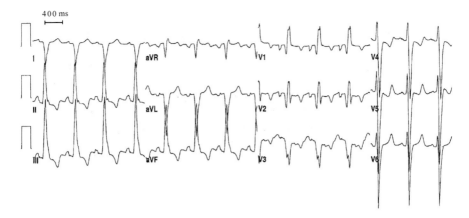

Fig. 1.19 A standard 12-lead ECG from an individual with a large anteroseptal myocardial infarction complicated by congestive heart failure and right bundle branch block with right axis deviation, presumably due to left posterior fascicular block. The patient developed transient high-degree atrioventricular block 72 h after admission (a class I indication) and subsequently underwent permanent pacemaker implantation.

MI is usually reversible and rarely requires permanent pacing. In contrast, conduction defects after an anterior wall MI usually warrant a permanent pacemaker or an ICD with appropriate pacing function insertion, although mortality remains extremely high because of pump failure (Fig. 1.19).

A class I recommendation (level of evidence: C) is that all patients who have an indication for permanent pacing after ST elevation MI should be evaluated for ICD indication. Likewise, class IIa recommendations (level of evidence: C) suggest that biventricular pacing should be evaluated if permanent pacing is indicated and that permanent dual-chamber pacing should be considered if the patient is in sinus rhythm.

The indications for permanent pacing following acute MI are:

Class I
1 Persistent second-degree AV block in the His–Purkinje system with bundle branch block or third-degree AV block within or below the His–Purkinje system after acute MI. (Level of evidence: B.)
2 Transient advanced (second- or third-degree) infranodal AV block and associated bundle branch block. If the site of block is uncertain, an electrophysiology study may be necessary. (Level of evidence: B.)
3 Persistent and symptomatic second- or third-degree AV block. (Level of evidence: C.)

Class IIb
1 Persistent second- or third-degree AV block at the AV node level. (Level of evidence: B.)

Class III
1 Transient AV block in the absence of intraventricular conduction defects. (Level of evidence: B.)
2 Transient AV block in the presence of isolated left anterior fascicular block. (Level of evidence: B.)
3 Acquired left anterior fascicular block in the absence of AV block. (Level of evidence: B.)
4 Persistent first-degree AV block in the presence of bundle branch block that is old or age indeterminate. (Level of evidence: B.)

European guidelines
Class I
Persistent third-degree heart block preceded or not by intraventricular conduction delay.
Persistent Mobitz II second-degree heart block associated with bundle branch block, with or without PR prolongation.
Transient Mobitz II second- or third-degree heart block associated with new-onset bundle branch block.

Class IIa
None.

Class IIb
None.

Class III
Similar to above.

Indications for temporary cardiac pacing

The following section reviews the clinical settings in which temporary cardiac pacing is indicated. Chapter 4 presents a review of the techniques and complications of temporary cardiac pacing. A summary of the general indications for temporary pacing is given in Table 1.7.

Acute myocardial infarction
In the setting of an acute MI, several different types of conduction disturbance may become manifest. They include abnormalities of sinus impulse formation or conduction, disorders of AV conduction, and disorders of intraventricular conduction. In general, any patient with bradyarrhythmias that are associated with symptoms or cause hemodynamic compromise must be treated. The ways of identifying the patient populations at greatest risk for the development of a significant bradyarrhythmia during acute MI, and in whom temporary pacing should be performed prophylactically, are discussed below. It is important to

Table 1.7 Indications for temporary pacing in the ABSENCE of acute myocardial infarction

---

In acute myocardial infarction
See Tables 1.8 and 1.9

In absence of acute myocardial infarction
Medically refractory symptomatic bradycardia
• sinus node dysfunction
• second- or third-degree AV block
Third-degree AV block with wide QRS escape or ventricular rate <50 bpm

Prophylactic
Swan–Ganz catheterization or endocardial biopsy in patient with left bundle branch block
Cardioversion in setting of sick sinus syndrome
New AV or bundle branch block with acute endocarditis (especially aortic valve endocarditis)
Perioperatively in patient with bifascicular block and history of syncope
To allow pharmacological treatment with drugs that worsen bradycardia

Treatment of tachyarrhythmias
Termination of recurrent ventricular or supraventricular tachycardia
Suppression of bradycardia-dependent ventricular tachyarrhythmias including torsades de pointes

---

realize that the indications for temporary pacing in the setting of acute MI are different from those for permanent pacing following infarction.

Sinus node abnormalities

Sinus node dysfunction may include sinus bradycardia, sinus arrest and/or sinoatrial exit block. The incidence of these electrocardiographic abnormalities is quite variable, ranging from 5% to 30% in different series. Abnormalities of sinus rhythm are more common, with inferoposterior infarction because either the right or left circumflex coronary artery is occluded—these arteries most commonly supply the sinus node. Another potential reason is chemically mediated activation of receptors on the posterior left ventricular wall—these receptors are supplied by vagal afferent fibers. Treatment of sinus bradycardia is not necessary, unless symptoms such as worsening myocardial ischemia, heart failure or hypotension are documented. Atropine may be administered for vagally mediated bradycardia. If bradycardia is prolonged and severe, or is not responsive to atropine, temporary cardiac pacing is indicated.

Disorders of atrioventricular conduction

AV block occurs without associated intraventricular conduction system abnormalities in 12–25% of patients with acute MI. The incidence of this finding depends largely on the patient population and the site of infarction. First-degree AV block occurs in 2–12% of patients, second-degree AV block in 3–10%, and third-degree AV block in 3–7% of patients. The majority of patients with abnormalities of AV conduction without bundle branch block have evidence of an inferoposterior infarction (approximately 70%). The reasons for the increased incidence of AV conduction abnormalities are related to the coronary blood supply to the AV node. The coronary artery supplying the inferoposterior wall of the left ventricle is typically the right or left circumflex coronary, which is occluded during an inferior infarction. In addition, activation of cardiac reflexes with augmentation of parasympathetic tone during inferior ischemia (infarction) may also be responsible. In some cases, AV block may be due to release of adenosine caused by inferior ischemia or during inferior infarction.

The risk of progression from first-degree AV block to high-grade AV block (during inferior infarction) varies from 10% to 30%, and that of second-degree AV block to complete heart block is approximately 35%. As would be expected, the development of high-grade AV block in the setting of acute inferoposterior infarction is usually associated with narrow QRS complex escape rhythms (Figs 1.20 and 1.21). The junctional escape rhythm usually remains stable at 50–60 pulses per minute and can be increased by intravenous atropine, so even complete AV block may not require temporary pacing in this situation.

Type I second-degree AV block with a narrow QRS almost always represents a conduction block in the AV node, and temporary cardiac pacing is rarely required unless the patient has concomitant symptoms. Type I second-degree AV block with a wide QRS complex may represent a conduction block in the AV node or His bundle or contralateral bundle branch block. In these

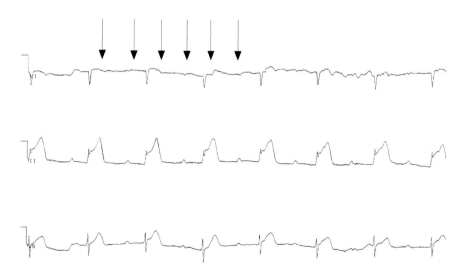

Fig. 1.20 A three-lead (standard leads V$_1$, II and V$_5$) rhythm strip in a 58-year-old man with an acute inferior wall myocardial infarction and complete atrioventricular block (the arrows in lead V$_1$ identify the P waves) with an escape rate of 45 ppm. Despite the slow rate, the patient did not exhibit signs or symptoms of hemodynamic compromise, so no therapy was required. Normal conduction resumed approximately 24 h later.

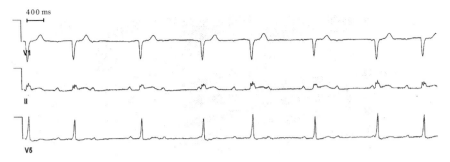

Fig. 1.21 Rhythm strips recorded from a 63-year-old woman with an acute inferior wall myocardial infarction showing high-grade atrioventricular (AV) block with junctional escape beats. The second, fourth and sixth QRS complexes are conducted with a prolonged PR interval (note shortening of the R–R interval with the conducted beats). The presence of junctional escape beats precludes typical Wenckebach conduction. Because the patient was asymptomatic, no therapy was administered. Normal AV conduction resumed spontaneously by the next morning.

patients, especially in the setting of anterior MI, temporary prophylactic pacing must be considered. In patients with type II second-degree AV block and a wide QRS complex in the setting of inferior infarction, or with a wide or narrow QRS complex during an anterior MI, a temporary pacemaker should be inserted. Patients with a narrow QRS complex and type II second-degree AV block in the setting of inferior infarction rarely progress to complete heart block.

Several special situations are worthy of consideration. Patients with high-grade AV block occurring in the setting of right ventricular infarction tend to be less responsive to intravenous atropine and may demonstrate markedly improved hemodynamics during AV sequential pacing. The mechanism for this hemodynamic improvement is probably a reflection of the restrictive physiology that the infarcted right ventricle demonstrates. Another group of patients who may benefit from prophylactic temporary pacing are those with acute inferior wall infarction with alternating Wenckebach periods. This electrocardiographic finding is rare (2%), but without temporary pacing it frequently leads to hemodynamic embarrassment.

In contrast to inferior wall infarction, high-grade AV block complicating an anterior wall infarction is usually located within the His–Purkinje system. The transition from the first non-conducted P wave to high-grade AV block is often abrupt, and the resulting escape rhythm is typically slow and unreliable. Conducted beats usually have a wide QRS complex. In general, an interruption of the blood supply to the anterior wall and the interventricular septum severe enough to cause AV block usually causes severe LV dysfunction and results in high mortality. Emergency temporary pacing and prophylactic pacing are indicated, although survival may not be significantly improved because of the extent of myocardial damage.

Disorders of the intraventricular conduction system

A number of studies have examined the incidence of development of new bundle branch block in the setting of acute MI and have determined that it varies between 5% and 15%, depending on the site of infarction. New bundle branch block is three times more likely during anterior infarction than during inferior infarction, because the left anterior descending coronary artery provides the major blood supply to the His bundle and the bundle branches. Not surprisingly, there is a high incidence of heart failure in this setting, and the associated high cardiac mortality leads to controversy as to whether temporary or permanent pacing improves the poor prognosis in these patients. As with anterior MI and complete heart block, new bundle branch block reflects extensive myocardial damage.

Multiple studies have shown that patients with acute infarction and bundle branch block have a fourfold to fivefold increased risk of progression to high-grade AV block (e.g. an increase from 4% to 18%).[20,21] Both in-hospital and out-of-hospital mortality are higher for patients presenting with bundle branch block during acute infarction. The basis of this increased mortality may be a variety of causes, including heart failure, infarct extension, ventricular tachycardia and heart block. The mortality of patients with bundle branch block and acute infarction is 30–40%, compared with 10–15% in patients without bundle branch block. Most of the increase in cardiac mortality appears to be related to the degree of heart failure.

Several small retrospective studies have attempted to identify groups of patients who may be at increased risk of progression to high-grade heart block. Unfortunately, many of these studies are limited by their retrospective nature, their small sample size, or their ascertainment bias. On the basis of the results of several studies, patients with conduction system abnormalities who should have temporary pacemakers inserted prophylactically are listed in Table 1.8.

Patients with a new bundle branch block and first-degree AV block or old bifascicular block and first-degree AV block are at intermediate risk of progression (19–29%) to high-grade AV block; they may undergo prophylactic pacing depending on the availability of facilities for emergency placement of a temporary pacemaker. Because the greatest risk of progression to complete heart block occurs in the first 5 days following infarction, these decisions should be made promptly so that temporary pacing may be instituted.

The Multicenter Investigation of the Limitation of Infarct Size (MILIS) study has suggested a simpler method of risk stratification.[22] A "risk score" for the development of complete heart block was devised. Patients with any of the following conduction disturbances were given one point: first-degree AV block, type I second-degree AV block, type II second-degree AV block, left anterior fascicular block, left posterior fascicular block, RBBB, and LBBB. The presence of no risk factors was associated with a 1.2% risk of third-degree AV block, one risk factor with a 7.8% risk, two risk factors with a 25% risk, and three risk factors with a 36.4% risk of complete heart block. These findings were validated by testing the risk score in over 3000 patients from previously published

Table 1.8 Risk of high-grade atrioventricular (AV) block during acute myocardial infarction

Patient group	Risk of high-grade AV block
First-degree AV block and new bifascicular BBB	38–43%
First-degree AV block and old bifascicular BBB	20–50%
New bifascicular BBB	15–31%
Alternating BBB	44%
MILIS risk score[a]	
0	1.2%
1	7.8%
2	25%
3	36.4%

[a]One point each for first-degree AV block, Mobitz I second-degree AV block, Mobitz II second-degree AV block, left anterior fascicular block, left posterior fascicular block, right bundle branch block, left bundle branch block.
BBB, bundle branch block; MILIS, Multicenter Investigation of the Limitation of Infarct Size.

studies. The risk score appears to be an alternative to risk stratification using combinations of conduction disorders.

The effect of thrombolytic and early interventional therapies on the subsequent development of high-grade AV block in patients presenting with acute infarction and intraventricular conduction system disease has been poorly studied. Although the incidence of complete AV block in acute MI has decreased following thrombolytic therapy, mortality remains high.[23]

The most recent AHA guidelines for temporary transvenous pacing in the setting of acute MI are as shown in Table 1.9.[24]

Pacing during cardiac catheterization

During catheterization of the right side of the heart, manipulation of the catheter may induce a transient RBBB in up to 10% of patients. This block generally lasts for seconds or minutes, but can occasionally last for hours or days. Trauma induced by right ventricular endomyocardial biopsy also may result in temporary, or rarely long-lasting, RBBB. This is a problem only in patients with preexisting LBBB, in whom complete heart block may result. We therefore recommend consideration of placement of a temporary transvenous pacing wire in patients who are undergoing right heart catheterization or biopsy in the presence of previously known LBBB. Catheterization of the left side of the heart in patients with known preexisting RBBB only rarely gives rise to complete heart block because of the short length of the left bundle branch. Significant bradycardia and asystole can occur during injection of the right coronary artery. This complication is extremely rare, and the placement of a temporary pacing catheter does not alter the morbidity or mortality of cath-

Table 1.9 Indications for temporary pacing in acute myocardial infarction

Class I
1. Asystole
2. Symptomatic bradycardia (includes sinus bradycardia with hypotension and type I second-degree AV block with hypotension not responsive to atropine)
3. Bilateral bundle branch block [BBB; alternating BBB or right BBB (RBBB) with alternating left anterior fascicular block (LAFB)/left posterior fascicular block (LPFB)] (any age)
4. New bundle branch block with Mobitz II second-degree AV block
5. RBBB plus fascicular block with Mobitz II second-degree AV block

Class IIa
1. Narrow QRS plus Mobitz II second-degree AV block
2. Old or new fascicular block with Mobitz II second-degree AV block and anterior MI
3. Old bundle branch block and Mobitz II second-degree AV block
4. New bundle branch block plus first-degree AV block
5. New bundle branch block plus Mobitz I second-degree AV block
6. RBBB plus LAFB or LPFB (new or indeterminate) with first-degree AV block
7. RBBB plus LAFB or LPFB (new or indeterminate) with Mobitz I second-degree AV block

Class IIb
1. Bifascicular block of indeterminate age and Mobitz II second-degree AV block
2. Old bundle branch block and first-degree AV block or second-degree AV block

Class III
1. First-degree heart block
2. Type I second-degree AV block
3. Accelerated idioventricular rhythm
4. BBB or fascicular block known to exist before acute myocardial infarction without conduction system disease

eterization. The bradycardia usually resolves after several seconds. The same comments apply in general to placement of a temporary pacing wire during angioplasty.

Preoperative pacing

One of the questions most frequently asked of a consulting cardiologist by both surgeons and anesthesiologists is whether it is necessary to insert a temporary pacing catheter in patients with bifascicular block undergoing general anesthesia. The results of several studies have shown that the incidence of intraoperative and perioperative complete heart block is quite low. There does not appear to be any benefit from preoperative prophylactic pacemaker insertion. Even in patients with first-degree AV block and bifascicular block, there is a very low incidence of perioperative high-grade heart block.

However, in patients who have bifascicular block and also type II second-degree AV block or a history of unexplained syncope or presyncope, the risk of development of high-grade AV block is higher, and a temporary pacemaker should be inserted. The appearance of new bifascicular block in the immediate postoperative period should also lead to insertion of a temporary pacemaker and should raise suspicion of an intraoperative MI. The general availability of transcutaneous pacing may make it an acceptable alternative to temporary transvenous pacing in lower risk individuals, although poor patient tolerance is often a limitation.

Open-heart surgery tends to be associated with a somewhat higher incidence of postoperative bradyarrhythmias than does non-cardiac surgery, due to the direct trauma to the conduction system and interference with blood supply. Cardiac surgeons generally implant temporary epicardial pacing wires at the time of surgery to facilitate temporary pacing. The major problem then becomes determining how long to wait for resumption of AV conduction and normalization of sinus node function before implanting a permanent pacemaker. Conventionally, a permanent pacemaker is recommended if the problem persists longer than 5–7 days after the operation. Although normal conduction may resume after this period of time, in the absence of definitive information about the natural history of these disorders, permanent pacing seems to be a prudent choice.

Other temporary pacing

Temporary pacing is indicated in patients with new AV or BBB in the setting of acute bacterial endocarditis. The development of a new conduction system abnormality generally suggests that there is a perivalvular (ring) abscess that has extended to involve the conduction system near the AV node and/or the His bundle. The endocarditis generally involves the non-coronary cusp of the aortic valve. In one study, high-grade or complete heart block developed in 22% of patients with aortic valve endocarditis and new first-degree AV block. Although these studies are retrospective, the patient with development of new AV block or BBB, especially in the setting of aortic valve endocarditis, should probably undergo temporary pacing while cardiac evaluation continues.

Treatment of tumors of the head and/or neck or around the carotid sinus may in some circumstances give rise to high-grade AV block. Temporary pacing may be required during surgical treatment, radiation therapy or chemotherapy. If the tumor responds poorly, permanent pacing may be necessary in some cases. The long-term risk for subsequent heart block due to tumor recurrence is difficult to predict in some cases.

Lyme disease, a tick-borne spirochete infection, causes a systemic infection with arthritis, skin lesions, myalgias, meningoencephalitis and cardiac involvement in 5–10% of patients. Lyme disease is epidemic in the summer months in the northeastern USA. Carditis typically occurs relatively late in the course of the illness, usually 4–8 weeks after the onset of symptoms. AV block is the most common manifestation of carditis and tends to be transient. Block is most common at the level of the AV node, and fluctuation between first-degree and higher degrees of AV block is frequent. Temporary cardiac pacing may be required, but the conduction disturbances usually resolve spontaneously, especially with antibiotic treatment, so permanent cardiac pacing is rarely necessary. Similar conduction disturbances can occasionally be seen in patients with viral myocarditis, as well as with other tick-borne infections.

A number of medications may produce transient bradycardia that may require temporary pacing until the drug has been stopped (see Table 1.5). These drugs may cause sinus node dysfunction and/or AV block; if used in combination, their effects may become more potent and exacerbate mild or latent conduction system disease. If long-term therapy with these agents is necessary for an underlying disorder and a substitute cannot be found, permanent pacing may be required. Recent studies have suggested that at least some patients with transient drug-related bradycardia may experience recurrent bradycardia requiring a pacemaker, even after the drug related to the bradycardia is stopped.

Treatment of tachycardias with temporary pacing

Temporary cardiac pacing has been used for the termination and/or prevention of a variety of arrhythmias. Pacing-termination of ventricular tachycardia is discussed in detail in Chapter 8 on the ICD and will not be dealt with here. Type I atrial flutter can be successfully pace-terminated approximately 65% of the time in an unselected population and in >90% of patients in whom atrial flutter develops after surgery. Due to the development of radiofrequency catheter ablation techniques, there is currently less interest in pace-termination of atrial flutter. Similarly, the most common varieties of paroxysmal supraventricular tachycardia are usually pace-terminable, but tend to be equally amenable to radiofrequency ablation.

Torsades de pointes is a polymorphic ventricular tachycardia with a sinusoidal electrocardiographic appearance, due to the QRS complex undulating about the baseline. It results from prolongation and dispersion (inequality in different parts of the ventricle) of myocardial repolarization, and is often reflected on the surface ECG by a prolonged QT or QT–U interval. Episodes of tachycardia are often preceded by a short–long–short series of changes in cycle length. Importantly, episodes tend to be recurrent, paroxysmal, and non-sustained initially, but may become sustained later unless the underlying condition is identified and corrected. Therefore, it is critical that the clinical syndrome be recognized, any offending toxins or drugs be stopped, and any electrolyte deficiencies be corrected. (A summary of the causes of torsades de pointes is provided in Table 1.6.) In some patients these treatments will be adequate; in some patients, other forms of therapy must be considered. Overdrive atrial and/or ventricular pacing may be effective in suppressing torsades de pointes because it provides more uniform repolarization and an increased heart rate, which will shorten the QT interval. Intravenous magnesium and isoproterenol (which also increases heart rate and shortens repolarization) may also be effective in suppressing torsades de pointes, although the latter is associated with troubling side effects. For individuals who have recurrent symptoms refractory to conventional management, implantation of an ICD should be strongly considered.

Summary

Updated AHA/ACC guidelines for pacemaker and defibrillator implantation are currently in progress. Recently, the European Society of Cardiology has published their updated guidelines for cardiac pacing and cardiac resynchronization therapy.[25]

References

1 Gregorators G, Abrams J, Epstein AE. ACC/AHA/NASPE 2002 Guideline Update for Implantation of Cardiac Pacemakers and Antiarrhythmia Devices: Summary Article: A Report of the American Heart College of Cardiology/American Heart Association Task Force on Practice Guidelines (ACC/AHA/NASPE Committee to Update the 1998 Pacemaker Guidelines). Circulation 2002; 106:2145–61.

2 Salukhe TV, Francis DP, Sutton R. Comparison of medical therapy, pacing and defibrillation in heart failure (COMPANION) trial terminated early; combined biventricular pacemaker-defibrillators reduce all-cause mortality and hospitalization. Int J Cardiol 2003; 87:119–20.

3 Barold SS. ACC/AHA guidelines for implantation of cardiac pacemakers: how accurate are the definitions of atrioventricular and intraventricular conduction blocks? Pacing Clin Electrophysiol 1993; 16:1221–6.

4 Lazarus A, Varin J, Babuty D *et al*. Long-term follow-up of arrhythmias in patients with myotonic dystrophy treated by pacing. J Am Coll Cardiol 2002; 40:1645-52.

5 Shah KB, Inoue Y, Mehra MR. Amyloidosis and the heart: a comprehensive review. Arch Intern Med 2006; 166:1805–13.

6 Lamas GA, Orav EJ, Stambler BS *et al*. Quality of life and clinical outcomes in elderly patients treated with ventricular pacing as compared with dual-chamber pacing. N Engl J Med 1998; 338:1097–104.

7 Lamas GA, Kerry LE, Sweeny MO *et al*. Ventricular pacing or dual chamber pacing for sinus node dysfunction. N Engl J Med 2002; 346:1854–62.

8 Connolly SJ, Sheldon R, Roberts RS, Gent M. Vasovagal Pacemaker Study Investigators. The North American Vasovagal Pacemaker Study (VPS): a randomized trial of permanent cardiac pacing for the prevention of vasovagal syncope. J Am Coll Cardiol 1999; 33:16–20.

9 Connolly SJ, Sheldon R, Thorpe KE *et al*. Pacemaker therapy for prevention of syncope in patients with recurrent severe vasovagal syncope: Second Vasovagal Pacemaker Study (VPS II): a randomized trial. JAMA 2003; 289:2224–9.

10 Weissmann P, Chin MT, Moss AJ. Cardiac tachypacing for severe refractory idiopathic orthostatic hypotension. Ann Intern Med 1992; 116:650.

11 Fananapazir L, Epstein ND, Curiel RV *et al*. Long-term results of dual-chamber (DDD) pacing in hypertrophic cardiomyopathy: evidence for progressive symptomatic and hemodynamic improvement and reduction of left ventricular hypertrophy. Circulation 1994; 90:2731–42.

12 Maron BJ, Nishimura RA, McKenna WJ *et al*. For the M-PATHY Study Investigators. Assessment of permanent dual-chamber pacing as a treatment for drug-refractory symp-

tomatic patients with obstructive hypertrophic cardiomyopathy: a randomized double-blind crossover study. Circulation 1999; 99:2927–33.

13 Linde C, Gadler F, Kappenberger L, Ryden L, PIC Study Group. Placebo effect of pacemaker implantation in obstructive hypertrophic cardiomyopathy. Am J Cardiol 1999; 83:903–7.

14 Gold MR, Feliciano Z, Gottlieb SS, Fisher ML. Dual-chamber pacing with a short atrioventricular delay in congestive heart failure: a randomized study. J Am Coll Cardiol 1995; 26:967–73.

15 Stambler BS, Ellenbogen K, Zhang X et al. Right ventricular outflow versus apical pacing in pacemaker patients with congestive heart failure and atrial fibrillation. J Cardiovasc Electrophysiol 2003; 14:1180–6.

16 Abraham WT, Fisher WG, Smith AL et al. Cardiac resynchronization in chronic heart failure. N Engl J Med 2002; 346:1845–53.

17 Friedman RA. Congenital AV block. Pace me now or pace me later? Circulation 1995; 92:283–5.

18 Michaelsson M, Jonzon A, Riesenfeld T. Isolated congenital complete atrio-ventricular block in adult life. A prospective study. Circulation 1995; 92:442–9.

19 Simons GR, Sgarbosa E, Wagner G et al. Atrioventricular and intraventricular conduction disorders in acute myocardial infarction: a reappraisal in the thrombolytic era. Pacing Clin Electrophysiol 1998; 21:2651–61.

20 Hindman MC, Wagner GS, JaRo M et al. The clinical significance of bundle branch block complicating acute myocardial infarction. 1. Clinical characteristics, hospital mortality, and one year follow up. Circulation 1978; 58:679–88.

21 Hindman MC, Wagner GS, JaRo M et al. The clinical significance of bundle branch block complicating acute myocardial infarction. 2. Indications for temporary and permanent pacemaker insertion. Circulation 1978; 58:689–99.

22 Lamas GA, Muller JE, Turi ZG et al. A simplified method to predict occurrence of complete heart block during acute myocardial infarction. Am J Cardiol 1986; 57:1213–9.

23 Harpaz D, Behar S, Gottlieb S et al. Complete atrioventricular block complicating acute myocardial infarction in the thrombolytic era. J Am Coll Cardiol 1999; 34:1721–8.

24 Antman EM, Anbe DT, Armstrong PW et al. American College of Cardiology, American Heart Association, Canadian Cardiovascular Society. ACC/AHA guidelines for the management of patients with ST-elevation myocardial infarction. J Am Coll Cardiol 2004; 44:671–719.

25 Vardas PE, Auricchhio A, Bland J-J et al. Guidelines for cardiac pacing and cardiac resynchronization therapy. The Task Force for Cardiac Pacing and Cardiac Resynchronization Therapy of the European Society of Cardiology. Developed in collaboration with the European Heart Rhythm Association. Eur Heart J 2007; 28:2256–95.

## CHAPTER 2

Basic concepts of pacing

Joshua M Cooper, G Neal Kay

Myocardial stimulation

An artificial electrical pacing stimulus excites cardiac tissue by the creation of an electrical field at the interface of the stimulating electrode and the underlying myocardium. Although a pacing stimulus can be applied to any portion of the body, a tissue response occurs only in cells that are excitable. For an artificial polarizing pulse to induce a response in excitable tissue, the stimulus must be of sufficient amplitude and duration to initiate a self-regenerating wavefront of action potentials that propagate away from the site of stimulation. Myocardial stimulation depends on an intact source of the electrical pulse (the pulse generator), a conductor between the source of the electrical pulse and the stimulating electrode (the lead conductor), an electrode for delivery of the pulse, and an area of myocardium that is excitable. In this section, the basic properties of myocardial stimulation are reviewed in detail.

Basic electrophysiology

The property of biological tissues such as nerve and muscle to respond to a stimulus with a response that is out of proportion to the strength of the stimulus is known as excitability.[1] Excitable tissues are characterized by a separation of charge across the cell membrane that results in a resting transmembrane electrical potential. For cardiac myocytes, the concentration of Na^+ ions outside the cell exceeds the concentration inside the cell. In contrast, the inside of the cell has a 35-fold greater concentration of K^+ ions than the outside of the cell. The resting transmembrane potential is maintained by the high resistance to ion flow, which is an intrinsic property of the lipid bilayer of the cell membrane. Because there is a passive leak of ions through membrane-bound ion channels, the resting potential is further maintained by two active transport mechanisms that exchange Na^+ ions for K^+ and Ca^{2+} ions. The Na^+–K^+ ATPase exchange "pump" extrudes three Na^+ ions for every two K^+ ions that are moved into the cell. The Na^+–Ca^{2+} transport mechanism exchanges three Na^+ ions toward the outside of the cell for each Ca^{2+} ion that is moved into the

Cardiac Pacing and ICDs, 5th edition. Edited by Kenneth A. Ellenbogen and Mark A. Wood. © 2008 Blackwell Publishing, ISBN: 978-1-4051-6350-7

cell. Because both of these transport mechanisms result in the net movement of three positive charges out of the cell in exchange for two positive charges that are moved in, a net polarization of the cell membrane is produced so that the inside of the cell is maintained electrically negative with respect to the outside. These transport mechanisms depend on the expenditure of energy in the form of high-energy phosphates and are susceptible to disruptions in aerobic cellular metabolism during myocardial ischemia.

Excitable tissues are further characterized by their ability to generate and propagate a transmembrane action potential.[1] The action potential is triggered by depolarization of the membrane from a resting potential of approximately −90 mV to a threshold potential of approximately −70 to −60 mV. Upon reaching the threshold transmembrane potential, specialized membrane-bound protein channels change conformation from an inactive state to an active state, which allows the free movement of Na^+ ions through the channel. The upstroke of the action potential (phase 0) is a consequence of this sudden influx of Na^+ into the myocyte and is associated with a change in transmembrane potential from −90 mV to approximately −20 mV (Fig. 2.1). It is estimated that the opening of a single Na^+ channel allows approximately 10^4 Na^+ ions to enter the cardiac myocyte. The number of Na^+ channels is estimated to be on the order of five to

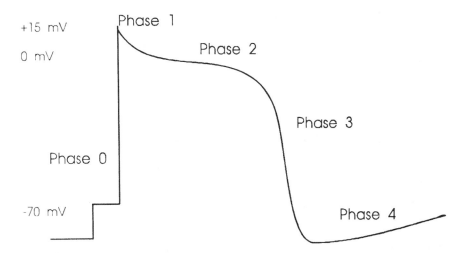

Fig. 2.1 The action potential of a Purkinje fiber is illustrated. The resting transmembrane potential is approximately −90 mV. Upon depolarization of the membrane to a threshold potential of −70 to −60 mV, the upstroke of the action potential is triggered (phase 0), carried predominantly by an influx of Na^+ ions into the cell. The transmembrane potential reaches approximately 15 mV (overshoot potential) and is repolarized to approximately 0 mV during phase 1. The plateau phase of the action potential (phase 2) is produced by a complex interaction of inward Ca^{2+} and Na^+ currents and outward K^+ currents. Repolarization of the cell occurs during phase 3, during which the cell regains the capability of responding to a polarizing electrical stimulus with another action potential. Phase 4 of the action potential is characterized by a slow upward drift in the transmembrane potential.

10 channels per square micrometer of cell membrane. In addition to Na^+ channels, specialized proteins are also suspended in the membrane that have differential selectivity for K^+, Ca^{2+} and Cl^- ions. The channels may remain in the open configuration for < 1 ms (characteristic of the Na^+ channel) to hundreds of milliseconds (typical of K^+ channels). The rapid upstroke of the action potential is followed by a short period of hyperpolarization when the transmembrane potential is transiently positively charged. The overshoot potential is quickly abolished (phase 1) by a transient outward K^+ current (I_{to}); and the cell enters the plateau phase (phase 2), during which Ca^{2+} and Na^+ are triggered to enter the cell and outward K^+ currents are activated. The cardiac cell is refractory to further electrical stimulation by a stimulus of any strength during the plateau phase. The net membrane voltage is maintained at approximately 0 mV as the inward Na^+ and Ca^{2+} currents are balanced by at least three outward K^+ currents having different time constants (slow, rapid, and ultrarapid: I_{KS}, I_{KR} and I_{KUR}). These K^+ currents have the property of delayed rectification. After the plateau phase, which lasts several hundred milliseconds, the cardiac cell begins the process of repolarization as the outward currents exceed the inward currents with regeneration of the resting membrane potential and the capability for responding to an electrical stimulus with another action potential (phase 3). The repolarization phase is characterized by the continuation of outward K^+ currents with inactivation of the inward Na^+ and Ca^{2+} currents, which results in a net negative polarization of the inside of the cell. During the repolarization phase an action potential may be induced if the myocyte is challenged by an electrical stimulus of sufficient strength. Following complete repolarization of the membrane, the cell enters a diastolic period during which it is fully excitable (phase 4).[2] Tissues demonstrating spontaneous automaticity exhibit a gradual upward drift in transmembrane potential until threshold is reached.

The response of excitable membranes to electrical stimuli is an active process that results in a response exceeding that of simple passive conductance along the membrane. Gap junctions that provide low-resistance intercellular connections conduct the action potential between myocytes.[3] The action potential at the site of stimulation results in the depolarization of neighboring areas of the myocyte membrane to threshold voltage, which triggers the Na^+ channels to open and results in regeneration of the action potential. The action potential is not only passively conducted, but also actively regenerated at each segment of membrane. However, propagation of the action potential away from the site of electrical stimulation also depends on certain passive cable properties of the myocardium, including the axis of myofiber orientation and the geometry of the connections between fibers. For example, a wavefront of depolarization is conducted with a conduction velocity that is three to five times greater along the longitudinal axis of a myofiber than along the transverse axis.[4] These anisotropic conduction properties may be further exaggerated in the presence of myocardial fibrosis, in which the intercellular collagen matrix is increased with decreased cell-to-cell communication. Such fibrosis is often present in patients with disorders of the cardiac conduction system. In addition, the safety factor for successful propagation is greater at sites where sheets of myocardium of similar size are joined than where a narrow isthmus of tissue joins a larger mass. Thus, as the structure of cardiac tissue is affected by pathological conditions such as fibrosis or infarction, the physiological properties of conduction and excitability may be significantly altered.

Stimulation threshold

Cardiac pacing involves the delivery of a polarizing electrical impulse from an electrode in contact with the myocardium with the generation of an electrical field of sufficient intensity to induce a propagating wave of cardiac action potentials.[5] The stimulating pulse may be either anodal or cathodal in polarity, although they demonstrate different stimulation characteristics. In addition, the stimulation characteristics are related to the source of the stimulating pulse, with constant-voltage and constant-current generators exhibiting somewhat different stimulation properties. The minimum stimulus intensity and duration necessary to reliably initiate a propagated depolarizing wavefront from an electrode is defined as the stimulation threshold. The stimulation threshold is a fundamental concept that is crucial to programming and troubleshooting permanent pacemakers and pacing leads. In this section, the factors that determine the stimulation threshold will be discussed.[6]

Strength–duration relation

For a pacing stimulus to produce a self-regenerating wave of depolarization in a cardiac chamber ("capture"), the stimulus must exceed a critical amplitude (measured in volts or milliamperes) and must be applied for a sufficient duration. These factors of stimulus amplitude and duration interact so that the minimal amplitude that is required to capture atrial or ventricular myocardium depends on the duration of the stimulating pulse (pulse duration).[7] The stimulus amplitude for endocardial stimulation has an exponential relation to the duration of the pulse, with a rapidly rising strength–duration curve at pulse durations < 0.25 ms and a relatively flat curve at pulse durations > 1.0 ms (Fig. 2.2). As can be appreciated by examining the hyperbolic strength–duration curve, a small change in pulse duration is associated with a significant change in the threshold amplitude at short pulse durations; however, only a small change at longer pulse durations. Because of the exponential relationship between stimulus amplitude and pulse duration, the entire strength–duration curve can be described relatively accurately by two points on the curve: rheobase and chronaxie. The rheobase of a strength–duration curve is defined as the lowest stimulus voltage that will electrically stimulate the myocardium at any pulse duration. For practical purposes, the rheobase voltage is usually determined as the threshold stimulus voltage at a pulse duration of 2.0 ms. Pulse durations > 2.0 ms provide a negligible lowering of the threshold stimulus voltage. One exception to this rule is with field stimulation, such as with transcutaneous or transesophageal pacing, in which the

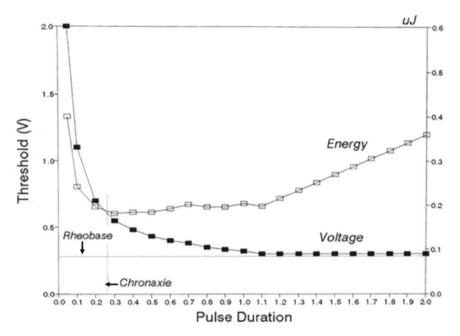

Fig. 2.2 Strength–duration curve for constant-voltage stimulation obtained at the time of permanent pacing lead implantation in a patient with complete atrioventricular block. The strength–duration relation is characterized by a steeply rising portion at short pulse durations and a relatively flat portion at pulse durations > 1 ms. The stimulus energy at each point on the strength–duration curve is also demonstrated. The rheobase voltage of a constant-voltage strength–duration curve is defined as the lowest stimulation voltage at any pulse duration. Because the curve is essentially flat at a pulse duration of 2 ms, rheobase can be accurately approximated as the threshold voltage at this point. Chronaxie, the threshold pulse duration at twice rheobase voltage, closely approximates the point of minimum threshold stimulation energy.

rheobase voltage is reached at much wider pulse durations (as long as 40 ms for transcutaneous pacing). The chronaxie is defined as the threshold pulse duration at a stimulus amplitude that is twice the rheobase voltage. Using the rheobase and chronaxie points, Lapicque, in 1909, described the following mathematical equation, which can be used to derive the strength–duration curve for constant-current stimulation:

$$I = I_r(1 + t_c/t) \tag{2.1}$$

where I is the threshold current at pulse duration t, I_r is the rheobase current, and t_c is the chronaxie pulse duration.

The relation of stimulus voltage, current, and pulse duration to stimulus energy is provided by the formula:

$$E = V^2/R \times t \tag{2.2}$$

where E is the stimulus energy, V is the stimulus voltage, R is the total pacing impedance, and t is the pulse duration. The chronaxie pulse duration is important in the clinical application of pacing, as it approximates the point of minimum threshold energy on the strength–duration curve, as can be appreciated from Fig. 2.2. With pulse durations greater than chronaxie, there is relatively little reduction in the threshold voltage. Rather, the wider pulse duration results in the wasting of stimulation energy without providing a substantial increase in safety margin. At pulse durations less than chronaxie, there is a steep increase in threshold voltage and stimulation energy. From the energy equation (Eq. 2.2), note that, whereas the energy of a pacing stimulus increases in direct relation to the pulse duration, the energy increases by the square of the voltage. Thus, doubling the pulse duration results in a twofold increase in stimulation energy, whereas doubling the stimulus voltage results in a fourfold increase.

An appreciation of the threshold strength–duration relation is important for the proper programming of the stimulus amplitude and pulse duration. Modern pulse generators offer two major methods for evaluating the stimulation threshold: either automatic decrementation of the stimulus voltage at a constant pulse duration, or automatic decrementation of the pulse duration at a constant stimulus voltage. To provide an adequate margin of safety, when the stimulation threshold is determined by decrementing the stimulus amplitude, the stimulus voltage is usually programmed to approximately twice the threshold value. Similarly, for pulse generators that determine threshold by automatically decrementing the pulse duration, the pulse duration is usually programmed to at least three times the threshold value. It should be recognized that the hyperbolic shape of the strength–duration curve has important implications for interpreting the results of threshold testing (Fig. 2.3). Although these methods provide comparable margins of safety when the threshold pulse duration is low (i.e. ≤ 0.15 ms), tripling a threshold pulse duration that is > 0.3 ms may not provide an adequate stimulation safety margin due to the flat nature of this part of the curve.

The threshold strength–duration curve is influenced by several factors, including the method of measurement, the nature of the electrode, the health of the tissue in contact with the electrode, the distance between the electrode and excitable myocardium, and the duration of lead implantation. Stimulation thresholds that are measured by decrementing the stimulus voltage until loss of capture are usually 0.1–0.2 V lower than when the stimulus intensity is gradually increased from subthreshold until capture is achieved.[8] This empiric observation, known as the Wedensky effect, must be considered when accurate measurements of the stimulation threshold are required. The Wedensky effect may be greater at narrow pulse durations, potentially reaching clinical significance. When the pacing rate is maintained as a constant during experimental conditions, the Wedensky effect is of marginal significance. This result suggests that this clinical phenomenon is probably explained by the ef-

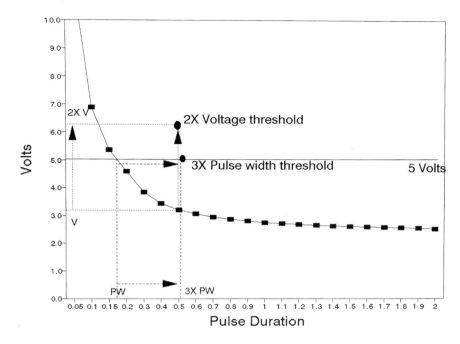

Fig. 2.3 The clinical use of the strength–duration relation to determine an adequate margin of safety for stimulation is demonstrated for a patient with a chronically implanted pacing lead. Note that when the stimulation threshold is determined by decrementing the pulse duration at a constant voltage (5 V), the strength–duration curve is encountered at the start of the rapidly rising portion of the curve. Tripling of the pulse duration provides an adequate safety margin. When the stimulation threshold is determined by decrementing the stimulus voltage at a constant pulse duration (0.5 ms), the strength–duration curve is encountered at a relatively flat portion of the curve. Doubling the stimulation voltage results in a somewhat greater margin of safety than with the alternative method.

fects of a varying cardiac rate during the gain or loss of capture as the stimulus amplitude is increased or decreased, respectively.

Strength–duration curves for constant-voltage and constant-current stimulation

There are several differences in the shape of the strength–duration curves for constant-current and constant-voltage stimulation (Fig. 2.4). For example, constant-voltage stimulation usually results in a flat curve at pulse durations > 1.5 ms, whereas the constant-current stimulation curve may be slowly downsloping beyond this pulse duration. The strength–duration curve with constant-current stimulation increases more steeply at short pulse durations than it does with constant-voltage stimulation. Small changes in pulse duration < 0.5 ms may result in a significantly greater reduction in the stimulation safety margin for constant-current than for constant-voltage pulse generators.

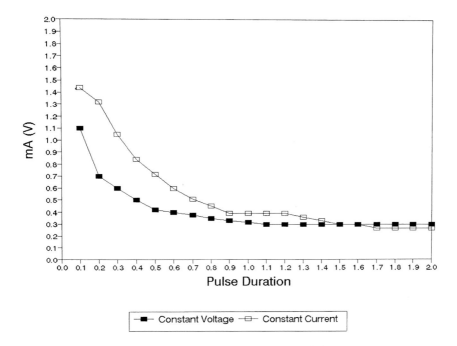

Fig. 2.4 Strength–duration curves determined with constant-current and constant-voltage stimulation in a single individual are demonstrated. Note that the constant-current stimulation curve continues to decline gradually at greater pulse durations than that obtained with constant-voltage stimulation.

Because of this difference in the shape of the strength–duration curves, the chronaxie pulse duration of a constant-current strength–duration relation is significantly greater than that observed with constant-voltage stimulation. Because the most efficient pulse duration for electrical stimulation is at chronaxie (in terms of threshold energy), a constant-voltage pulse generator can be set to deliver a narrower pulse duration than a constant-current generator and yet provide the same safety margin. Virtually all permanent pacemakers presently in use are constant-voltage generators. In contrast, most temporary pacemakers use constant-current generators.

Time-dependent changes in the stimulation threshold

Myocardial stimulation thresholds may change dramatically following positioning of a permanent pacing lead.[9] The typical course of events following implantation of a non-steroid eluting endocardial pacing lead starts with an acute rise in threshold that begins within the first 24 h (Fig. 2.5). The threshold usually continues to rise over the next several days, usually peaking at approximately 1 week. The typical stimulation threshold then gradually declines over the next several weeks. By 6 weeks, the myocardial stimulation threshold has usually stabilized at a value that is significantly greater than

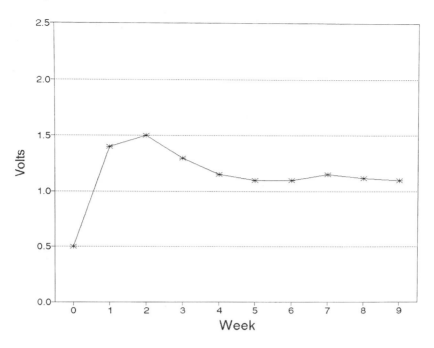

Fig. 2.5 Typical evolution of the stimulation threshold over the first 2 months following implantation of a platinum–iridium pacing lead. The stimulation threshold increases from implantation, peaking at 1–2 weeks. The chronic stimulation threshold has stabilized by 6 weeks in this individual. Although this curve is typical of those obtained with standard (non-steroid) permanent pacing leads, there is considerable variability among individuals in the absolute values and slope. With steroid eluting leads, the stimulation threshold rise is significantly blunted, and a lower final plateau is typically seen.

that measured at implantation of the lead, but less than the acute peak. The magnitude of the change in threshold varies widely between individuals and relates to the electrode's size, shape, chemical composition and surface structure. The stability of the electrode–myocardial interface and the flexibility of the lead also influence the acute-to-chronic change in threshold. In addition to the typical evolution of the stimulation threshold following lead implantation, certain leads may exhibit a hyperacute phase of threshold evolution. For example, active fixation electrodes using a screw helix as the active electrode may produce, immediately following implantation, an increased stimulation threshold that gradually decreases over the course of minutes. This transient high threshold is probably related to acute injury at the myocardial–electrode interface and is generally not observed with atraumatic passive fixation leads. Clinically, the hyperacute phase may be manifested by a current of injury in the electrogram. Both the current of injury and the stimulation threshold usually decline rapidly over the first several minutes before pursuing the typical acute-to-chronic threshold evolution, shown in Fig. 2.5. Thus, comparisons of changes in stimulation threshold between varying lead designs require an appreciation of the acute effects of the fixation mechanism. The addition of steroid elution to a pacing electrode (or a steroid-eluting collar around the electrode) markedly attenuates the gradual evolutionary effects, resulting in a much more constant stimulation threshold over time. Several other factors may affect the change in stimulation threshold that occurs with lead maturation, such as the mass of the lead tip, the stability of the electrode in relation to the myocardial interface, and the force with which the electrode is held in contact with the myocardium. In general, the more stable and the less traumatic the interaction of the electrode and lead with the myocardium, the lower the rise in threshold over time.

Proper programming of the stimulus amplitude of a permanent pacemaker requires an understanding of several factors. First, the strength–duration relation must be appreciated. Second, the safety margin that is chosen for a particular patient must be based on the degree of pacemaker dependency—that is, the likelihood of the patient's developing symptoms should loss of effective pacing occur. For patients judged to be highly pacemaker-dependent, a higher stimulation safety margin may be prudent. As an example, a patient with complete atrioventricular (AV) block with an unreliable ventricular escape rhythm may be more likely to develop symptoms with loss of ventricular capture than may a patient with intermittent sinus node dysfunction. On the other hand, the patient with AV block is likely to be less dependent on atrial than ventricular capture. Thus, a higher safety margin may be needed for the ventricular stimulus than for the atrial stimulus in such an individual. Third, an appreciation of the effect of stimulus amplitude and duration on battery longevity is required. As discussed later in this chapter in the section on output circuits, programming the stimulus intensity > 2.8 V results in a marked increase in current drain from the battery. Fourth, the overall metabolic and pharmacological history of the patient must be considered. For example, patients requiring the addition of certain antiarrhythmic drugs to their medication regimen may experience a small increase in pacing threshold. Similarly, patients subject to major shifts in potassium concentration or acid–base balance, such as those with renal failure, may have transient increases in pacing threshold. The safety margin that is chosen for these individuals may need to be greater than that for other patients.

Several investigators have reported that the pacing threshold varies inversely with the surface area of the stimulating electrode.[10] For spherical electrodes, the smaller the surface area of the electrode, the lower the pacing threshold. The explanation for this observation relates to the intensity of the electric field that is generated at the surface of the electrode. For a constant-voltage pulse, the smaller the electrode, the greater the intensity of the electric field and the current density at the surface. The threshold maturation process has been shown to be caused by the growth of an inexcitable capsule of fibrous tissue surrounding the electrode (Fig. 2.6).[11] This fibrous capsule effectively

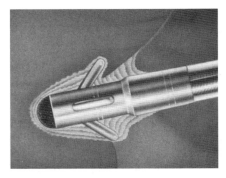

Fig. 2.6 Diagram of a fibrous capsule surrounding a chronically implanted passive fixation pacing electrode. The inexcitable capsule increases the effective radius of the stimulating electrode, reducing the current density at the interface of the capsule and excitable myocardium and increasing the stimulation threshold. (Courtesy of Medtronic, Inc.)

increases the surface area of the electrode, thereby decreasing the intensity of the electric field at the junction of the fibrous capsule and the more normal, excitable myocardium.

The cellular events that result in the development of a fibrous capsule have been intensively studied. The initial tissue reaction to the implantation of a permanent pacing lead involves acute injury to cell membranes. This damage is rapidly followed by the development of myocardial edema and coating of the electrode by platelets and fibrin. These events are followed by the release of chemotactic factors and the development of a typical cellular inflammatory reaction with the infiltration of polymorphonuclear leukocytes and mononuclear cells. Following the acute polymorphonuclear response, the myocardium at the interface with the stimulating electrode is invaded by macrophages. The extracellular release of proteolytic enzymes and toxic free oxygen radicals results in an acceleration of tissue injury underlying the electrode. The acute inflammatory response is followed by the accumulation of more macrophages and the influx of fibroblasts into the myocardium. The fibroblasts in the myocardium begin producing collagen, leading to the development of the fibrotic capsule surrounding the electrode.

The influences of several pharmacological agents on the electrode–myocardial maturation process have been studied. Non-steroidal anti-inflammatory drugs have been shown to have minimal influence on the evolution of pacing thresholds. In contrast, corticosteroids, either systemically or locally administered, may have dramatic effects on the evolution of pacing thresholds. By the use of an infusion pump to deliver dexamethasone sodium phosphate from the center of a ring-shaped electrode, Stokes has demonstrated a dramatic decrease in the expected acute-to-chronic rise in pacing threshold with both atrial and ventricular pacing leads in canines. Clinical studies have confirmed these findings and have led to the development of leads that gradually elute dexamethasone from a reservoir beneath the stimulating electrode.[12] These corticosteroid-eluting leads have been associated with stable pacing thresholds from the time of implantation and through the follow-up period of several years. Other designs incorporate dexamethasone into a drug-eluting collar that surrounds the stimulating electrode. The application of corticosteroid-eluting collars to active fixation leads has demonstrated that the nature of the electrode remains important to the evolution of pacing thresholds, even in the presence of anti-inflammatory drugs. Nevertheless, steroid elution has been shown to be an effective means of lowering the long-term pacing threshold for leads of virtually all designs, including active and passive fixation endocardial leads as well as epimyocardial screw-in leads.

Strength–interval relation

The stimulation threshold is influenced significantly by the coupling interval of electrical stimuli and the frequency of stimulation.[13] Figure 2.7 demonstrates a typical ventricular strength–interval curve for both cathodal and anodal stimulation. Note that the stimulus intensity required to capture the ventricle remains quite constant at long extrastimulus coupling intervals, but rises exponentially at shorter intervals. The rise in stimulation threshold at short coupling intervals is related to impingement of the stimulus on the relative refractory period of the ventricular myocardium. As discussed

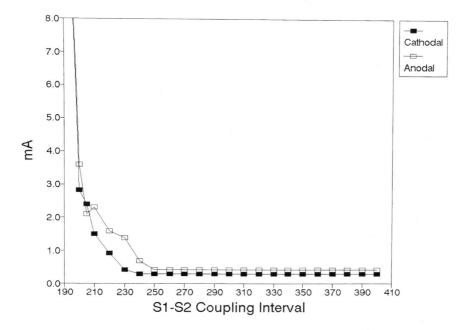

Fig. 2.7 The strength–interval relationship for constant current with unipolar anodal and cathodal stimulation is demonstrated in a normal individual. Note that the shape of the curve is relatively flat at long extrastimulus coupling intervals and rises exponentially at short coupling intervals. Also note that cathodal stimulation results in a lower stimulation threshold at long coupling intervals than does anodal stimulation. At short coupling intervals, the anodal stimulation curve may transiently "dip" before rapidly rising.

previously, an electrical stimulus applied during the repolarization phase of the cardiac action potential will result in a propagated action potential only if it is of sufficient intensity. However, during the plateau phase of the action potential, electrical stimuli of any intensity will not be able to generate an action potential as the absolute refractory period is encountered. Figure 2.7 also illustrates the important differences in anodal and cathodal stimulation. Late diastolic stimulation thresholds are lower with cathodal than with anodal stimulation. However, at relatively short extrastimulus coupling intervals, the anodal stimulation threshold may be less than the cathodal threshold. During the relative refractory period, the anodal threshold may actually decline ("dip") before abruptly rising at shorter coupling intervals. With bipolar cardiac pacing, the stimulation threshold is generally determined by the cathode. However, with short extrastimulus coupling intervals, the bipolar stimulation threshold may actually be determined by the anode. If the stimulus intensity exceeds both the cathodal and anodal thresholds, bipolar pacing may result in stimulation at both electrode–myocardial interfaces (both anodal and cathodal stimulation).

Effects of pacing rate on myocardial stimulation

The stimulation frequency may have an important influence on pacing threshold, although increases in threshold have been demonstrated only at very rapid pacing rates.[14] At shorter stimulation cycle lengths, the action potential of atrial and ventricular myocardium shortens, resulting in a proportional decrease in the relative refractory period. At rapid pacing rates, these factors are manifested by a shift in the strength–interval curve to the left. However, at pacing rates exceeding 250 beats per minute (bpm), pacing stimuli may be delivered during the relative refractory period, resulting in an increase in threshold. The strength–duration curve is shifted upward and to the right at very rapid pacing rates (Fig. 2.8), which may have important implications for antitachycardia pacing. Thus, a stimulation amplitude that provides an adequate safety margin for pacing at slow rates may not be sufficient at rapid pacing rates. Antitachycardia devices provide for this possible increase in stimulation threshold by an automatic increase in the amplitude of pacing stimuli that are delivered at rapid pacing rates. In recognition of the rate dependence of the pacing threshold, implantable cardioverter defibrillators (ICDs) typically provide greater stimulus intensity during antitachycardia pacing than during antibradycardia pacing.

Pharmacological and metabolic effects on the stimulation threshold

The stimulation threshold may demonstrate considerable variability over the normal 24-h period, generally increasing during sleep and falling during the waking hours (Table 2.1).[15] The changes in threshold parallel fluctuations in autonomic tone and circulating catecholamines, and consequently there is a decreased threshold during exercise. The stimulation threshold is inversely

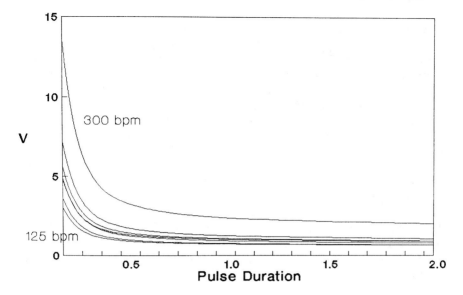

Fig. 2.8 The effect of pacing rate on the atrial strength–duration relation for a normal individual is demonstrated. Threshold curves were obtained at pacing rates of 125–300 ppm in increments of 25 ppm. Note that the strength–duration curves largely overlap at pacing rates of 125–250 ppm. At pacing rates of 275–300 ppm, the curve is shifted upward and to the right.

Table 2.1 Pharmacological and metabolic effects on stimulation threshold

	Increase threshold	*Decrease threshold*
Antiarrhythmic drugs	Class I Quinidine Procainamide Flecainide Propafenone Class III Amiodarone (?)	
Other drugs	β-Blockers	Catecholamines Isoproterenol Corticosteroids
Metabolic conditions	Hyperkalemia Hyperglycemia Hypoxemia Hypercarbia Metabolic acidosis Metabolic alkalosis	
Activity/other conditions	Sleeping Eating Viral illness Vagal tone	Exercise Sympathetic tone

related to the level of circulating corticosteroids. The stimulation threshold may increase following eating, during hyperglycemia, hypoxemia, hypercarbia, and metabolic acidosis or alkalosis. The stimulation threshold may increase dramatically during acute viral illnesses, especially in children. The concentration of serum electrolytes may also influence the stimulation threshold, with the most common clinical scenario being a rise in the stimulation threshold in the setting of hyperkalemia.

Drugs may also influence the stimulation threshold. As mentioned above, catecholamines reduce the threshold, and the infusion of isoproterenol may restore capture in some patients with exit block. In contrast, β-blocking drugs increase the stimulation threshold. Corticosteroids, either orally or parenterally administered, may produce a dramatic decrease in the stimulation threshold and are occasionally useful for the management of the acute increase in threshold that may be observed following lead implantation. The list of drugs that raise the stimulation threshold includes the type I antiarrhythmic drugs quinidine, procainamide, flecainide and propafenone. It is not clear whether the type III drug amiodarone has similar effects. Virtually all antiarrhythmic drugs may influence the pacing threshold, although they are usually clinically important only at high serum concentrations.

Occasional patients exhibit a progressive rise in the stimulation threshold over time, a clinical syndrome known as "exit block." Exit block seems to occur despite optimal lead positioning, as it recurs with the subsequent implantation of new pacing leads. In patients with exit block, the threshold changes in the atrium tend to parallel those in the ventricle. Exit block is best managed by the use of steroid-eluting ventricular leads, which have been associated with low thresholds in patients with this syndrome (Fig. 2.9).

Impedance

Impedance is the sum of all factors that oppose the flow of current in an electric circuit. Impedance is not necessarily the same as resistance. The relationship between voltage (V), current (I) and resistance (R) in an electrical circuit is estimated by Ohm's law, $V = IR$. For circuits that follow Ohm's law, impedance and resistance are equal. If voltage is held constant, the current flow is inversely related to the resistance of the circuit ($I = V/R$). The leading-edge voltage of a constant-voltage pulse generator is fixed, and the lower the resistance, the greater the current flow. In contrast, the greater the resistance, the lower the current flow. Because implantable pulse generators are powered by lithium iodine batteries with a fixed amount of charge, pacing impedance is an important determinant of battery longevity.

The total pacing impedance is determined by factors that are related to the lead conductor (resistance), the resistance to current flow from the electrode to the myocardium (electrode resistance) and the accumulation of charges of opposite polarity in the myocardium at the electrode–tissue interface (polarization). Thus, the total pacing impedance (Z_{total}) = $Z_c + Z_e + Z_p$, where Z_c is the

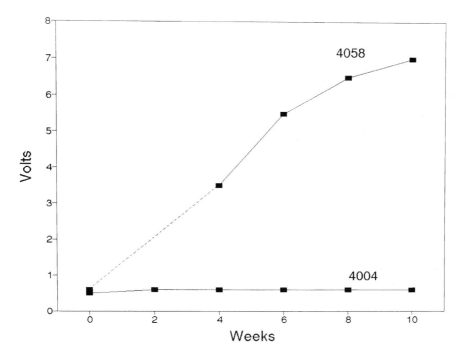

Fig. 2.9 The evolution of the stimulation threshold voltage (pulse duration 0.5 ms) in the right ventricular apex is demonstrated for an individual with a history of exit block. Note that the stimulation threshold increases progressively from implantation with an active fixation ventricular lead (model 4058). Following implantation of a corticosteroid-eluting electrode (model 4004) in the same patient, the stimulation threshold remains low. Exit block occurs infrequently, but usually occurs with standard (non-steroid) pacing leads.

conductor resistance, Z_e is the electrode resistance, and Z_p is the polarization impedance. The resistance to current flow provided by the lead conductor results in a voltage drop across the lead with a portion of the pacing pulse converted into heat. Thus, this component of the total pacing impedance is an inefficient use of electrical energy and does not contribute to myocardial stimulation. The ideal pacing lead would have a very low conductor resistance (Z_c). In contrast, the ideal pacing lead would also have a relatively high electrode resistance (Z_e) to minimize current flow and maximize battery life. The electrode resistance is largely a function of the electrode radius, with higher resistance provided by a smaller electrode. An electrode with a small radius minimizes current flow in an efficient manner. In addition to providing greater electrode resistance, pacing electrodes with a small radius provide increased current density and lower stimulation thresholds. Because of these properties, modern pacing and ICD leads take advantage of smaller electrodes to increase electrode resistance, allowing the total pacing impedance to exceed 1000 Ω. Compared with a pacing lead with a total impedance of 500 Ω, a lead with

1000 Ω of impedance would decrease the current drain of each pacing pulse by 50%, thereby prolonging the usable battery life of the implantable pulse generator. The routine use of these leads has allowed implantable devices to become smaller while maintaining battery longevity. There is a practical lower limit to the size of the electrode, which is related to the likelihood of maintaining stable contact of the electrode with the endocardium throughout the cardiac and respiratory cycles. For example, pacing leads with a very small distal electrode may be associated with a relatively high pacing threshold in a small proportion of patients (< 5%), probably as a result of radiographically imperceptible "microdislodgement" of the electrode at the point of contact with the endocardium.

The third component of pacing impedance, polarization impedance, is an effect of electrical stimulation and is related to the movement of charged ions in the myocardium toward the cathode. When an electrical current is applied to the myocardium, the cathode attracts positively charged ions and repels negatively charged ions in the extracellular space. The cathode rapidly becomes surrounded by a layer of hydrated Na^+ and H_3O^+ ions. Farther away from the cathode, a second layer forms of negatively charged ions (Cl^-, HPO_4^{2-}, and OH^-). Thus, the negatively charged cathode induces the accumulation of two layers of oppositely charged ions in the myocardium. Initially, the movement of charged ions results in the flow of current in the myocardium. As the cathode becomes surrounded by an inside layer of positive charges and an outside layer of negative charges, a functional capacitor develops that impedes the further movement of charge (Fig. 2.10). The capacitive effect of polarization increases throughout the application of the pulse, peaking at the trailing edge and decaying exponentially following the pulse as the charged layers dissolve into electrical neutrality (Fig. 2.11). Because polarization impedes the movement of charge in the myocardium, it creates inefficiency and results in an increased voltage requirement for stimulation. Thus, polarization impedance reduces the effectiveness of a pacing stimulus to stimulate the myocardium and wastes current. Polarization impedance is directly related to the duration of the pulse and can be minimized by the use of relatively short pulse durations. Polarization is inversely related to the surface area of the electrode. To minimize the effect of polarization (Z_p) but maximize electrode resistance (Z_e), a complex, porous surface can be used to coat the electrode in order to maintain a small geometric radius, yet greatly increase the microscopic sur-

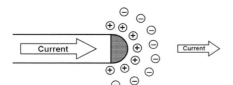

Fig. 2.10 When current is applied to the myocardium, the pacing cathode becomes surrounded by a layer of positively charged ions, which in turn attracts a layer of negatively charged ions. This effect is known as polarization, where the layers of ions serve as a functional capacitor, impeding current flow into the myocardium.

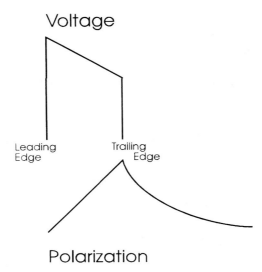

Voltage

Leading
Edge

Trailing
Edge

Polarization

Fig. 2.11 The relationship between the voltage waveform of a constant-voltage pulse and the development of polarization effect at the electrode–myocardial interface is illustrated. Note that the polarization effect rises during application of the stimulating pulse and decays exponentially. The trailing edge of the output pulse is less than the leading edge, as the output capacitor loses charge during discharge of the pulse.

face area.[16] Electrodes constructed with activated carbon or coated with platinum black or iridium oxide are effective in minimizing the wasteful effects of polarization and in diminishing afterpotentials, which can interfere with sensing.

The evolution of pacing impedance is usually characterized by a fall over the first 1–2 weeks following implantation. The chronic pacing impedance then rises to a stable value that is, on average, approximately 15% higher than that at implant. Serial measurements of pacing impedance are extremely valuable for the assessment of lead integrity; low impedance measurements usually reflect a failure of conductor insulation, and high values often suggest conductor fracture or a loose set-screw at the proximal connector. It should be emphasized that the method of measurement greatly influences the impedance value. For example, if the pacing impedance is measured at the leading edge of the pulse, the value reflects Z_c and Z_e, but not Z_p. In contrast, measurements near the midpoint of the pulse are a more accurate reflection of the total pacing impedance. For clinical purposes, serial assessments of impedance should use a consistent method of measurement.

Bipolar vs. unipolar stimulation

The term unipolar pacing is technically a misnomer, as both bipolar and unipolar configurations require an anode and a cathode to complete the electrical circuit. Because both unipolar and bipolar pacing use an electrode in contact with the myocardium (usually as the cathode), the difference in these configurations lies in the location of the other electrode (usually the anode). For a unipolar pacing stimulus, the anode is extracardiac, being the metal casing or "can" of the pulse generator (Fig. 2.12). The anode for bipolar stimulation is located on the pacing lead within the heart, either in contact with the endocardium or lying free within the blood pool of the cardiac chamber. The pacing impedance is slightly higher with bipolar than with unipolar pacing, because two conducting wires are required. The stimulation threshold is slightly lower with unipolar than with bipolar pacing, but this difference is of a small magnitude that is rarely of any clinical significance.

The clinically important differences between bipolar and unipolar pacing relate to the fact that the pacemaker can, which acts as the anode in the unipolar configuration, lies adjacent to the pectoral muscle. During unipolar sensing, pectoral myopotentials may be sensed, resulting in inappropriate pacing inhibition during muscle contraction. With unipolar pacing at higher outputs, pectoral muscle stimulation may be encountered with paced stimuli, resulting in muscle twitching. Because the distance between cathode and anode is so much greater during unipolar pacing, the pacing stimulus on the surface electrocardiogram (ECG) is much larger than during bipolar pacing. The increased size of the "pacer spike" may be visually helpful to determine proper pacemaker function when interpreting cardiac telemetry recordings or transtelephonic ECG tracings during remote pacemaker monitoring. Conversely,

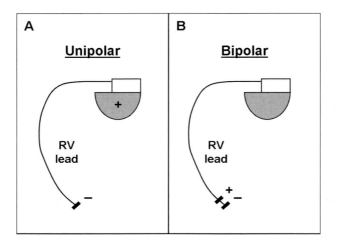

Fig. 2.12 (A) A unipolar pacing configuration uses the distal pacemaker electrode as the circuit cathode and the metal of the pacemaker can as the circuit anode. (B) A bipolar pacing configuration requires a pacemaker lead with two separate conductors, one leading to the distal "tip" electrode, which is the pacing cathode, and the second leading to the closely spaced, but more proximal "ring" electrode, which is the pacing anode. RV, right ventricular.

the larger amplitude signal from unipolar pacing is far more likely to interfere with appropriate sensing of the cardiac rhythm by an ICD in the rare instance that a patient has a separate pacemaker and ICD implanted. Because of the autogain sensing algorithms found in ICDs, a sensed large-amplitude unipolar pacing stimulus will result in subsequent underdetection of low-amplitude intracardiac signals, such as those that occur during ventricular fibrillation (VF). It is for this reason that the use of bipolar pacing is critical when a separate pacemaker is present in an ICD patient. Bipolar pacing leads are also necessary for some rate-adaptive sensors, such as the minute-ventilation sensor, as well as for some types of automatic threshold algorithms, where the ring electrode is used to sense myocardial capture.

Biventricular pacing

In the early days of cardiac resynchronization therapy (CRT) pacing, implantable devices were not manufactured with separate pacing circuits for the right and left ventricular leads. In addition, only unipolar leads were manufactured for the purpose of pacing the left ventricle via a cardiac vein. Because of these limitations, unique pacing issues arose related to the configuration of a pacing circuit for biventricular stimulation (Fig. 2.13). The most common configuration usually involved electrically linking the tip electrodes of the right ventricular (RV) and left ventricular (LV) leads as a split cathode, and using either the RV ring electrode (if a bipolar RV lead was present) or the pulse generator as the common anode. An alternative, less-used configuration was to create a widely spaced bipole with the RV tip electrode as the cathode (or anode) and the LV tip electrode as the anode (or cathode), relying on both anodal and cathodal capture for biventricular stimulation. In the split cathodal configuration, the leads were electrically linked either with a separate Y-adaptor component or a "built-in" Y-adaptor in the device header. Because the two ventricular leads essentially function as circuits in parallel, the total impedance decreases, current drain increases, and stimulation thresholds are higher, compared with the measured parameters of each lead alone. The combined ventricular output had to be programmed above the higher of the two stimulation thresholds in order to maintain biventricular pacing. Additionally, lead parameter assessment was more challenging. Separate RV and LV thresholds could not be performed, and so a change in the paced QRS morphology had to be appreciated during threshold testing to signify loss of capture of one of the ventricular leads. Conductor fractures and insulation breaks were also more difficult to diagnose, as their effect on the common ventricular impedance was less prominent, being only one limb of a parallel circuit configuration. Some of these early-model biventricular devices remain in use, and the above-mentioned characteristics of parallel circuits should be appreciated with regard to assessment of lead parameters and lead integrity.

Almost all modern biventricular devices include separate RV and LV pacing circuits, with separately programmable pacing parameters, which greatly

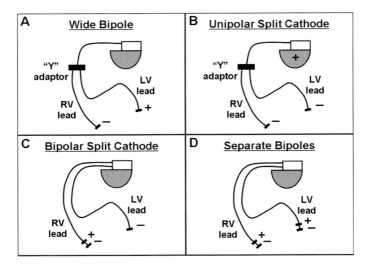

Fig. 2.13 (A) Extended bipolar configuration for biventricular pacing where the right ventricular (RV) tip electrode serves as the cathode and the left ventricular (LV) tip electrode serves as the anode. A "Y" adaptor converts two unipolar leads into a bipolar connector pin that is inserted into the pacemaker header. Sufficient pacing output must be delivered to permit both cathodal and anodal capture in order for biventricular stimulation to occur. (B) Unipolar split cathode configuration where the RV and LV tip electrodes are electrically "linked" via a separate "Y" adaptor or one that is integrated into the pacemaker header. Both lead distal electrodes serve as cathodes and the pacemaker can serves as the common anode. The two leads are connected in parallel, and the pacing circuit therefore displays electrical properties of resistors in parallel, which has implications for interpreting pacing impedance measurements (see text). (C) Bipolar split cathode configuration, also described as an "extended bipole" LV pacing configuration when separate pacing circuits are present. The distal RV and LV tip electrodes serve as cathodes and the RV ring electrode serves as the common anode. Modern biventricular devices give the option for this pacing configuration, even when a bipolar LV lead is present. (D) Separate bipolar pacing configurations for RV and LV leads, which each have tip (cathode) and ring (anode) electrodes. The two pacing circuits can be separately tested, and each circuit has its own pacing impedance characteristics.

simplifies lead assessment and also reduces battery current drain. Coronary sinus leads are currently manufactured in both unipolar and bipolar varieties. A unipolar LV lead can be configured either unipolar (where the pacemaker generator is the anode), or extended bipolar (where the RV ring or RV coil electrode—in the setting of some ICD leads—is the anode). A bipolar LV lead allows for even more possible pacing configurations, which can be of clinical utility when phrenic nerve stimulation is an issue. Because the LV lead is frequently positioned near the left phrenic nerve, which runs along the pericardium on its way to the left hemidiaphragm, rhythmic stimulation of the phrenic nerve may occur with LV pacing. With a unipolar LV lead, reduction in pacing output is the only non-invasive option for eliminating diaphragmatic pacing, and this option may be limited when the phrenic nerve stimulation threshold is not much higher than the myocardial stimulation threshold. With a bipolar LV lead, aside from the option of trying unipolar and bipolar pacing configurations, some device manufacturers allow for extended bipolar pacing configurations using either the LV tip or LV ring electrode as the cathode, which may further increase the chance that a programming change can eliminate phrenic nerve capture, thereby avoiding the need to reposition the LV lead.

Sensing

Sensing of the cardiac electrogram is essential to the proper function of permanent pacemakers. In addition to responding to appropriate intrinsic atrial or ventricular electrograms, permanent pacing systems must be able to discriminate these signals from unwanted electrical interference: far-field cardiac events, diastolic potentials, skeletal muscle signals, and pacing stimuli. In this section, the basic determinants of electrogram sensing will be discussed.

Intracardiac electrograms

Intracardiac electrical signals are produced by the movement of electrical current through the myocardium. An electrode that overlies a region of resting myocardium records from the outside of cardiac myocytes, which are positively charged with respect to the inside of the cell. An electrode sitting in one region of resting myocardium will record a charge similar to that recorded by an electrode in another region of resting myocardium (no potential voltage difference between the electrodes). During depolarization, the outside of the cell becomes electrically negative with respect to the inside. Therefore, as a wavefront of depolarization travels toward an endocardial electrode that is in contact with resting myocardium, the electrode becomes positively charged relative to the depolarized region. This is manifested in the intracardiac electrogram as a positive deflection. As the wavefront of depolarization passes under the recording electrode, the outside of the cell suddenly becomes negatively charged relative to resting myocardium, and a brisk negative deflection is inscribed in the intracardiac electrogram. The peak negative deflection in the intracardiac electrogram, known as the intrinsic deflection (Fig. 2.14), is considered the moment of myocardial activation underlying the recording electrode.

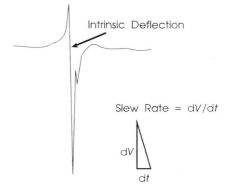

Fig. 2.14 A typical bipolar ventricular electrogram in a normal individual. The sharp downward deflection in the electrogram represents the intrinsic deflection and indicates the moment of activation under the recording electrode. The slope of the intrinsic deflection (dV/dt) is expressed in volts per second and is referred to as the slew rate. For an electrogram to be sensed by a sensing amplifier, the amplitude and slew rate must exceed the sensing thresholds.

The positive and negative deflections that precede and follow the intrinsic deflection represent activation in neighboring regions of myocardium relative to the recording electrode. In clinical practice, the intrinsic deflection in the intracardiac electrogram is usually biphasic, with predominantly negative or positive deflections less frequently observed.[17] Because of the greater mass of myocardium, a normal ventricular electrogram is usually of far greater amplitude than a normal atrial electrogram.

Characteristics of intracardiac electrograms

The frequency content of atrial and ventricular electrograms has been demonstrated to be similar. By using Fourier transformation, one can express the frequency spectrum of an electrical signal as a series of sine waves of varying frequency and amplitude. Fourier transformation of ventricular electrograms demonstrates that the maximum density of frequencies for R waves is usually found between 10 and 30 Hz. The effects of filtering the ventricular electrogram are shown in Fig. 2.15. As can be appreciated from the figure, removing frequencies below 10 Hz markedly attenuates the repolarization artifact, which is usually a slow, broad signal composed of lower frequencies (< 5 Hz),

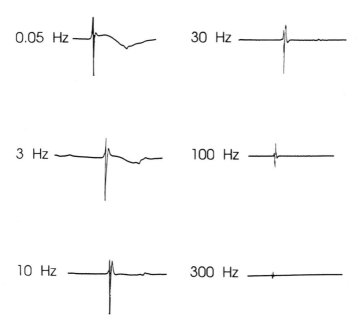

Fig. 2.15 The effects of filtering on the bipolar ventricular electrogram are demonstrated. Note that high-pass filtering of the electrogram to eliminate frequencies below 10 Hz has the effect of attenuating the repolarization artifact. Filtering of frequencies > 30 Hz results in marked attenuation of the electrogram amplitude. The center frequency of most sensing amplifiers is approximately 30 Hz, consistent with the typical frequency spectra of intracardiac electrograms.

without significantly influencing the R wave. Similarly, the far-field R wave in the atrial electrogram is composed predominantly of low-frequency signals, and can be removed, along with other unwanted low-frequency components, with a high-pass filter. In contrast, the frequency spectrum of skeletal myopotentials, such as those of the pectoral muscle or diaphragm, ranges from approximately 10 to 200 Hz, with considerable overlap with the intrinsic R and P waves. Although some high-frequency components can be removed with filtering, inappropriate sensing of myopotentials remains an issue with the unipolar configuration.

For the intracardiac electrogram to be sensed by the sense amplifier of an implantable pulse generator, the signal must be of sufficient amplitude, measured in peak-to-peak voltage. In addition, the intrinsic deflection of the electrogram must have sufficient slope. The intrinsic deflection is the rapid biphasic part of the endocardial electrogram, which represents the time that the myocardium under the electrode is depolarized as the wavefront passes through the tissue. The peak slope (dV/dt) of the intrinsic deflection of the electrogram (also known as the slew rate) is of critical importance to proper sensing (see Fig. 2.14). The sense amplifier of most pulse generators has a center frequency (the frequency for which the amplifier is most sensitive) in the range of 30–40 Hz, so frequencies greater than this are attenuated and less likely to be sensed. Components of the electrogram less than the center frequency are also attenuated, with the output of the filter proportional to the slew rate of the waveform. In general, the higher the slew rate of an electrogram, the higher the frequency content. Thus, slow and broad signals with a low slew rate may not be sensed, even if the peak-to-peak amplitude of the electrogram is large. In clinical practice, the slew rate and amplitude of intracardiac electrograms are only modestly proportional. Because of this, both the slew rate and the amplitude of the intracardiac electrogram need to be considered with regard to device sensing.

Unipolar and bipolar sensing

As both unipolar and bipolar sensing configurations detect the difference in electrical potential between two electrodes, the inter-electrode distance has a considerable influence on the nature of the electrogram. If a transvenous bipolar lead is used for sensing, both electrodes are located in the heart with an inter-electrode distance that is almost always < 3 cm. A unipolar lead uses one electrode in contact with the heart and the other in contact with the pulse generator, often with an inter-electrode distance of 30–50 cm. Because both electrodes may contribute to the electrical signal that is sensed, the bipolar electrode configuration is minimally influenced by electrical signals that originate outside the heart, while the unipolar configuration may detect electrical signals that originate near the pulse generator pocket. These features of unipolar sensing make this electrode configuration much more susceptible to interference by electrical signals originating in skeletal muscle (myopotentials). The myopotentials associated with pectoral muscle contraction may be sensed by unipolar pacemakers, resulting in inappropriate inhibition (if sensed in the ventricular channel) or triggering of pacing output (if sensed in the atrial channel). Bipolar sensing is relatively immune to myopotentials, which is a significant clinical advantage. Bipolar sensing is less likely to be influenced by electromagnetic signals from the environment, such as those due to electrocautery or other sources of electromagnetic interference, than is unipolar sensing. Bipolar sensing is also less likely to sense far-field signals (e.g. an atrial bipolar lead is less likely than an atrial unipolar lead to sense a ventricular "far-field" signal). Typical amplitudes for ventricular electrograms are 3–30 mV and for atrial electrograms are 1–6 mV.

A bipolar electrogram is actually the instantaneous difference in electrical voltage between the two electrodes. Thus, a bipolar electrogram can be constructed by subtracting the absolute unipolar voltage recorded at the cathode (vs. ground) from the unipolar voltage recorded at the anode (vs. ground). Because the bipolar configuration represents the signal at the cathode minus the signal at the anode, the net electrogram may be considerably different from that of either unipolar electrogram alone. For example, if an advancing wavefront of depolarization is perpendicular to the inter-electrode axis of a bipolar lead, each electrode will be activated at exactly the same time, and the instantaneous difference in voltage will be minimal. In this situation, the bipolar electrogram will be markedly attenuated. In contrast, a wavefront of depolarization traveling parallel to the electrode axis of a bipolar lead will activate one electrode before the other, and the resulting bipolar electrogram may have significantly greater amplitude than either unipolar electrogram alone. From these examples, it should be recognized that bipolar sensing is more sensitive to the direction in which the depolarizing wavefront travels than is unipolar sensing. Bipolar electrograms are more likely to be influenced by phasic changes in orientation of the lead with respiration than are unipolar electrograms. Because of these considerations, the electrogram measured at the time of lead implantation should be recorded in the configuration that will be used for sensing by the pulse generator.

Another significant difference between unipolar and bipolar sensing relates to the amplitude of far-field signals. Because of the significantly greater mass of the ventricles, the atrial unipolar electrogram often records a far-field R wave that can sometimes be equal to or of greater amplitude than the atrial deflection itself (Fig. 2.16). In contrast, the bipolar atrial electrogram usually records an atrial deflection that is considerably larger than the far-field R wave. The use of an atrial blanking period after a paced or sensed ventricular event can effectively reduce inappropriate sensing of far-field R waves in the atrial channel, but ventricular oversensing can still be an issue, even with a bipolar sensing configuration, occasionally leading to inappropriate pacemaker behavior and inaccurate reporting of atrial high-rate episodes.

The problem of far-field R-wave detection in the atrial electrogram has been addressed by the development of leads incorporating a pair of closely spaced electrodes placed circumferentially around the lead body, separated by 180°,

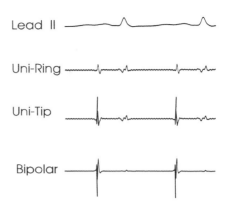

Lead II

Uni-Ring

Uni-Tip

Bipolar

Fig. 2.16 Simultaneously recorded unipolar and bipolar atrial electrograms from the ring and tip electrodes of a permanent pacing lead. Note that both of the unipolar electrograms record a far-field R wave. The bipolar electrogram records a sharp atrial deflection and markedly attenuates the far-field R wave. Bipolar sensing is characterized by relative immunity to far-field electrical events.

known as an orthogonal electrode array. These electrodes do not contact the atrial myocardium directly but "float" free within the right atrium. The advantage of orthogonal sensing is that ventricular signals approach the atrial bipole perpendicular to its axis, resulting in marked attenuation of the far-field R wave, whereas atrial signals approach from various directions, including parallel to the bipole, resulting in a much larger atrial electrogram. The improved signal-to-noise characteristics of orthogonal atrial electrodes have allowed the use of more sensitive atrial amplifiers and increased reliability of atrial sensing. The orthogonal electrode concept has also provided a method for dual-chamber pacing that uses a single lead (known as a "VDD" lead because of the associated required pacing mode). This lead uses a standard electrode at the tip, which is placed at the right ventricular apex for ventricular pacing and sensing, and the orthogonal electrode array is located proximally on the body of the lead where it traverses the right atrium. As this proximal bipole is not in contact with atrial muscle, it can be used only for atrial sensing and not for pacing.

The first generation of CRT devices did not have separate pacing and sensing circuits for the RV and LV leads, which were instead integrated into the same circuit using an external or internal Y-connector. As a consequence, the ventricular channel would receive electrogram information from both leads, which were typically located on opposite sides of the heart. The resulting composite electrogram from each single ventricular event therefore consisted of two distinct components (Fig. 2.17). If the width of the combined electrogram exceeded the ventricular blanking period, the potential existed for double-counting of the ventricular rate. From a tachyarrhythmia detection perspective, the composite biventricular electrogram created the potential for inappropriate detection of ventricular "tachycardias" by an ICD. When double-counting occurred, the rate identified by the ICD would be double the actual ventricular rate and ICD therapies could be delivered inappropriately. The most common scenario was for sinus tachycardia to be sensed as ventricular tachycardia or VF. In addition, a relatively slow ventricular tachycardia could be sensed at a rate double that of the actual rate, so that it was falsely classified and treated as

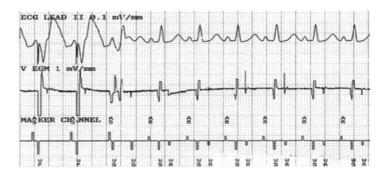

Fig. 2.17 An example of loss of atrial tracking in a biventricular device with a ventricular "Y" adaptor that routes electrogram signals from both right ventricular (RV) and left ventricular (LV) leads into the single ventricular sensing channel. A premature ventricular complex (PVC) inhibits ventricular pacing for one beat, which is then followed by double-counting of the intrinsically conducted ventricular electrogram, with separate sensing of both RV and LV components. Because of the long interventricular conduction delay (RV to LV) during sinus rhythm, double-counting of the ventricular electrogram results in resetting of the post-ventricular atrial refractory period (PVARP) such that the next sinus atrial electrogram is ignored. As a result, there is perpetuation of intrinsic conduction and failure to maintain consistent biventricular pacing. During sinus tachycardia, such double-counting of ventricular electrograms can result in inappropriate shocks from a biventricular defibrillator, which will falsely conclude that the ventricular rate is double the actual ventricular rate.

VF. From a pacing standpoint, the second ventricular electrogram component would reset the post-ventricular atrial blanking period, leading to underdetection of atrial events that otherwise should have triggered ventricular pacing output. To address these sensing problems, modern CRT devices detect ventricular events only from the RV lead and not from the LV lead, which has a separate, dedicated pacing and sensing circuit.

Polarization

Following application of a polarizing pulse, an afterpotential of opposite charge is induced in the myocardium at the interface of the stimulating electrode (Fig. 2.18). Immediately after cathodal stimulation, an excess of positive charges surrounds the electrode, which then exponentially decays to electrical neutrality. This positively charged afterpotential can be inappropriately sensed by the sensing circuit of the pulse generator with resulting inhibition or delay of the next pacing pulse. The amplitude of afterdepolarization is directly related to the amplitude and duration of the pacing stimulus, as well as the properties of the pacing electrode. Thus, afterdepolarizations are most likely to be sensed with use of particular leads, during conditions of maximum stimulus voltage and pulse duration, combined with the maximum sensitivity setting of the pulse generator. Inappropriate sensing of afterpotentials has been eliminated by the use of sensing refractory periods that prevent the sensing circuit from responding to electrical signals for a programmable peri-

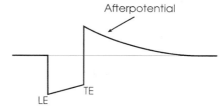

Fig. 2.18 Diagram of a constant-voltage output pulse (downward deflection) and a resultant afterpotential of opposite polarity. LE, leading edge; TE, trailing edge.

od following the pacing stimulus. However, for dual-chamber pacing systems, afterdepolarizations of sufficient amplitude in one chamber may be sensed by the sensing amplifier in the other chamber. This is most likely to occur with the sensing of atrial afterpotentials by the ventricular sensing circuit, resulting in inappropriate inhibition of ventricular stimulus output (crosstalk). Because of the potential for inhibition of ventricular pacing by the far-field sensing of atrial afterdepolarizations, the ventricular sensing circuit is inactivated for a period (blanking period) following the delivery of an atrial pacing stimulus. Crosstalk is a very rare clinical problem in the current era of predominantly bipolar pacing and sensing, along with the design of pacing electrodes that minimize the polarization phenomenon.

Time-related changes in intracardiac electrograms

Immediately following implantation of a transvenous lead, the electrogram usually demonstrates a typical injury current. The current of injury is caused by the pressure that is exerted by the distal electrode on myocardial cell membranes, and is observed with both atrial and ventricular leads. Absence of the typical acute injury electrogram immediately after lead implantation suggests either poor contact between the distal electrode and the endocardium, or placement of the lead in an area of fibrotic myocardium. The injury current is observed with both active and passive fixation electrodes, and usually disappears over a period ranging from several minutes to several hours.

With passive fixation leads, the amplitude of the intracardiac electrogram typically declines abruptly within several days following implantation, with a gradual increase back toward the acute value by 6–8 weeks. The chronic R-wave amplitude of passive fixation electrodes has been shown to be approximately 85% of the acute value. The attenuation of the slew rate is considerably greater, with chronic values averaging approximately 50–60% of the acute measurement. Modern corticosteroid-eluting leads have demonstrated minimal deterioration of the electrogram from implantation through regular follow-up assessments.

Active fixation leads may be associated with a different time course than passive fixation leads in the evolution of the intracardiac electrogram, with more markedly attenuated amplitude and slew rate immediately following lead positioning. Over the next 20–30 min, the electrogram amplitude typically increases. It is likely that the trauma caused by extension of a screw helix into the myocardium is responsible for this hyperacute evolution of the intra-cardiac electrogram. Recognition of this phenomenon may prevent the unnecessary repositioning of an active fixation lead. In general, active and passive fixation leads are associated with similar chronic electrogram amplitudes.

Sensing impedance

The intracardiac electrogram must be transmitted by the pacing lead from its source in the myocardium to the sensing amplifier of the pulse generator. The voltage drop that occurs from the origin of the electrical signal in the heart to the proximal portion of the lead depends on the source impedance. The components of the source impedance include the resistance between the electrode and the myocardium, the resistance offered by the lead conductor, and the effect of polarization. The electrode resistance is inversely related to the surface area of the electrode. The polarization impedance is also inversely related to the electrode surface area. Thus, electrodes with large surface area minimize the source impedance and contribute to improved sensing.

The electrogram that is sensed by the pulse generator can also be attenuated by a mismatch in impedance between the lead (the source impedance) and the sensing amplifier (the input impedance). The greater the ratio of the input impedance to the source impedance, the less the electrogram is attenuated and the more accurately it reflects the true amplitude and morphology of the signal in the myocardium. Thus the drop in electrogram amplitude from the actual voltage in the myocardium to the signal that is sensed by the pulse generator is minimized by a low source impedance and a high input impedance. The source impedance of current pacing leads ranges from approximately 400 to 1500 Ω. The sensing amplifiers of currently available pulse generators typically have an input impedance > 25 000 Ω. The clinical significance of impedance mismatch (too low a ratio of input impedance to source impedance) is the failure of sensing with insulation failure or conductor fracture. Insulation failure (low pacing impedance, typically < 200 Ω) between the conductors of a bipolar lead results in shunting across the amplifier and an effective fall in input impedance. In this situation the electrogram amplitude may be attenuated, with loss of appropriate sensing. Conductor fracture (high pacing impedance, typically > 1500–2000 Ω) leads to a marked increase in source impedance and a similar impedance mismatch and sensing failure.

Automated capture features

There is a fundamental conflict with regard to programming pacing output—the desire to guarantee myocardial capture, which argues for a higher programmed output, and the desire to maximize battery longevity, which argues for a lower pacing output. The standard compromise is expressed in the concept of a "safety margin," which describes an output setting that is likely always to exceed the capture threshold, even taking into account fluctuations that may occur over time. When programming a fixed pacing output, it is common to set the pulse amplitude two to three times that of the pacing threshold, at a particular pulse duration, in order to ensure myocardial capture, while avoiding the excessive battery current drain that would result from even higher outputs. Electrode design and steroid elution have resulted in lower acute and chronic pacing thresholds, but late threshold rise may still occur. Automatic capture algorithms have been developed which allow the pacemaker to determine the pacing threshold automatically and program pacing output accordingly.

The key feature of automatic capture algorithms is the ability of the pacemaker to detect the presence or absence of an "evoked response" (ER), which is the electrical event that results from myocardial capture after an output pulse. A second electrical event that occurs immediately following a paced event is the polarization phenomenon at the electrode–myocardial interface. The success of an automatic threshold algorithm is critically dependent on the pacemaker being able to differentiate reliably between the ER and polarization artifact. The development of pacing electrodes that minimize the polarization effect, along with specific pacemaker algorithms and sensing circuits, has allowed for reliable automatic confirmation of pacing capture and automated programming of pacing output. The more frequently the pacing threshold is measured, the lower the necessary margin of safety because of the reduced chance for an undetected rise in threshold. If capture is assessed with every beat, then pacing output need only be marginally higher than threshold, and the opportunity then exists for delivery of a backup, higher output pulse with any non-capture event.

The AutoCapture™ algorithm found in St. Jude pacemakers verifies capture on a beat-to-beat basis and provides an illustrative example of an automatic capture algorithm. To first verify that ER can be reliably differentiated from the polarization signal, five paired pulses are delivered with an amplitude of 4.5 V and a minimum pulse width of 0.5 ms. The paired pulses are separated by 100 ms, with the first capturing the myocardium and creating ER, and the second falling into the absolute refractory period of the myocardium, with no ER and only polarization artifact created. If the ER amplitude is sufficient, the polarization signal not too great, and there is sufficient difference between the two, then a reliable ER sensitivity can be set and AutoCapture™ can be recommended. Once the capture threshold is determined by the pacemaker, the pacing output is automatically set at 0.25 V above the measured threshold, and ER is assessed with each paced beat thereafter. After the pacing output, there is a 14-ms blanking period, followed by a 47-ms ER detection window. If ER is not detected, a backup pulse of 5 V is delivered 100 ms after the first pulse, and the next pulse will again be delivered at 0.25 V above the last capture threshold. Two sequential "non-capture" pulses (with associated backup pulses of 5 V) define a rise in threshold and will result in an increase in output of the third pulse by 0.25 V. This process of sequential output increase continues until an ER is detected, in a sequence called "loss of capture recovery." When two consecutive primary pulses both produce an ER, this output is the new capture threshold. A full automatic threshold test will be performed every 8 h, after every magnet application including after pacemaker interrogation, and after a loss of capture recovery sequence. During automated threshold testing, the paced and sensed AV delays are shortened to 50 and 25 ms, respectively, to preclude the possibility for fusion beats in the setting of preserved intrinsic AV conduction. The algorithm works by reducing the pacing output in 0.25-V steps with consecutive pairs of beats until loss of capture occurs on two consecutive beats, with a 5-V backup pulse delivered with each loss of capture event. The output is then increased in 0.125-V steps until two consecutive capture beats are seen, thereby defining capture threshold. The 0.25-V margin is then added to this threshold for subsequent pacing until loss of capture is seen or the next threshold test is performed. Because fusion or pseudofusion may occur in the setting of intact AV conduction, resulting in difficulty detecting ER in the ER sensing window, a separate algorithm is used to investigate this possibility. When a non-capture event is seen, a backup pulse is delivered and the AV delay will be extended by 100 ms for the next cycle in order to search for intrinsic conduction. If a native R wave is sensed on the subsequent cycle, the pacing output is not incremented and the longer AV delay is left in place to permit intrinsic conduction to occur. If the second pulse again shows lack of capture, then another backup pulse is delivered and capture recovery is initiated. The end result of the AutoCapture™ algorithm is that myocardial capture is ensured with each beat, while permitting a slim margin between capture threshold and pacing output in order to minimize unnecessary battery current drain. The AutoCapture™ algorithm will only work with a unipolar pacing output configuration and a bipolar lead with low polarization properties. It is important to know when this algorithm is being used and how it works, in order to interpret correctly electrocardiograms that may demonstrate unusual pacing behavior due to the pacemaker performing a threshold test or a capture recovery sequence (Fig. 2.19).

Other manufacturers offer variants of the automatic capture algorithm, some of which deliver backup pulses on a beat-to-beat basis, and others do not, but provide automatic determination of pacing threshold at programmed intervals during the day. Guidant/Boston Scientific pacemakers make use of a coupling capacitor to "absorb" polarization energy, allowing their beat-to-beat capture algorithm to be used with a wide range of pacing leads. The Ventricular Capture Management™ feature of Medtronic also works with a wide range of leads, but rather than looking for beat-to-beat capture, the algorithm performs a strength duration threshold test at a programmable interval (nominal is once per day). With this algorithm, the amplitude threshold is first determined at a fixed pulse duration (0.4 ms), and then the pulse amplitude is doubled and a pulse duration threshold is measured. The permanent ventricular stimulation amplitude is then automatically set using a preprogrammed amplitude safety margin (usually twice threshold, which is the nominal setting) or a programmable minimum amplitude (whichever is higher, nominal value is 2.5 V). During measurement of the pacing threshold, each test pulse is followed by a backup pulse 110 ms later to ensure that a pacing pause does not occur.

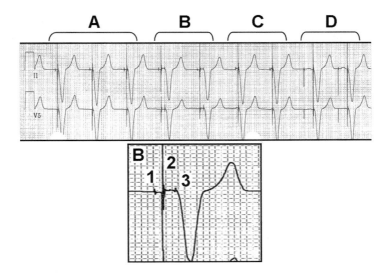

Fig. 2.19 Pacemaker automatic capture test being performed while a 12-lead ECG was coincidentally being recorded. Top panel: (A) While the automatic capture algorithm systematically decrements unipolar pacing output to assess the capture threshold, the atrioventricular (AV) delay is dramatically shortened to minimize the opportunity for intrinsic conduction and pseudofusion. (B) When an evoked response is no longer seen, signifying that ventricular capture is lost, a 5-V backup pacing stimulus is delivered to avoid any pauses that would otherwise result from loss of capture. (C) After two sequential losses of capture events, the ventricular pacing output is incrementally increased by 0.125 V, resulting in recovery of myocardial capture. (D) After two consecutive capture events, the pacemaker has re-established the ventricular capture threshold, a 0.25-V margin is added, and routine dual-chamber pacing is restored, with the baseline programmed AV delay. The bottom panel shows the three pacing "spikes" that are seen when ventricular capture is lost—the first spike is an atrial bipolar pacing output, the second spike is a ventricular unipolar pacing output that fails to capture the myocardium (note the short AV delay during automatic capture testing), and the third spike is a ventricular 5-V backup bipolar pacing output to ensure ventricular stimulation after loss of evoked response is noted with the decrementing unipolar output (note the difference in amplitude of unipolar and bipolar pacing spikes on surface ECG).

In general, automatic capture algorithms function quite effectively and may reduce the risk of loss of capture due to fluctuations in pacing threshold caused by drugs, metabolic derangement or lead dislodgement. The capability for reducing the programmed margin of safety is effective for prolonging battery life and may reduce the frequency of clinic follow-ups. It is important to understand how each manufacturer-specific automatic capture algorithm works before activating it, particularly when used in a pacemaker-dependent patient.

Autosensing functions

The amplitude of the atrial and ventricular electrogram can vary with the cardiac rhythm, patient activity, medications, or changes at the electrode–myocardial interface. Atrial electrograms, for example, are generally smaller in atrial fibrillation than in sinus rhythm, whereas the ventricular electrogram amplitude can decrease in the setting of infarction or fibrosis of the myocardium near the ventricular electrode. In pacemakers, a fixed sensitivity setting is used, and electrograms that surpass this cut-off are sensed, and those of smaller amplitude fail to be sensed. To minimize the chance of undersensing intrinsic electrograms, while avoiding oversensing of far-field events, typical nominal sensitivity settings are in the 0.3–0.5 mV range. Because the most common cause of anomalous pacemaker behavior relates to problems with sensing, several manufacturers have introduced pacemakers that regularly determine the amplitude of P and R waves, and automatically reprogram the atrial and ventricular sensitivity settings to maintain an acceptable sensing safety margin. The clinical utility of an autosensitivity algorithm is highlighted by the observation that programming a 100% sensing safety margin based on a single P-wave measurement provides reliable atrial sensing in only 72% of patients with dual-chamber pacemakers.

The Medtronic Sensing Assurance™ feature repeatedly measures the amplitude of P and R waves and classifies each as low, high or adequate based on a non-programmable target safety margin. This feature reprograms the bipolar atrial sensitivity value so that the atrial electrogram is maintained within a range that is 4.0–5.6 times the programmed sensitivity value, and for atrial unipolar leads and all ventricular leads the target safety margin is 2.8–4.0 times the programmed sensitivity. For example, if the atrial sensitivity value is programmed to 0.5 mV and the atrial electrogram amplitude is measured between 0.5 and 2.0 mV, the sensing margin is classified as low (between 1.0 and 4.0 times the sensitivity value) and the sensitivity is automatically increased (i.e. programmed to a lower numerical value). Conversely, a series of high-amplitude events (> 5.6 times the sensitivity value) would permit the Sensing Assurance algorithm to program a less sensitive setting (i.e. a higher numerical value).

Ventricular sensing in ICDs is far more complex, and includes a time-dependent increase in sensitivity after each sensed event. Because electrogram amplitude during VF may be quite small and highly variable, this automatic sensitivity gain increase is essential to avoid underdetection of VF. Different sensitivity decay algorithms are used by different manufacturers, with varying degrees of programmability. Sensitivity might need to be adjusted to ensure detection of VF or to reduce oversensing of the T wave during sinus rhythm. Defibrillator sensing and programming are reviewed in detail in the chapter on ICDs.

Lead design

Permanent pacing leads have five major components: (i) the electrode(s); (ii) the conductor(s); (iii) insulation; (iv) the connector pin; and (v) the fixation mechanism. Each of these components has critical design considerations, as well as failure modes. In this section, the factors that are important for the design of leads are reviewed.

Electrodes

As discussed previously in this chapter, the stimulation threshold is a function of the current density generated at the electrode. In general, the smaller the radius of the electrode, the greater the current density, and the lower the pacing threshold. In addition, the resistance at the electrode–myocardial interface is higher with smaller electrodes, which results in less current drain for each constant-voltage pacing pulse ($V = IR$) and greater battery longevity. Both of these factors favor electrodes with a small radius for myocardial stimulation. In contrast, sensing impedance and electrode polarization are increased with electrodes of smaller surface area, which can impair myocardial electrogram sensing. Although a higher sensing impedance with a small electrode is easily compensated by a higher input impedance of the sensing amplifier, the issue of polarization at the electrode–tissue interface favors the use of a larger electrode to minimize afterpotentials. The ideal pacing lead would therefore have an electrode with a small radius (to increase current density and improve pacing) and yet have a large surface area (to reduce polarization and improve sensing). The solution to these conflicting considerations for optimal stimulation and sensing characteristics has been addressed by the development of electrodes that have a small radius but a very complex surface structure that results in a large exposed surface area.[19]

Electrode shape

The effect of electrode shape on current density has been studied extensively by Irnich and colleagues. Electrodes with a smooth, hemispherical shape produce a uniform current density. In contrast, electrodes with more complex shapes typically produce an irregular pattern of current density, with "hot spots" at the edges and points of the electrode. Electrodes with an irregular shape enable a high current density to be maintained at these hot spots while presenting a larger overall surface area for sensing. For example, a ring-tipped electrode resulted in better stimulation thresholds and sensing characteristics than did the older hemispherical electrode designs. Other electrode shapes that were introduced to produce areas of high current density included a grooved hemispherical design and a dish-shaped design with holes bored into the electrode. Leads with helical, screw-shaped electrodes, hooks and barbs have all been demonstrated to provide areas of increased current density and acceptable stimulation thresholds. Most modern leads use a small electrode with a complex surface structure to achieve improved stimulation and sensing characteristics.

Surface structure

Early pacing leads used electrodes with a polished metal surface. The use of electrodes with a textured surface has resulted in a dramatic increase in the surface area of the electrode without an increase in radius. The complex, textured surface of modern leads minimizes the polarization effect and improves both sensing and stimulation efficiency (Fig. 2.20). The microscopic surface of a modern electrode will typically be extremely porous, with thousands of microscopic pores ranging in size from 20 to 100 μm. The same type of textured surface is sometimes achieved by coating the electrode with sintered microspheres of Elgiloy, platinum or iridium oxide, or by constructing the electrode with a woven mesh of microscopic metallic fibers enclosed within a screened basket of wire. The performance of carbon electrodes has been improved by roughening of the surface, a process known as activation. Each of these porous or roughened surface structures has been shown to minimize polarization greatly after a pacing stimulus is delivered. It should also be noted that porous surfaces also allow for the ingrowth of tissue into the electrode.

The ability to differentiate a true evoked myocardial electrogram from polarization-induced afterpotentials has dramatically improved with the development of low-polarization electrodes. The ability of a pacing system to properly detect a myocardial electrogram immediately following a pacing stimulus has strong implications with regard to automatic capture algorithms. Once the pacemaker is able to confirm myocardial capture accurately, then automatic pacing threshold testing can be performed, with the potential for automated programming of appropriate pacing output. Additionally, beat-to-beat verification of capture is also possible, with higher output backup pulse

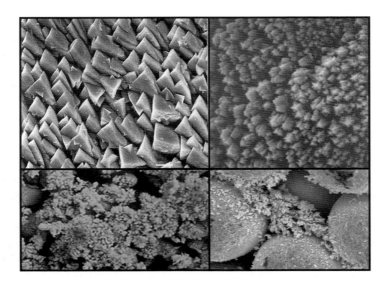

Fig. 2.20 Scanning electron micrographs of four different pacing electrodes, all demonstrating a complex, porous microscopic texture, which increases surface area in order to reduce polarization and improve sensing and stimulation efficiency. [Courtesy of St. Jude Medical, Inc. (top two) and Medtronic, Inc. (bottom two).]

delivery when loss of capture is seen. This latter pacemaker feature might be particularly useful for patients who are pacemaker-dependent, where a chronic rise in pacing threshold might otherwise result in symptomatic loss of capture. These automatic capture algorithms are currently available in many pacemaker models, but will not function properly with a lead that has high-amplitude afterpotentials related to polarization at the electrode.

Chemical composition

To minimize inflammation and subsequent fibrosis at the tissue interface, electrodes for permanent pacing leads should be biologically inert and resistant to chemical degradation. Certain metals, such as zinc, copper, mercury, nickel, lead and silver, are associated with toxic reactions in the myocardium and are unsuitable for use in the electrodes of chronically implanted leads. In addition to these materials with direct tissue toxicity, metals that are susceptible to corrosion have been demonstrated to result in increased chronic stimulation thresholds. Stainless steel alloys are variably associated with the potential for corrosion. Titanium and tantalum have been shown to acquire a surface coating of oxides, which may impede charge transfer at the electrode interface. However, titanium that is coated with microscopic particles of platinum or vitreous carbon has been found to have excellent long-term performance as a pacing electrode. The polarity of the electrode may also have an important influence on its chemical stability. For example, cobalt–chromium–nickel (Elgiloy) is a quite acceptable electrode material when used as the cathode. However, when used as the anode, Elgiloy is susceptible to a significant degree of corrosion.

The materials presently in use for the electrodes of permanent pacing leads include platinum–iridium, Elgiloy, platinum coated with platinized titanium, vitreous or pyrolytic carbon coating a titanium or graphite core, platinum, titanium–nitride, or iridium oxide. The platinized-platinum, iridium-oxide and titanium-nitride electrodes have been associated with a reduced degree of polarization. Although a small degree of corrosion may occur with any of these materials, the carbon electrodes appear to be less susceptible.

Steroid-eluting electrodes

Pacing thresholds of implanted leads tend to have two peaks—an acute rise immediately after implantation related to tissue injury, and a more gradual, chronic rise over time that probably results from an inflammatory cellular response with fibrous capsule formation around the lead electrode. A major advance in permanent pacing lead technology has been the development of electrodes that gradually elute small amounts of the corticosteroid dexamethasone sodium phosphate, which has a significant impact on reducing the chronic pacing threshold increase that is seen with non-steroid-eluting leads. Steroid-eluting electrodes incorporate a silicone core or collar that is impregnated with a small quantity of dexamethasone that is very gradually released to the surrounding tissue (Figs. 2.21 and 2.22). These steroid-eluting leads

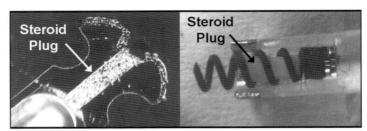

Fig. 2.21 Cutaway views of passive fixation (left) and active fixation (right) pacing electrodes, each containing a steroid reservoir at the distal tip. Steroid-eluting electrodes demonstrate a dramatic reduction in the rise in stimulation threshold that is a prominent characteristic of non-steroid-eluting electrodes. (Courtesy of St. Jude Medical, Inc.)

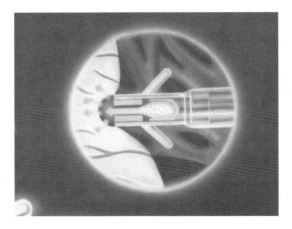

Fig. 2.22 Diagram of a steroid-eluting electrode with a reservoir of dexamethasone sodium phosphate that slowly elutes through the electrode into the underlying myocardium. (Courtesy of Medtronic, Inc.)

are characterized by a minimal change, if any, in stimulation threshold from implantation to a follow-up period of several years. The suppression of the variable rise in chronic thresholds that is otherwise seen allows for the confident use of lower pacing amplitudes, and provides increased reliability and safety for patients who are pacemaker-dependent. It should be emphasized that the corticosteroid eluted from the lead does not affect acute stimulation thresholds; rather, dexamethasone controls the chronic elevation of the pacing threshold. Corticosteroid leads are now routinely used for both active and passive fixation designs and have dramatically reduced the risk of exit block (an excessive increase in chronic stimulation threshold, also referred to as "loss of capture," when the pacing threshold exceeds the programmed output) for endocardial pacing and ICD leads as well as for epimyocardial leads.

The studies of Stokes and Bornzin have indicated that the mechanism by which dexamethasone sodium phosphate prevents a rise in chronic stimulation threshold remains to be fully explained. Although the thickness of the fibrous capsule that surrounds the electrode is reduced, the magnitude is less than would be expected by the evolution in stimulation threshold. This suggests that other mechanisms may be involved. The duration of drug elution required for sustained low thresholds remains to be fully defined. Nevertheless, long-term follow-up for > 10 years has indicated that the impressively low chronic thresholds observed with steroid-eluting electrodes appear to be maintained over the usable entire service life of most pacing leads. The routine use of steroid-eluting leads, coupled with smaller pacing electrodes and high electrode resistance, has allowed pulse generators to be reduced in size. Low chronic pacing thresholds allow for lower chronic pulse amplitudes, and battery longevity can therefore be maintained even while reducing battery capacity.

Fixation mechanism
The chronic performance of permanent pacing leads is critically dependent on stable positioning of the electrode(s). Although early pacing leads were associated with an unacceptably high risk of dislodgment, the development of active and passive fixation mechanisms has dramatically reduced the need for lead repositioning. Previous generations of permanent transvenous pacing leads included several appendages at the distal end that were designed to lodge within the trabeculae of the right atrium or ventricle. However, tines have become the predominant fixation mechanism currently used for passive permanent pacing leads (Fig. 2.23). Passive fixation leads are typically entrapped within the trabeculae of the right heart chambers immediately upon correct positioning of the lead. Effective fixation of the lead can be confirmed at the time of implantation by gentle traction or rotation of the lead. Tines generally add minimal technical difficulty to the implantation procedure, although they may occasionally become entrapped in the tricuspid valve apparatus. The passive fixation devices are rapidly covered by fibrous tissue, making later removal of the lead by simple traction difficult or impossible in as short a time as 6 months. Besides the effectiveness of passive fixation devices to prevent dislodgment, the increased stability that is provided for the distal electrode serves to minimize trauma at the myocardial interface caused by motion. This added stability is likely to result in a smaller fibrous capsule surrounding the electrode and improvement of the chronic stimulation threshold. The passive fixation devices have the relative disadvantage of increasing the maximum external diameter of the lead, requiring the use of a larger venous introducer when the subclavian vein puncture technique is used. Removability of pacing leads is an important consideration. In general, passive fixation leads are more difficult to extract than active fixation leads.

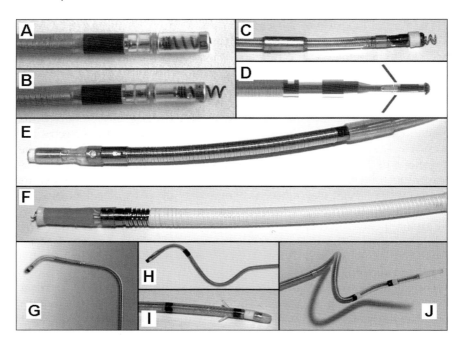

Fig. 2.23 Common types of transvenous pacing and defibrillation leads. (A) Active fixation lead with extendable–retractable helix, helix retracted. (B) Active fixation lead with extendable–retractable helix, helix extended. (C) Active fixation lead with fixed, non-retractable helix. The entire lead is rotated to affix the helix into the myocardium; the helix is initially covered by a dissolvable mannitol coating to permit easy passage through the vasculature (absent in photo). (D) Passive fixation tined lead. The four flexible tines are designed to lodge between myocardial trabeculae, anchoring the lead in place. (E) Active fixation implantable cardioverter defibrillator (ICD) lead with helix retracted. The distal high-voltage electrode is clearly seen, as this shocking coil is wound around the body of the lead. (F) Active fixation ICD lead with a sleeve of expanded polytetrafluoroethylene (GORE-TEX®) covering the distal high-voltage electrode. This sleeve is designed to reduce tissue ingrowth for ease of future lead extraction, if necessary. (G) Angled curve bipolar pacing lead for left ventricular pacing; the curve is designed to anchor the lead within a coronary vein. (H) "S" curve bipolar pacing lead for left ventricular pacing and fixation within a coronary vein. (I) Straight bipolar pacing lead for left ventricular pacing, with fins designed to anchor the lead within a smaller coronary vein. (J) Spiral curve bipolar pacing lead for left ventricular pacing, designed to anchor the lead within the lumen of larger coronary vein branches. [Courtesy of St. Jude Medical, Inc. (D,H), Medtronic, Inc. (G), Boston Scientific, Inc. (J).]

Active fixation leads

Although several different fixation methods such as screws, barbs, or hooks have been developed, the present generation of active fixation pacing leads largely relies on a screw helix that is extended into the endocardium. The screw helix may be fixed and permanently exposed at the tip of the lead (a fixed-screw), requiring the lead to be rotated in a clockwise direction to affix the lead to the myocardium, and counterclockwise rotation is needed during lead manipulation and advancement through the vasculature to prevent fixation at an undesired site. Other leads allow the screw helix to be extended from the tip once the lead has been atraumatically passed through the venous system to the heart, and positioned at the desired intracardiac fixation location (Figs 2.23 and 2.24). The design of Bisping and colleagues incorporates an extendable–retractable helical screw that is well suited for positioning at several sites in the atrium or ventricle at the time of implantation. Active fixation leads may use the screw helix as both the fixation mechanism and the electrically active electrode (see Fig. 2.24). Other designs use a separate electrode at the distal end of the lead for stimulation and sensing with an electrically inactive helix. Although both devices provide similar long-term thresholds, the inactive helix leads are associated with lower acute thresholds. One method of preventing premature fixation of an exposed helix involves using a cap of mannitol or polyethylene glycol over the screw helix to facilitate introduction of the lead through the vasculature. After approximately 5 min in the blood pool, the mannitol or polyethylene glycol completely dissolves, exposing the screw and allowing it to engage the endocardium.

The extendable–retractable design has become the most widely prescribed active fixation mechanism because of its ease of implantation and because the fixation mechanism can be retracted long after implantation, thereby allowing for an easier extraction procedure. Active fixation leads offer the implanting physician the capability for stable positioning of the lead at many sites in either the atrium or the ventricle, including spots that are not as heavily trabeculated, and the rate of atrial lead dislodgement is significantly reduced compared with passive fixation leads. Although historically the chronic pacing thresholds of active fixation leads were higher than those of passive fixation leads, this difference has largely been eliminated with the routine use of corticosteroid elution in active fixation leads. Although active fixation leads are potentially easier to extract than passive fixation leads, the risk of myocardial perforation during implantation is higher. Because the stimulation thresholds, sensing and dislodgement rates of modern active fixation leads tend to be

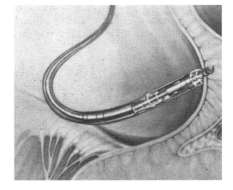

Fig. 2.24 A bipolar Bisping-type active fixation that uses the screw helix as the active distal electrode. The screw helix is extended into the endocardium by rotating the proximal connector of the lead. The screw helix is both extendable and retractable, allowing atraumatic passage through the vasculature. (Courtesy of Medtronic, Inc.)

similar to those observed with passive fixation leads, the choice of active or passive fixation has become largely a matter of preference by the implanting physician.

Mostly of historic interest, a particular fixation feature should be mentioned: that of the J retention wire. Certain models of atrial leads have been manufactured with a thin, flexible metal ribbon that was welded to the proximal electrode and was positioned longitudinally underneath the outer insulation layer. This retention wire gave the lead a permanent "J" shape, which allowed for ease of implantation in the atrium. In one particular model, known as the Accufix lead, the J retention wire had an increased risk of fracture over time, due to metal fatigue during cardiac motion. The fractured, sharp end of wire could then perforate through the lead insulation and then through the myocardium, leading occasionally to pericardial tamponade or injury to adjacent structures. The decision of whether to monitor or extract these leads was made on a case-by-case basis, with regular monitoring performed via fluoroscopy.

Coronary sinus lead fixation

In the era of dual-site ventricular pacing for cardiac resynchronization pacing, new leads have been specifically designed for placement into the branches of the coronary venous system (Fig. 2.23). Because these leads are positioned within the lumen of a vein, rather than advanced against the endocardium within a cardiac chamber, their fixation mechanism is fundamentally different. Use of a potentially traumatic anchoring mechanism at the lead tip, such as an active fixation helix, could potentially result in perforation or rupture of the fragile venous wall, with the possible consequence of pericardial effusion and tamponade. Most coronary sinus pacing leads rely instead on creating several points of contact between the lead and the venous wall, to allow friction to act as the anchoring force. Leads have been designed with small fins or various curves of the lead body (angled curve, "S" curve, spiral curve) in order to apply gentle lateral force against the lead wall and prevent forward or backward migration of the lead after its precise positioning. When a guidewire or stylet is advanced through the central lumen of these leads, the curves disappear, allowing the operator to advance and navigate the lead along a potentially tortuous route within the coronary venous system. When the lead is positioned at its desired location, the guidewire or stylet is withdrawn in order to deploy the natural curve of the lead, gently anchoring it in place.

Conductors

The conducting wire that connects the stimulating and sensing electrode(s) to the proximal connector pin of the lead is a critical determinant of the usable service life of permanent pacing leads. At a minimum pacing rate of 70 ppm (pulses per minute), the heart contracts and relaxes at least 36 million times a year, producing substantial mechanical stress on a permanent pacing lead.

If one considers that the lead must flex with each heartbeat in a complex manner having longitudinal, transverse and rotational components, one can appreciate the potential for metal fatigue and fracture of the conductor. The most common site for lead fracture is at the fulcrum of a freely moving conductor with a stationary point. Thus the junction of the subclavian vein and the first rib is a common site of conductor failure. In addition, leads may fail at the site of mechanical injury, such as with excessively tight fixation sutures, especially when an anchoring sleeve is not used. Although early pacing leads were made of a single conductor wire and were associated with a high rate of fracture, modern leads use multiple wires that are coiled. The use of multiple conducting coils has dramatically improved the conductor's resistance to metal fatigue and tensile strength.

Stainless steel was used for the conducting coils of early multifilar leads. Stainless steel was eventually abandoned because of the potential for corrosion, and was replaced by Elgiloy or MP35N, an alloy of nickel. More recently, conductors manufactured with the drawn-brazed-strand (DBS) technique have been introduced. The DBS conductor is made of six nickel alloy wires that are drawn together with heated silver. The silver forms the matrix of the conductor, occupying the central core and the spaces between the nickel alloy wires. Silver also forms a thin outer layer that coats the conductor. DBS conductors are characterized by excellent resistance to flexion-related fracture. This conductor also has a very low ohmic resistance, allowing more efficient delivery of the stimulating pulse to the electrode and reduced sensing impedance. The silver chloride in these conductors, however, has been found to cause oxidation of polyurethane, and this reaction has resulted in insulation failure of particular lead models with DBS conductors and polyurethane insulation. Because of the potential for internal oxidation of polyurethane by silver complexes, DBS conductors are no longer used with polyurethane-insulated leads.

Unipolar pacemaker leads have one conductor, bipolar pacemaker leads have two conductors, integrated bipolar ICD leads have three conductors, and true bipolar ICD leads have four conductors. Each conductor may consist of one or more strands, called filars (unifilar vs. multifilar, Fig. 2.25). The conductors within a lead must be insulated from the outside environment as well as from each other. Unipolar leads consist of one coil of wire surrounded by a layer of insulation. Bipolar leads are usually constructed with a coaxial design, with an inner conductor coil leading to the distal tip electrode, surrounded by a layer of insulation, which in turn is wrapped in the outer conductor coil that leads to the proximal ring electrode, which is surrounded by a second layer of insulation (Fig. 2.26). Alternatively, some bipolar leads are constructed with a coradial conductor design. With this design, the two conductors are wrapped in parallel, side by side, around the central lumen, with one layer of surrounding insulation (Fig. 2.27). To insulate the conductors from each other, they are bonded with an insulating coating, such as ethylene tetrafluoroethylene (ETFE, a molecular relative of

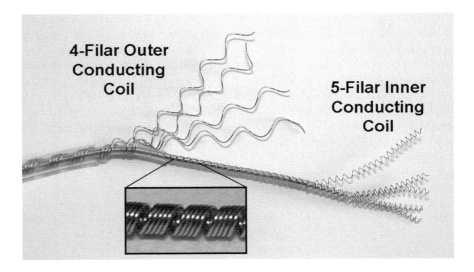

Fig. 2.25 A bipolar pacemaker lead, with the two coil conductors partially unwound to reveal their multifilar construction. The inner conducting coil has five filars (inset shows the five filars wound together), while the outer conducting coil has four filars.

Teflon). The coradial design has shown excellent durability and allows for a smaller external diameter, as there is no second coil or second sleeve of insulation.

ICD leads typically have a multilumen design to accommodate the three or four conductors, as a pure coaxial design would result in a lead with a prohibitively large diameter (Fig. 2.28). The distal pacing and sensing conductor is wound around a central lumen, in coil fashion, as in pacemaker leads.

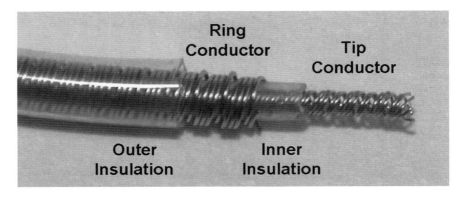

Fig. 2.26 A coaxial bipolar pacemaker lead. The inner conducting coil (which connects to the tip electrode) is surrounded by an inner layer of insulation, which is in turn wrapped in the outer conducting coil (which connects to the ring electrode), and then a second outer layer of insulation.

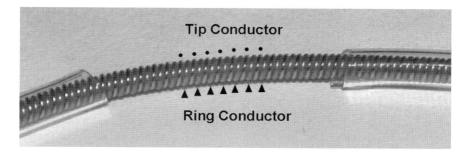

Fig. 2.27 A coradial bipolar pacemaker lead. The two unifilar conductors are wound side by side around the central lead lumen, with the tip conductor (dots) and ring conductor (arrowheads) seen in alternating turns. The two conductors are insulated from one another by an insulating coating of ethylene tetrafluoroethylene, and a single sleeve of insulation surrounds the coradial coil to provide redundant protection from the outside environment.

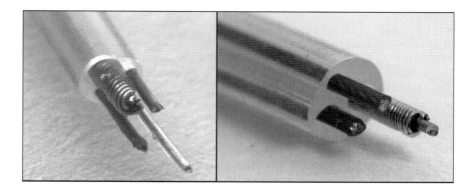

Fig. 2.28 Two multilumen implantable cardioverter defibrillator (ICD) leads. In the left panel, a true bipolar ICD lead has four conductors, including a distal pacing/sensing coil conductor that contains the central lead lumen and connects to the distal tip electrode, a second pacing/sensing conductor that connects to the ring electrode, and two high-voltage conductors that connect to the right ventricular (RV) and superior vena cava (SVC) shocking coils. In the right panel, an integrated bipolar ICD lead has three conductors, including a pacing/sensing coil conductor that connects to the distal tip electrode (a cut stylet is seen within the lumen of this pace/sense coil conductor), and two high-voltage conductors that connect to the RV and SVC shocking coils. The RV high-voltage coil also serves as the anode for pacing and sensing.

The high-voltage conductors, which connect to the one or two shocking coils, typically have a cable (longitudinal woven multifilament) design, are independently insulated with ETFE or some equivalent, and run lengthwise down the ICD lead in separate lumens within the lead body (Fig. 2.29). Each longitudinal lumen is designed to resist compression or crush of the conductors contained within.

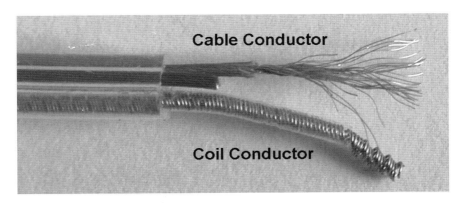

Fig. 2.29 An integrated bipolar implantable cardioverter defibrillator lead with partially unraveled conductors. The pace/sense conductor is a four-filar coil with a central lumen, whereas the high-voltage conductors are multifilament woven cables without a lumen. Each conductor has an individual layer of insulation in addition to the multilumen housing of the outer insulation.

Insulation

The materials used for the insulation of permanent pacing leads are of two varieties: silicone rubber and polyurethane (Table 2.2). Silicone rubber has proven to be a reliable insulating material over decades of clinical experience, being biologically inert and demonstrating minimal degradation over time. Silicone is a relatively soft material, however, with a low tear strength, and can be easily nicked or damaged when manipulated during implantation (Fig. 2.30). Silicone insulation must therefore be thicker than it would be if it

Table 2.2 Pacemaker lead insulation

	Advantages	Disadvantages
Silicone rubber	• 30-year proven history • Repairable • Low process sensitivity • Easy fabrication/molding • Very flexible	• Tears easily (nicks, ligatures) • Cuts easily • Low abrasion resistance • High friction in blood • Requires thicker walls (large diameter) • More thrombogenic and fibrotic • Subject to cold flow failure • Absorbs lipids (calcification)
Polyurethane	• 10-year proven history (P55D) • High tear strength • High cut resistance • Low friction in blood • High abrasion resistance • Thinner walls possible (small diameter) • Relatively non-thrombogenic	• Relatively stiff (especially P55D) • Not repairable • Manufacturing process sensitive • Environmental stress cracking (ESC) • Metal ion oxidation (MIO) • History of clinical failures (P80A)

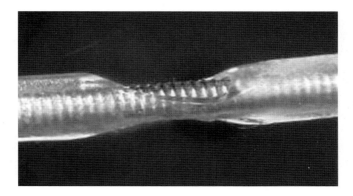

Fig. 2.30 A photograph of a silicone-insulated lead showing severe abrasion damage 4 years after implantation. Silicone is prone to abrasion injury either at the time of lead implantation, or from gradual friction-induced wear as a result of contact with other leads or the pulse generator. (Courtesy of St. Jude Medical, Inc.)

were stronger and more resistant to abrasion. In addition, silicone rubber is "sticky," with a high coefficient of friction, making the manipulation of two leads in a single vein difficult. These disadvantages have been addressed by the introduction of platinum-cured silicone rubber, which is characterized by improved mechanical strength. The coefficient of friction has been greatly reduced by the development of a lubricious, "fast-pass" coating. These improved silicone leads are of smaller external diameter and are far easier to manipulate when in contact with another lead.

Polyurethane was introduced as an insulation material because of its superior tear strength and low coefficient of friction. These properties allow polyurethane leads to be constructed with smaller external diameter than those made with conventional silicone rubber. Two major forms of polyurethane, known as P80A and P55D, have been used to insulate permanent pacing leads. The P80A polymer, which is less stiff than the P55D variety, was used in the first polyurethane-insulated cardiac pacing leads. The P55D polymer, although stiffer, has greater tensile and tear strength, and is therefore the predominant form of polyurethane used for pacing leads.

Within 4 years of the first human implant, polyurethane insulation failures became clinically apparent, with evidence of microscopic surface cracks in the outer surface of the P80A polyurethane insulation and clinical insulation failure (Fig. 2.31). Extensive investigation has shown that the surface cracks are likely to be related to environmental stresses rather than to biological degradation. The surface cracks in the polyurethane develop in the manufacturing process as the heated polyurethane cools more rapidly than the inner core, leading to opposing stresses within the insulation. Although microscopic cracks in the outer surface of the polyurethane are usually clinically unimportant, these cracks may predispose the insulation to further degradation by

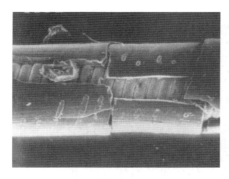

Fig. 2.31 Cracking of polyurethane insulation (P80A) covering a bipolar permanent pacing lead 2 years after implantation. (Courtesy of St. Jude Medical, Inc.)

trauma during or after lead implantation. At sites of additional mechanical stress, such as at the anchoring suture or during stylet insertion, the surface cracks may propagate deeper into the polyurethane, leading to insulation failure. Polyurethane has also been shown to undergo degradation by metal ion oxidation, notably by the silver chloride contained in DBS conductors. The mechanisms of polyurethane failure have been addressed by changes in the manufacturing process (slower cooling of the heated polyurethane and the elimination of solvents) and by the recognition that conductors made with silver should not be used with leads insulated with this material. Nevertheless, the P80A polymer has an unacceptable risk of insulation failure when used for permanent pacing leads, prompting an industry shift to the use of the P55D polyurethane polymer, which is more resistant to damage and degradation.

Although both silicone and P55D polyurethane remain the most common materials for lead insulation, with some leads manufactured with segments of each at different parts of the lead, new compounds are being developed with the goal of achieving the advantages of each. One such compound is a silicone–polyurethane co-polymer that also contains polyhexamethylene oxide. Early testing suggests that this polymer is more abrasion resistant and lubricious than silicone, and more flexible and crack resistant than polyurethane. As with all new lead components and designs, clinical experience over time will be the true test of lead performance and durability.

Epimyocardial leads

Permanent epicardial pacing leads are used when tricuspid valve abnormalities, central venous obstruction, congenital heart disease or technical issues preclude transvenous lead placement, when recurrent bloodstream infection is an issue, or when there is a need for lead implantation coincident with another intrathoracic surgical procedure. Epicardial pacing leads are either sutured to the epicardial surface or screwed into the epimyocardium of the atrium or ventricle (Fig. 2.32). Fixation mechanisms include a fishhook-shaped electrode that is stabbed into the atrial myocardium and a large screw helix that is rotated into the ventricular myocardium. These leads are typically unipolar and are frequently non-steroid eluting, with chronic stimulation thresholds that

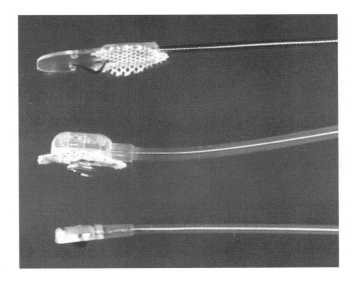

Fig. 2.32 Epimyocardial leads. Top: Fishhook-like atrial epimyocardial lead, unipolar. Middle: Large screw helix ventricular epimyocardial lead, unipolar. Bottom: Steroid-eluting epimyocardial lead, with non-penetrating electrode that is sutured in place against the myocardial surface. This steroid-eluting lead is available in both unipolar and bipolar designs. (Courtesy of Medtronic, Inc.)

tend to run higher than modern endocardial electrodes. A newer epicardial lead design does not involve penetration of the electrode into the myocardium, but, instead, a steroid-eluting electrode rests against the epicardium and is sutured in place. This lead design, which is available in unipolar and bipolar models, has the advantage of lower chronic pacing thresholds and better long-term performance, but it may require greater cardiac exposure, can be technically more difficult to place, and the presence of regions of epicardial fat can limit effective implant locations. Because epicardial leads have a higher rate of developing unacceptably high pacing thresholds, it is the practice of some cardiothoracic surgeons to implant two leads in a given cardiac chamber, with the second lead either connected to a different pacemaker port or left capped in the pacemaker pocket, in case the first lead fails and must be substituted. In the era of CRT, epicardial leads have experienced a resurgence, and are frequently used when a functional LV lead cannot be placed transvenously due to limitations imposed by the coronary venous anatomy.

Connectors
Over the first three decades of pacing, a major problem for pacemaker and lead manufacturers, as well as for implanting physicians, was the incompatibility of lead connectors and pulse generator headers that resulted from the lack of a consistent standard. Permanent pacing leads have evolved from a standard

5–6-mm connector pin for unipolar and bifurcated bipolar models to an "in-line" bipolar connector with a 3.2-mm diameter (Fig. 2.33). The considerable variability in the design of the in-line bipolar connector led to considerable confusion among physicians as to whether a particular lead of one manufacturer would match the pulse generator of another. Much of this confusion was related to the location of sealing rings; some manufacturers preferred to place the sealing rings in the header of the pulse generator, and others preferred the sealing rings to be on the connector of the lead. Because of this chaotic situation (Fig. 2.34), an international meeting of manufacturers agreed on a voluntary standard for leads and connectors incorporating the sealing rings on a 3.2-mm lead connector (VS-1). After continued problems with universal acceptance of the VS-1 connector, the incompatibility problem has been largely resolved with an industry-wide standard configuration known as IS-1 (Fig. 2.35).

Although modern leads and devices are now fully interchangeable and compatible, when a generator change is planned, the implanting physician must be aware of the type of leads that are present to ensure that the appropriate device header or adaptor is available, if needed, to accommodate an old lead with a non-IS-1 connector pin. A similar compatibility issue more recently arose in the early days of cardiac resynchronization pacing, with both IS-1 and LV-1 connector pins used, the latter being developed by Guidant to fit through a component of their early transvenous LV lead implantation system. The device industry quickly reverted to universal use of IS-1 connectors for all LV leads, although compatibility issues may again arise at the time of Guidant biventricular device generator change.

ICD leads currently have a yoke that leads to two or three connector pins: an IS-1 connector for the pace/sense component of the lead, and one or two

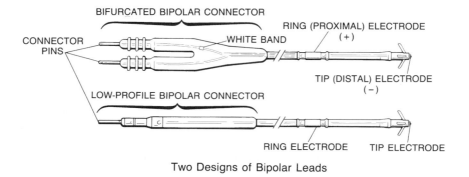

Two Designs of Bipolar Leads

Fig. 2.33 Old bifurcated bipolar connector vs. a more modern single-pin bipolar connector. Top: A white band marks the conductor leading to the distal electrode on a standard bifurcated bipolar lead connector with two connector pins. Bottom: A low-profile "Medtronic"-type bipolar connector has a single pin, with the distal electrode connecting to the terminal connector pin and the ring electrode connecting to the more proximal ring connector.

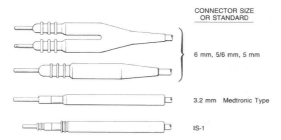

Fig. 2.34 Four varieties of lead connectors. (1) The upper connector is a bifurcated bipolar design with two connector pins, each 5–6 mm in diameter, with sealing rings on the lead. (2) The second connector is a standard unipolar design of 5 or 6 mm in diameter incorporating sealing rings. (3) The Medtronic-type, low-profile connector has a 3.2 mm diameter and no sealing rings. (4) The IS-1 connectors are incompatible with the other designs and include sealing rings on the proximal portion of the lead. Currently manufactured leads universally use the IS-1 type connector pin, but patients who require pacemaker generator change may have functional leads with older generation connectors, and the implanting physician must be prepared to implant a new pulse generator that is compatible.

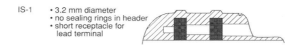

Fig. 2.35 Currently manufactured pulse generators universally use the IS-1 type header, pictured here, although some manufacturers continue to produce a limited supply of pulse generators with older header designs to be used at the time of generator change for a patient with older pacing leads in place.

DF-1 connectors for the high-voltage coils, which are separately connected to the device header. Future ICD leads will not have a yoke, but will use a new single IS-4 connector pin that is secured into a single compatible IS-4 channel in a new device header design.

Reducing tissue binding and ingrowth

Because pacing and ICD leads may need to be extracted, newer leads are being designed so that the trauma of lead extraction can be minimized. Scar tissue binds leads to the endocardial and venous walls at points of contact, with more vigorous binding in younger patients and progressively greater binding with time. The high-voltage coils of ICD leads provide a very large, complex surface for scar ingrowth, and these coils frequently represent the sites of greatest tissue binding, and thereby the greatest challenge to removal at the time of lead extraction. Whenever possible, leads are designed to be isodiametric, which means that they either remain the same diameter or become smaller down the length of the lead. If there are ridges or areas of increased diameter, these regions may provide a shelf for scar binding and impede the ability to slide the lead back through a tube of circumferential scar tissue. With regard to ICD coils, two separate strategies have been used to reduce binding and facilitate future extraction, if needed. The first involves applying a silicone "backfill" to the coils, which fills the spaces between the coil filars, greatly reducing the exposed surface area for tissue ingrowth. The second novel strategy is the application of a sleeve of ePTFE (expanded polytetrafluoroethylene, or Goretex^{Tm}) over each coil (see Fig. 2.23). The ePTFE sleeve has been shown to prevent tissue ingrowth between the coil filars, while having no significant effect on the conduction of electrical energy during shock delivery. These coil coatings or coverings are likely to reduce the difficulty and risk of later lead extraction.

Pulse generators

All pulse generators presently used in permanent pacing systems have several basic functional elements that are critical to the operation of the device. These include a power source, an output circuit, a sensing circuit and a timing circuit. Pulse generators also contain a telemetry coil for sending and receiving programming instructions and diagnostic information. In addition to these basic elements, almost all pulse generators contain circuits for sensing the output of an artificial, rate-adaptive sensor. The integrated circuit of most pulse generators also contains the capability of storing information in memory—either read-only memory (ROM) or random access memory (RAM)—which can be used to process diagnostic data or alter the feature set of the device following its implantation. In this section, the important aspects of each of these basic elements of pulse generators are reviewed.

Power source

The power source of all pulse generators presently in use is a chemical battery. Modern pulse generators almost exclusively use lithium as the anodal element and iodine as the cathodal element (Fig. 2.36). The energy provided by a chemical battery is generated by the transfer of electrons from the anodal element to the cathodal element of the battery. In the case of lithium batteries, lithium is the anodal element and provides the supply of electrons. The cathodal element of the battery receives the electrons. In a lithium–iodine cell, iodine serves as the cathodal element and accepts electrons from lithium. Poly-2-vinyl pyridine is combined with the cathodal element to assist in the transfer of electrons to iodine. At the battery terminals, the anode gives up electrons and is negatively charged, and the cathode accepts electrons and is positively charged. Internally, the anodal reaction proceeds as $2Li \rightarrow 2Li^+ + 2e^-$, with the cathodal reaction being $2I + 2e^- \rightarrow 2I^-$. Thus, within the battery, the anode is positively charged and the cathode is negatively charged; the overall chemical reaction is $2Li + 2I \rightarrow 2LiI$. The electrons are carried from the anodal terminal of the battery to the cathodal terminal when the circuit is completed through the external load. For a stimulating pulse,

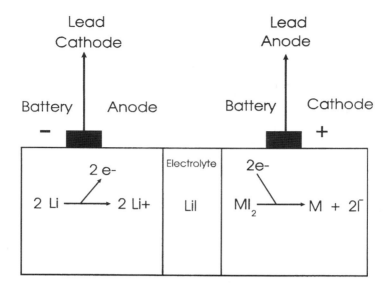

Fig. 2.36 Schematic of a lithium–iodine battery. The anodal terminal of the battery is negatively charged as lithium releases electrons to the lead. The battery anode leads to the cathode of the pacing lead (which is also negatively charged). The anodal portion of the battery itself becomes positively charged with the reaction $2Li \rightarrow 2Li^+ + 2e^-$. The cathodal terminal of the battery is positively charged and connects to the anode of the lead. The cathodal reaction is $MI_2 + 2e^- \rightarrow M + 2I^-$, where M represents poly-2-vinyl pyridine.

the output circuit of the pulse generator, the pacing lead, and the myocardium provide the external load.

The battery also contains an electrolyte, the material separating the anodal and cathodal elements; this material serves as a conductor of ionic movement, but is a barrier to the transfer of electrons. The electrolyte for a lithium–iodine battery is composed of a semisolid layer of lithium iodide that gradually increases in thickness over the life of the cell. Lithium iodide is not a good electrical conductor, and as the LiI layer grows the internal impedance of the battery increases. A major advantage of the lithium–iodine battery is the solid nature of the material, allowing the cell to be hermetically sealed and relatively resistant to corrosion.

The battery voltage depends on the chemistry of the cell. For example, the lithium–iodine cell generates approximately 2.8 V at the beginning of its life. The lithium–silver-chromate cell generates 3.2 V and the lithium–thionyl-chloride cell produces 3.6 V at the beginning of life, whereas the lithium–lead-iodide cell has a voltage of only 1.9 V. Because the voltage of each of these cells is less than that which may be required for chronic myocardial stimulation, a voltage multiplier in the output circuit must be used to allow output pulses of greater amplitude than the cell voltage. If the lithium–iodine battery potential is 2.8 V, how is it possible for a pacemaker to deliver an amplitude of 5 V? There are two potential methods for delivering a stimulus with an amplitude that is greater than that generated by the chemical reaction of the battery.

First, the pacemaker could use two batteries placed in series. Using cells in series increases the output voltage of the battery, but does not increase battery capacity. Electrochemical cells may also be connected in parallel to increase capacity. However, cells in parallel do not generate an increased voltage. The alternative method is to use the battery charge of two capacitors in parallel and then to discharge the two capacitors to the lead in series. In this way a single battery with a potential of 2.8 V could generate 5.6 V with two capacitors, or 8.4 V with three capacitors. The total capacitance (C_T) of two capacitors (C_1 and C_2) charged in parallel is equal to $C_T = C_1 + C_2$. Because the total charge (Q) is related to the voltage (V) and capacitance (C) of the capacitor by the equation $Q = CV$, a double amount of charge is drawn from the battery. However, when these two capacitors are then discharged in series onto the lead, the capacitance is given by the equation

$$(1/C_T) = (1/C_1) + (1/C_2)$$

Thus, the discharge of these two capacitors in series results in a capacitance that is equal to one-half that for a single capacitor. Because an equal amount of charge must flow from each capacitor in series, the remaining voltage on the capacitor after discharge is $V_f/2$, where V_f is the final voltage. The net result is that by programming the pacemaker to a voltage that is double the battery voltage, the charge taken from the battery is equal to twice that delivered to the lead and the total amount of charge drained from the battery increases fourfold.

The longevity of a battery is determined by several factors, including the chemical elements of the battery, the size of the battery, the amount of internal discharge, and the voltage decay characteristics of the cell. To maximize battery life, the ideal electrochemical cell would have no internal discharge. However, batteries used for permanent pacemakers have been associated with internal discharge of variable degrees. For example, the initial zinc–mercury cells were associated with an internal rate of self-discharge of > 15% per year. The lithium–iodine cell is associated with a low rate of self-discharge following the initial reaction of lithium and iodine in the cell, generally < 1% per year in chronic use.

For a battery to be suitable for use in permanent pacemakers, the decay characteristics of the cell should be predictable (Fig. 2.37). The ideal battery should have a predictable fall in voltage near end of life, yet provide sufficient service life after the initial voltage decay to allow time for the elective replacement indicator to be detected and for replacement to be performed. The early zinc–mercury batteries were associated with a nearly constant cell voltage until the end of life, when the voltage declined abruptly. These characteristics were generally unacceptable because of the difficulty of anticipating battery depletion. Lithium cells are associated with a more predictable behavior at end of life. The lithium–silver-chromate cell is characterized by two distinct plateau phases of voltage, the first phase (3.2 V) representing approximately

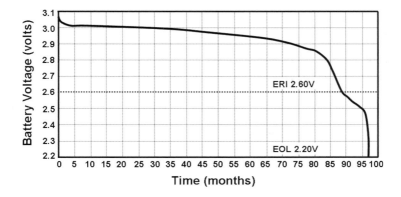

Fig. 2.37 Voltage decay characteristics of a pacemaker battery. At beginning of life, the cell generates 3.1 V. When the battery voltage decreases to 2.6 V, the elective replacement indicator (ERI) is reached, and the pulse generator should be changed, as the battery is approaching the predictable steep decline in voltage that occurs at the end of its usable life. When the battery voltage decreases to 2.2 V, this cell is at end of life (EOL). Different batteries have different voltage cut-offs for ERI and EOL, and a universal device encyclopedia is available as a reference, with battery voltage information on all models of pacemakers and implantable cardioverter defibrillators that are currently in use.

70% of the service life and a second phase of approximately 2.5 V. This two-phase decay characteristic is an attractive feature of this cell and allows a wide period in which to detect the elective replacement indicator.

Another battery that has been used for permanent pacemakers is the lithium–thionyl-chloride cell. This battery was associated with instances of an abrupt fall in battery voltage related to a sudden rise in cell impedance and unexpected end-of-life behavior. The voltage produced by a lithium–iodine cell is inversely related to the internal battery impedance. The internal impedance of the battery increases with the thickness of the lithium-iodide electrolyte layer, from < 1 kΩ at the beginning of life to > 15 kΩ at the extreme end of life. The voltage generated by the cell declines almost linearly from the initial value of 2.8 V to 2.4 V at approximately 90% of the usable battery life. Following this, the voltage declines exponentially to 1.8 V at the end of life. The magnet-related pacing rate of the pulse generator is related to the cell voltage, usually declining once the voltage falls below 2.4 V. The end-of-life indicator of pulse generators is usually signaled by a decrease in the magnet-related pacing rate to a fixed percentage of the beginning-of-life rate. Unfortunately, the end-of-life magnet rate is variable between manufacturers and between models. Some manufacturers signal the end of life by a two-step process, with an initial decrease in the magnet rate to an intermediate value, followed by a stepwise decrease in rate to a second, lower value in association with a change in pacing mode, such as from DDD to VVI. In addition to a decrease in the magnet rate, the cell impedance can be directly measured and retrieved during a device interrogation, allowing a more precise estimation of the usable service life. Some manufacturers also include an automatic increase in the pulse duration of the output circuit so that the total energy of the pulse delivered remains constant. Although the output energy may remain constant by the stretching of the pulse duration, loss of capture will occur if the stimulus voltage falls below rheobase.

The usable service life of a pulse generator not only depends on the characteristics of the battery, but is greatly influenced by the current drain of the integrated circuit, the amplitude and duration of the output pulse, the frequency of stimulation, the total impedance of the pacing lead and the additional energy required to monitor and generate the output of a rate-adaptive sensor. Advances in the design of integrated circuits have greatly minimized the static current drain required to operate the circuit to $< 2\,\mu A$. The major source of current drain for the present generation of pulse generators is the output pulse. Thus, the amplitude, duration and frequency of stimulating pulses are major contributors to the life of the power source. The pacing impedance is another critical influence on the current drain of the output pulse. Advances in pacing leads that have improved pulse generator longevity while providing an adequate safety margin have included the use of electrodes with steroid elution, high electrode–tissue impedance, and low polarization. With the use of these high-performance leads, the nominal output energy has been significantly reduced. The addition of automatic threshold testing and capture verification also increases pulse generator longevity by permitting lower stimulus outputs in the setting of ongoing automatic verification of pacing capture.

The implantable defibrillator battery is designed to be able to deliver a shock within about 10 s after a ventricular arrhythmia is detected. The ICD must charge a high-voltage capacitor, and thus the battery needs to sustain a high current while maintaining a high voltage. ICDs require a battery with high peak power and therefore the battery must have small and thick electrodes. Instead of a single central anode, the battery has wound layers of anode and cathode material separated by a small thin porous film. Today, ICD batteries have lithium–silver vanadium oxide cathodes. Generally, ICD batteries have a beginning-of-life voltage of about 3.15 V, and over time show a gradual decline in voltage to a plateau, and then a final more rapidly declining voltage as the battery approaches elective replacement.

Output circuits

The output pulse of the pulse generator is generated from the discharge of a capacitor to the anode and cathode of the pacing leads. The output capacitor is charged from the battery at a relatively slow rate to the programmed output voltage. Because the battery voltage of lithium–iodine cells is approximately 2.8 V, delivery of a stimulus of amplitude greater than this requires the use of a voltage multiplier. The voltage multiplier involves charging more than one capacitor from the battery. For example, if a stimulus voltage of 5.6 V is programmed, two capacitors must be charged from the battery in parallel and discharged in series. The cost of doubling the output voltage is a fourfold increase in current drain from the battery. If the stimulus amplitude is programmed to 8.4 V (three times the voltage of a lithium–iodine cell), three capacitors must be charged. In this case, a threefold increase in stimulus voltage results in a ninefold increase in current drain from the battery, markedly shortening the battery life.

Output pulse waveforms

Most pulse generators used for permanent cardiac pacing deliver a capacitively coupled, constant-voltage pulse of programmable duration. When the fully charged capacitor is discharged, the resulting voltage at the leading edge of the pulse is independent of the pacing impedance. However, the trailing edge voltage of the pulse is less than that of the leading edge, with the magnitude of the voltage drop being a function of the pacing impedance (Fig. 2.38). Because the capacitor stores a charge of fixed quantity, the greater the current flow, the smaller the charge (and voltage) remaining on the capacitor at the end of the pulse. Therefore, the lower the impedance, the greater the current delivered and the greater the drop in voltage from leading edge to trailing edge during the pulse. Thus, even though the term constant voltage is used to describe the stimulus waveform of permanent pacemakers, in reality the output voltage of the pulse is not constant from beginning to end.

Constant-current generators are no longer being implanted for permanent pacing. However, constant-current pulse generators are typical of many external pacing systems. The constant-current pulse is typically flat, with little or no change in current from leading edge to trailing edge. However, as the polarization impedance rises during the pulse, the resulting voltage must also rise proportionally to maintain the current at a constant level. Although either constant-current or constant-voltage pulse generators are capable of providing reliable pacing in the vast majority of clinical circumstances, at extremely high lead impedances the voltage required to maintain a constant-current pulse may exceed the capabilities of the battery.

Fig. 2.38 Output voltage and current waveforms for constant-voltage (left) and constant-current (right) stimulation. With a constant-voltage pulse, the leading-edge voltage is independent of load. The trailing-edge voltage depends on the total pacing impedance. The delivered current also declines from leading edge to trailing edge. With constant-current stimulation, the current remains constant throughout the pulse (provided that the cell can generate the required voltage). The delivered voltage increases with rising impedance during the pulse.

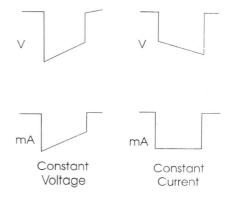

The output waveform of the pulse generator is followed by a low-amplitude, long-duration wave of opposite polarity known as the afterpotential. The afterpotential is caused by polarization at the electrode–tissue interface and is dependent on the stimulus amplitude and duration. The afterpotential is also influenced by the polarization characteristics of the electrode. Afterpotentials may be inappropriately sensed by the sensing circuit if the stimulus amplitude and pulse duration are great and the sensing threshold is low. To reduce the afterpotential, the output circuit of some manufacturers incorporates a fast recharge pulse, during which the electrode polarity is reversed for a short period following the output pulse. This diminishes the polarization at the electrode–tissue interface, although it does not eliminate the need for low-polarization electrodes. As mentioned previously, the major clinical impact of afterpotentials relates to the ability of the pulse generator to automatically determine myocardial capture.

Sensing circuits

The intracardiac electrogram is conducted from the electrodes to the sensing circuit of the pulse generator, where it is amplified and filtered. As discussed previously in this chapter, to minimize attenuation of the signal the sensing amplifier must have an input impedance greatly in excess of the sensing impedance. The greater the input impedance, the less the electrogram is attenuated by the amplifier. The input impedances of the sense amplifiers used in permanent pacing systems are > 25 000 Ω. The intracardiac electrogram is filtered to remove unwanted frequencies, a process that markedly affects the amplitude of the processed signal. A bandpass filter attenuates components of the electrogram on either side of the center frequency (the frequency with least attenuation) (Fig. 2.39). The bandpass filters of different manufacturers vary significantly with regard to center frequency (from approximately 20 to 40 Hz), so intracardiac electrograms measured with a pacing system analyzer of one manufacturer may produce considerably different electrogram amplitudes than will the pulse generator sensing amplifier of another manufacturer. It is also somewhat difficult to compare the sense amplifiers of different manufacturers because the shape of the test waveform has an important influence on the amplitude of the filtered electrogram, such that square-wave and sinusoidal test pulses may produce frequency attenuation spectra that differ from those of intracardiac electrograms. Following filtering of the intracardiac signal, the processed signal is compared with a reference voltage to determine if the signal exceeds a threshold detection level. Signals with amplitudes greater than the sensitivity threshold level are sensed as intracardiac events, whereas signals of lower amplitude are discarded as noise. Signals that exceed the threshold level are marked by an output voltage pulse that is sent to the timing circuit.

Some permanent pacemakers also contain noise reversion circuits that change the pulse generator to an asynchronous pacing mode when the sensing threshold level is exceeded at a rate faster than the noise reversion rate.

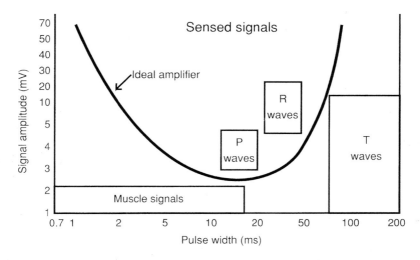

Fig. 2.39 Signal processing with bandpass filtering of a sine-squared test waveform by a ventricular sensing amplifier. The curve denotes the signal amplitude required to be detected by the sensing amplifier with a threshold sensitivity value of 2.5 mV. Note that the amplitude of the signal that is needed for appropriate sensing is markedly increased at frequencies below and above the center frequency.

The noise reversion mode prevents inhibition of pacing in the presence of electromagnetic interference. The electronic circuitry of the pulse generator must also be protected from damage caused by overwhelming electrical energy generated in the clinical environment. The input voltage to the sensing amplifier is limited by a Zener diode that is designed to protect the integrated circuit from high external voltages such as may occur during defibrillation shocks or electrocautery. When the input voltage carried by the pacing leads exceeds the Zener voltage, the excess energy is shunted back to the myocardium through the leads. In addition to these features, which are designed to manage external electromagnetic interference, the sensing amplifier must prevent the detection of unwanted intracardiac signals such as far-field R waves in the atrial electrogram, afterpotentials, T waves, and retrogradely conducted P waves.

The potential for inappropriate inhibition of the ventricular output of a dual-chamber pacemaker by far-field ventricular sensing of the atrial pacing stimulus or its afterpotential can be effectively reduced by the use of a ventricular blanking period. During the ventricular blanking period, the ventricular sensing amplifier is turned off immediately following the atrial pacing pulse. Although the blanking period has been quite effective in decreasing the frequency of ventricular crosstalk (inappropriate inhibition of ventricular pacing by far-field atrial pacing stimuli), several manufacturers also provide a short, non-physiological AV delay with delivery of a ventricular pacing pulse upon sensing a ventricular event of uncertain origin early in the AV interval, following an atrial pacing output (known as "safety pacing" in Medtronic devices). The inappropriate detection of intracardiac signals is also managed by the use of sensing refractory periods, during which the sense amplifier is not responsive to events such as T waves or retrogradely conducted P waves. The initial portion of the refractory period is a blanking period during which the sense amplifier is totally insensitive to electrical signals.

The remainder of the refractory period is typically a noise sampling period. Events in this portion of the refractory period do not reset the timing circuit, but initiate a new blanking period. Although sensing refractory periods are extremely effective for the management of unwanted signals, there are relative disadvantages to this approach, such as the inability of a DDD pacing system to track rapid atrial rates when a prolonged atrial refractory period is required to manage retrograde ventriculoatrial conduction. Pacing systems that incorporate variable refractory periods that change in proportion to the output of a metabolic sensor may reduce the importance of these disadvantages.

Timing circuits

The pacing cycle length, sensing refractory and alert periods, pulse duration and AV interval are precisely regulated by the timing circuit of the pulse generator. The timing circuit of a pulse generator is a crystal oscillator that generates a very accurate signal with a frequency in the kHz range. The output of the crystal oscillator is sent to a digital timing and logic control circuit that operates internally generated clocks at divisions of the oscillator frequency. The output of the logic control circuit is a logic pulse that triggers the output pacing pulse, the blanking and refractory intervals, and the AV delay. The timing circuit also receives input from the sense amplifier to reset the escape intervals of an inhibited pacing system or trigger initiation of an AV delay for triggered pacing modes. The pulse generator also contains a rate-limiting circuit that prevents the pacing rate from exceeding an upper limit in the case of a random component failure. This runaway protection rate is typically in the range of 180–200 ppm.

Telemetry circuits

Programmable pulse generators have the capability of responding to radiofrequency signals emitted from the programmer as well as sending information in the reverse direction, from the pulse generator to the programmer. The pulse generator is capable of both transmitting information from a radiofrequency antenna and receiving information with a radiofrequency decoder. Telemetry information may be sent as radiofrequency signals or as a pulsed magnetic field. Information that is sent from an external programmer to the pulse generator is sent in coded programming sequences with a preset frequency spectrum. Most pulse generators require the radiofrequency signal to be pulsed with a specific frequency in a sequence that is typically 16 pulses in duration. Thus the radiofrequency signal is quite precise, decreasing the likelihood of inappropriate alteration of the program by environmental sources of radiofrequency energy or magnetic fields. This characteristic also prevents

the programmers of one manufacturer from programming the pulse generator of another. The detected telemetry bursts from the programmer are sent
as digital information from the radiofrequency demodulator to the telemetry
control logic circuit of the pulse generator. This logic circuit also provides for
properly timed pulses to be sent from the antenna of the pulse generator to the
programmer. "Real-time telemetry" is the term used to describe the capability of a pulse generator to transmit information to the programmer regarding
measurements of pulse amplitude and duration, lead impedance, battery impedance, and delivered current, charge and energy.

Reed switch

Implantable devices have a reed switch which normally is open until a magnet or magnetic field (e.g. a magnetic resonance imaging scanner) comes into
close contact with the device. The magnet will close the reed switch and the
device will be switched to the "magnet mode." The magnet mode is typically
asynchronous pacing for a pacemaker (e.g. VOO, DOO, AOO) and for most defibrillators is deactivation of tachycardia therapy, but not bradycardia pacing
and sensing functions. The magnet may be unable to close the reed switch if it
is not powerful enough or the magnet function is programmed off.

Microprocessors

Microprocessors have become the standard control circuits of implantable
pacemakers and ICDs. Microprocessors have several advantages over older
integrated circuits, including a far greater circuit density and greatly reduced
current drain. Microprocessors also allow very sophisticated algorithms,
requiring multiple calculations to be incorporated into implantable devices,
and have vastly increased data storage. The microprocessor can respond to
changes in programming instructions that allow functions to be added or
changed after implantation. The integrated circuit of pulse generators may
contain both read-only memory (ROM) and random access memory (RAM).

ROM (typically 1–2 kb of 8–32 bits) is used to guide the sensing and output
circuits. Critical pacemaker codes, such as those used for reset routines and
program storage, are stored in ROM. Devices with 8- or 16-bit processors usually require several clock cycles to decode an instruction from memory. The
processors operating with larger instruction words (such as 32 bits) may load
and execute an instruction in a single clock cycle, improving the efficiency of
the repetitive tasks that are required for pacing and sensing.

In addition, RAM is used to store diagnostic information regarding pacing
rate, intrinsic heart rates and sensor output. The amount of RAM that is included in the pulse generator varies between models and manufacturers. The
amount of RAM in modern pulse generators has rapidly increased, allowing
for a far greater amount of diagnostic information that can be stored in the
pulse generator. Such data include histograms of paced and intrinsic heart
rate, sensor function, trends of heart rate and sensor function over time, storage of intracardiac electrograms from episodes of high atrial or ventricular

rates, and mode-switching events. The rapidly expanding diagnostic capabilities of pacemakers has allowed for improved assessment of the physiological condition of the patient, including stored information about heart rate variability, respiration, intracardiac pressure, patient activity, lung water, and arrhythmia logs.

Almost all manufacturers offer fully RAM-based pulse generators. There are several important advantages to microprocessor-based pacemakers, including decreased production costs for an entire product line, increased flexibility to upgrade features in subsequent pacemaker models, and the capability for downloading new features into previously implanted pacemakers by telemetry. It is important to emphasize that the microprocessors used in permanent pacemakers must be custom designed to minimize current drain and operate with a lithium–iodine battery. Thus, a microprocessor that is used in a microcomputer and has access to a virtually unlimited power supply (AC current operating at 110 V) would not be feasible for inclusion in a permanent pacemaker.

Rate-adaptive sensors

Whereas the prevention of symptomatic or life-threatening bradycardia is the principal purpose of a pacemaker, augmentation of heart rate in response to a variety of physiological conditions that call for increased cardiac output is an important secondary pacemaker function that has important implications for a patient's quality of life. An intact sinus node is the ideal rate-responsive sensor, adjusting heart rate according to biological need under the direct influence of the autonomic nervous system. It is partially for this reason that dual-chamber pacemakers are used in patients with atrioventricular block; the electronic pacemaker, via atrial sensing, adjusts the ventricular pacing rate to match the output of the intact sinus node. When the sinus node does not function properly, as in sinus node dysfunction, or is not accessible to the electronic pacemaker, in the setting of a single-chamber pacemaker or atrial fibrillation, the pacemaker must rely on an alternative cue to determine the appropriate heart rate. It is for this reason that several different types of rate-adaptive artificial sensors have been developed.[19,20]

Because the primary situation in which heart rate augmentation is needed is with physical activity, most pacemaker sensors are designed to detect patient movement or an increased respiratory rate. Other conditions, such as emotional stress, hypovolemia, febrile illness, or hypermetabolic states, are less easily translated into an electrical or physical parameter that could be sensed by a pacemaker. Temperature sensors, QT-interval sensors and electrical sensors to detect local myocardial contractility are examples of rate-responsive sensors that have been designed to respond to non-activity-related conditions that call for an increase in heart rate, but accelerometers (that detect movement) and minute-ventilation sensors (that detect respiratory rate) dominate the pacemaker market and generally work well to reproduce the heart rate changes that would ordinarily occur throughout the day.

The sensors themselves only detect the physical or electrical parameters they were designed to track; how this information is translated into a specific heart rate is dependent on additional programmable and non-programmable algorithms that control the degree to which the pacing rate is increased. The sensor threshold, slope of increase in heart rate, target heart rate, duration of accelerated pacing, and slope of decline in heart rate are some of the parameters that must be tailored to each patient to ensure adequate heart rate support, but avoid excessive heart rates when more rapid pacing is not appropriate.

Technical considerations also arise with regard to sensor implementation. The sensor must have durability, especially considering that some motion sensors have moving parts, it must not result in excessive drain on the battery that would lead to significant shortening of the life span of the pulse generator, and it ideally should not require the implantation of additional hardware that could increase the risk of a procedural complication or sensor failure due to increased system complexity. An effective sensor should demonstrate high sensitivity to exercise or other physiological conditions in which the heart rate should be increased, but also high specificity to avoid the detection of stimuli that should not result in faster pacing.

Activity or vibration sensors

There are two main types of motion sensors that have been used in modern devices: piezoelectric crystals and accelerometers (Fig. 2.40). The piezoelectric

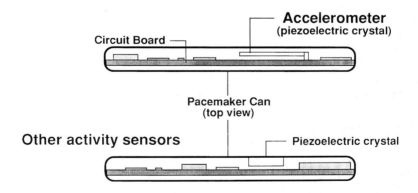

Fig. 2.40 Schematic of two motion-sensing, rate-adaptive pacing systems. Top: An accelerometer is mounted on the circuit board of the pulse generator. Similar to a pedometer, the accelerometer arm moves with anteroposterior movement of the chest, which deforms a piezoresistive material and alerts the pacemaker that physical activity is occurring. Bottom: A piezoelectric crystal is bonded to the inside of the pulse generator case. The crystal detects vibrations, which include those generated during physical activity, as well as those resulting from pressure on the pacemaker case or vibrations from the environment, such as a motor vehicle. (Courtesy of Intermedics, Inc.)

crystal sensor detects mechanical vibration and pressure, and is bonded to the inside of the pulse generator can. Flexion and deformation of the crystal result in the production of a small electric current, which occurs when vibrations are transmitted throughout the human body (which has a resonant frequency of approximately 4 Hz), such as during stair-climbing or walking. Greater frequency and amplitude of vibrations result in a greater degree of crystal flexion, and a larger current is thereby generated. The electrical output from the crystal sensor is processed electronically and used by the device to modulate the pacing rate proportionally when the sensor is programmed to be active. Vibration or distortion of any sort will deform the piezoelectric crystal, so direct pressure on the can will activate this sensor, even if the device is otherwise motionless. Consequently, certain activities, such as lying in the prone position or riding in a vibrating motor vehicle, can result in sensor activation at a time when increased heart rate is not needed. Conversely, the piezoelectric crystal sensor does not respond well to certain types of activity, such as swimming or isometric exercise, where the vibrations the sensor detects are less prominent. Both the activity and vibration sensors respond promptly to the onset of activity and thus are capable of early exercise detection.

Accelerometer sensors

Because of the above-mentioned limitations, use of the piezoelectric vibration sensor to detect body motion has largely been supplanted by use of the second type of motion sensor, the accelerometer. Acceleration sensors consist of a diving-board-like arm that is mounted on the circuit board. Movement of the pulse generator in the anterior–posterior axis results in movement and flexion of the accelerometer arm and deformation of an attached piezoelectric or piezoresistive material. Because the accelerometer is mounted on the circuit board, it is mechanically insulated from the device can, and so simple pressure on the device will not result in sensor activation. Instead, it is the change in velocity of the accelerometer mass (acceleration = dV/dt) that creates output from the sensor. Accelerometers have been shown to deliver a remarkably consistent response to varying degrees and types of activity, across a wide range of individuals with different size, body weight, age and physiological condition. These devices have better resolution to detect small changes in motion when compared with vibration sensors, and are thereby able to offer rate modulation that is more proportional to exercise workload. In addition, because the accelerometer detects lower frequencies than vibration sensors, environmental noise, which typically has a higher frequency range, is more easily filtered out and ignored. Accelerometers are also characterized by their ability to detect and respond rapidly to the onset of activity, and they tend to fare well when evaluated during stair climbing, walking and treadmill exercise testing.[21]

Minute-ventilation sensors

In some activity settings, the anterior–posterior movement of the chest does not sufficiently correlate with the level of metabolic demand. For example, during bicycle racing, where the movement of the torso may not be proportional to the degree of exertion, an accelerometer sensor might underestimate the appropriate heart rate. A more common scenario occurs in patients who are elderly or are restricted in mobility, where metabolic demand during ambulation outstrips the physical movement of the torso. In such settings, motion sensors might not provide adequate heart rate response, so other types of sensors might be necessary to more closely approximate heart rate needs. Respiratory rate and tidal volume increase in proportion to changes in carbon dioxide production (VCO_2) and oxygen consumption (VO_2), and minute-ventilation sensors have been developed and demonstrated to provide rate modulation that is closely correlated with VO_2 in most patients.[22]

The minute-ventilation sensor relies on changes in transthoracic impedance that occur during inspiration and expiration (Fig. 2.41). Changes in transthoracic impedance are proportional to changes in minute ventilation. Low-energy, subthreshold pulses are rapidly delivered in a unipolar con-

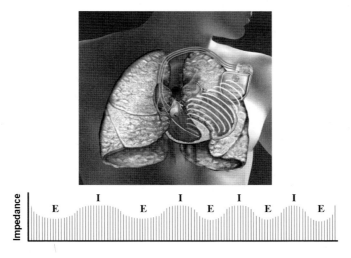

Fig. 2.41 Schematic of how a minute-ventilation sensor works. Top: Rapid, low-energy pulses are delivered between the intracardiac pacing lead and the pacemaker can in the pectoral region, spanning lung tissue. The transthoracic impedance will vary, depending on how much air (insulator) is in the lungs. Bottom: Hypothetical graph of impedance measurements during slow, then faster respirations. When the lungs are more deflated during expiration (E), transthoracic impedance falls due to relatively less air and relatively more tissue fluid present within the minute-ventilation circuit. When the lungs are more inflated during inspiration (I), transthoracic impedance rises. By tracking the rate of rise and fall in transthoracic impedance over a time frame of seconds, the minute-ventilation sensor can determine the respiratory rate, and this information can be used for rate-responsive pacing. Over a time frame of days to weeks, more gradual trends in transthoracic impedance may reflect changes in lung water due to congestive heart failure, and some devices use this information to track heart failure status. [Courtesy of Medtronic, Inc. (top).]

figuration from the intracardiac pacing lead, with the pectoral pulse generator can acting as the second electrode. If a pulse of known amplitude is delivered, and the resultant voltage between the lead electrode and the pulse generator can is measured, the impedance can be calculated. When the lungs are inflated during inspiration, there is more insulating air interposed between the lead and the can, which raises the impedance in the circuit. When the lungs deflate during expiration, there is less air and proportionally more tissue water in the circuit, and the impedance decreases. Pulses are delivered at high frequency, every 50 ms, which allows the sensor to detect fluctuations in transthoracic impedance with regard to both frequency (correlates to respiratory rate) and amplitude (correlates to tidal volume), and thereby calculate minute ventilation (the product of respiratory rate and tidal volume). A bipolar pacing lead is needed for the minute-ventilation sensor to work, as the ring electrode is used for pulse delivery and the tip electrode is used to simultaneously measure voltage in order to calculate impedance. Either a bipolar atrial or ventricular lead can be used, but a pacing system with exclusive unipolar leads cannot accommodate a minute-ventilation sensor. Because transthoracic impedance fluctuates during the cardiac cycle, and with thoracic and arm movements, a low-pass filter is used to eliminate impedance fluctuations with frequencies that exceed the typical range of respiratory rates.

At the onset of activity, minute ventilation tends to increase more slowly than heart rate in the setting of an intact sinus node, whereas during sustained exercise at high workloads, minute ventilation increases out of proportion to heart rate and oxygen consumption, particularly if the anaerobic threshold is crossed. Because of this changing relationship between minute ventilation, oxygen consumption and heart rate throughout exercise, the minute-ventilation sensor will typically use a steeper slope at the onset of exercise and a flatter slope at high levels of exercise when calculating the target pacing rate. In this fashion, a slight increase in respiration will translate into a greater degree of heart rate increase early on during exercise, but more dramatic increases in minute ventilation at peak exercise will result in a lesser degree of heart rate increase, in order to prevent overpacing.

Most pulse generators with minute-ventilation sensors will also have an activity sensor, and measured data from both sensors can be combined to form a "blended sensor" that may provide an even better rate-adaptive response to exercise than either sensor alone (Fig. 2.42). Information from the activity sensor is typically weighted more heavily at the onset of exercise, when physical motion is more prominent than increased respiration, and the minute-ventilation sensor is more prominent after more sustained activity and in recovery, when metabolic needs remain elevated after physical motion has slowed or stopped. With this sensor combination, the rapid increase in pacing rate with the onset of activity and the more gradual decline of heart rate in recovery can closely approximate the physiological heart rate response pattern of the intact sinus node, and the utility of the blended sensor has been demonstrated.[23]

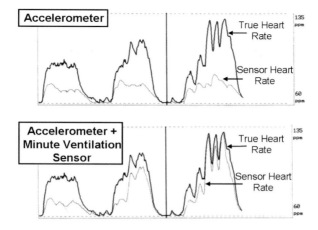

Fig. 2.42 Comparison of rate-responsive pacing with accelerometer vs. blended sensor in a patient with a rate-responsive pacemaker and an intact sinus node. Top: The dark line represents the patient's actual heart rate (normal sinus node) during three sequential episodes of exertion. The lighter line represents the projected heart rate that the pacemaker would have provided if rate-responsive pacing were activated using the accelerometer sensor at current sensor programmed settings. Bottom: The dark line again shows the patient's actual heart rate for the same time period. The lighter line now represents the projected heart rate that the pacemaker would have provided with both the accelerometer and the minute-ventilation sensor active in a "blended sensor" configuration. The sensor-driven heart rate more closely approximates the physiological heart rate when the minute-ventilation sensor is added. It should be noted that improved rate-responsive pacing could also potentially be achieved by increasing the sensitivity and/or aggressiveness of the accelerometer sensor settings. (Courtesy of Boston Scientific, Inc.)

Sensor programmability

There is variability in the relationship between sensor input and appropriate heart rate in different individuals, with factors such as age, body size, weight, degree of fitness, device location and orientation, and types of exertion playing a role. It is for this reason that rate modulation sensors have several programmable and non-programmable parameters and algorithms that are used to tailor heart rate response to the individual. The terminology for sensor parameters varies from one device company to the next, but the principles are the same. Typical programmable sensor parameters include base rate, maximum sensor rate, activity threshold, reaction time, slope, recovery time and lifestyle. The activity threshold parameter is used to determine how much sensor input is needed before rate modulation initiates—with an accelerometer, for example, this setting determines how much movement of the device is needed before the pacemaker starts increasing the pacing rate. If the sensor threshold is too low, the patient may notice a faster pulse rate during low-level activities, whereas, if it is too high, poor augmentation of heart rate will result and the patient may experience exercise intolerance (Fig. 2.43). The reaction time and slope are used to determine how soon to start increasing the heart

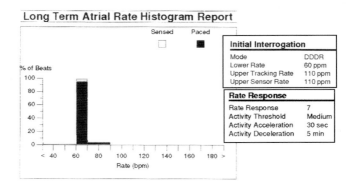

Fig. 2.43 Example of a patient with chronotropic incompetence, whose rate-responsive pacemaker has failed to provide adequate heart rate augmentation with exertion. The atrial rate histogram shows that the pacemaker is pacing in the atrium at the lower rate limit (60 ppm) virtually all the time despite an upper sensor rate of 110 ppm, and rate-responsive pacing active (DDDR mode). Changes in sensor settings that would be likely to improve rate-responsive pacing include increasing the rate response setting (currently set at "7"), lowering the activity threshold (currently set to "medium"), and raising the upper sensor rate. If the patient continued to note initial fatigue with activity that improved with continued exertion, the activity acceleration time could be shortened as well.

rate in response to sensor activation, and how rapidly the heart rate should be increased (Fig. 2.44). The lifestyle input is used to help determine an optimal heart rate profile, which will depend on the degree to which the patient typically exerts him or herself.

Many devices have automatic algorithms that self-adjust many of the programmable sensor parameters, taking into account the patient's age, activity profile and heart rate histogram. Parameters such as the threshold, slope, and target heart rate may be automatically adjusted in order to create a heart

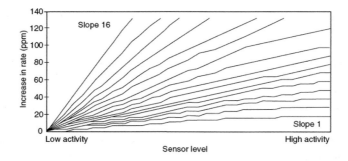

Fig. 2.44 Graph demonstrating the behavior of different "slope" settings in a St. Jude rate-responsive pacemaker. A lower slope setting will augment the pacing rate less than a higher slope setting for a given amount of sensor input. (Courtesy of St. Jude Medical, Inc.)

rate profile that is consistent with typical patterns of heart rate in patients with normal sinus node activity. It should be noted that the calculated target heart rate for a given level of sensor input is dependent on the maximum programmed sensor rate, so increasing this rate from 120 to 160 ppm, for example, can have a marked influence on the rate-adaptive profile of the pacemaker, even if the other parameters, such as threshold and slope, are left unchanged. Finding the optimal sensor parameters for an individual might involve several programming adjustments, after the patient has the opportunity to evaluate activity-related symptoms either at home between visits or during repeated exercise treadmill testing in the office. Because different types of activity may activate the activity sensor in different ways, programming adjustments are best made after the patient engages in the activities that reproduce their most profound symptoms related to either excessive or inadequate pacing rates. Because different vendors use different nomenclature and different numeric designations for the various sensor settings, it is important to be certain of the meaning of each setting before making programming changes. A higher numeric value for a particular parameter might either increase or decrease the aggressiveness of rate-responsive pacing, depending on that particular parameter or device model.

Other sensors

With an intact sinus node, the heart rate will increase in response to sympathetic tone and catecholamines even outside the setting of activity. Emotional stress, illness and hemodynamic derangement, for example, call for an increased heart rate, yet motion and minute-ventilation sensors will be inadequate to detect these cues. Other sensors have been developed to try to reproduce the increases in heart rate that are needed outside the setting of physical activity.

Alternative sensors that do not require a specialized pacing lead include those that measure the QT interval (Vitatron) and those that detect small changes in impedance at the lead tip in the setting of increased myocardial contractility ("Closed Loop System," Biotronik). The QT interval will shorten in response to increased heart rate and sympathetic tone. For a device to measure the QT interval, a pacing stimulus must be delivered to generate a QRS–T complex, and then the evoked electrical response that follows must be filtered in a way to permit detection of the lower amplitude, lower slew rate repolarization (T-wave) signal. The QT interval can be markedly influenced by medications and electrolyte disturbances, which may confound its use as a rate-responsive parameter at times. The QT sensor can be blended with an accelerometer for more optimal performance. The closed loop system (CLS) relies on small changes in the electrical environment of the lead–myocardial interface at times of increased cardiac contractility. A bipolar lead is required for this sensor, and pacing stimulation is also needed. The CLS sensor cannot be blended with an accelerometer, although pulse generators will also have an accelerometer that could be substituted by simply reprogramming the device if the CLS does not provide adequate rate response for that individual. The advantages of these alternative sensors are that they are compatible with standard pacing leads and may provide better rate response in certain situations. The disadvantages are that cardiac stimulation is required, and they may not always respond as reliably as the more traditional sensors in the setting of physical activity.

More esoteric sensors have also been developed, such as those that measure central venous temperature, mixed venous oxygen saturation, right ventricular dP/dt, peak endocardial acceleration and intracardiac impedance. These sensors have been shown to demonstrate excellent physiological rate response characteristics. Each of these sensors, however, requires specialized pacing leads, which has greatly limited their clinical utility and has prevented widespread acceptance.

References

1 Hodgkin AL, Huxley AF. A quantitative description of membrane current and its application to conduction and excitation in nerves. J Physiol (Lond) 1952; 117:500–44.
2 DiFrancesco D, Ferroni A, Mozzanti M et al. Properties of the hyperpolarizing activated current (I_f) in cells isolated from the rabbit sinoatrial node. J Physiol 1986; 377:61–88.
3 DeMello WC. Intracellular communication in cardiac muscle. Circ Res 1982; 51:1–9.
4 Spach MS, Dolber PC, Heidlage JR et al. Propagating depolarization in anisotropic human and canine cardiac muscle: apparent directional differences in membrane capacitance. A simplified model for selective directional effects of modifying the sodium conductance on Vmax, tau foot, and the propagation safety factor. Circ Res 1987; 60:206–19.
5 Winfree AT. The electrical thresholds of ventricular myocardium. J Cardiovasc Electrophysiol 1990; 1:393–410.
6 Irnich W. The fundamental law of electrostimulation and its application to defibrillation. Pacing Clin Electrophysiol 1990; 13:1433–77.
7 Blair HA. On the intensity–time relations for stimulation by electric currents. J Gen Physiol 1932; 15:709–29.
8 Sylven JC, Hellerstedt M, Levander-Lingren M. Pacing threshold interval with decreasing and increasing output. Pacing Clin Electrophysiol 1982; 5:646–9.
9 Platia EV, Brinker JA. Time course of transvenous pacemaker stimulation impedance, capture threshold, and electrogram amplitude. Pacing Clin Electrophysiol 1986; 9:620–5.
10 Smyth NPD, Tarjan PP, Chernoff E et al. The significance of electrode surface area and stimulation thresholds in permanent cardiac pacing. J Thorac Cardiovasc Surg 1976; 71:559–65.
11 Beyersdorf F, Schneider M, Kreuzer J et al. Studies of the tissue reaction induced by transvenous pacemaker electrodes. I. Microscopic examination of the extent of connective tissue around the electrode tip in the human right ventricle. Pacing Clin Electrophysiol 1988; 11:1753–9.
12 Mond H, Stokes K, Helland J et al. The porous titanium steroid eluting electrode: a double blind study assessing the stimulation threshold effects of steroid. Pacing Clin Electrophysiol 1988; 11:214–9.

13 Buxton AE, Marchlinski FE, Miller JM *et al*. The human atrial strength–interval relation. Influence of cycle length and procainamide. Circulation 1989; 79:271–80.

14 Kay GN, Mulholland DH, Epstein AE, Plumb VJ. Effect of pacing rate on the human–strength duration curve. J Am Coll Cardiol 1990; 15:1618–23.

15 Preston TA, Fletcher RD, Lucchesi BR, Judge RD. Changes in myocardial threshold. Physiologic and pharmacologic factors in patients with implanted pace-makers. Am Heart J 1967; 74:235.

16 Amundson D, McArthur W, MacCarter D *et al*. Porous electrode–tissue interface. Pacing Clin Electrophysiol 1979; 2:40–50.

17 Furman S, Hurzeler P, DeCaprio V. The ventricular endocardial electrogram and pacemaker sensing. J Thorac Cardiovasc Surg 1977; 73:258.

18 Brummer SB, Robblee LS, Hambrecht FT. Criteria for selecting electrodes for electrical stimulation: theoretical and practical considerations. Ann NY Acad Sci 1983; 405:159–71.

19 Benditt DG, Mianulli M, Fetter J *et al*. Single chamber cardiac pacing with activity-initiated chronotropic response. Evaluation by cardiopulmonary exercise testing. Circulation 1987; 75:184–91.

20 Lau CP, Butrous G, Ward DE, Camm AJ. Comparison of exercise performance of six rate-adaptive right ventricular cardiac pacemakers. Am J Cardiol 1989; 63:833–8.

21 Bacharach DW, Hilden RS, Millerhagen JO *et al*. Activity-based pacing: comparison of a device using an accelerometer versus a piezo-electric crystal. Pacing Clin Electrophysiol 1992; 15:188–96.

22 Kay GN, Bubien RS, Epstein AE, Plumb VJ. Rate-modulated cardiac pacing based on transthoracic impedance measurements of minute ventilation: correlation with exercise gas exchange. J Am Coll Cardiol 1989; 14:1283–9.

23 Alt E, Theres H, Heinz M *et al*. A new rate-modulated pacemaker system optimized by combination of two sensors. Pacing Clin Electrophysiol 1988; 11:1119–29.

CHAPTER 3

Hemodynamics of cardiac pacing and pacing mode selection

Bruce S Stambler, Dwight W Reynolds

Cardiac pacing in an individual patient can have either beneficial or detrimental effects on hemodynamic function and clinical outcomes. Appropriate selection of a cardiac rhythm management device for a given patient and optimal management of a patient with a permanent pacing device require proper understanding of the major factors that influence hemodynamic function. Knowledge of, as well as interest in, the hemodynamics of cardiac pacing has evolved substantially over the last five decades, essentially *pari passu* with the technology of cardiac pacing. Although a general knowledge of this subject has played an important role in the evolution of sophisticated pacing capabilities, the technology itself has facilitated the expansion of the knowledge of cardiovascular hemodynamics generally and as it relates to pacing.

While early generations of cardiac pacemakers were sufficient technologically to prevent symptomatic bradycardia, the goal of cardiac pacing over the last few decades has been the accomplishment of "physiological" pacing. Many variables in pacing systems can affect cardiac hemodynamic function. The ideal pacemaker should maintain and optimize heart rate, atrioventricular (AV) synchrony and ventricular activation to enable cardiac output to meet the metabolic needs of the patient, whether at rest or during exercise. The concept and definition of physiological pacing have evolved over time in concert with our understanding of pacing-related cardiovascular hemodynamics, as well as with technological sophistication. In the current era, the goals of physiological pacing include maintaining and optimizing AV synchrony, minimizing right ventricular (RV) pacing to avoid ventricular desynchronization, using alternative RV pacing sites for improved hemodynamic performance, and selecting patients with heart failure for cardiac resynchronization therapy. Optimization of hemodynamic function in the pacemaker patient is determined to a large extent by a complex interaction between device-related variables (e.g. pacing mode, pacing lead position, pacing rate, rate responsiveness, AV relationships, atrial and ventricular activation sequences, frequency of RV pacing, etc.) and the underlying patient substrate (e.g. atrial rhythm,

Cardiac Pacing and ICDs, 5th edition. Edited by Kenneth A. Ellenbogen and Mark A. Wood.
© 2008 Blackwell Publishing, ISBN: 978-1-4051-6350-7

chronotropic competence, AV and ventricular conduction, ventricular function, history of heart failure and/or myocardial infarction, etc.).[1]

The key concepts of physiological pacing, considered most broadly, include the proper sequencing of atrial and ventricular contraction and physiological rate modulation. These topics are discussed in this chapter along with a practical guide for the selection of pacing mode as it relates to these physiological and hemodynamic issues. By no means is our understanding of the hemodynamics of cardiac pacing complete. Knowledge in this field will continue to evolve over time and be applied to pacemaker patient management. Even after 50 years of cardiac pacing, the pursuit of the ideal or physiological cardiac pacemaker has still not been fully achieved.

Atrioventricular synchrony

The hemodynamics of AV synchrony have been examined for centuries, but most extensively since the 1960s, especially related to the development of AV sequential pacing.[2–4] The introduction of dual-chamber (AV sequential) pacing in 1962 was designed to avoid AV desynchronization imposed during ventricular only pacing and resulted in improved hemodynamics.[5] Enthusiasm for AV sequential (DDD) pacing and the importance of maintaining AV synchrony was so high in the 1980s that a number of clinicians in the field at that time believed that these pacemakers could permit the restoration of normal cardiac physiology.[6] However, subsequent studies and randomized clinical trials of pacemaker therapy have provided important new insights into the hemodynamics of AV synchrony and pacing mode selection. The widespread recognition of the potential deleterious effects of frequent RV pacing along with the introduction of left ventricular (LV)-based pacing and cardiac resynchronization therapy have further complicated consideration of the hemodynamics of AV synchrony, optimal pacemaker mode selection and dual-chamber pacemaker programming.

The hemodynamics of AV synchrony are discussed in the context of advantages that might accrue from maintaining AV synchrony. The physiological basis of these hemodynamic benefits results from the ability of AV synchrony to: (i) maximize ventricular preload and therefore contractility; (ii) close AV valves before ventricular systole, limiting AV valvular regurgitation; (iii) maintain low mean atrial pressures, thus facilitating venous return; and (iv) regulate autonomic and neurohumoral reflexes involving atrial pressure and volume.

Advantages of atrioventricular synchrony

The loss of AV synchrony during ventricular pacing in the presence of sinus rhythm is associated most consistently with increases in atrial pressures, alterations in pulmonary and systemic venous flow patterns and AV valvular regurgitation.[7] Effects of AV desynchronization on systemic blood pressure and cardiac output are more variable between patients. Autonomic activation associated with atrial distension can result in an inappropriate decrease in peripheral vascular resistance. Rarely, VVI pacing with loss of appropriate AV synchrony can produce dramatic responses and disabling symptomatology with severe symptomatic hypotension, decreased cardiac output and syncope in occasional patients.

Atrial pressures

An increase in right and left atrial pressures during ventricular pacing is probably the most common mechanism by which symptoms are produced when AV synchrony is not maintained. Increases in atrial pressure during ventricular pacing (VVI) are related primarily to the contraction of the atria against the closed AV valves during ventricular systole. During AV synchrony, atrial contraction augments ventricular end-diastolic filling pressure while maintaining a low mean atrial pressure throughout diastole. In the absence of AV synchrony, a higher mean atrial pressure is required to achieve the same degree of ventricular filling. By this mechanism, AV synchrony is associated with lower venous and left atrial pressures (Fig. 3.1).

In Fig. 3.1, the left panel shows recordings of the pulmonary capillary wedge pressure in one patient during AV-synchronous pacing [80 pulses per minute (ppm), AV interval 150 ms]. The right panel shows the pulmonary capillary wedge pressure during ventricular pacing (80 ppm) with intact ventriculoatrial (VA) conduction. A relatively normal pulmonary capillary wedge pressure tracing is produced during AV pacing with mean pressures between 4 and 8 mmHg and without significant phasic aberration. In contrast, during ventricular pacing, the mean pressures are elevated to between 8 and 12 mmHg with large A waves (or VA waves) that, at times, exceed 16 mmHg. This eleva-

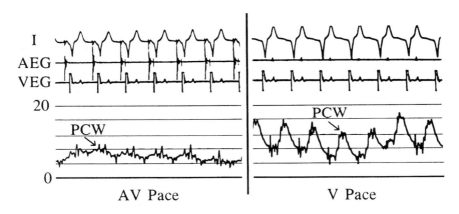

Fig. 3.1 Pulmonary capillary wedge (PCW) pressure recordings from a single patient during (left) atrioventricular (AV) pacing (AV Pace) and (right) ventricular pacing (V Pace) at 80 ppm with AV interval = 150 ms. (Scale = mmHg; I, ECG lead I; AEG, atrial electrogram; VEG, ventricular electrogram.)

tion in atrial pressures, and specifically the production of giant or "cannon" A waves, occurs because of left atrial contraction against a closed mitral valve; the increased pressure wave is present not only in the left atrium, but also in the pulmonary veins and pulmonary capillary wedge position. The same phenomenon occurs on the right side of the heart.

Figures 3.2 and 3.3 display simultaneous right atrial and pulmonary capillary wedge recordings during ventricular pacing (80 ppm) in which VA conduction is intact. In Fig. 3.2, 1 : 1 VA conduction is present, whereas in Fig. 3.3, there is 2 : 1 VA conduction. Intact VA conduction produces consistent elevations in pressure in the left atrium and right atrium due to the contraction of the atria against closed AV valves. Even when VA conduction is not intact, because of unequal atrial and ventricular rates there will be frequent periods when atrial contraction occurs during ventricular systole, during which the AV valves are closed; hence the problems of elevated pressures in the atria and pulmonary veins occur. Some patients are actually more symptomatic

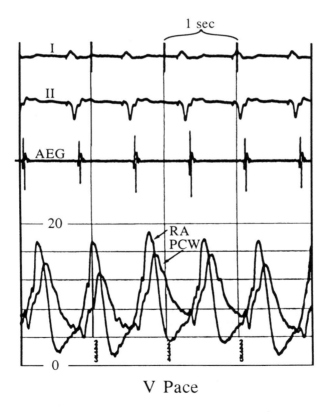

V Pace

Fig. 3.2 Right atrial (RA) and pulmonary capillary wedge (PCW) pressure recordings during ventricular pacing (V Pace) at 80 ppm with 1 : 1 ventriculoatrial conduction. (Scale = mmHg; I, II standard ECG leads; AEG, atrial electrogram.)

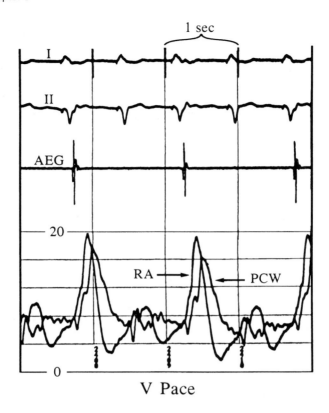

Fig. 3.3 Right atrial (RA) and pulmonary capillary wedge (PCW) pressure recordings during ventricular pacing (V Pace) at 80 ppm with 2 : 1 ventriculoatrial conduction. Scale = mmHg; I, II standard ECG leads; AEG, atrial electrogram.

when VA conduction is not intact, due to the intermittency of these elevated pressures, thus preventing patients from establishing tolerance of this phenomenon.

The relationship of the phasic changes in the pulmonary capillary wedge (and left atrial) pressures to LV pressures can be seen in Figs 3.4, 3.5 and 3.6. Figure 3.4 is a display of normal LV and pulmonary capillary wedge pressure recordings during AV pacing (80 ppm, AV interval of 150 ms). The appropriately timed A wave can be seen in both the LV and pulmonary capillary wedge pressure recordings. In contrast, as Fig. 3.5 shows, during ventricular pacing (80 ppm) with a consistent 1 : 1 VA relationship, the loss of the A-wave contribution to the upstroke of the LV pressure recording and the giant A wave, late in ventricular systole, can be seen consistently in the pulmonary capillary wedge pressure recording. Figure 3.6 displays this relationship when the atrial contraction is random in relation to ventricular contraction.

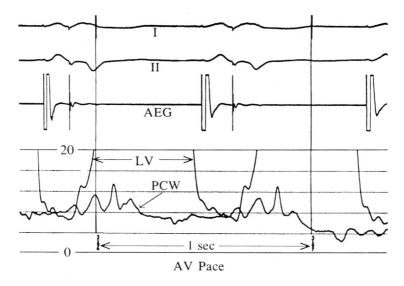

Fig. 3.4 Left ventricular (LV) and pulmonary capillary wedge (PCW) pressure recordings during atrioventricular (AV) pacing at 80 ppm with AV interval = 150 ms. Scale = mm Hg; I, II = standard ECG leads; AEG, atrial electrogram.

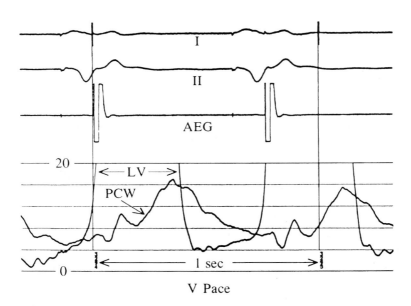

Fig. 3.5 Left ventricular (LV) and pulmonary capillary wedge (PCW) pressure recordings during ventricular pacing at 80 ppm with a 1 : 1 ventriculoatrial (VA) relationship (VA interval = 150 ms). Scale = mmHg; I, II = standard ECG leads; AEG, atrial electrogram.

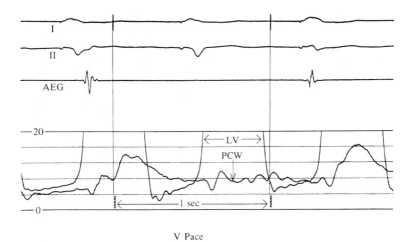

V Pace

Fig. 3.6 Left ventricular (LV) and pulmonary capillary wedge (PCW) pressure recordings during ventricular pacing at 80 ppm with ventriculoatrial dissociation. Scale = mmHg; I, II = standard ECG leads; AEG, atrial electrogram.

Pulmonary venous flow patterns

Doppler echocardiography is a particularly valuable methodology that can provide non-invasive insight into physiological, pacemaker-related changes in paced patients, including alterations in pulmonary vein flow and left atrial mechanical function (Figs 3.7 and 3.8). Ventriculoatrial (retrograde) conduction produces a contraction of the atria against closed AV valves, which induces a reversal of blood flow from the left atrium toward the pulmonary veins. This can be recognized by retrograde flow into the pulmonary vein (z wave) on the pulsed-Doppler echocardiographic recording (Fig. 3.7). Even when retrograde conduction during ventricular pacing is absent, atrial contraction may still occur shortly after ventricular activation by chance, resulting in intermittent regurgitation into the pulmonary veins (Fig. 3.8). Inappropriately timed atrial reverse flow at the time of ventricular systole markedly decreases the systolic flow velocities of pulmonary veins and reverses flow into the pulmonary veins. A study using transesophageal Doppler echocardiography has demonstrated that atrial reverse flow into the pulmonary veins is a consistent finding in patients during VVI pacing when VA conduction is present. Furthermore, during ventricular pacing (VVI) with VA conduction, patients with clinical signs and symptoms of pacemaker syndrome (i.e. hypotension with dizziness, dyspnea, fatigue) have significantly higher atrial reverse flow velocities into their pulmonary veins than patients without pacemaker syndrome (Figs 3.9 and 3.10).

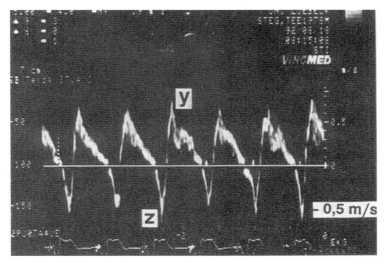

Fig. 3.7 Ventricular pacing with 1 : 1 retrograde conduction. In this transesophageal pulsed-Doppler echocardiographic recording, positive values depict antegrade flow in a pulmonary vein, whereas negative values depict retrograde flow. After each ventricular stimulus (see ECG at the bottom of the tracing), a retrograde P wave appears, resulting in regurgitation into the pulmonary vein (z wave). (Reproduced by permission from Stierle U, Krüger D, Mitusch R, Potratz J, Taubert G, Sheikhzadeh A. Adverse pacemaker hemodynamics evaluated by pulmonary venous flow monitoring. Pacing Clin Electrophysiol 1995; 18:2028–34.)

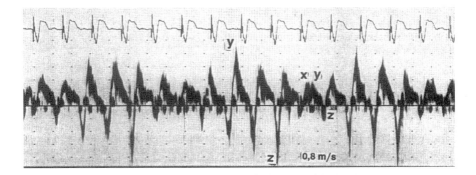

Fig. 3.8 Ventricular pacing without retrograde conduction. Transesophageal pulsed-Doppler echocardiographic recording as in Fig. 3.7. With a VVI pacing rate (75 bpm) different from the sinus rate, P waves appear shortly after the ventricular stimulus in three out of the five cycles, resulting in regurgitation into the pulmonary vein (z wave as in Fig. 3.7). (Reproduced by permission from Stierle U, Krüger D, Mitusch R, Potratz J, Taubert G, Sheikhzadeh A. Adverse pacemaker hemodynamics evaluated by pulmonary venous flow monitoring. Pacing Clin Electrophysiol 1995; 18:2028–34.)

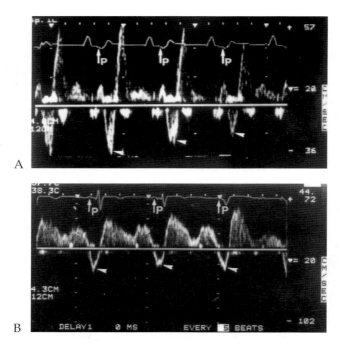

A

B

Fig. 3.9 Representative Doppler tracings of left pulmonary vein flow in a patient with clinical pacemaker syndrome before (A) and after (B) reprogramming to DDD mode. A, Atrial reverse flow (arrowhead) of the pulmonary vein regularly occurs after the electrocardiographically retrograde P wave. B, Atrial reverse flow (arrowhead) of the pulmonary vein is noted after the electrocardiographically antegrade P wave. Systolic flow velocities of the pulmonary vein are increased compared with those in A. (Reproduced by permission from Lee TM, Su SF, Lin YJ, Chen WJ, Chen MF, Liau CS, Lee YT. Role of transesophageal echocardiography in the evaluation of patients with clinical pacemaker syndrome. Am Heart J 1998; 135:634–40.)

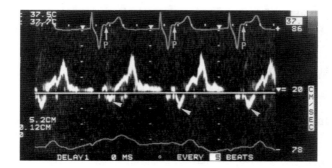

Fig. 3.10 Representative Doppler tracings of left pulmonary vein flow together with respiration in an asymptomatic patient during VVI pacing. Atrial reverse flow (arrowhead) of the pulmonary vein is noted after the electrocardiographically retrograde P wave, similar to Fig. 3.9A. The magnitude of atrial reverse flow is significantly lower than that in Fig. 3.9A. (Reproduced by permission from Lee TM, Su SF, Lin YJ, Chen WJ, Chen MF, Liau CS, Lee YT. Role of transesophageal echocardiography in the evaluation of patients with clinical pacemaker syndrome. Am Heart J 1998; 135:634–40.)

Atrioventricular valvular regurgitation

Effective and properly timed atrial and ventricular contraction is functionally important for complete mitral valve leaflet closure.[8] Thus, it is not surprising that RV pacing (VVI) is associated with substantial worsening or production of significant mitral and/or tricuspid regurgitation (MR) in some patients due to the loss of AV synchrony or an inappropriately timed AV interval.[9] In an experimental model in sheep, ventricular pacing was associated with delayed mitral valve leaflet closure and increased mitral valve regurgitant volume compared with baseline in sinus rhythm. In contrast, during AV pacing, mitral regurgitant volume and leaflet and annular dynamics were unchanged from baseline.

A number of case reports have described dramatic reductions in the severity of MR in patients with severe MR during ventricular pacing after upgrading to a dual-chamber device and/or adjustment of the AV interval (Fig. 3.11).

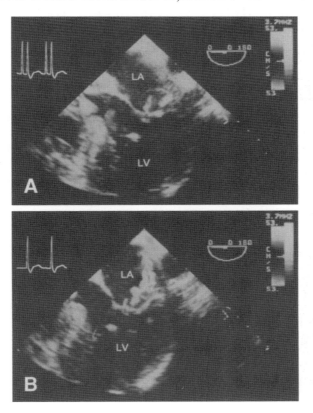

Fig. 3.11 (A) Transesophageal Doppler flow image showing mitral regurgitant jet. During atrioventricular sequential pacing, there was mild mitral regurgitation. (B) Transesophageal Doppler flow image showing mitral regurgitation jet during ventricular pacing (10 s after image shown in A). With ventricular pacing, mitral regurgitation is severe. LA, left atrium; LV, left ventricle. (Reproduced by permission from Berglund H, Nishioka T, Hackner E *et al.* Ventricular pacing: a cause of reversible severe mitral regurgitation. Am Heart J 1996; 131:1035–7.)

In one study, the majority of patients (67%) with signs and symptoms of pacemaker syndrome during ventricular pacing (VVI) with retrograde conduction had significant MR (≥ moderate) documented. Strikingly, MR disappeared in these patients after reprogramming to DDD mode. Other investigators likewise have demonstrated that the extent of valve regurgitation may be an important factor in the genesis of subclinical pacemaker syndrome. Thus, RV pacing can cause AV valve regurgitation in some patients that may resolve with the resumption of AV synchrony using AAI pacing or AV pacing programming to DDD mode.

When atrial contraction is not followed by an adequately synchronized ventricular contraction, the AV pressure gradient reverses during atrial relaxation and diastolic ventricular pressures exceed those in the atria (VA pressure gradient).[10] This results in diastolic AV valve regurgitation because the mitral and tricuspid valves are incompletely closed. The presence of diastolic MR highlights the importance of adequately timed AV synchrony for optimal diastolic filling of the ventricle. Diastolic mitral and tricuspid regurgitation is a relatively common finding when AV synchrony is lost, such as during ventricular only pacing (e.g. VVI) in the presence of sinus rhythm or in the presence of AV conduction abnormalities (Fig. 3.12). Significant elevation of LV end-diastolic filling pressures will contribute to worsening of diastolic MR during AV dyssynchrony.

In the presence of first-degree AV block and LV systolic dysfunction, dual-chamber pacing at a short AV interval may improve hemodynamics by optimization of atrial and ventricular synchrony and elimination of diastolic MR.[10] Elimination or reduction of diastolic regurgitation results in lengthening of the diastolic LV filling time and augmentation of the stroke volume and cardiac output (Fig. 3.13). Although controversial, this approach has been suggested as a potential therapeutic option in a subset of patients with severe LV dysfunction. Appropriate patients for this therapy may be symptomatic heart failure patients in sinus rhythm with a long PR interval, prolonged functional diastolic MR (≥ 450 ms) and a ventricular filling time of < 200 ms at rest.

In most pacemaker patients, however, worsening of AV regurgitation appears to play a lesser role in elevating atrial pressure than does the contraction of the atria against closed AV valves during ventricular pacing. Furthermore, in the absence of ventricular dysfunction or structural heart disease, diastolic MR during AV desynchronization is usually a benign phenomenon without significant therapeutic clinical implications. In a study by Reynolds et al., pacemaker patients underwent LV cineangiography for assessment of MR during both AV and ventricular pacing.[11] Of the 16 patients who underwent paired LV cineangiograms, five (approximately 30%) had slight worsening in the degree of MR during ventricular pacing compared with AV pacing. Similarly, in the study by Lee et al. using transesophageal Doppler echocardiography, significant MR was found only during VVI pacing with VA conduction in 8% of a group of patients without clinical pacemaker syndrome.

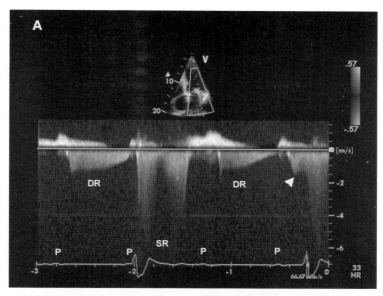

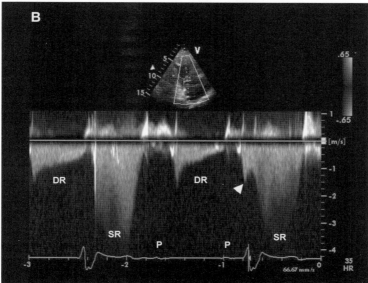

Fig. 3.12 Mitral valve (A) and tricuspid valve (B) continuous-wave Doppler recordings from an apical transducer position obtained in an 80-year-old male with complete atrioventricular (AV) block. There is a ventricular escape rhythm at 33–35 bpm (QRS complexes). Note the diastolic AV valve regurgitation that occurs when the P wave is not followed by an appropriately timed ventricular contraction. Also note that diastolic AV regurgitation is reduced (arrowhead) when the ventricular contraction (QRS complex at the right side of each image) happens by chance to fall at an appropriate interval after the P wave (simulating a more synchronized AV relationship). DR, diastolic regurgitation; SR, systolic regurgitation; P, P wave.

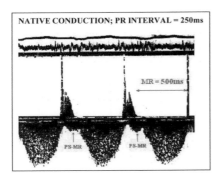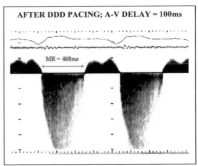

Fig. 3.13 Continuous-wave Doppler recordings show mitral regurgitation (MR) in a patient with DCM and prolonged PR interval, before and after DDD pacing with A–V delay optimization. MR is of long duration (500 ms) during native conduction with a distinct pre-systolic component (PS-MR), impinging into and abbreviating the left ventricular (LV) filling time. Shortening the A–V delay with DDD pacing eliminates PS-MR, shortens the total MR duration and increases the LV filling time. (Reproduced by permission from Salukhe TV, Henein MY, Sutton R. Pacing in heart failure: patient and pacing mode selection. Eur Heart J 2003; 24:977–86.)

Blood pressure

For grouped patient data, AV synchrony generally provides similar or slightly greater systolic and mean blood pressures than ventricular pacing. A typical example of the blood pressure comparison among atrial, AV and ventricular pacing is shown in Fig. 3.14. In this case, essentially no differences exist between the blood pressures when comparing atrial with AV pacing. The blood pressure during ventricular pacing is slightly lower than during either atrial or AV pacing. A heterogeneous group of pacemaker patients studied at the University of Oklahoma showed statistically significant differences in their femoral artery systolic pressure, but not in their diastolic and mean pressures (Table 3.1).

Although not the typical response, some individuals do have dramatic and symptomatic decreases in systemic blood pressure when ventricular pacing is instituted (Fig. 3.15). Several mechanisms may be responsible for this phenomenon. Loss of LV preload volume from mistimed atrial contraction (loss of atrial "kick") and loss of inhibitory cardiac reflexes (due also to inappropriately timed atrial contraction) have been the mechanisms most commonly implicated. This marked hypotension can produce dramatic symptoms, including syncope. In a clinical setting, if this problem is suspected but hypotension with symptoms cannot be reproduced in a supine position, an upright or semiupright posture may unmask the problem, especially if it is related to a left ventricular preload deficiency caused by loss of atrial contribution to ventricular filling. An important consideration in the hemodynamic response to ventricular pacing is VA conduction. VA conduction, the ability to conduct electrical impulses retrograde from the ventricles through the AV junction to the atria, can lead to atrial contraction during ventricular systole or, in cases of

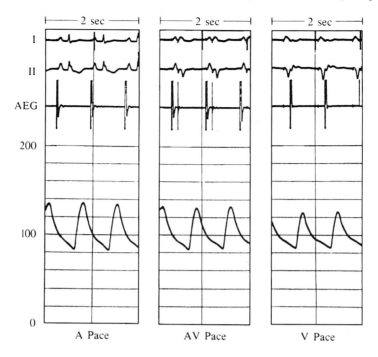

Fig. 3.14 Femoral artery pressure recordings from one patient. Left: During atrial pacing (A Pace). Center: During atrioventricular (AV) sequential pacing (AV Pace). Right: During ventricular pacing (V Pace). All tracings are at 80 ppm with an AV interval of 150 ms during AV pacing. Scale in mmHg. I, II, III = standard ECG leads; AEG, atrial electrogram.

long VA conduction, early diastole. This can cause loss of the atrial contribution to ventricular filling as well as other hemodynamic problems. VA conduction has been found in as many as 90% of patients with sick sinus syndrome and in 15–35% of individuals with a variety of degrees of AV block. This is an important issue in the use of hysteresis in VVI pacemakers, a feature available in single-chamber pacemakers since 1980. During ventricular pacing, even when VA conduction is not intact, if the ventricular pacing rate is unequal to the atrial rate, there will be periods of time when atrial contraction occurs during ventricular systole with the resulting disadvantageous hemodynamics.

Cardiac output

Properly timed atrial contraction provides a significant increase in ventricular end-diastolic volume and is responsible for the so-called atrial kick (Fig. 3.16). Studies have shown a wide range in the actual importance of the atrial contribution to ventricular filling depending on the patient population and study conditions. By increasing the end-diastolic volumes (right and left ventricles), the cardiac output is, in turn, increased. The average increase in cardiac out-

Table 3.1 Hemodynamic evaluation of atrioventricular and ventricular pacing

Parameter	AV*	V*	N	p†
RA mean (mmHg)	6.0 ± 0.6	8.1 ± 0.6	22	< 0.001
PA systolic (mmHg)	24.5 ± 1.6	28.3 ± 1.7	23	< 0.001
PA diastolic (mmHg)	12.6 ± 1.0	14.3 ± 1.1	23	< 0.02
PA mean (mmHg)	17.1 ± 1.1	20.6 ± 1.2	23	< 0.001
PCW mean (mmHg)	7.7 ± 1.0	13.4 ± 1.2	22	< 0.001
LV systolic (mmHg)	141.3 ± 5.2	132.0 ± 5.1	23	<.01
LV end-diastolic (mmHg)	9.8 ± 1.4	10.1 ± 0.8	22	NS
FA systolic (mmHg)	141.4 ± 5.1	133.4 ± 5.1	23	< 0.01
FA diastolic (mmHg)	80.3 ± 2.0	80.9 ± 2.4	23	NS
FA mean (mmHg)	105.6 ± 2.8	103.1 ± 3.4	23	NS
CI.TD (l min^{-1} m^{-2})	2.575 ± 0.148	2.073 ± 0.126	23	< 0.001
CT.Angio (l min^{-1} m^{-2})	3.337 ± 0.210	2.878 ± 0.157	19	< 0.001
LV.EDVI (ml m^{-2})	85.7 ± 7.4	76.6 ± 6.8	19	< 0.001
LV.ESVI (ml m^{-2})	46.2 ± 5.9	42.2 ± 5.4	19	< 0.05
LV.SVI (ml m^{-2})	39.7 ± 2.6	34.3 ± 2.0	19	< 0.001
LV.EF (%)	48.9 ± 2.8	47.6 ± 2.8	19	NS
SVR (dyne s^{-1} cm^{-5})	1856.1 ± 160.3	2178.0 ± 180.6	23	< 0.001
PVR (dyne s^{-1} cm^{-5})	169.0 ± 16.3	152.1 ± 15.0	22	NS

*Mean ± SEM.
†Paired *t*-test.
Angio, angiography; CI, cardiac index; EDVI, end-diastolic volume index; EF, ejection fraction; ESVI, end-systolic volume index; FA, femoral artery; LV, left ventricle; NS, not statistically significant; PA, pulmonary artery; PCW, pulmonary capillary wedge; PVR, pulmonary vascular resistance; RA, right atrium; SVI, stroke volume index; SVR, systemic vascular resistance; TD, thermodilution.

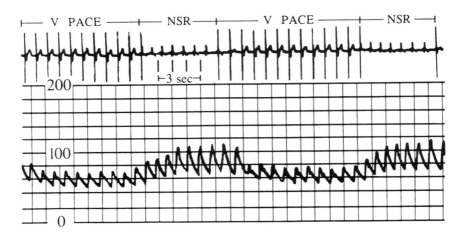

Fig. 3.15 Radial artery pressure recording from a patient during right ventricular pacing (V PACE) at 80 ppm and normal sinus rhythm (NSR) (scale in mmHg). This patient's blood pressure, measured by radial artery line, drops from approximately 110/70 mmHg during sinus rhythm to approximately 75/55 mmHg during ventricular pacing.

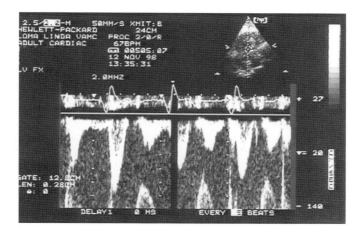

Fig. 3.16 Doppler echocardiographic evaluation of the velocity time integral in the left ventricular outflow tract obtained from a patient with a VVI pacemaker originally implanted for complete heart block. The sinus mechanism was intact and the patient had palpitations and symptoms consistent with a low cardiac output. There is marked beat-to-beat fluctuation in the stroke volume in accord with waxing and waning coincidental atrioventricular (AV) synchrony clearly demonstrating a benefit of restoring AV synchrony and providing justification for replacement of an otherwise normally functioning VVI pacemaker with a more appropriate dual-chamber system. (Courtesy of Paul A. Levine, MD.)

put in a pacing population, if AV synchrony is maintained, is between 15% and 25% in comparison with non-AV-synchronized ventricular pacing.

The benefits of AV synchrony on cardiac output were confirmed in a broad-based pacing population (Table 3.1). AV pacing at 80 ppm with an AV interval of 150 ms was compared with ventricular pacing at 80 ppm during which VA conduction was intact or was created by VA pacing. Consistently higher cardiac outputs maintained by AV synchrony were seen in both thermodilution and angiographic evaluations. The patients were supine when examined; an upright posture might have amplified these differences, because in that position ventricular diastolic filling depends more on atrial kick due to loss of venous return of blood to the heart (lower extremity pooling).[12]

The hemodynamic benefits of AV-synchronized vs. ventricular pacing have also been demonstrated for patients after myocardial infarction and cardiac surgery. Patients with reduced cardiac output—especially if such reduced function is due to relative volume depletion or only mild to moderately depressed LV function—frequently benefit significantly from maintenance of AV synchrony; this should be kept in mind when dealing with patients in these situations. In a group of patients with severe LV systolic dysfunction (mean LV ejection fraction, 0.21 ± 0.07) and New York Heart Association (NYHA) class II to IV heart failure, there were significant reductions in cardiac index (~12%) with single-chamber VVI pacing compared with pacing modes that

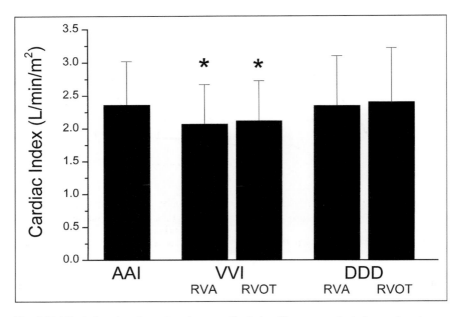

Fig. 3.17 Effect of pacing site and mode on cardiac index. Measurements during pacing at a fixed rate were compared in each patient. Pacing was performed in AAI, VVI and DDD modes from the RV apex (RVA) or outflow tract (RVOT). Means ± SD are shown. *$P < 0.05$ vs. AAI. (Reproduced by permission from Gold MR, Brockman R, Peters RW, Olsovsky MR, Shorofsky SR. Acute hemodynamic effects of right ventricular pacing site and pacing mode in patients with congestive heart failure secondary to either ischemic or idiopathic dilated cardiomyopathy. Am J Cardiol 2000; 85:1106–9.)

maintained AV synchrony (AAI or DDD with ventricular pacing from the RV apex or outflow tract)[13] (Fig. 3.17).

There is a general perception that patients with abnormal cardiac function benefit most from maintenance of AV synchrony. This may be true, but the reasons are frequently not due to better cardiac output. In fact, if cardiac output were the only consideration hemodynamically, it is patients with very poor ventricular function (markedly increased end-diastolic volume and depressed ejection fraction) that benefit least from AV synchrony. This can be best understood by using the concept of ventricular function curves that compare stroke volume or cardiac output with LV end-diastolic volume or preload.

Figure 3.18 shows hypothetical ventricular function curves for a patient with normal ventricular function (curve 1), one with moderate LV dysfunction (curve 2), one with very poor LV function and a markedly dilated ventricle (curve 3), and a patient with hypertrophic cardiomyopathy (curve 4). These curves describe the performance of the left ventricle in generating stroke volume (or cardiac output) in relation to the end-diastolic volume (or preload). In patients with normal LV function (curve 1), as end-diastolic volume increases, stroke volume (and cardiac output) increases until the flat or descending por-

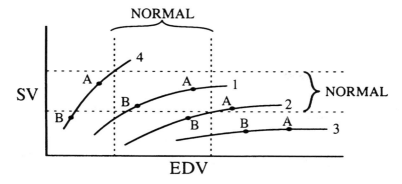

Fig. 3.18 Hypothetical ventricular function curves comparing (1) stroke volume (SV) and left ventricular end-diastolic volume (EDV) in patients with normal ventricular function; (2) moderately depressed ventricular function; (3) severely depressed ventricular function; and (4) hyperdynamic ventricular function. Point A = with normal atrioventricular (AV) sequence. Point B = without normal AV sequence.

tion of the curve is reached. In patients with depressed LV function (curves 2 and 3), there is a lesser increase in stroke volume that depends on end-diastolic volume to the point that, in patients with poor LV function (curve 3), there is negligible improvement in stroke volume with further increases in end-diastolic volume. On the other hand, patients with hypertrophic or hypertensive cardiomyopathy tend to have small ventricles that are normal (i.e. normal systolic function) or hyperdynamic in function (curve 4). Small increases in end-diastolic volume can significantly increase stroke volume in this situation. As has been discussed, AV synchrony provides the atrial kick that increases end-diastolic volume. Point A on these curves represents the hypothetical stroke volume and end-diastolic volume during AV pacing. Point B represents stroke volume and end-diastolic volume during ventricular pacing (with associated loss of atrial kick). In the normal situation (curve 1), although end-diastolic volume is greater and hence stroke volume is greater during AV-synchronized pacing, the loss of AV synchrony during ventricular pacing does not drop the end-diastolic volume and the stroke volume significantly. This, however, might not be the case if the filling volume were otherwise reduced by volume depletion due to blood loss, diuresis, and so on. In these situations, even with normal LV function, the higher end-diastolic volumes and stroke volumes provided by properly timed atrial contraction might be important. With depressed LV function of a moderate degree (curve 2), although maintenance of AV synchrony provides for a greater end-diastolic volume, the stroke volume advantage is diminished. It is possible that, due to overall reduction in stroke volume (and cardiac output), even this modest increment in stroke volume would be of important benefit. In patients with more severely depressed LV function and extremely flat LV function curves (curve 3), end-diastolic volume can be augmented with maintenance of AV synchrony, but there is little advantage in stroke volume.

With regard to patients with hypertrophic cardiomyopathy or highly non-compliant ventricles (curve 4), maintenance of AV synchrony may be very important in enhancing stroke volume and cardiac output because of the relatively small end-diastolic volumes. This is because small increments in end-diastolic volume may substantially increase the stroke volume due to the steep slope of the curve. This relatively steep-sloped ventricular function curve is also characteristic of patients with ventricular diastolic dysfunction, a group for whom maintenance of AV synchrony is also very important. Figure 3.19 displays this concept in a group of patients studied using quantitative nuclear techniques.[14] Although only data from the supine position at 80 ppm are shown (AV interval 150 ms during AV-synchronized pacing), the same situation hemodynamically was found to be present at a faster pacing rate (100 ppm) and in an upright posture.

The conceptual approach of ventricular function curves is useful for practical understanding of the benefits of AV synchrony. However, movement along single ventricular function curves probably is overly simplistic. A number of variables that can affect hemodynamic function, such as afterload, can be modulated by other factors that might cause shifting from one curve to another as well as movement along a given curve. In this regard, systemic vascular resistance may be significantly higher during ventricular pacing. The increase in systemic vascular resistance is related mechanistically to an increase in neural reflexes. These autonomic responses to ventricular pacing include increased peripheral sympathetic nerve tone and circulating catecholamine levels supportive of blood pressure when cardiac output is diminished.

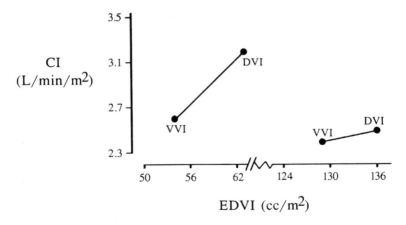

Fig. 3.19 Ventricular function curves comparing cardiac index (CI) and left ventricular end-diastolic volume index (EDVI) from (left) a group of nine patients with relatively normal ventricular function and (right) a group of four patients with markedly depressed ventricular function. The patients were studied in the supine position at a pacing rate = 80 ppm; atrioventricular (AV) interval during DVI pacing = 150 ms. Points are group mean. VVI, ventricular pacing (no AV synchrony); DVI, AV sequential pacing (AV synchrony).

A hemodynamic variable that is usually not significantly affected in most individuals (AV vs. ventricular pacing) is ejection fraction (see Table 3.1). Although the components of ejection fraction—both end-diastolic volume and stroke volume—are significantly lower during ventricular pacing, ejection fraction is unaffected because both the numerator (stroke volume) and the denominator (end-diastolic volume) of the ejection fraction vary in the same proportion. Ejection fraction is a crude measurement of contractile performance, so it is not surprising that the presence or absence of AV synchrony, which primarily affects preload and cardiac output, has no effect on ejection fraction.

Autonomic neural and neurohormone level alterations

Single-chamber RV pacing is associated with higher levels of sympathetic nerve activity, cardiac norepinephrine spillover and plasma epinephrine and norepinephrine levels than AV synchronous pacing.[15] Catecholamine levels increase most during VVI pacing with retrograde conduction. The enhanced sympathetic outflow appears to be mediated by the arterial and cardiopulmonary baroreflexes.

Plasma levels of natriuretic peptides, including atrial and brain natriuretic peptides (ANP and BNP, respectively), appear to reflect the presence of appropriate AV synchrony and the hemodynamic changes produced by different cardiac pacing modes. A number of studies have demonstrated that RV pacing without AV synchrony (VVI) is associated with higher levels of plasma ANP and BNP, when compared with pacing modes with AV synchrony (AAI or DDD).[16] Increased natriuretic peptide levels develop within several minutes after AV synchrony is lost, both at rest and during exercise. These hormonal alterations persist over the long term, but return toward normal after AV synchrony is restored. The release of these hormones occurs in response to worsened cardiac hemodynamics reflecting atrial distension, higher atrial pressures and increased LV filling pressures with AV desynchronization. Low levels of natriuretic peptides might be used as a cardiac biomarker reflective of the presence of a physiological pacing mode.

Mortality and cardiovascular outcomes

At least five prospective randomized trials have compared AV synchronous pacing modes (AAI or DDD with or without rate response) with the ventricular only pacing mode (VVI) on mortality and important cardiovascular outcomes in patients with bradycardia indications for permanent pacemaker implantation[17–21] (Table 3.2). A recent meta-analysis has summarized the results of these five trials in over 7000 patients.[22] The major conclusions of this systematic review of these important clinical trials in the field of cardiac pacing were that: (i) atrial-based pacing does not reduce all-cause mortality, cardiovascular death or heart failure; (ii) atrial-based pacing does reduce the incidence of atrial fibrillation (AF) [hazard ratio (HR) 0.80; 95% confidence interval (CI) 0.72–0.89; $P = 0.00003$); (iii) atrial-based pacing is associated with a reduction of borderline significance in stroke (HR 0.81; 95% CI 0.67–0.99; $P = 0.035$); and (iv)

Table 3.2 Randomized controlled trials of pacemaker mode selection

Trial (Ref. no.)	Date	No. of patients	Avg F/U, years	Indication	Pacing modes	Mean age, years	Primary end-point	Summary of results; P value (hazard ratio; 95% CI)	Mortality %/year	AF %/year	Thromboembolism %/year
Danish[17]	1994	225	5.5	Sinus node dysfunction	AAI vs. VVI	76	Mortality, AF, thromboembolism	Mortality: 0.045 (0.66; 0.44–0.99) AF: 0.012 (0.54; 0.33, 0.89) Thromboembolism: 0.023 (0.47; 0.24–0.92)	5.8 vs. 6.8	4.1 vs. 7.1	1.7 vs. 5.4
PASE[18]	1998	407	1.5	All pacemaker patients ≥ 65 yo	DDDR vs. VVIR	76	Quality of life	No overall group differences between pacing modes	10.7 vs. 11.3	11.3 vs. 12.7	1.3 vs. 2.3
CTOPP[19]	2000	2568	6.0	All pacemaker patients	DDD/DDDR or AAI/AAIR vs. VVI/VVIR	73	Cardiovascular death or stroke	0.26 (0.91; 0.78–1.05); (AF less frequent in atrial-based group)	6.3 vs. 6.6	5.3 vs. 6.6	1.0 vs. 1.1
MOST[20]	2002	2010	4.5	Sinus node dysfunction	DDDR vs. VVIR	74	Death or non-fatal stroke	0.40 (0.97; 0.80–1.18); (AF and heart failure reduced in DDDR)	7.0 vs. 7.3	7.9 vs. 10.0	1.4 vs. 1.8
UKPACE[21]	2005	2021	4.6	AV block ≥ 70 yo	DDD vs. VVI/VVIR	80	Death	0.56 (0.96; 0.83–1.11)	7.4 vs. 7.2	2.8 vs. 3.0	1.7 vs. 2.1

Date, date of study publication; AVG, average; F/U, follow-up; P, P-value; CI, confidence interval; AF, atrial fibrillation; AAI, atrial pacing; VVI, ventricular pacing; DDD, dual-chamber pacing; AAIR, atrial pacing with rate adaptation; DDDR, dual-chamber pacing with rate adaptation; VVIR, ventricular pacing with rate adaptation; yo, years old; AV, atrioventricular. (The annual incidences of death, atrial fibrillation and thromboembolism were obtained from the primary publications along with reference 22 and Nielsen JC. Pacing mode selection in patients with sick sinus syndrome. Dan Med Bull 2007; 54:1–17.)

no patient subgroups derived a special benefit from atrial-based pacing. Aside from these conclusions, there is evidence derived from the clinical trials that dual-chamber devices modestly improve quality of life and are less likely to be associated with pacemaker syndrome.[23] Thus, most clinicians believe that the clinical evidence is sufficient to justify routine use of pacing modes that provide AV synchrony. In addition, there is hope that the use of algorithms that minimize ventricular pacing in dual-chamber pacemakers and alternative ventricular pacing sites will enhance the benefits of atrial-based pacing. These are areas of active interest and investigation (see later discussion).

Effects of atrioventricular interval timing

An optimally timed AV interval maximizes LV filling and stroke volume by the Frank–Starling mechanism. The mere presence of a consistent AV relationship does not ensure the best possible hemodynamics in an individual patient (Fig. 3.20). Atrial contraction should occur before the isovolumic contraction phase. Some AV timing relationships are detrimental, such as during 1 : 1 VA conduction. Similarly, inappropriately short or long AV delays can be detrimental. An excessively long AV delay may inadequately fill the ventricle by causing early mitral valve closure and truncating the diastolic filling time. This causes a loss of the booster pump function of the atrium. In addition, diastolic AV valvular regurgitation may occur with re-opening of the valve before ventricular systole. An excessively short AV delay may limit active filling of the ventricle and promote systolic AV valvular regurgitation as ventricular contraction begins while the AV valves are still open.

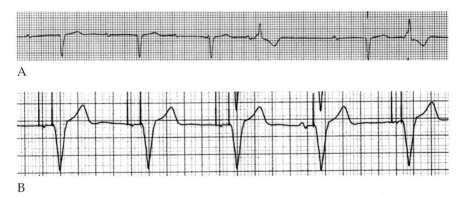

A

B

Fig. 3.20 ECG tracings from a 74-year-old male with complaints of fatigue and exercise intolerance without syncope or dizziness. A, Marked first-degree atrioventricular (AV) block is present (PR interval > 500 ms) with a normal QRS duration and PVCs. The Holter monitor from this patient demonstrated first-degree, second-degree (type I) and 2 : 1 AV block with heart rates from 36 to 150 bpm. The longest pause was 2.7 s. There were also very frequent PVCs (> 9000 in 24 h). B, DDD rhythm with appropriate AV intervals (150/120 ms). Following dual-chamber pacemaker implantation, the patient noted a marked improvement in his symptoms with improvement in his functional capacity, more energy and overall improved quality of life.

Programming of an optimal AV interval in a patient with a dual-chamber pacemaker is required to maximize hemodynamics. The potential contribution of a correctly timed AV delay to cardiac output varies from 13% to 40%.[24] Some authors have suggested that when the AV delay is selected empirically, it is incorrectly programmed in approximately two-thirds of patients.[25] Thus, dual-chamber pacemaker programming must be tailored to the individual patient. Leaving a device at the nominal settings at the time of implant is not acceptable for ensuring optimal cardiac hemodynamics. The optimal range for the AV interval when the right atrium and ventricle are paced is on average between 150 and 200 ms in patients at rest with normal ventricular function (Fig. 3.21). However, this interval may vary considerably from patient to patient and from time to time in a specific patient (i.e. as short as 100 ms and up to 250 ms). This variation is mostly dependent on the degree of interatrial and interventricular conduction delays in response to DDD pacing. With conventional right heart pacing systems, the activation sequence of the left-sided chambers may be quite different from the programmed values in situations where there are marked interatrial and interventricular conduction delays. Long AV intervals (250–350 ms) may be required to provide effective left atrial systole in occasional patients with high-grade interatrial conduction delay in the presence of atrial disease and either sick sinus syndrome or heart block.

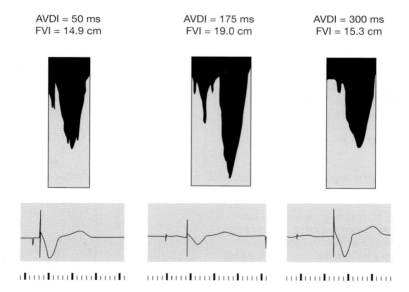

AVDI = 50 ms
FVI = 14.9 cm

AVDI = 175 ms
FVI = 19.0 cm

AVDI = 300 ms
FVI = 15.3 cm

Fig. 3.21 Doppler aortic flow velocity integrals (FVI) recorded at varying atrioventricular (AV) pacing intervals. Note the maximal aortic flow velocity at AV interval (AVI) of 175 ms. (Reproduced with permission from Janosik DL, Pearson AC, Buckingham TA *et al*. The hemodynamic benefit of differential atrioventricular delay intervals for sensed and paced atrial events during physiologic pacing. J Am Coll Cardiol 1989; 14:499–507.)

A variety of invasive and non-invasive techniques have been used to determine the optimal AV interval. Echocardiography has been used widely to analyze diastolic transmitral Doppler flow velocity (e and a waves), stroke volume assessed by aortic velocity time integral (VTI) and AV valve regurgitation for optimization of AV intervals. Ritter's method of AV interval optimization, which uses Doppler echocardiography of the mitral valve inflow profile, is the most widely applied technique. This technique is based on the assumption that the AV delay that maximizes cardiac output is the one that provides the longest LV filling time without interruption of the A wave (atrial contraction wave) and allows ventricular systole to begin immediately subsequent to maximum diastolic ventricular filling, thus avoiding cannon A waves and diastolic MR (Fig. 3.22). An alternative simplified approach has been proposed that uses the surface ECG alone and defines the optimal AV delay based on a delay of 100 ms from the end of the surface P wave to the peak/nadir of the paced ventricular complex (Fig. 3.23).[26] The end of the surface P wave represents the end of left atrial activation, whereas the peak/nadir of the paced ventricular complex coincides with the onset of the isometric contraction period. The AV delay is considered optimal when the end of left atrial contraction (A

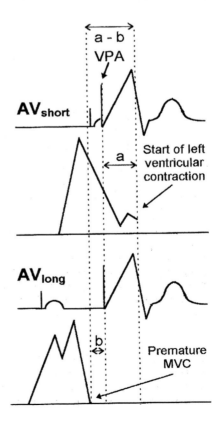

Fig. 3.22 Doppler technique for optimizing the atrioventricular (AV) interval. The surface ECG and Doppler mitral inflow pattern are depicted schematically for a very short AV interval (e.g. 50 ms) in the top of the figure and a very long AV interval (e.g. 250 ms) in the bottom of the tracing. Interval "a" represents the longest time between the ventricular pacing artifact (VPA) and the mitral valve closure (MVC) for the short AV interval. Interval "b" represents the time between ventricular pacing and mitral valve closure during the long AV interval and may be a negative value due to diastolic regurgitation. The optimal AV delay is calculated as the long AV delay minus the difference between intervals a and b. (Adapted from Kinderman M *et al.* Optimizing the AV delay in DDD pacemaker patients with high degree AV block: mitral valve Doppler versus impedance cardiography. PACE 1997; 20:2453–62.)

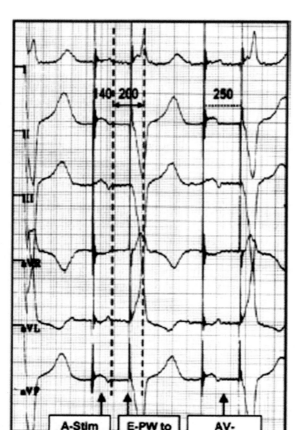

Fig. 3.23 Determination of optimal paced atrioventricular (AV) delay (AVD$_{opt}$) by surface ECG. First, a long AV delay of 250 ms was programmed (AVD$_{prog}$, programmed interval from atrial to ventricular stimulus). The interval from the end of the P wave to the peak/nadir of the paced ventricular complex (T) was 200 ms. The interval from the atrial stimulus to the end of the P wave (=global atrial conduction time) was 140 ms. According to the algorithm [AVD$_{opt}$ = AVD$_{prog}$ + 100 − T] the optimized AV delay was 150 ms. A-Stim to E-PW = The interval between the pacing stimulus and the end of P wave deflection; E-PW to QRS$_{nadir}$ = end of P wave (E-PW) to peak/nadir of paced QRS; AV-interval$_{prog}$ = long AV delay programmed for testing. (Reproduced with permission from Strohmer B, Pichler M, Froemmel M, Migschitz M, Hintringer F; ELVIS Study Group. Evaluation of atrial conduction time at various sites of right atrial pacing and influence on atrioventricular delay optimization by surface electrocardiography. Pacing Clin Electrophysiol 2004; 27:468–74.)

wave) coincides with complete mitral valve closure and the onset of the isometric contraction period.

There is some predictability in certain aspects of AV interval optimization. It is consistent that optimal hemodynamics at higher heart rates require shorter AV delays than are optimal at lower rates. With exercise, there is a relatively linear decrease in the normal PR interval as exercise increases from the resting state to near maximal exertion. The total reduction in spontaneous PR interval in normal individuals is about 20–50 ms or approximately 4 ms for each 10-beat increment in heart rate. Rate-adaptive AV interval shortening or automatic rate-adaptive AV delay is a programmable feature on many DDD pacemaker generators, which is designed to mimic the normal physiological response of the PR interval to increasing heart rates. Cardiac output can be more effectively increased and pulmonary capillary wedge pressures (and presumably atrial pressures) can be effectively maintained at lower levels using rate-variable AV intervals rather than fixed AV intervals.

Atrial sensed vs. atrial paced atrioventricular intervals
Appropriate programming of the AV interval may depend on whether the atrium is sensed or paced. Programming differential AV intervals for sensing and pacing may give rise to small but significant increases in cardiac output in patients with LV dysfunction, due to differences in paced vs. sensed atrial conduction times.[27] If atrial activity is sensed, this marks the initiation of the pacemaker AV interval. Because some atrial activation has already occurred at this time, the AV interval based on sensed atrial activity should be shorter than when the atrium is paced to begin both the AV interval and atrial electrical activation (Fig. 3.24). Generally, an atrial sensed AV interval of 20–50 ms less than the atrial paced AV interval is used, but the most appropriate difference is probably variable in different patients.

Atrial vs. atrioventricular pacing
Both atrial and AV pacing have the advantage of providing AV synchrony.

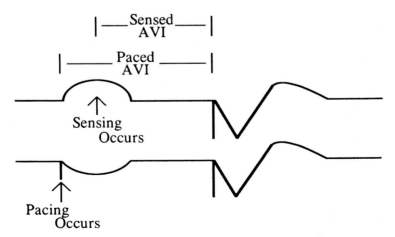

Fig. 3.24 Hypothetical relationship of appropriate atrioventricular intervals (AVI) during atrial sensing vs. atrial pacing at initiation of the AVI.

Aside from differing AV intervals, the major difference between atrial and AV sequential pacing is the ectopic ventricular activation with RV pacing in the dual-chamber mode vs. intrinsic AV conduction during atrial only pacing. In recent years, there has been widespread recognition of the detrimental effects of RV pacing on hemodynamic function. Numerous studies have shown acute improvements in cardiac output, ejection fraction and pulmonary capillary wedge pressure with AAI compared with DDD pacing. RV pacing compared with intrinsic ventricular activation produces increases in LV filling pressures and end-systolic volume as well as reductions in regional septal ejection fraction, ventricular dP/dt, stroke volume, and indices of diastolic function. Chronic RV pacing is associated with an increased risk of AF, heart failure and mortality.[17,20,28,29] Thus, as a result of the concern over the long-term consequences of chronic RV pacing, there has been a major shift away from imposed AV sequential pacing in the dual-chamber mode to the use of programmed AV intervals and pacemaker algorithms that allow for maintenance of AV synchrony but minimize RV pacing.

It should be recognized, however, that in order to minimize RV pacing while maintaining the dual-chamber mode, it may be necessary in some patients to program the device to very long paced and sensed AV delays, sometimes near the available maximal programmable values. Very long AV delays, even when followed by intrinsic ventricular conduction or fusion, may compromise atrial transport function and promote diastolic MR and possibly AF. Thus, a low percentage of ventricular pacing may not be desirable when it is associated with very prolonged AV intervals (i.e. AV > 300 ms), especially at higher heart rates. Rate-adaptive AV delay programming allows long AV delays to be programmed at lower heart rates, but more appropriate AV intervals at higher heart rates. Algorithms that switch from an atrial-based mode (AAI or AAIR) to a dual-chamber mode when the device detects AV block are being increasingly utilized in pacemakers and implantable cardioverter defibrillators (ICDs). Clinical experience with these algorithms that promote intrinsic AV conduction has shown dramatic reductions in ventricular pacing frequency and, most significantly, a reduced risk of AF without an increased risk of heart failure or mortality[1] (see discussion below).

Pacemaker syndrome

Pacemaker syndrome is a term proposed in 1974 to describe a condition comprising a variety of symptoms and signs produced by ventricular pacing.[32] Pacemaker syndrome has been defined variably, but the broadest definition is probably most appropriate. It is best thought of as any combination of the variety of symptoms and signs occurring with ventricular pacing that are relieved by restoration of AV synchrony. Although it is most often the result of VVI pacing, pacemaker syndrome can result from any pacing mode that results in AV dyssynchrony, even AAI pacing with long PR intervals.[33]

Two difficulties in ascribing symptoms and signs specifically to pacemaker syndrome are commonly encountered. First, patients who have pacemakers implanted are frequently patients with other cardiovascular problems that produce the symptoms and signs described. Second, many pacemaker patients unfortunately have the belief that having the pacemaker, *de facto*, forces them to accept a less than normal sense of well-being. An extreme symptom frequently associated with pacemaker syndrome is syncope. Syncope is very uncommon and is most likely related to profound hypotension—and, in some, a decrease in cardiac output—associated with loss of AV synchrony. Additional symptoms related to blood pressure and cardiac output include malaise, easy fatigability, a sense of weakness, lightheadedness, and dizziness. Symptoms related to higher atrial and venous pressures include dyspnea (frequently at rest), orthopnea, paroxysmal nocturnal dyspnea, a sensation of fullness and/or pulsations in the neck and chest, as well as palpitations, chest pain, nausea and peripheral edema. Experience has shown that careful questioning is frequently necessary to elucidate these symptoms. It is not uncommon for patients who have had a pacemaker implanted for some time to deny symptoms, but, on specific questioning, to admit to having experienced symptoms that can be directly related to ventricular pacing with loss of AV synchrony. Careful examination is necessary to find physical signs related to ventricular pacing. Some of these signs include relative or absolute hypotension that can be continuous or fluctuating, neck vein distension with prominent "cannon" A waves, pulmonary rales, and rarely peripheral edema.

The incidence of pacemaker syndrome during ventricular pacing is quite variable in the literature, ranging from 2% to 83% depending in part on the definition used to diagnose this clinical entity.[17] The Mode Selection Trial (MOST) was a randomized trial of pacing mode selection (DDDR vs. VVIR) in 2010 patients with sick sinus syndrome.[20] Pacemaker syndrome was defined in MOST as either new or worsened dyspnea, orthopnea, elevated jugular pressure, rales, and edema with VA conduction during ventricular pacing, or symptoms of dizziness, weakness, presyncope, or syncope and a 20-mmHg reduction of systolic blood pressure when the patient was ventricular paced compared with atrial pacing or sinus rhythm.[34] Based on this definition, pacemaker syndrome occurred in 18.3% of the patients treated with VVIR pacing ($n = 996$) in the trial. This incidence is similar to the 26% found in the Pacemaker Selection in the Elderly (PASE) trial, which studied pacemaker recipients > 65 years without chronic AF randomly assigned to VVIR vs. DDDR pacing.[35] The strongest predictor of pacemaker syndrome in the MOST trial was a higher percentage of ventricular paced beats. Pacemaker syndrome caused a marked decrease in quality of life, which improved significantly after reprogramming to the DDDR pacing mode.

In a substudy of the PASE trial, development of pacemaker syndrome in patients programmed to the VVIR pacing mode was associated with elevated plasma ANP levels (> 90 pgml^{-1}) reflective of the non-physiological pacing mode. The diagnosis of pacemaker syndrome was made within the first week after pacemaker implantation and programming to VVIR pacing mode. After crossover from VVIR to DDDR pacing mode in these patients, there was prompt resolution of the symptoms that led to the diagnosis and a decline in plasma ANP levels (< 90 pgml^{-1}). Physiologically, increased release of ANP during VVI pacing may reduce arterial pressure because of its potent vasodilator effects and reflexly result in enhanced sympathetic nervous outflow. This may account for or worsen the signs and symptoms of pacemaker syndrome in this setting. These findings support a role for ANP release in the pathogenesis of pacemaker syndrome and as a clinical marker of this syndrome in VVIR-paced patients.

Pacemaker syndrome results from a complex interaction of hemodynamic, neurohumoral and vascular changes induced by the loss of AV synchrony (Fig. 3.25). It has been speculated that patients who develop pacemaker syn-

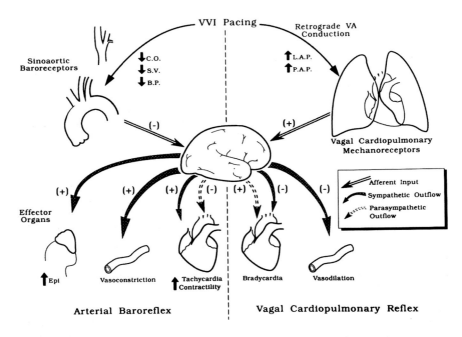

Fig. 3.25 Diagrammatic representation of the multiple reflex pathways involved in pacemaker syndrome. The arterial baroreflexes detect a decrease in stroke volume when atrioventricular (AV) dyssynchrony occurs, leading to sympathetic activation and vasoconstriction. Conversely, AV dyssynchrony leads to increased atrial wall tension and activation of reflex pathways, leading to vagally mediated vasodilation as well as release of humoral substances, such as atrial natriuretic peptide (ANP), which further facilitate baroreflex-mediated vasoconstriction. LAP, left atrial pressure; PAP, pulmonary artery pressure; CO, cardiac output; SV, stroke volume; BP, blood pressure; EPI, epinephrine. (Reproduced with permission from Ellenbogen KA, Stambler BS. Pacemaker syndrome. In: Clinical cardiac pacing, 1st edn. Eds Ellenbogen KA, Kay, Wilkoff, Philadelphia: W.B. Saunders, 1995:419–31.)

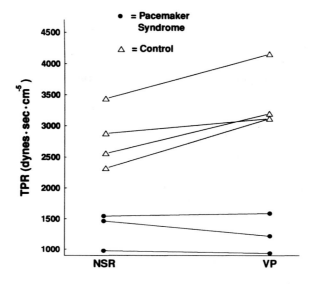

Fig. 3.26 Changes in total peripheral vascular resistance (dynes s⁻¹ cm⁻⁵) during normal sinus rhythm and ventricular pacing (VP) in four control patients and in three patients with pacemaker syndrome. In control subjects, there was an approximately 20% increase in peripheral resistance, whereas peripheral resistance failed to increase in the patients with pacemaker syndrome. (Reproduced with permission from Ellenbogen KA, Wood MA, Stambler BS. Pacemaker syndrome: clinical, hemodynamic and neurohumoral features. In: Barold SS, Mugica J, eds. *New Perspectives in Cardiac Pacing 3*. Armonk, NY: Futura Publishing, 1993:85–112.)

drome during ventricular pacing may have a failure to increase systemic vascular resistance adequately despite elevated peripheral sympathetic nerve traffic and circulating catecholamines (Fig. 3.26). Sympathetic nervous system activation is a normal physiological response during ventricular pacing.[15] Besides the reduced stroke volume and cardiac output resulting from the loss of atrial kick during ventricular pacing, pacemaker syndrome may result in some patients from an inadequate sympathetic response to ventricular pacing, with a failure to compensate for upright posture with augmentation in sympathetic tone. In other patients, the elevated venous pressures resulting from atrial contraction against closed AV valves may activate inhibitory atrial and cardiopulmonary vagal afferent nerves that can counteract the protective vasoconstrictive reflex, resulting in peripheral vasodilation and hypotension.

Based on this understanding, it has been speculated that pacemaker syndrome might be predicted by a simple hemodynamic evaluation at the time of pacemaker implant. Pacemaker syndrome may be more likely to result from VVI pacing if the systolic blood pressure drops by > 20 mmHg during ventricular pacing (Fig. 3.15). In the PASE trial, the need for future crossover to dual-chamber mode was predicted by a decrease in supine systolic blood pressure during VVI pacing at the time of pacemaker implantation to < 110 mmHg (relative risk 2.6; 95% CI 1.5, 4.5; $P \leq 0.001$).[35] The sensitivity of a decrease in paced systolic blood pressure to < 110 mmHg at the time of implantation for predicting intolerance to VVIR pacing was 36%, specificity was 86%, positive predictive power was 48%, and negative predictive power was 79%. In contrast, however, in MOST, systolic blood pressure drop with VVIR pacing at implantation was not associated with the development of pacemaker syndrome.[34]

It has often been thought that pacemaker syndrome is more likely to occur and be more severe when intact retrograde VA conduction is present. In this regard, it should be noted that although retrograde conduction is common, even in patients with complete heart block, it may be intermittent and not consistently present at implant. Thus, the absence of retrograde conduction at implant during sedation may not preclude subsequent development of signs and symptoms of pacemaker syndrome. In the PASE trial, VA conduction or cannon A waves were present in almost 50% of patients who required crossover from VVIR to DDDR pacing. However, in both the MOST and PASE trials, the presence of VA conduction at implant was not a significant predictor of the development of intolerance to VVIR pacing.[34,35]

Therefore, despite attempts to identify clinical variables that predict intolerance to ventricular pacing, multiple studies have failed to identify any that consistently predict the development of pacemaker syndrome. In clinical practice, the vast majority of pacemaker implanters have concluded that because prediction of pacemaker syndrome in an individual patient on clinical criteria alone is imprecise, the most effective way to prevent pacemaker syndrome is to implant atrial-based pacemakers in all patients. Undoubtedly, as a consequence of this major shift away from the use of VVI/VVIR pacing in clinical practice over the past 20 years in the USA, there has been a reduced prevalence of pacemaker syndrome.

The management of patients with VVI pacemaker syndrome after VVI pacemaker implantation includes upgrading to a DDD system, reducing the lower pacing rate to encourage conduction of native rhythm, use of hysteresis, or withdrawal of medications that impair sinus node function. For the rare patients with pacemaker syndrome and dual-chamber systems, appropriate programming to ensure atrial capture and the avoidance of atrial non-pacing modes (VDD) or atrial non-tracking modes (DDI or DVI) may be useful.

Detrimental effects of right ventricular pacing

RV pacing can have detrimental effects on myocardial function and result in progression of heart failure in patients with LV dysfunction.[1] RV pacing produces an asynchronous pattern of activation, contraction and relaxation within and between the left and right ventricles. RV pacing reduces systolic and diastolic function. These hemodynamic derangements occur whether or not normal AV synchrony is present and probably are most pronounced when the ventricular pacing site is the RV apex. Ventricular pacing may compromise effective forward stroke volume further by inducing functional mitral valve regurgitation.[36] RV pacing results in significant regional differences in perfusion and oxygen consumption and reduced myocardial mechanical efficiency.[37] In a group of patients with complete AV block and normal ventricular function at the time of permanent lead implantation, chronic RV pacing induced regional myocardial perfusion defects, wall motion abnormalities, and impaired left ventricular systolic and diastolic function.[38]

Asynchronous activation during chronic RV apical pacing leads to long-term adaptations of the myocardium, referred to as remodeling. Experimental and clinical studies have shown that chronic RV pacing induces ventricular dilation, asymmetric LV hypertrophy and thinning, altered perfusion distribution, increased myocardial catecholamine concentrations, abnormal histological changes including myofiber disarray and impairment of LV function.[39–42] These alterations are due to the LV dyssynchronous contraction present during chronic RV apical pacing. Thus, preservation of a normal ventricular activation sequence during permanent cardiac pacing is of enormous importance for optimization of hemodynamic function.

Recent studies have observed a high prevalence of asymptomatic LV dysfunction in pacemaker patients.[43–45] In a single-center study, a history of having a permanent pacemaker with a right ventricular apical (RVA) pacing lead was the strongest predictor (HR 6.6, $P = 0.002$) of a decrease in LV ejection fraction (LVEF decrease of > 7 points) over 18 months' follow-up.[44]

In the MOST trial in a large pacemaker population of sinus node disease patients, there was a strong association between the percentage of (single- as well as dual-chamber) ventricular pacing and the development of heart failure.[20,43] Chronic RV apical pacing was associated with an increased risk of heart failure and AF, even among patients with preserved AV synchrony and normal baseline QRS duration. Ventricular desynchronization imposed by RVA pacing in the DDDR mode $> 40\%$ of the time conferred a 2.6-fold increased risk of heart failure hospitalization compared with lesser pacing among similar patients with a normal baseline QRS duration. Ventricular pacing in the VVIR mode $> 80\%$ of the time was also associated with increased heart failure risk. In absolute terms, the average risk of heart failure in those receiving RVA pacing was approximately 10%; however, the risk was approximately 2% if RVA pacing was minimal ($< 10\%$ of the time). The risk of AF increased linearly with cumulative RVA pacing in both groups. The investigators concluded that both heart failure progression and AF can be reduced by implementing strategies that minimize ventricular pacing and preserve normal ventricular activation.

Clinical evidence of the deleterious effects of chronic RV pacing was also demonstrated in the Dual Chamber and VVI Implantable Defibrillator (DAVID) trial, performed in patients with impaired ventricular systolic function and an ICD.[28] DAVID tested the hypothesis that dual-chamber pacing for rate support would be more efficacious than backup pacing in patients receiving ICDs. The trial was a multicenter study of patients with standard indications for ICD implantation (VT/VF, LVEF ≤ 40%), but without indications for antibradycardia pacing. All patients had a dual-chamber, rate-responsive pacing ICD implanted and were randomized to ventricular backup pacing (VVI 40) or dual-chamber rate-responsive pacing (DDDR 70, average AV delay 180 ms). The study was prematurely discontinued because of increased mortality and hospitalization in patients treated with dual-chamber pacing (73.3% 1-year survival and 22.6% requiring hospitalization) compared with backup ventricular pacing (83.9% survival and 13.3% hospitalization).

A subsequent analysis of the DAVID trial has demonstrated that percent RV pacing predicted the primary clinical outcomes (composite end-point of death or hospitalization for congestive heart failure).[46] Patients with DDDR RV pacing ≤ 40% had similar or better outcomes compared with the VVI backup group, whereas outcomes were worse among patients with DDDR RV pacing > 40%. Thus, continuous RV pacing is a risk factor for heart failure progression.

Hemodynamics of alternative site right ventricular pacing

Based on the findings of adverse events occurring in patients receiving frequent cumulative RV pacing, attempts should be made to minimize RV pacing when intrinsic AV conduction is present (see discussion). However, in patients with AV conduction disease in whom reducing the percentage of ventricular pacing is not feasible because of the requirement for ventricular pacing support, more physiological alternatives to RV apical pacing should be considered. Pacing from the right ventricular outflow tract (RVOT), RV septum or para-Hisian region may offer theoretical advantages over the RV apex that could result in a more synchronous ventricular activation sequence. Despite these potential advantages, the clinical benefits of alternative site RV pacing have not yet been demonstrated conclusively.

Several small studies have investigated the feasibility of permanent para-Hisian pacing to produce a narrow paced QRS complex identical to that in sinus rhythm.[47–51] The criteria for direct His-bundle pacing (DHBP) include 12-lead surface ECG equivalence between native and paced QRS and an HV interval of the spontaneous rhythm equal to that of the pace ventricular interval. Although it has been clearly demonstrated that chronic DHBP can be performed in some patients, the major disadvantages of this approach that limit its widespread application are the technical limitations in being able to achieve DHBP in > 90% of patients. Among five published studies that included 126 patients, DHBP was achieved in < 70% of patients in whom it was attempted.

Most studies of alternative RV site pacing have focused on the RV outflow tract (RVOT), and in particular on the septal portion of the outflow tract. It has been speculated that septal or RVOT pacing will not be associated with the deleterious effects on hemodynamic function seen with RV apical pacing. Most of the data comparing alternative pacing sites to RVA pacing, however, have been equivocal. Some studies have found significant acute hemodynamic advantages, but several randomized controlled chronic studies have demonstrated either modest or negligible benefit of RVOT pacing compared with RVA pacing.[52–58] It should be noted that among the numerous acute and chronic clinical studies, in only one study was RVOT pacing hemodynamically worse than RVA pacing.

The Right Ventricular Outflow Versus Apical Pacing (ROVA) trial was the largest study designed to examine differences between single-site RVA pacing and alternative site RVOT pacing as well as dual-site (RVA and RVOT) pacing.[58] This multicenter, prospective, randomized crossover trial enrolled 103 patients with indications for VVIR pacing, a history of heart failure (NYHA class II or III), LV dysfunction (LVEF ≤ 40%), and chronic AF (AF > 7 days). The primary end-point was health-related quality of life after 3 months. Secondary end-points were NYHA functional class, LVEF, severity of MR by echocardiography, exercise capacity, and lead-related complications. QRS duration was significantly shorter during RVOT (149 ± 19 ms) and dual-site RV pacing (164 ± 18 ms) compared with RVA pacing (180 ± 23 ms). At 3 months' follow-up, no significant differences in quality of life or other clinical outcomes were observed with RVOT or dual-site RV pacing compared with RVA pacing.

One of the difficulties in evaluating the potential benefits of RVOT pacing is that this region is somewhat difficult to identify using fluoroscopy and therefore is not standardized anatomically with respect to pacing sites. Thus, confirmation of anatomical lead location remains challenging and not well validated. In addition, many studies of alternative site RV pacing are difficult to interpret because of the small number of patients, wide range of baseline LV function, varying spectrum of underlying heart disease and varying durations of follow-up. Few randomized trials comparing RVA pacing with alternative RV sites have followed patients over extended periods beyond 1 year. Tse and colleagues have evaluated the long-term effects of RVOT vs. RVA pacing on myocardial function and perfusion in 24 patients.[57] The LVEF was higher and there were fewer regional wall motion abnormalities and myocardial perfusion defects after 18 months of follow-up between patients paced in the RVOT vs. RVA. These differences were not apparent after 6 months of follow-up. The observed benefits in the RVOT group seemed to result from prevention of the deterioration of LV function that developed in the RVA group.

Further complicating the evaluation of alternative RV pacing sites, some studies have suggested that the hemodynamically optimal RV pacing site may vary from patient to patient and may not always reside on the RV septum.[56,59] One study in 14 patients has attempted to find the best RV pacing site, defined as the site with the shortest paced QRS duration.[56] The study found that a shorter QRS duration positively correlated with a higher LVEF, but that the RV septal pacing site did not necessarily produce the shortest QRS or consistently result in improved LV function. QRS duration was shorter in nine patients, longer in four patients and no different in one patient between RV septal and apical pacing. Overall, the QRS duration was not significantly different between RV septal and apical pacing (156 ± 10 vs. 166 ± 18 ms, respectively). Thus, anatomical lead optimization may not be as critical as hemodynamic lead optimization, and the optimal RV site may not be anatomically defined but may vary from patient to patient. In summary, the optimal RV pacing site remains not well defined, and whether the detrimental hemodynamic effects of RVA pacing can be attenuated by selecting the optimal RV pacing site continues to be of clinical interest. A number of ongoing, long-term pacemaker studies continue to evaluate this issue.

Strategies to minimize right ventricular pacing

Although the maintenance of physiological AV intervals has hemodynamic benefits, recent clinical studies have shown that frequent or unnecessary RVA pacing, particularly dual-chamber pacing, increases the risk of AF, progression of heart failure, or death.[28,43] Of note, the majority of patients who received dual-chamber (DDDR) pacing in these trials utilized "physiological AV delays" in the range of 120–200 ms, resulting in a high percentage of ventricular pacing. Thus, the preponderance of evidence indicates that preservation of a normal ventricular activation sequence is of greater importance than maintenance of AV synchrony when attempting to promote physiological pacing.

The risks of frequent or continuous RV stimulation may be reduced by using "minimal ventricular pacing" strategies that use backup ventricular pacing (VVI or VVIR) when AV synchrony is not required, or extended AV intervals during dual-chamber pacing, to allow for intrinsic ventricular activation (see Fig. 3.27). Simple measures that are often employed to reduce ventricular pacing include lengthening the programmed AV intervals to avoid ventricular pacing, programming a lower pacing rate below the resting sinus rate, adding hysteresis for periods of inactivity, and adjusting drugs that affect AV nodal conduction. Rate-adaptive AV interval pacing is usually reserved for patients who are symptomatic with long AV delays or high-grade AV block. However, many dual-chamber pacemakers impose limitations on maximum allowable AV intervals in order to maintain atrial tracking at elevated rates and adequate sensing windows for atrial tachyarrhythmia mode switch algorithms. In ICDs, allowable AV intervals are more restricted to prevent VT underdetection due to cross-chamber blanking periods. Furthermore, long AV delays increase the risk for development of pacemaker-mediated tachycardias. Finally, if RV pacing continues to occur at long programmed AV delays (> 300 ms), this imposes both AV and ventricular desynchronization resulting in reduced cardiac output, diastolic MR and impaired left atrial function. To deal with the issues and limitations related to DDD/R pacing with long AV delays, many newer dual-chamber bradyarrhythmia devices as well as some dual-chamber ICDs use algorithms that essentially provide AAIR pacing with ventricular monitoring and backup DDDR pacing as needed during

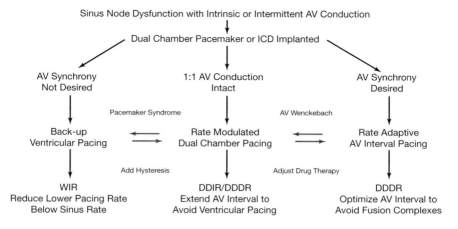

Fig. 3.27 Minimal ventricular pacing strategy to promote intrinsic atrioventricular (AV) conduction after implant of a dual-chamber pacemaker or implantable cardioverter defibrillator for treatment of sinus node dysfunction with impaired AV conduction (present or anticipated). Left: Backup VVIR pacing is used if AV synchrony is not required. The lower pacing rate is programmed below sinus rate and rest hysteresis is added when appropriate. Change to dual-chamber pacing if pacemaker syndrome (due to retrograde VA conduction) develops. Middle: Rate-modulated dual-chamber pacing is preferred for patients with intrinsic AV conduction. The programmed AV interval is extended to promote normal ventricular activation in patients capable of maintaining 1 : 1 AV conduction. Discontinue or adjust drugs that affect AV conduction when appropriate. Add rate-adaptive pacing if patient is symptomatic with extended AV delays. Right: Rate-varied AV interval pacing is used for patients requiring physiological AV intervals. During programming, sensed and paced AV intervals should be optimized to avoid ventricular fusion complexes.

AV block, and can extend AV delays beyond 300 ms.[60] These algorithms are highly effective in reducing the frequency of ventricular pacing to very low levels (< 5–10%).[61]

Hemodynamics of left ventricular pacing and cardiac resynchronization therapy

Over the last decade, cardiac resynchronization therapy (CRT) has been established as a major therapeutic advance in the management of patients with LV systolic dysfunction, heart failure and ventricular dyssynchrony.[62–64] Recent guidelines promote CRT as a class I indication for patients with class III or ambulatory class IV heart failure and prolonged QRS duration (> 130 ms).[64] CRT involves ventricular stimulation of both the right and left ventricles (biventricular pacing) or the LV lateral wall alone. Biventricular devices incorporate pacing leads capable of stimulating the RV and LV via the coronary sinus transvenously or from the epicardium surgically. Univentricular LV pacing (without RV pacing) can be beneficial hemodynamically, with studies demonstrating acute improvements during LV pacing that are similar to biventricular pacing.[65] The long-term effects of univentricular LV pacing have not been well studied, however, especially when compared with the numerous, large clinical trials evaluating biventricular resynchronization pacing. The benefit of LV pacing may be due to fusion between a wavefront produced by intrinsic conduction down the AV node and the intact right bundle and a second wavefront stimulated by LV pacing.

The ventricular pacing site has a significant impact on cardiac hemodynamics and ventricular function. As discussed above, RVA pacing results in nonphysiological LV activation. Chronic RVA pacing can lead to LV dyssynchrony, deleterious ventricular remodeling and adverse clinical outcomes. In contrast, biventricular and LV-based resynchronization pacing improves systolic ventricular in patients with heart failure and intraventricular conduction delay. Sustained therapy can result in reverse remodeling in heart failure patients with dyssynchrony leading to improvements in LVEF, reduction in MR and reduction in LV chamber dilation. Many clinical trials have demonstrated the benefits of CRT on hemodynamics, quality of life, heart failure symptoms and functional class, exercise tolerance, heart failure hospitalization and mortality. However, individual responses are variable with as many as one-third of patients considered as "non-responders." Studies to date have focused primarily on patients with severely reduced LV systolic function, refractory heart failure, markedly prolonged QRS durations (usually due to left bundle branch block), and no bradycardia indication for pacing. A recent comprehensive summary of CRT in patients with LV systolic dysfunction using pooled data from 14 randomized trials (4420 patients) found that CRT decreased hospitalizations by 37% (95% CI 7, 57) and all-cause mortality by 22% (95% CI 9, 33).[66]

CRT seeks to optimize LV contraction by normalizing the dysfunctional activation patterns associated with ventricular conduction delays present in patients with cardiomyopathy or produced by RVA pacing. With marked intraventricular conduction delays, regions of the ventricle may still be actively contracting while other regions are relaxing and filling in diastole. The result is that part of the contractile effort does not contribute to cardiac ejection. In addition, interventricular conduction delays may impair the synergy provided by simultaneous RV and LV contraction. A variety of mechanisms contribute to the hemodynamic improvements associated with CRT.[65,67,68] By pacing both the right and left ventricles, CRT results in a more synchronous electrical activation sequence and mechanical contraction. CRT resynchronizes the severely uncoordinated and dysfunctional patterns of ventricular contraction in patients with prolonged native QRS complexes. CRT improves systolic function acutely within one beat of initiation of pacing, with immediate improvements in LV contractility, cardiac output and arterial pulse pressure. Chronic therapy is required to produce reverse remodeling with reductions in end-diastolic volume. Reduction of the severity or duration of MR is a further benefit of CRT in many patients. Optimization of the AV timing and contraction sequence prolongs the diastolic filling time and reduces diastolic MR. Shortening of ventricular activation (QRS duration) with biventricular pacing also optimizes diastolic filling times. Single-site LV lateral wall pacing results in hemodynamic benefits that are similar to biventricular pacing despite persistently prolonged and abnormal ventricular electrical activation. This suggests that CRT pacing can result in mechanical resynchronization without a requirement that electrical synchrony be produced. Thus, institution of mechanical synchrony may be most critical to the hemodynamic benefit of CRT and may help to identify responders vs. non-responders.

A more complete discussion of biventricular and LV pacing is provided in the chapter on cardiac resynchronization therapy. Most importantly in the context of current discussion of the hemodynamics of cardiac pacing, there is now definitive evidence that LV-based ventricular pacing avoids the detrimental effects of RV pacing. Therefore, it seems likely that in the future the use of CRT will continue to expand in patients with advanced heart failure or possibly in any patient who requires ventricular-based pacing.

Rate-adaptive pacing

A variety of terms have been used to describe the capacity of a pacing system to respond to physiological need by increasing or decreasing pacing rate. The earliest term used to describe this physiological property of pacing systems was rate responsive. Significant objection to this term (for grammatical reasons) has led to the more acceptable use of the terms rate adaptive and rate modulating. However, all these terms are used interchangeably. When the chronotropic function of the sinus node is impaired, the capability of a pacing system to provide rate adaptation depends on the presence of physiological sensors that monitor the need for heart rate modulation. Rate-adaptive pacing is available in almost all modern pulse generators. Rate-adaptive pacing sensors detect physical or physiological indices to mimic the rate response of the normal sinus node. A variety of sensors have been developed to modulate pacing rate according to metabolic demands and to correct chronotropic incompetence.[69] Activity, accelerometer, minute-ventilation and QT-interval sensors are commercially available in the USA and Europe. There is no single sensor that ideally mimics normal cardiac physiology and perfectly modulates heart rate according to metabolic demands. A detailed review of the technology of physiological sensors is given elsewhere.

The sinus node should be given priority as the primary modulator of heart rate when its chronotropic function is unimpaired. Thus, for patients with complete AV block and preserved sinoatrial nodal function, an artificial sensor is not required for rate-adaptive pacing. The VDD and DDD pacing modes provide rate modulation and AV synchrony in this setting. Patients with sinus node dysfunction and an inadequate chronotropic response to exercise are candidates for AAIR or DDDR pacemakers, depending on AV conduction status. In dual-chamber devices programmed in the DDDR mode, rate-adaptive pacing might result from ventricular tracking of the atrial rhythm or be sensor driven (atrial or AV sequential pacing). When rate adaptation is activated, a sensor-driven rate is recorded. If the sensor-driven rate exceeds both the intrinsic atrial rate and the lower rate limit, rate-adaptive pacing occurs. A programmed maximum sensor rate determines the fastest rate at which pacing can occur. For patients with paroxysmal or chronic atrial arrhythmias, a rate-adaptive pacing system is often preferred. Patients with chronic AF or flutter and inappropriately slow ventricular rates during exercise are managed best with VVIR pacing.

Exercise physiology

The importance of rate modulation in pacing systems is related directly and specifically to the importance of matching cardiac output with physiological need. The predominant need for rate modulation derives from physical activity or exertion. There are other physiological situations in which normally there are modulations of heart rate—e.g. during fever and emotional stress. These situations, however, have received much less attention, especially in the context of pacing systems.

During exercise—or "work," as it is frequently referred to by physiologists—the body tissues increase their demand for oxygen.[12] In addition, there is increased need for removal of metabolic by-products, such as CO_2, from the tissues. The body has a number of physiological mechanisms in place to provide for the increased metabolic demands during exercise. Redistribution of blood flow to working tissues, increased ability of working tissues to extract oxygen from the blood, and, most important, increased cardiac output are these mechanisms. Here, we focus on the last of these, the body's ability to increase cardiac output with exercise, as this is what rate adaptation provides.

The importance of cardiac output during work must be appreciated. A direct, relatively linear relationship exists between the amount of work accomplished and oxygen consumption. Maximal work capacity, therefore, is specifically related to maximum oxygen consumption. Further, consistent with the Fick principle,

$$\text{cardiac output} = O_2 \text{ consumption} / AV\ O_2 \text{ difference}$$

where AV means arterial–venous. Also,

$$\text{cardiac output} = \text{stroke volume} \times \text{heart rate}$$

By substitution in these equations,

$$O_2 \text{ consumption} = \text{stroke volume} \times \text{heart rate} \times AV\ O_2 \text{ difference}$$

Because oxygen consumption is directly linearly proportional to work (Fig. 3.28),

$$\text{work} = \text{stroke volume} \times \text{heart rate} \times AV\ O_2 \text{ difference}$$

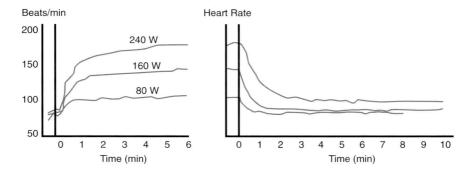

Fig. 3.28 Heart rate response at onset and termination of exercise in eight healthy young men at different workloads. W, watts. At onset of exercise, the majority of the total increment in heart rate occurs in the first minute of effort. (Reproduced with permission from Linnarsson D. Dynamics of pulmonary gas exchange and heart rate changes at start and end of exercise. Acta Physiol Scand 1974; 415:1–68.)

Increasing any of these variables will support an increased ability to do work, but the increase in heart rate is the most important. Maximum work, in normal individuals, is accomplished by an increase in stroke volume to approximately 150% of the resting value, an increase in heart rate to approximately 300% of the resting value, and an increase in AV O_2 difference to approximately 250% of the resting value. These changes allow an increase in work to over 10 times resting levels. In normal individuals, peak cardiac output can be increased to 300% of resting values simply by an increase in heart rate. During peak exercise, the stroke volume is increased to approximately 150% of the resting value. This increase in stroke volume is not linear and is achieved at approximately the halfway point between the rest and maximal exercise levels. The increased stroke volume is accomplished by an increase in venous return, ventricular filling, and contractility. Loss of AV synchrony can compromise stroke volume, even with exercise, although it appears that AV synchrony is usually less important in providing ventricular filling during exercise than at rest. It is ideal, however, to optimize stroke volume, because this is a more energy-efficient way of accomplishing cardiac output (milliliters of cardiac output/milliliters of O_2 consumption) than by an increase in heart rate.

Clearly, the most important mechanism by which cardiac output is increased during exercise is by increasing heart rate. The normal heart rate response to exercise follows a triphasic response (Fig. 3.28).[70] Heart rate increases most rapidly within the first 10–15 s of exercise and reaches 70% of the total heart rate increase in this phase. A slower exponential rise in heart rate follows during the next 60–90 s. Finally, a slow linear increase or plateau phase results from sustained activity. Heart rate deceleration with cessation of exercise is generally slower than the rate of acceleration and also follows a biphasic or triphasic response.

Chronotropic incompetence

The inability to increase and maintain heart rate appropriately with exercise is called chronotropic incompetence.[71] A number of criteria have been proposed to diagnose chronotropic incompetence, including the inability to increase heart rate with exercise to at least 70–85% of the maximum predicted heart rate (maximum predicted heart rate = 220 – age in years). This is a useful criterion for diagnosing chronotropic incompetence, but it cannot be used in individuals with limitations on their exercise function unrelated to cardiopulmonary status. Thus, the diagnosis of chronotropic incompetence is difficult if the patient cannot undergo formal exercise testing or perform a simple hall walk test. Further, there are patients with delayed chronotropic responses who could benefit from rate-modulating pacing systems but might be missed by this criterion. More complicated formulas have been developed to allow determination of the presence of chronotropic incompetence by exercise testing with assessments made by stage.[72] The Wilkoff chronotropic assessment exercise protocol (CAEP) is an easily performed treadmill test that has become widely used for chronotropic competency evaluation (Table 3.3). It uses gradual increases in both elevation and speed, and can be used for the evaluation of devices with a variety of sensor types. It is also noted that making predictions regarding the future need for rate-adaptive pacing is unreliable at the time of implantation. This is usually not a clinical issue, because rate-adaptive pacing is available in almost all modern pacemaker generators and can be programmed on if needed after implantation.

Chronotropic incompetence is common among pacemaker patients. However, the frequency of chronotropic incompetence in part depends on the definition used and method of assessment. Among a cohort of pacemaker patients (42% AV block, 56% sinus node disease and 59% AF), 51% were diagnosed as having chronotropic incompetence based on the Wilkoff chronotropic index.[73]

Table 3.3 Chronotropic assessment exercise protocol

Stage		Speed (mph)	Grade (%)	Time (min)	Cumulative time	METs
Warm-up	0	1.0	0	—	—	1.5
	1	1.0	2	2.0	2.0	2.0
	2	1.5	3	2.0	4.0	2.8
	3	2.0	4	2.0	6.0	3.6
	4	2.5	5	2.0	8.0	4.6
	5	3.0	6	2.0	10.0	5.8
	6	3.5	8	2.0	12.0	7.5
	7	4.0	10	2.0	14.0	9.6
	8	5.0	10	2.0	16.0	12.1
	9	6.0	10	2.0	18.0	14.3
	10	7.0	10	2.0	20.0	16.5
	11	7.0	15	2.0	22.0	19.0

METs, metabolic equivalents.

Among patients in whom sinoatrial disease is the primary indication for pacing, not all will manifest chronotropic incompetence during formal exercise testing. Some individuals with sinus node dysfunction may demonstrate normal chronotropic response to exercise, whereas others with sinus node dysfunction may have little or no ability to increase heart rate during exercise. Thus, the need for rate-adaptive pacing is unpredictable in sinoatrial disease. The overall pattern of chronotropic response in an individual is variable and may evolve over time. Some patients are able to achieve the appropriate heart rate for the level of exercise, but do so more slowly than is normal. Patients with any form of chronotropic incompetence are candidates for pacing systems with rate-modulation capabilities.

Chronotropic incompetence may be provoked by disease, most commonly ischemic heart disease, valvular heart disease and heart failure, or induced by drugs. In a study of pacemaker patients, significant predictors of chronotropic incompetence included the existence of coronary artery disease, presence of an acquired valvular heart disease, former cardiac surgery, and therapy with digitalis, β-blockers, or amiodarone.[73] Chronotropic incompetence has important prognostic implications in patients with coronary artery disease. Chronotropic incompetence predicts all-cause mortality independent of angiographic severity of coronary artery disease.[74] The prevalence of chronotropic impairment in heart failure patients also is variably reported (25–70%), possibly due to a lack of a standardized definition and/or differing assessment methodologies.[75] Chronotropic impairment impacts the physical function and quality of life of heart failure patients.

Advantages of rate modulation

As is obvious from the foregoing discussion of exercise physiology, the ability of patients to increase heart rate with exercise is the primary means of meeting metabolic demands. Thus, exertional intolerance is inevitable if heart rate cannot be increased appropriately. The ability to increase rate is the most important determinant of cardiac output and exercise capacity, especially at higher levels of exertion. A positive linear correlation between improvement of exercise capacity and heart rate is observed. An inappropriate chronotropic response to exercise can decrease peak exercise oxygen uptake by as much as 15–20%.

It should be recognized that most pacemaker recipients are elderly and function at submaximal levels of exertion during virtually all of their daily activities. Rarely does the typical pacemaker patient require improvement in maximal work capacity, and few patients are expected to stress to the point of their maximal heart rate, except for young or extremely vigorous patients. References are available that provide normal ranges of heart rates in response to moderate exercise according to age, sex and body surface area, which have relevance to rate-adaptive pacemaker programming. However, such rates are often inappropriate for some patients, such as those with coronary artery disease, valvular heart disease or diastolic dysfunction. Optimization of heart rate by providing rate modulation at submaximal levels of exertion during activities of daily living should be the therapeutic goal during pacemaker programming. This often requires highly individualized programming to suit the unique needs of each patient.

Quantification of the improvement in work capacity in pacemaker populations comparing non-rate-modulating with rate-modulating modes has shown the advantages of the rate-modulating systems. Rate-modulating pacing systems have been shown not only to improve the heart rate response with exercise but also to increase work capacity. For every 40% increase in paced rate during rate-modulated pacing compared with non-rate-modulated pacing, there is a 10% increase in work capacity. Compared with VVI pacing, VVIR mode improves exercise duration and cardiac index in patients undergoing paired stress testing. These improvements are independent of patient age and ejection fraction. Even greater improvements in exercise hemodynamics are documented with DDDR pacing compared with either VVIR or DDD modes.[130] Compared with VVIR, DDDR pacing has demonstrated improved exercise capacity, cardiac output, and cardiac metabolic indices, suggesting more efficient cardiac work. In patients with sick sinus syndrome, DDDR pacing provides greater maximal heart rates, exercise times, higher maximal oxygen

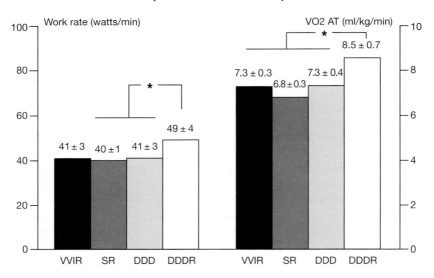

Work rate and oxygen uptake at anaerobic threshold (sinus node disease)

Fig. 3.29 Work rate vs. oxygen uptake at anaerobic threshold in nine patients with sinus node dysfunction. Each patient underwent testing in sinus rhythm (SR), VVIR, DDD and DDDR pacing modes using a respiratory sensor pacemaker. Oxygen uptake was greater in DDDR mode compared with all others at anaerobic threshold. (Reproduced with permission from Lemke B *et al.* Aerobic capacity in rate modulated pacing. PACE 1992; 15:1914–8.)

uptake and higher oxygen uptake at anaerobic threshold than DDD pacing (Fig. 3.29). These benefits are attributed largely to the increased heart rate in the rate-adaptive mode.

Despite the physiological basis for rate-adaptive pacing and acute improvements in exercise hemodynamics with the use of this technology, it has not been clearly and consistently established that rate-adaptive pacing provides clinically relevant improvements in symptoms, quality of life or other important cardiovascular outcomes. In a small trial of patients with the tachy–brady syndrome, symptomatic improvement was demonstrated in patients programmed to the DDDR compared with the DDD mode.[76] The improvement in symptoms in the DDDR group was mostly due to reduced palpitations related to less mode switching episodes. The Advanced Elements of Pacing Trial (ADEPT) studied 872 patients with at least mild chronotropic incompetence and found no significant improvements in quality of life in patients assigned to rate-modulated compared with fixed-rate pacemakers (DDDR vs. DDD).[77,78] Furthermore, there were no differences in the composite end-point of death, non-fatal myocardial infarction, stroke, hospitalization for heart failure or AF between the two groups. Interestingly, the DDDR group was significantly more likely to experience hospitalization for heart failure compared with the DDD group (7.3% vs. 3.5%). Thus it should be concluded that the addition of rate modulation, in spite of attempting to replicate the normal response to exercise, does not have a positive impact on quality of life or cardiovascular outcomes in pacemaker recipients. It may be that the increased frequency of RV pacing at higher heart rates during rate-modulated pacing, with the resultant forced ventricular dyssynchrony, may increase the risk of heart failure and negate the potential benefits of restoring chronotropic competence. The clinical utility of rate modulation during biventricular pacing has not been established.

Although there are a variety of sensors that can be used for rate modulation in currently available pacemakers, there is little evidence to support a major clinical difference in outcomes between sensors and their combinations. Interestingly, when three of the most commonly utilized rate-adaptive sensors (accelerometer, piezoelectric and blended sensors) were compared in DDDR-paced patients with sinus node dysfunction in the Mode Selection Trial (MOST), quality of life analyses demonstrated that patients with blended sensors had significantly worse physical function than did patients with the other two sensor systems.[79] There were no significant differences, after adjustment for baseline differences, among the three sensors in clinical end-points after long-term follow-up, including no significant differences in the risk of death, heart failure hospitalization, AF, and the combined end-point of mortality and stroke.

Dual-chamber devices allow rate-responsive AV delays to be programmed. This feature is designed to simulate normal shortening of the PR interval during exercise and allow AV synchrony to be maintained at higher heart rates. The importance of AV synchrony, however, may diminish at higher heart rates as the early and late diastolic filling phases converge. In Figs 3.30 and 3.31, the relative hemodynamic benefits of rate modulation and stroke volume and rate

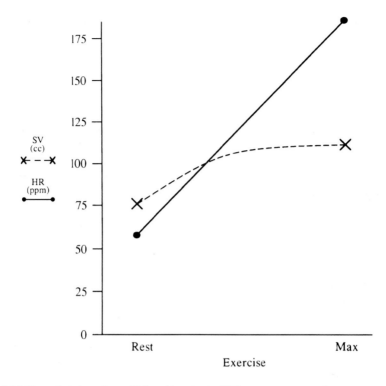

Fig. 3.30 Normal stroke volume (SV) and heart-rate (HR) response to exercise.

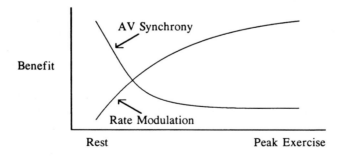

Fig. 3.31 Hypothetical, general relationship between atrioventricular synchrony and rate modulation with respect to hemodynamic benefit, both at rest and during exercise.

modulation and AV synchrony scaled from rest to maximum exertion can be seen for a general population. At rest, AV synchrony is of pre-eminent benefit, whereas this benefit is diminished as one approaches maximal exercise, especially in relation to rate modulation. Rate modulation is of very little value at rest, but becomes quite important early in exercise and increases in relative benefit approaching maximal exercise. Rate modulation and AV synchrony are complementary, not competitive, physiological concepts.

Hemodynamics of pacing in hypertrophic obstructive cardiomyopathy

Hypertrophic obstructive cardiomyopathy (HOCM) represents a special clinical situation in which cardiac pacing has been proposed to have a therapeutic role in selected patients. These patients have obstruction to LV outflow caused by hypertrophy of the interventricular septum, typically in the subaortic valve area, combined with systolic anterior motion of the mitral valve. In this select subset of patients with LV outflow tract (LVOT) obstruction and refractory symptoms despite pharmacological therapy, DDD pacing with a short AV delay may be of benefit. It is speculated that by producing dyssynchrony of LV contraction and paradoxical septal movement, dual-chamber pacing with ventricular pacing from the RV apex will reduce the degree of outflow obstruction and symptoms. An AV delay of < 100 ms is usually necessary to ensure full RV apical pre-excitation and AV delays ranging from 80 to 100 ms probably are optimal for gradient reduction. An example of modest improvement in LV outflow gradient is shown in Fig. 3.32.

Retrospective studies have suggested that AV synchronous pacing with a short AV delay decreases LVOT gradient and symptoms. Other investigators have documented objective as well as subjective improvement in such parameters as oxygen consumption at peak exercise. These studies have generated interest in the role of pacing in HOCM, but subsequent studies of dual-chamber pacing have yielded conflicting results.[80–82] Results varied from patient to patient and were inconsistent. Some patients had marginal benefit, whereas others obtained complete gradient abolition. Shorter AV delays allow for more complete apical pre-excitation and minimal basal septal activation through the His–Purkinje system. In addition, apical pre-excitation with short AV delays must be maintained at higher heart rates and during exercise. However, delays that are too short can be detrimental to diastolic filling and can worsen symptoms. If interatrial conduction is impaired, then short AV delays will result in left atrial contraction occurring after mitral valve closure, which can elevate left atrial pressure and promote atrial arrhythmias. Reduction in LVOT gradient may require AV interval optimization with Doppler echocardiographic guidance assessing both LV outflow gradient and mitral inflow velocities.

At least three randomized, controlled, crossover trials of pacing in HOCM patients refractory to medical therapy have been performed and have found that the benefits of this therapy are less than that suggested by earlier reports. These studies included a total of about 140 patients and suggested that pacing can reduce the LVOT gradient and lead to a modest reduction in symptoms, but does not improve exercise capacity. The M-PATHY trial was a randomized,

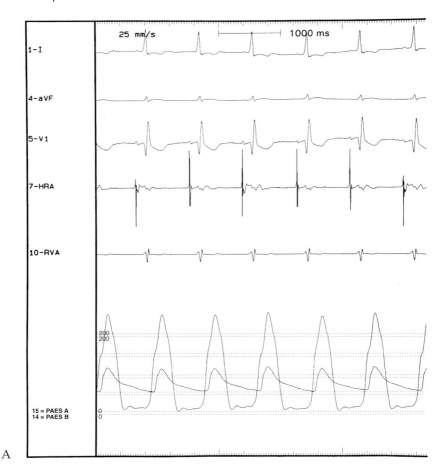

Fig. 3.32 Tracings showing the impact of atrioventricular (AV) sequential pacing on left ventricular and femoral arterial pressure in a selected patient with hypertrophic obstructive cardiomyopathy. A, The presence of a nearly 150 mmHg pressure gradient at baseline during sinus rhythm. B, With AV sequential pacing at an AV interval of 75 ms, the pressure gradient decreases to 50–90 mmHg. The beat-to-beat variability of the measurement of this gradient is highlighted by the bottom tracing. Top to bottom: I, aVf, V₁ = surface ECG leads; RA, right atrial intracardiac recording; RV, right ventricular intracardiac recording and femoral and left ventricular pressure tracings (in mmHg) superimposed on each other. (Reproduced by permission from Sweeney MO, Ellenbogen KA. Implantable devices for the electrical management of heart disease: overview of indications for therapy and selected recent advances. In: Antman EM, ed. Cardiovascular therapeutics, 2nd edn. Philadelphia: WB Saunders, 2002.)

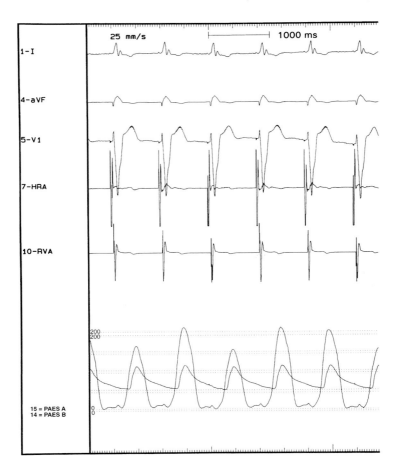

Figure 3.32 (*Continued.*)

double-blind, crossover multicenter North American trial of 48 patients with drug-refractory HOCM.[82] An average reduction in LVOT gradient of 40 mmHg was seen, but there was no significant effect on quality of life, exercise capacity, peak oxygen consumption or septal wall thickness noted. A small subgroup of patients over the age of 65 showed consistent improvement in functional capacity. Likewise, the Pacing in Cardiomyopathy (PIC) study, which was a multicenter European study, also suggested that elderly patients (> 65 years) are most likely to respond to pacing.[81] However, the placebo effect of pacing system implantation appears to play an important role in overall subjective improvement. Therefore, pacing cannot be regarded as primary therapy for obstruction because of inconsistent results.

A non-randomized comparison of dual-chamber pacing and septal myectomy for patients with drug-refractory symptoms has been performed.[83] This concurrent cohort study analyzed LVOT gradients, symptoms, and exercise testing in 39 patients who underwent surgery or pacemaker implantation based on physician preference. Although both groups showed subjective improvement, myectomy patients had a greater reduction in LVOT gradients and larger improvements in functional status.

In summary, despite observations that some patients derive benefit, DDD pacing with short AV delays cannot be regarded as a primary treatment modality for LVOT obstruction in HOCM and is not routinely indicated for the alleviation of symptoms. There may be benefit of pacing therapy in selected subgroups, such as those > 65 years old or patients who are not candidates for myectomy or septal ablation because of comorbidities. American College of Cardiology/American Heart Association/Heart Rhythm Society guidelines give pacing in patients with HOCM who are refractory to pharmacological therapy a class IIb indication.[84] Pacing is indicated in HOCM patients with sinus node dysfunction or AV block and may have utility in preventing bradycardia and allowing more aggressive drug therapy with β-blockers or verapamil. The European Society of Cardiology Guidelines are also consistent, and give pacing in patients with drug-refractory HOCM a class IIb indication as well.[85] There is no evidence that pacing reduces the risk of sudden death or overall mortality in HOCM.[86] Whether incorporating DDD pacing with short AV delays into implantable defibrillators plays a role in the treatment of HOCM patients has not been well defined.

Pacemaker mode selection

The long-standing common clinical practice of using dual-chamber pacemakers to achieve physiological pacing in an attempt to preserve AV synchrony and provide rate adaptation has come under intense scrutiny over the past decade with the publication of several important randomized controlled trials of pacemaker mode selection (Table 3.2). Clearly, these trials have demonstrated that the conventional dual-chamber pacemaker does not truly mimic normal cardiovascular physiology. Thus, pacemaker technology will continue to need to evolve and be refined. The lessons from the past decade of evidence-based medicine in the field of cardiac pacing are that carefully designed, controlled clinical trials will continue to be required to evaluate any new advances designed to achieve physiological pacing.

At the present time, the logical approach to pacemaker selection is to choose a mode of pacing that targets the underlying bradycardia and to avoid modes that electrically stimulate chambers that have appropriate intrinsic electrical and conduction properties. Selection of the appropriate bradyarrhythmia pacing mode should fit the patient's electrical and hemodynamic status. This decision should incorporate consideration of the patient's electrical conduction status, including the atrial rhythm, AV conduction, ventricular conduction (i.e. QRS duration) and chronotropic competence, and hemodynamic status including the patient's LV systolic function and whether there is a history of heart failure. Pacemaker mode selection should be consistent with evidence from clinical trials indicating at least a lack of harm of a particular pacing mode and preferably supporting a potential benefit on important clinical outcomes.[148] Striving to provide both AV synchrony and rate modulation, when clinical evidence supports a benefit, assists in this decision-making process.[87] A pacemaker mode selection flow chart is shown in Fig. 3.33.

In pure sinus node dysfunction with normal AV conduction, atrial pacing should be the primary mode of pacing and RV stimulation should be avoided as much as possible. This can be accomplished either by using atrial pacing (AAI) alone or with a dual-chamber pacing (DDD) system, preferably one that incorporates an algorithm that reduces the frequency of unnecessary ventricular pacing. These pacing mode selections are supported by evidence from clinical trials indicating a reduction in the incidence of AF and progression to chronic AF, a lower risk of developing pacemaker syndrome and small improvements in quality of life with atrial-based pacing compared with single-chamber RV pacing. In patients with sinus node dysfunction as the primary indication for pacemaker implantation, determination of AV conduction status and the likelihood of future development of AV conduction disturbances are important considerations in selection between single-chamber atrial vs. dual-chamber pacing systems. Careful evaluation of AV conduction status dramatically reduces the likelihood that subsequent AV conduction problems will develop, but a small risk remains. Pre-existing PR interval prolongation (> 200 ms), left bundle branch block or a low Wenckebach rate (< 100 bpm) are predictors for subsequent requirement for implantation of a ventricular lead.[149-152] Symptomatic high-degree AV block subsequently developed at a rate of 1.7% per year (range < 1% to 4.5% per year) in studies in patients with an atrial pacemaker for sinus node disease.[17,88-92] It is for this reason that most implanters in the USA usually implant a dual-chamber pacing system in patients with sinus node disease and normal AV conduction, but may initially program an atrial pacing mode.

In patients with AV block, both dual-chamber and single-chamber ventricular pacing systems will prevent bradycardia, but only dual-chamber pacemakers will maintain AV synchrony. The importance of maintaining AV synchrony, however, is even less well established in patients with AV block than in those with sinus node dysfunction. The United Kingdom Pacing and Cardiovascular Events (UKPACE) trial randomized patients > 70 years old with high-grade AV block to dual-chamber or ventricular pacing.[21] Over 4.6 years of follow-up, no significant differences between the two groups in all-cause death, AF, heart failure or thromboembolic events were detected. Selection of an appropriate pacing mode in a patient with AV block as the primary indication for pacemaker implantation should be based on whether the AV block is intermittent or permanent, whether LV systolic function is

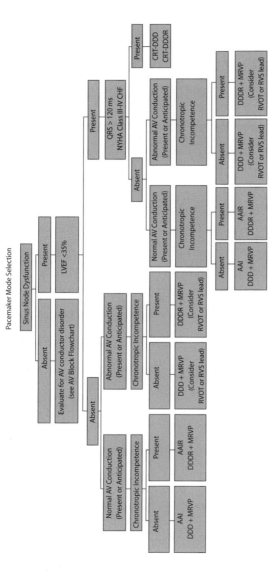

Fig. 3.33 Pacemaker mode selection algorithm for sinus node dysfunction. DDD, dual-chamber pacing; DDDR, dual-chamber rate-adaptive pacing; AAI, atrial demand pacing; AAIR, atrial demand rate-adaptive pacing; AV, atrioventricular; NYHA, New York Heart Association; CHF, congestive heart failure; CRT, cardiac resynchronization therapy; MRVP, minimize right ventricular pacing; RVOT, right ventricular outflow tract; RVS, right ventricular septal. Pacemaker codes are discussed in detail in Chapter 6.

normal or abnormal and the atrial rhythm status (sinus rhythm or paroxysmal or permanent atrial tachyarrhythmias). For patients in sinus rhythm or with paroxysmal atrial tachyarrhythmias and intermittent AV block, dual-chamber pacemakers with algorithms to minimize ventricular pacing can be utilized. Back-up VVI pacing (40–50 ppm) could also be considered in these AV block patients, especially if the AV block is expected to be infrequent (< 5% ventricular pacing) and there is no evidence of chronotropic incompetence. In patients with complete AV block or advanced ventricular conduction system disease, dual-chamber pacing systems are usually implanted. Because of the need for frequent ventricular pacing in these patients, alternatives to RVA pacing should be considered to address the issue of forced ventricular desynchronization. If symptomatic LV dysfunction (LVEF < 35% and NYHA class III or IV) and AV block are present, then cardiac resynchronization therapy should be utilized. For patients with complete heart block and normal LV systolic function, alternative RV pacing sites (RVOT, RV septum) should be considered, as is the case in patients with impaired LV systolic function but in whom the LVEF is > 35%. However, in the latter group of patients, an LV lead might be implanted, but support for biventricular pacing in this subgroup is limited. In addition, the existing clinical data are equivocal in support of alternative RV pacing sites in these patients; there is no evidence to suggest an increase in detrimental effects, but no definitive evidence of improved clinical outcomes over the RV apex. In patients with intermittent or complete AV block and chronic, persistent atrial tachyarrhythmias, ventricular only pacing systems should be implanted with the choice of VVI, VVIR or BiV-VVI(R) based on the presence of chronotropic incompetence and the need for cardiac resynchronization therapy. A pacemaker mode selection chart is shown in Fig. 3.34.

When chronotropic incompetence accompanies sinus node dysfunction or AV block, as it often does in the pacemaker population, then rate-adaptive pacing might be considered. However, the rate-adaptive pacing mode should not be programmed at the expense of a greater frequency of ventricular pacing and promotion of ventricular dyssynchrony. Rate-adaptive pacing may promote ventricular pacing, particularly if rate-adaptive AV delays are programmed. Furthermore, it must be recognized that there is an absence of conclusive data showing that DDDR pacing is superior to DDD with regard to improved quality of life and reduced symptoms.[87] Thus, rate-adaptive pacing should not be used routinely in pacemaker patients unless there is a strong clinical need (i.e. highly symptomatic patients with inadequate chronotropic response to exercise).

In patients who require bradycardia pacing support and also have symptomatic heart failure (NYHA class III or IV), LV systolic dysfunction (LVEF < 35%) and a widened QRS complex (> 120 ms), an LV pacing lead should be implanted so that cardiac resynchronization therapy (BiV-DDD[R]) can be provided. In most clinical trials of CRT, patients who required pacing for bradycardia were not included except in some studies after AV junction abla-

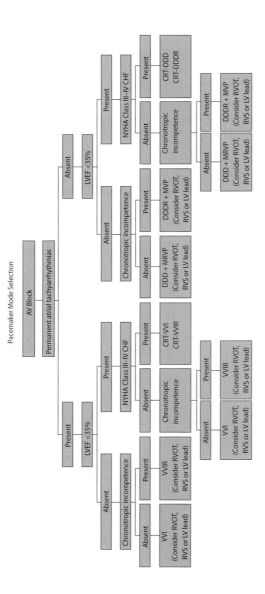

Fig. 3.34 Pacemaker mode selection algorithm for atrioventricular block. DDD, dual-chamber pacing; DDDR, dual-chamber rate-adaptive pacing; VVI, ventricular demand pacing; VVIR, ventricular demand rate-adaptive pacing; LVEF, left ventricular ejection fraction; AV, atrioventricular; NYHA, New York Heart Association; CHF, congestive heart failure; CRT, cardiac resynchronization therapy; MRVP, minimize right ventricular pacing; RVOT, right ventricular outflow tract; RVS, right ventricular septal; LV, left ventricular. Pacemaker codes are discussed in detail in Chapter 6.

tion. However, there is substantial evidence that CRT reduces mortality and heart failure hospitalization, and improves quality of life in heart failure patients with ventricular dyssynchrony.

References

1 Sweeney MO, Hellkamp AS. Heart failure during cardiac pacing. Circulation 2006; 113:2082–8.

2 Harvey W. Exercitatio anatomica de motu cordis et sanguinis in animalibus (1628). R Willis, translator. England: Barnes Survey, 1874.

3 Lewis T. Fibrillation of the auricles: its effects upon the circulation. J Exp Med 1912; 16:395–8.

4 Gesel RA. Auricular systole and its relation to ventricular output. Am J Physiol 1911; 29:32–63.

5 Furman S. The present status of cardiac pacing. Herz 1991; 16:171–81.

6 Lamas GA. Physiological consequences of normal atrioventricular conduction: applicability to modern cardiac pacing. J Card Surg 1989; 4:89–98.

7 Panidis IP, Ross J, Munley B *et al*. Diastolic mitral regurgitation in patients with atrioventricular conduction abnormalities: a common finding by Doppler echocardiography. J Am Coll Cardiol 1986; 7:768–74.

8 Timek T, Dagum P, Lai DT *et al*. The role of atrial contraction in mitral valve closure. J Heart Valve Dis 2001; 10:312–9.

9 Barold SS, Ovsyshcher IE. Pacemaker-induced mitral regurgitation. Pacing Clin Electrophysiol 2005; 28:357–60.

10 Salukhe TV, Henein MY, Sutton R. Pacing in heart failure: patient and pacing mode selection. Eur Heart J 2003; 24:977–86.

11 Reynolds DW, Olson EG, Burrow RD *et al*. Mitral regurgitation during atrioventricular and ventriculoatrial pacing. Pacing Clin Electrophysiol 1984; 7:476 (abstract).

12 Astrand PO, Rodahl K. Textbook of work physiology, 2nd edn. New York: McGraw-Hill, 1977.

13 Gold MR, Brockman R, Peters RW, Olsovsky MR, Shorofsky SR. Acute hemodynamic effects of right ventricular pacing site and pacing mode in patients with congestive heart failure secondary to either ischemic or idiopathic dilated cardiomyopathy. Am J Cardiol 2000; 85:1106–9.

14 Reynolds DW, Wilson MF, Burow RD *et al*. Hemodynamic evaluation of atrioventricular sequential vs. ventricular pacing in patients with normal and poor ventricular function at variable heart rates and posture. J Am Coll Cardiol 1983; 1:636 (abstract).

15 Taylor JA, Morillo CA, Eckberg DL, Ellenbogen KA. Higher sympathetic nerve activity during ventricular (VVI) than during dual-chamber (DDD) pacing. J Am Coll Cardiol 1996; 28:1753–8.

16 Horie H, Tsutamoto T, Ishimoto N *et al*. Plasma brain natriuretic peptide as a biochemical marker for atrioventricular sequence in patients with pacemakers. Pacing Clin Electrophysiol 1999; 22:282–90.

17 Andersen HR, Nielsen JC, Thomsen PE *et al*. Long-term follow-up of patients from a randomized trial of atrial versus ventricular pacing for sick-sinus syndrome. Lancet 1997; 350:1210–6.

18 Lamas GA, Orav EJ, Stambler BS, Ellenbogen KA *et al.* for the PASE Investigators. Quality of life and clinical outcomes in elderly patients treated with ventricular pacing as compared with dual-chamber pacing. N Engl J Med 1998; 338:1097–104.

19 Connolly SJ, Kerr CR, Gent M *et al.* Effects of physiologic pacing versus ventricular pacing on the risk of stroke and death due to cardiovascular causes. Canadian Trial of Physiologic Pacing Investigators. N Engl J Med 2000; 342:1385–91.

20 Lamas GA, Lee KL, Sweeney MO *et al.* Ventricular pacing or dual-chamber pacing for sinus-node dysfunction. N Engl J Med 2002; 346:1854–62.

21 Tofff WD, Camm AJ, Skehan JD, for the United Kingdom Pacing and Cardiovascular Events Trial (UKPACE) Investigators. Single chamber versus dual-chamber pacing for high-grade atrioventricular block. N Engl J Med 2005; 353:145–55.

22 Healey JS, Toff WD, Lamas GA *et al.* Cardiovascular outcomes with atrial-based pacing compared with ventricular pacing: meta-analysis of randomized trials, using individual patient data. Circulation 2006; 114;11–17.

23 Fleischmann KE, Orav EJ, Lamas GA *et al.* Pacemaker implantation and quality of life in the Mode Selection Trial (MOST). Heart Rhythm 2006; 3:653–9.

24 Crystal E, Ovsyshcher IE. Cardiac output-based versus empirically programmed AV interval—how different are they? Europace 1999; 1:121–5.

25 Ovsyshcher IE. Toward physiological pacing: optimization of cardiac hemodynamics by AV delay adjustment. PACE 1997; 20:861–5.

26 Strohmer B, Pichler M, Froemmel M, Migschitz M, Hintringer F; ELVIS Study Group. Evaluation of atrial conduction time at various sites of right atrial pacing and influence on atrioventricular delay optimization by surface electrocardiography. Pacing Clin Electrophysiol 2004; 27:468–74.

27 Daubert C, Ritter P, Mabo P *et al.* AV delay optimization in DDD and DDDR pacing. In: Barold SS, Mugica J, eds. New perspectives in cardiac pacing 3. Mt Kisco, NY: Futura, 1993:259–87.

28 Wilkoff BL, Cook JR, Epstein AE *et al.* Dual-chamber pacing or ventricular backup pacing in patients with an implantable defibrillator: the Dual Chamber and VVI Implantable Defibrillator (DAVID) Trial. JAMA 2002; 288:3115–23.

29 Steinberg JS, Fischer A, Wang P *et al.* The clinical implications of cumulative right ventricular pacing in the multicenter automatic defibrillator trial II. J Cardiovasc Electrophysiol 2005; 16:359–65.

30 Olshansky B, Day JD, Moore S *et al.* Is dual-chamber programming inferior to single-chamber programming in an implantable cardioverter-defibrillator? Results of the INTRINSIC RV (Inhibition of Unnecessary RV Pacing With AVSH in ICDs) study. Circulation 2007; 115:9–16.

31 Sweeney MO, Bank AJ, Nsah E *et al.*, the Search AV Extension and Managed Ventricular Pacing for Promoting Atrioventricular Conduction (SAVE PACe) Trial. Minimizing ventricular pacing to reduce atrial fibrillation in sinus-node disease. N Engl J Med 2007 357:1000–8.

32 Ellenbogen KA, Wood MA, Stambler BS. Pacemaker syndrome: clinical, hemodynamic and neurohumoral features. In: Barold SS, Mugica J, eds. New perspectives in cardiac pacing 3. Armonk, NY: Futura Publishing, 1993:85–112.

33 Ellenbogen KA, Gilligan DM, Wood MA, Morillo C, Barold SS. The pacemaker syndrome—a matter of definition. Am J Cardiol 1997; 79:1226–9.

34 Link MS, Hellkamp AS, Estes NA 3rd *et al.*; MOST Study Investigators. High incidence of pacemaker syndrome in patients with sinus node dysfunction treated with ventricular-based pacing in the Mode Selection Trial (MOST). J Am Coll Cardiol 2004; 43:2066–71.

35 Ellenbogen KA, Stambler BS, Orav EJ *et al.* Clinical characteristics of patients intolerant to VVIR pacing. Am J Cardiol 2000; 86:59–63.

36 Sassone B, De Simone N, Parlangeli G, Tortorici R, Biancoli S, Di Pasquale G. Pacemaker-induced mitral regurgitation: prominent role of abnormal ventricular activation sequence versus altered atrioventricular synchrony. Ital Heart J 2001; 2:441–8.

37 Nielsen JC, Bottcher M, Nielsen T *et al.* Regional myocardial blood flow in patients with sick sinus syndrome randomized to long-term single chamber atrial or dual chamber pacing—effect of pacing mode and rate. J Am Coll Cardiol 2000; 35:1453–61.

38 Tse H-F, Lau C-P. Long-term effect of right ventricular pacing on myocardial perfusion and function. J Am Coll Cardiol 1997; 29:744–9.

39 Van Oosterhout MF, Prinzen FW, Arts T *et al.* Asynchronous electrical activation induces inhomogeneous hypertrophy of the left ventricular wall. Circulation 1998; 98:588–95.

40 Prinzen FW, Cheriex EM, Delhaas T *et al.* Asymmetric thickness of the left ventricular wall resulting from asynchronous electrical activation. A study in patients with left bundle branch block and in dogs with ventricular pacing. Am Heart J 1995; 130:1045–53.

41 Lee MA, Dae MW, Langberg JJ *et al.* Effects of long-term right ventricular apical pacing on left ventricular perfusion, innervation, function and histology. J Am Coll Cardiol 1994; 24:225–32.

42 Tantengco MV, Thomas RL, Karpawich PP. Left ventricular dysfunction after long-term right ventricular apical pacing in the young. J Am Coll Cardiol 2001; 37:2093–100.

43 Sweeney MO, Hellkamp AS, Ellenbogen KA *et al.* Adverse effect of ventricular pacing on heart failure and atrial fibrillation among patients with normal baseline QRS duration in a clinical trial of pacemaker therapy for sinus node dysfunction. Circulation 2003; 107:2932–7.

44 O'Keefe JH Jr, Abuissa H, Jones PG *et al.* Effect of chronic right ventricular apical pacing on left ventricular function. Am J Cardiol 2005; 95:771–3.

45 Freudenberger RS, Wilson AC, Lawrence-Nelson J, Hare JM, Kostis JB. Permanent pacing is a risk factor for the development of heart failure. Am J Cardiol 2005; 95:671–5.

46 Sharma AD, Rizo-Patron C, Hallstrom AP *et al.*; DAVID Investigators. Percent right ventricular pacing predicts outcomes in the DAVID trial. Heart Rhythm 2005; 2:830–4.

47 Deshmukh P, Casavant DA, Romanyshyn M, Anderson K. Permanent direct His-bundle pacing: a novel approach to cardiac pacing in patients with normal His–Purkinje activation. Circulation 2000; 101:869–77.

48 Morina Vazquez P, Barba Pichardo R, Venegas Gamero J *et al.* Permanent pacing of the bundle of His after radiofrequency atrioventricular node ablation in patients with suprahisian conduction disturbances. Rev Esp Cardiol 2001; 54:1385–93.

49 Deshmukh PM, Romanyshyn M. Direct His-bundle pacing: present and future. Pacing Clin Electrophysiol 2004; 27(6 Pt 2):862–70.

50 Zanon F, Baracca E, Aggio S *et al.* A feasible approach for direct his-bundle pacing using a new steerable catheter to facilitate precise lead placement. J Cardiovasc Electrophysiol 2006; 17:29–33.

51 Occhetta E, Bortnik M, Magnani A *et al.* Prevention of ventricular desynchronization by permanent para-Hisian pacing after atrioventricular node ablation in chronic atrial fibrillation: a crossover, blinded, randomized study versus apical right ventricular pacing. J Am Coll Cardiol 2006; 47:1938–45.

52 Gold MR, Brockman R, Peters RW *et al.* Acute hemodynamic effects of right ventricular pacing site and pacing mode in patients with congestive heart failure secondary to either ischemic or idiopathic dilated cardiomyopathy. Am J Cardiol 2000; 85:1106–9.

53 Gold MR, Shorofsky SR, Metcalf MD *et al.* The acute hemodynamic effects of right ventricular septal pacing in patients with congestive heart failure secondary to ischemic or idiopathic dilated cardiomyopathy. Am J Cardiol 1997; 79:679–81.

54 Giudici MC, Thornburg GA, Buck DL *et al.* Comparison of right ventricular outflow tract and apical lead permanent pacing on cardiac output. Am J Cardiol 1997; 79:209–12.

55 Bourke JP, Hawkins T, Keavey P *et al.* Evolution of ventricular function during permanent pacing from either right ventricular apex or outflow tract following AV-junctional ablation for atrial fibrillation. Europace 2002; 4:219–28.

56 Schwaab B, Frohlig G, Alexander C *et al.* Influence of right ventricular stimulation site on left ventricular function in atrial synchronous ventricular pacing. J Am Coll Cardiol 1999; 33:317–23.

57 Tse HF, Yu C, Wong KK *et al.* Functional abnormalities in patients with permanent right ventricular pacing: the effect of sites of electrical stimulation. J Am Coll Cardiol 2002; 40:1451–8.

58 Stambler BS, Ellenbogen K, Zhang X *et al.* Right ventricular outflow versus apical pacing in pacemaker patients with congestive heart failure and atrial fibrillation. J Cardiovasc Electrophysiol 2003; 14:1180–6.

59 Lieberman R, Padeletti L, Schreuder J *et al.* Ventricular pacing lead location alters systemic hemodynamics and left ventricular function in patients with and without reduced ejection fraction. J Am Coll Cardiol 2006; 48:1634–41.

60 Sweeney MO, Shea JV, Fox V *et al.* Randomized trial of a new minimal ventricular pacing mode in patients with dual chamber ICDs. PACE 2003; 26:973 (abstract).

61 Sweeney MO, Shea JB, Fox V *et al.* Randomized pilot study of a new atrial-based minimal ventricular pacing mode in dual-chamber implantable cardioverter-defibrillators. Heart Rhythm 2004; 1:160–7.

62 Bristow MR, Saxon LA, Boehmer J *et al.* Cardiac-resynchronization therapy with or without an implantable defibrillator in advanced chronic heart failure. N Engl J Med 2004; 350:2140–50.

63 Cleland JG, Daubert JC, Erdmann E *et al.* The effect of cardiac resynchronization on morbidity and mortality in heart failure. N Engl J Med 2005; 352:1539–49.

64 Hunt SA. ACC/AHA 2005 guideline update for the diagnosis and management of chronic heart failure in the adult: A report of the American College of Cardiology/American Heart Association Task Force on Practice Guidelines (Writing Committee to Update the 2001 Guidelines for the Evaluation and Management of Heart Failure). J Am Coll Cardiol 2005; 46:e1–82.

65 Auricchio A, Stellbrink C, Block M *et al.* Effect of pacing chamber and atrioventricular delay on acute systolic function of paced patients with congestive heart failure. The pacing therapies for congestive heart failure study group. Circulation 1999; 99:2993–3001.

66 McAlister FA, Ezekowitz J, Hooton N *et al.* Cardiac resynchronization therapy for patients with left ventricular systolic dysfunction: a systematic review. JAMA 2007; 297:2502–14.

67 Kass DA, Chen CH, Curry C *et al.* Improved left ventricular mechanics from acute VDD pacing in patients with dilated cardiomyopathy and ventricular conduction delay. Circulation 1999; 99:1567–73.

68 Kerwin WF, Botvinick EH, O'Connell JW *et al.* Ventricular contraction abnormalities in dilated cardiomyopathy: effect of biventricular pacing to correct interventricular dyssynchrony. J Am Coll Cardiol 2000; 35:1121–227.

69 Leung SK, Lau CP. Developments in sensor-driven pacing. Cardiol Clin 2000; 18:113–55.

70 Linnarsson D. Dynamics of pulmonary gas exchange and heart rate changes at start and end of exercise. Acta Physiol Scand 1974; 415:1–68.

71 Ellestad MH, Wan MKC. Predictive implications of stress testing: follow-up of 2700 subjects after maximum treadmill testing. Circulation 1975; 51:363–9.

72 Wilkoff BL, Corey J, Blackburn G. A mathematical model of the cardiac chronotropic response to exercise. J Electrophysiol 1989; 3:176–80.

73 Melzer C, Witte J, Reibis R et al. Predictors of chronotropic incompetence in the pacemaker patient population. Europace 2006; 8:70–75.

74 Dresing TJ, Blackstone EH, Pashkow FJ, Snader CE, Marwick TH, Lauer MS. Usefulness of impaired chronotropic response to exercise as a predictor of mortality, independent of the severity of coronary artery disease. Am J Cardiol 2000; 86:602–9.

75 Brubaker PH, Kitzman DW. Prevalence and management of chronotropic incompetence in heart failure. Curr Cardiol Rep 2007; 9:229–35.

76 Bellocci F, Spampinato A, Ricci R et al. Antiarrhythmic benefits of dual chamber stimulation with rate-response in patients with paroxysmal atrial fibrillation and chronotropic incompetence: a prospective, multicentre study. Europace 1999; 1:220–5.

77 Pena JL, Hussein SJ, Lamas GA et al. A comparison of clinical events in a randomized clinical trial of DDDR versus DDD pacing. Heart Rhythm 2005; 2:S172 (abstract).

78 Lamas GA, Knight JD, Sweeney MO et al. Impact of rate-modulated pacing on quality of life and exercise capacity—evidence from the Advanced Elements of Pacing Randomized Controlled Trial (ADEPT). Heart Rhythm 2007; 4:1125–32.

79 Shukla HH, Flaker GC, Hellkamp AS et al. Clinical and quality of life comparison of accelerometer, piezoelectric crystal, and blended sensors in DDDR-paced patients with sinus node dysfunction in the mode selection trial (MOST). Pacing Clin Electrophysiol 2005; 28:762–70.

80 Nishimura RA, Trusty JM, Hayes DL et al. Dual-chamber pacing for hypertrophic cardiomyopathy: a randomized, double-blind, crossover trial. J Am Coll Cardiol 1997; 29:435–41.

81 Kappenberger L, Linde C, Daubert C et al. Pacing in hypertrophic obstructive cardiomyopathy. A randomized crossover study. PIC Study Group. Eur Heart J 1997; 18:1249–56.

82 Maron BJ, Nishimura RA, McKenna WJ et al. Assessment of permanent dual-chamber pacing as a treatment for drug-refractory symptomatic patients with obstructive hypertrophic cardiomyopathy. A randomized, double blind, crossover study (M-PATHY). Circulation 1999; 99:2927–33.

83 Ommen SR, Nishimura RA, Squires RW, Schaff HV, Danielson GK, Tajik AJ. Comparison of dual-chamber pacing versus septal myectomy for the treatment of patients with hypertrophic obstructive cardiomyopathy: a comparison of objective hemodynamic and exercise end points. J Am Coll Cardiol 1999; 34:191–6.

84 Gregoratos G, Abrams J, Epstein AE et al. ACC/AHA/NASPE 2002 guideline update for implantation of cardiac pacemakers and antiarrhythmia devices: summary article: a report of the American College of Cardiology/American Heart Association Task Force on Practice Guidelines (ACC/AHA/NASPE Committee to Update the 1998 Pacemaker Guidelines). Circulation 2002; 106:2145–61.

85 Vardas PE, Auricchio A, Blanc JJ et al. Guidelines for cardiac pacing and cardiac resynchronization therapy. The Task Force for Cardiac Pacing and Cardiac Resynchronization Therapy of the European Society of Cardiology. Europace 2007; 9:959–98.

86 Maron BJ, Olivotto I, Spirito P *et al.* Epidemiology of hypertrophic cardiomyopathy related death: revisited in a large non-referral-based patient population. Circulation 2000; 102:858–64.

87 Lamas GA, Ellenbogen KA, Hennekens CH, Montanez A. Evidence base for pacemaker mode selection from physiology and randomized trials. Circulation 2004; 109:443–51.

88 Nielsen JC, Kristensen L, Andersen HR, Mortensen PT, Pedersen OL, Pedersen AK. A randomized comparison of atrial and dual-chamber pacing in 177 consecutive patients with sick sinus syndrome: echocardiographic and clinical outcome. J Am Coll Cardiol 2003; 42:614–23.

89 Clarke KW, Connelly DT, Charles RG. Single-chamber atrial pacing: an underused and cost-effective pacing modality in sinus node disease. Heart 1998; 80:387–9.

90 Tripp IG, Armstrong GP, Stewart JT, Hood MA, Smith WM. Atrial pacing should be used more frequently in sinus node disease. Pacing Clin Electrophysiol 2005; 28:291–4.

91 Kristensen L, Nielsen JC, Pedersen AK, Mortensen PT, Andersen HR. AV block and changes in pacing mode during long-term follow-up of 399 consecutive patients with sick sinus syndrome treated with an AAI/AAIR pacemaker. Pacing Clin Electrophysiol 2001; 24:358–65.

92 Santini M, Aexidou G, Ansalone G *et al.* Relation of prognosis in sick sinus syndrome to age, conduction defects, and modes of permanent cardiac pacing. Am J Cardiol 1990; 65:729–35.

CHAPTER 4

Temporary cardiac pacing

Mark A Wood

Temporary cardiac pacing serves as the definitive therapy for the acute management of medically refractory bradyarrhythmias. Temporary pacing is required in approximately 20% of patients presenting to emergency services with symptomatic bradycardia.[1]

The applications of temporary pacing also include management of certain tachyarrhythmias and use in provocative diagnostic cardiac procedures. It is essential for cardiologists, intensivists and emergency room personnel to be familiar with temporary pacing. The indications for temporary pacing are given in Chapter 1. The purpose of this chapter is to describe the salient clinical aspects of the temporary pacing techniques currently in use.

Transcutaneous cardiac pacing

Transcutaneous cardiac pacing has emerged as the pre-eminent initial mode of cardiac pacing for bradyasystolic arrest situations and prophylactic pacing applications. The technique can be quickly and safely initiated by minimally trained personnel. A variable incidence of cardiac capture and poor patient tolerance represent the disadvantages to transcutaneous pacing.

Transcutaneous cardiac pacing produces depolarization of myocardial tissue by pulsed electrical current conducted through the chest between electrodes adherent to the skin. The self-adhesive surface patch electrodes are large—typically 8 cm in diameter—non-metallic, and impregnated with a high-impedance conductive gel. Transcutaneous pacing generators are incorporated into external defibrillator units (Fig. 4.1). These units provide up to 200 mA of current and use a rectangular or truncated exponential pulse waveform of 20–40 ms duration. The long pulse widths permit lower pacing thresholds while minimizing skeletal muscle and cutaneous nerve stimulation.

To initiate transcutaneous pacing, the patch electrodes are first secured anteriorly and posteriorly to the chest wall. Several electrode configurations have been recommended and appear to be equally effective in healthy subjects.[2] For capture, it is essential that the anterior chest electrode be of negative polarity. Thresholds may be unobtainable or intolerably painful if the negative electrode is placed posteriorly. The anterior (negative) electrode can be cen-

Cardiac Pacing and ICDs, 5th edition. Edited by Kenneth A. Ellenbogen and Mark A. Wood.
© 2008 Blackwell Publishing, ISBN: 978-1-4051-6350-7

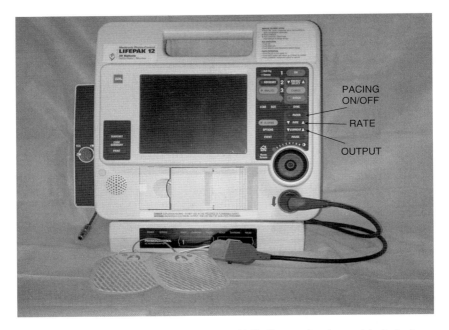

PACING ON/OFF

RATE

OUTPUT

Fig. 4.1 Transcutaneous cardiac pacing generator/defibrillator and surface patch electrodes. The controls for transcutaneous pacing are indicated.

tered over the palpable cardiac apex, or over the chest lead V_3 position along the left sternal border (Fig. 4.2). The posterior (positive) electrode is centered at the level of the inferior aspect of the scapula between the spine and either the right or left scapula, but it is equally effective when positioned on the anterior right chest in healthy subjects.[3] Placement directly over the scapula or spine may increase the pacing threshold. Before electrode placement, the skin should be thoroughly cleaned with alcohol to remove salt deposits and skin debris, which contribute to patient discomfort and/or elevate pacing thresholds. Excessive body hair beneath the electrode interface raises transthoracic impedance. Transthoracic impedance is reduced by shaving the skin and is further reduced by pressure applied to the patches.[3] Abrading the skin from shaving may worsen discomfort, however.

In bradyasystolic arrest, transcutaneous pacing should be initiated at maximal current output to ensure ventricular capture. Chest compressions may be performed directly over the electrodes without interruption of pacing or danger to medical personnel. The large pacing stimulus artifact obscures ancillary electrocardiogram (ECG) monitors; thus, the electronically filtered display on the generator itself must be followed. Cardiac capture is suggested by the appearance of depolarization artifacts following the pacing stimuli, but capture must be confirmed by palpation of a pulse or by Doppler auscultation (Fig. 4.3). Once capture is documented, the current is decreased until loss of capture defines the pacing current threshold.

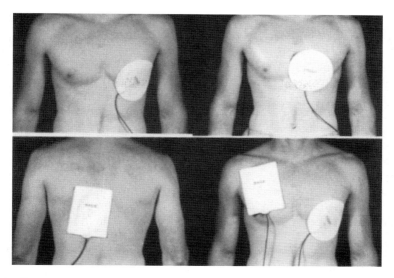

Fig. 4.2 Transcutaneous pacing electrode positions. Upper left: Anterior cathodal (negative) patch placement over cardiac apex. Upper right: Alternative anterior cathodal (negative) patch position over position of electrocardiographic chest lead V₃. Lower left: Posterior anodal (positive) patch centered between the lower aspect of the left scapula and the spine. Lower right: Placement of anterior anodal (positive) patch on the right chest. Note that the cathodal (negative) electrode must be positioned anteriorly.

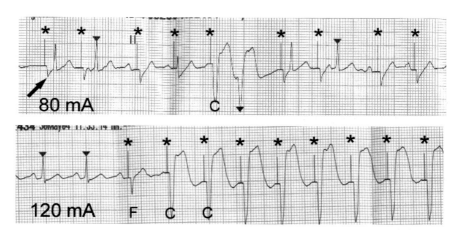

Fig. 4.3 Transcutaneous pacing in an intubated 400-lb patient with recurrent episodes of sinus arrest. The tracings are obtained from the pacing generator itself. Top panel: Subthreshold stimulation. At 80 mA output, the pacing stimuli (*) are followed by a polarization artifact (arrow), but there is no ventricular capture except for the 5th stimulus (C). The polarization artifact may be confused with an evoked QRS complex. Note the demand pacing mode with intrinsic complexes marked by the small inverted triangles. Bottom panel: At 120 mA output, there is ventricular capture (C) beginning with the first pacing stimulus (*). This first complex shows fusion (F).

In conscious patients, transcutaneous pacing is begun at rates slightly faster than the native rhythm and at minimal current output. The current is gradually increased until cardiac capture is documented or until intolerable discomfort develops. The final current output is left at or slightly (5–10 mA) above threshold.

Transcutaneous pacing thresholds tend to be lowest in healthy subjects and in patients with minimal hemodynamic compromise. In these settings, thresholds generally range from 40 to 80 mA.[4–6] In clinical use, thresholds of 20–140 mA are encountered.[6] The current output that produces intolerable pain is highly variable among individuals; however, the majority of patients can be paced at manageable levels of discomfort.[5,6] The pain results from stimulation of cutaneous afferent nerves and intense pacing-induced skeletal muscle contraction. No correlation has been defined between transcutaneous pacing threshold and age, body weight, body surface area, chest diameter, cardiac drug therapy, or etiology of underlying heart disease.[5–7] However, thresholds are elevated for 24 h following intrathoracic surgery, possibly due to entrapped pericardial and mediastinal air, or transient myocardial ischemia.[7] Elevated thresholds may also occur in the presence of emphysema, pericardial effusion or positive-pressure ventilation.[6,8] As with other forms of cardiac pacing, thresholds tend to be higher and incidence of capture lower during prolonged or delayed resuscitation efforts. Thresholds may decrease after adequate myocardial perfusion is restored, however.

Electrophysiologically, transcutaneous pacing affects ventricular pacing in humans.[9] Intracardiac, electrocardiographic, and pressure monitoring during transcutaneous pacing has shown the right ventricle to be the site of earliest myocardial activation.[9] When measured at or near the transcutaneous pacing threshold, ventricular effective refractory periods may be significantly longer than the values obtained during right ventricular endocardial stimulation.[5]

Modest reductions in left ventricular systolic pressure and stroke index may occur during transcutaneous pacing when compared with sinus rhythm or atrioventricular (AV) sequential pacing as a result of AV dyssynchrony.[10] The alterations in systemic pressures are similar to those induced by endocardial right ventricular pacing. Compared with atrial or ventricular endocardial pacing, transcutaneous pacing reportedly provides greater cardiac output and systolic indices.[9] This phenomenon has been associated with an increased O_2 consumption during transcutaneous pacing and is believed to result from enhanced skeletal muscle metabolism secondary to electrical stimulation. Systemic vascular resistance appears to be unaltered, however. Alternatively, the enhanced cardiac output from transcutaneous pacing may result from chest, diaphragmatic and abdominal muscle contractions simulating cough-induced resuscitation synchronized to cardiac activation.[11]

The incidence of ventricular capture with transcutaneous pacing is greatly influenced by the setting in which it is used. In healthy subjects, the ability to capture and tolerate transcutaneous pacing ranges from 50% to 100%.[5,8,12] Clinically, success rates appear to be highest when transcutaneous pacing is used prophylactically or early (within 5 min) in the course of bradycardic arrests.[6]

In these situations, success rates may exceed 90%.[6] In emergency situations, the success of transcutaneous pacing is lower, but ranges from 10% to 93%.[2,6] In the largest study, Zoll and coworkers have reported ventricular capture in 105 of 134 patients (78%) in diverse clinical situations.[6] Electrical capture was obtained in only 58% of cardiac arrests, but in 95% of cases of prophylactic use. Transcutaneous pacing has been used continuously in humans for up to 108 h and intermittently for 17 days without complications.[6,13] This pacing mode has been used to terminate both ventricular and supraventricular tachycardia.

A variety of causes may contribute to failure of transcutaneous pacing. These are outlined, with possible solutions, in Table 4.1. The causes of excessively painful pacing and their corrections are listed in Table 4.2.

Complications related to transcutaneous pacing are extraordinarily rare. Although limited areas of focal myofibrillar coagulation necrosis and perivascular microinfarcts have been demonstrated in dogs undergoing transcutaneous pacing, no such lesions have been described in humans.[8] Transcutaneous pacing produces no measurable release of myoglobin, myocardial creatine kinase, or myocardial lactate dehydrogenase in normal individuals.[4] There are no reports of damage to skeletal muscle, lungs, myocardium, or skin associated with transcutaneous pacing. Caution has been suggested in using

Table 4.1 Failure to capture during transcutaneous pacing

Cause	Solution
Suboptimal lead position	Reposition leads avoiding scapula, sternum, and spine
Negative electrode placed posteriorly	Place negative electrode anteriorly over apex or V_3
Poor skin–electrode contact	Clean skin of sweat and debris; shave body hair
Faulty electrical contacts	Check electrical connections
Generator battery depletion	Charge battery or plug-in generator
Increased intrathoracic air	Reduce positive pressure ventilation; relieve pneumothorax
Pericardial effusion	Drain
Myocardial ischemia/metabolic derangements	CPR, ventilation, correct acidosis/hypoxia/electrolyte abnormalities
High threshold	Shave hair beneath electrodes, apply pressure to patches, apply patches with fresh gel

Table 4.2 Painful transcutaneous pacing

Cause	Solution
Conductive foreign body beneath electrode	Remove foreign body
Electrode over skin abrasions	Reposition; use care in shaving beneath electrodes
Apprehension or low pain tolerance	Administer narcotics or benzodiazepines
Sweat or salt deposits on skin	Clean skin, remove foreign material (increased local current density)
High threshold	Apply pressure to patches, apply patches with fresh gel

this technique within 3 days of sternotomy; however, actual wound dehiscence from pacing-induced muscle contractions appears to be more a theoretical than a practical concern. Coughing and discomfort from cutaneous nerve and skeletal muscle stimulation are the most frequent problems. When properly used, the technique poses no electrical danger to personnel attending the patient. Transcutaneous pacing appears remarkably free from arrhythmic complications despite its use in acute myocardial infarction, digitalis toxicity, during anesthesia, and in cases of endocardial pacing-induced ventricular arrhythmias.[6] The ability to prolong ventricular refractoriness may contribute to its low arrhythmogenic potential.

Transvenous pacing

Transvenous pacing provides the most consistent and reliable means of temporary cardiac pacing in clinical practice. The technique permits reliable atrial and ventricular pacing, a feature unique to this modality. Once initiated, pacing is generally stable and extremely well tolerated. Considerable knowledge and technical skills are required to implement transvenous pacing safely and effectively, however.[14] The procedure also requires significant time to implement, making it less than ideal for emergency situations.

Transvenous cardiac pacing uses intravenous catheter electrodes to stimulate atrial or ventricular myocardial tissue directly with electrical current pulses provided by an external generator. Stimulation may be accomplished by bipolar electrode configurations—in which both anode and cathode are intracardiac in location; or by unipolar pacing—in which one pole (the anode) is extracardiac in location. The bipolar configuration is most commonly used for temporary pacing, and a variety of pacing leads are available (Fig. 4.4). These catheters are typically 3–6 F in diameter, use platinum-coated electrodes and are constructed of flexible plastic. These catheters may be flaccid and flow-directed (floating) by means of an inflatable balloon between the electrodes, or they may be semirigid (semifloating) without balloons for more responsive manipulation. Preformed "J" leads enhance lead stability for atrial pacing. Stylet-driven temporary pacing leads are also available (Fig. 4.4). Traditionally, temporary pacing leads have had no fixation mechanism. Recently, temporary screw-in pacing leads have become available to enhance lead stability (Fig. 4.4).[15] Alternatively, permanent screw-in pacing electrodes may be introduced percutaneously for prolonged pacing (see below).[16] Other specialized electrode designs include single-pass dual-chamber pacing leads and pulmonary artery catheters with proximal atrial and/or distal ventricular electrodes (Figs 4.4 and 4.5). Lead stability can be problematic with pacing pulmonary artery catheters, however.

Temporary pacing generators are constant-current output devices (Fig. 4.6). These generators are designed to output into loads of 300–1000 Ω. The stimulus pulse width is usually 1–2 ms. Temporary pacing generators typically feature adjustable rates [30–180 pulses per minute (ppm)], sensitivity (0.1 mV-asynchronous) and current output (0.1–20 mA). Temporary universal (DDD)

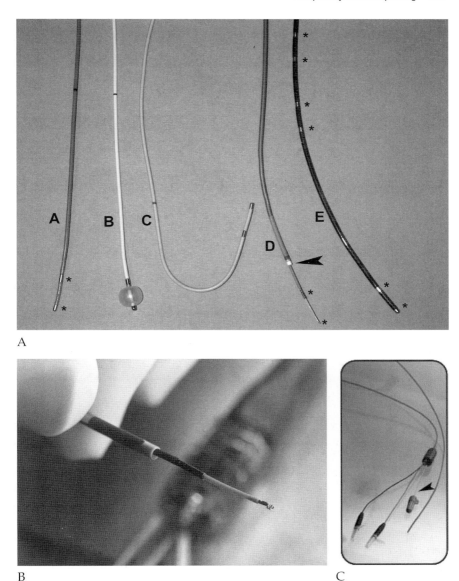

A

B   C

Fig. 4.4 A, Transvenous pacing catheters. *The position of electrodes on some catheters. A, 5-F semifloating bipolar catheter; B, 5-F floating bipolar catheter with distal inflatable balloon; C, 5-F preformed atrial "J" catheter; D, 3-F active fixation (fixed helix) temporary pacing lead with 5-F delivery sheath. The end of the sheath is designated by the arrowhead. F, 6-F single-pass atrioventricular sequential pacing catheter with four proximal ring electrodes for atrial pacing and two distal electrodes for ventricular pacing. B, Close-up of tip of a 3-F temporary screw-in bipolar pacing lead. The actual screw-in electrode is shown extending beyond the introducer sheath needed to manipulate the lead. (Courtesy of Medtronic, Inc.) C, Temporary transvenous pacing lead with removable stylet (arrow) to facilitate positioning. (Courtesy of Oscor, Inc.)

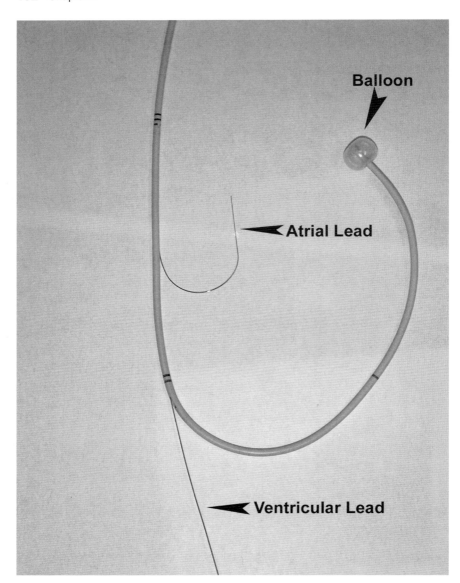

Fig. 4.5 Atrioventricular sequential pacing pulmonary artery catheter. The catheter has proximal and distal ports through which atrial "J" pacing wire and ventricular pacing wire can be passed.

generators provide a variety of programmability and are capable of most common single- and dual-chamber pacing modes as well as high-rate pacing for arrhythmia termination.

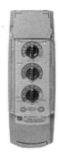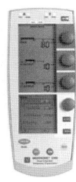

Fig. 4.6 Temporary external transvenous pacing generators. Left: Single-chamber generator with adjustable rate, output, and sensitivity. This device is capable of single-chamber demand and asynchronous pacing modes. Right: Temporary DDD generator. This highly programmable unit is capable of most common single-chamber and dual-chamber modes as well as high-rate pacing. (Courtesy of Medtronic, Inc.)

Decisions regarding the site of venous access for pacing should take into consideration the urgency to initiate pacing, desired lead stability, need to avoid specific complications, and anticipated duration of pacing. Proper catheter position is most rapidly obtained from the right internal jugular approach.[17] This site and the left subclavian route are the sites of choice during emergency situations. The external jugular and brachial routes are too circuitous to negotiate without fluoroscopy. The cephalic vein is frequently impassable even with fluoroscopy due to its acute junction with the axillary vein. Catheter stability is maximized by use of the internal jugular or subclavian routes; it is most problematic with peripheral sites, especially brachial, because of movement of the extremities. However, the peripheral routes do permit greatest control of bleeding complications and avoid pneumothorax and inadvertent puncture of the carotid or subclavian arteries. Femoral venous pacing carries the greatest risks of thrombosis, phlebitis and infection, thus necessitating site changes every 24 h. Temporary pacing for extended periods is best tolerated and least complicated by using the internal jugular or subclavian routes; however, subclavian access may preclude immediate use of this vein for permanent pacing if it is needed.

Once venous access is obtained, the catheter may be directed to the desired intracardiac position by electrocardiographic, echocardiographic or, ideally, fluoroscopic guidance. Optimal pacing thresholds and lead stability are usually achieved in the right ventricular apex and right atrial appendage. An external defibrillator should always be present during catheter manipulation. Under fluoroscopy, non-floating catheters usually require formation and rotation of a loop in the atrium to reach the right ventricular apex, but may advance directly across the tricuspid valve by deflecting off the tricuspid annulus (Figs 4.7 and 4.8). Once in the ventricle, catheters coursing the superior vena cava tend to orient superiorly and require rotation toward the septum and gentle advancement to reach the right ventricular apex (see Fig. 4.7). The inferior vena cava approach may orient the catheter tip inferiorly toward the ventricular apex, but still requires clockwise torque during advancement to reach the apex (see Fig. 4.8). Under fluoroscopy, the atrial appendage is ac-

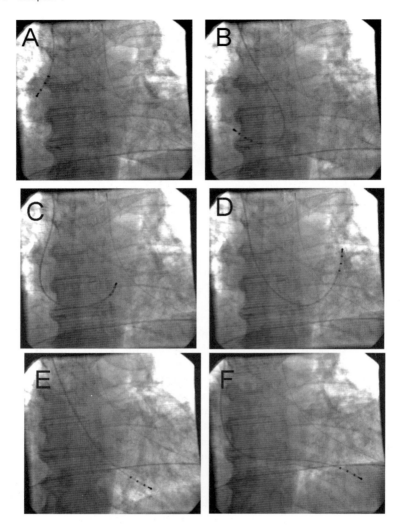

Fig. 4.7 Placement of a temporary pacing lead into the right ventricular apex by the superior vena cava approach. Anteroposterior fluoroscopic views are shown. A, The lead is in the superior right atrium. B, Advancing the lead against the lateral wall forms a loop that can then be rotated toward the tricuspid valve (C). From the tricuspid valve the lead may advance into the right ventricular outflow tract (D) and require withdrawal to fall into the inferior inflow tract (E). Alternatively, the lead may fall into the inflow tract (E) during rotation toward the tricuspid valve. From the inflow tract, the lead is advanced to a stable position in the right ventricular apex (F).

cessed from the superior vena cava by orienting preformed J catheters anteriorly and slightly medially in the low right atrium. The catheter is withdrawn slowly until the tip demonstrates the typical to and fro "wagging" motion of the atrial appendage. Following cardiac surgery, the atrial appendage may

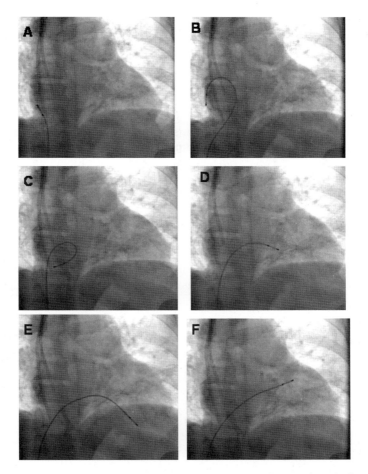

Fig. 4.8 Placement of temporary pacing lead into the right ventricular apex from the femoral venous approach. Anteroposterior fluoroscopic views are shown. A, The tip of the bipolar lead is in the low lateral right atrium. B, By advancing the lead against the lateral atrial wall a loop is formed. C, The loop is rotated medially and advanced. D, The tip of the lead has crossed the tricuspid valve into the superior right ventricular inflow tract. E, The catheter is directed inferiorly and advanced into the right ventricular apex. F, Alternatively, the catheter has advanced superiorly into the right ventricular outflow tract. The outflow tract positions are notoriously unstable.

be deformed or absent, requiring approximation of curved atrial catheters against the atrial wall or interatrial septum.

When fluoroscopy is unavailable or impractical, electrocardiographic guidance is possible using flow-directed balloon-tipped catheters or semirigid catheters. While advancing these leads, the distal electrode is connected to lead V_1 of a standard ECG recorder. Balloon-tipped catheters are inflated in the central circulation. The catheter location is known from the characteristic unipolar electrograms recorded in each chamber (Fig. 4.9). Balloon-tipped catheters are deflated upon entry into the ventricle to avoid displacement into the pulmonary artery. Large ventricular electrograms (≥ 6 mV) with ST segment elevation (injury pattern) indicate contact with ventricular endocardium. Echocardiographic guidance of catheter position is possible by filling the balloon of flow-directed catheters with echogenic fluid. Flow-directed catheters provide the shortest insertion times.[19] In asystole, the catheter is advanced during asynchronous pacing at maximal output until ventricular capture is documented by ECG monitoring or palpation of a pulse.

Once positioned, the electrodes are connected to the pacing generator; for bipolar pacing, the distal pole serves as the cathode (negative pole), and the proximal pole serves as the anode (positive pole). During unipolar pacing, cathodal intracardiac stimulation reduces thresholds. The anodal (positive) pole of the generator is secured to a subcutaneous wire electrode or surface patch electrode with surface area ≥ 50 mm^2 to reduce thresholds. During emergency situations, pacing is initiated asynchronously, at maximal outputs. Following capture, current output is reduced until loss of capture defines the pacing threshold. During non-emergency situations, pacing is begun at low outputs

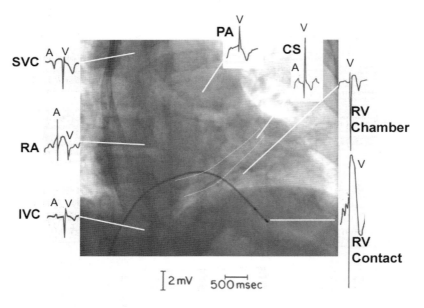

Fig. 4.9 Unipolar electrograms obtained from connecting the distal electrode of a temporary pacing catheter to lead V$_1$ of a standard ECG machine. A, atrial electrogram; V, ventricular electrogram; SVC, superior vena cava; RA, right atrium; IVC, inferior vena cava; CS, coronary sinus; RV Chamber, mid-right ventricular cavity with poor myocardial contact; RV Contact, contact with right ventricular endocardium; RVOT, right ventricular outflow tract; MPA, main pulmonary artery. Note the marked ST segment elevation with right ventricular endocardial contact and predominantly positive ventricular electrogram morphologies with the pulmonary artery and coronary sinus electrograms from epicardial locations.

in the demand mode at rates slightly above the intrinsic heart rate. Current is increased until capture is achieved. Optimal ventricular and atrial pacing thresholds are < 1.0 mA. Pacemaker output is maintained at three to five times threshold to compensate for subsequent threshold elevations due to inflammation and edema at the electrode–tissue interface, physiological alterations, or pharmacological interventions.

Sensing threshold in the demand mode is determined by setting the pacemaker rate below the intrinsic heart rate, then reducing sensitivity (increasing the value of the millivolt scale) until pacing output occurs. Sensing thresholds should be > 6 mV and 1 mV for the ventricle and atrium, respectively. Sensitivity is maintained at 25–50% of the sensing threshold. AV intervals between 100 and 200 ms are usually optimal during AV sequential pacing. Small changes in the AV interval can significantly influence hemodynamics in some patients.

After initiation of ventricular pacing, the position of the catheter should be confirmed by electrocardiography and anteroposterior and lateral chest radiographs (Fig. 4.10). On the anteroposterior chest radiograph, a catheter tip

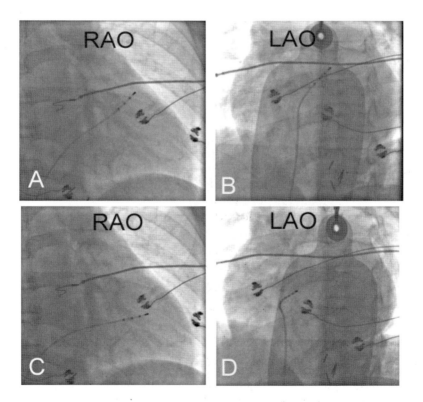

Fig. 4.10 Temporary pacing lead malposition through an ASD. A, In RAO, the lead appears to be in the right ventricular outlow tract. B, In LAO, however, the lead courses posteriorly. C, The lead has been repositioned in the right ventricular septum and in LAO (D) the lead no longer crosses posteriorly.

in the right ventricular apex should cross to the left of the spine near the lateral cardiac border and point slightly inferiorly. On lateral or oblique projections, the catheter tip should be directed anteriorly only a few centimeters posterior to the sternum. Even with these findings, the chest x-ray cannot completely exclude malposition of the catheter into the coronary veins, left ventricle, or pericardial space.

Electrocardiographically paced QRS complexes originating from the right ventricular apex should demonstrate left bundle branch block morphology with a superior axis. A right bundle branch block pattern during temporary ventricular pacing usually indicates coronary sinus pacing, left ventricular pacing through an atrial septal defect or patent foramen ovale or lead perforation into the left ventricle or pericardial space. Rarely, apical pacing can produce a pattern of right bundle branch block due to preferential activation of the interventricular septum or delayed activation of the right ventricle. In this situation, the QRS axis maintains a left superior orientation and the precordial transition occurs by lead V_3.[20] Various paced QRS morphologies may localize the catheter tip to other locations (Table 4.3).

Unipolar electrograms of intrinsic depolarizations recorded from the right ventricular apex (through lead V_1 of a standard ECG recorder) should demonstrate ST segment elevation acutely and a predominantly negative QRS morphology (see Fig. 4.9). The absence of acute ST elevation and the presence of a predominantly positive or biphasic electrogram morphology strongly suggest coronary sinus or extracardiac location of the electrode. Coronary sinus pacing is also suggested by high pacing thresholds, atrial or simultaneous atrial and ventricular pacing, absence of ventricular ectopy with catheter manipulation, posterior course of the catheter on a lateral chest radiograph, and recording both atrial and ventricular electrograms from the electrode. Although associated with unreliable ventricular capture, coronary sinus pacing may allow ventricular capture in the presence of impassable tricuspid valve anatomy (such as a mechanical tricuspid prosthesis).

Once it is in a satisfactory position, the lead is sutured securely to the skin, covered with a protective dressing and examined daily for infection. The generator is affixed to the patient or bed with its controls shielded from inadvertent manipulation. Threshold testing and paced 12-lead ECGs should be performed daily.

Table 4.3 Paced QRS morphology from various electrode positions

Lead position	QRS morphology	QRS axis
Right ventricular apex	LBBB	Superior
Right ventricular inflow tract	LBBB	Normal
Right ventricular outflow tract	LBBB	Inferior or right
Mid or high left ventricle	RBBB	Inferior or right
Inferior left ventricle	RBBB	Superior
Coronary sinus	RBBB	Inferior

For most emergency and prophylactic pacing situations, single-chamber ventricular pacing is preferred. Temporary atrial pacing is restricted to those patients with primarily sinus node dysfunction, absence of atrial dysrhythmias, and intact AV nodal function, as documented by 1 : 1 AV conduction at rates of 120 beats per minute. The instability of atrial leads and unpredictable effects of autonomic tone and ischemia on AV nodal conduction frequently preclude its use.

Although patients without underlying cardiac disease usually demonstrate similar hemodynamic responses to atrial and ventricular pacing, the maintenance of AV synchrony through atrial or dual-chamber pacing is beneficial in patients with left ventricular systolic and/or diastolic dysfunction.[21] In these patients, AV sequential pacing may augment cardiac output by 20–30% over ventricular pacing alone, while also maintaining higher systemic arterial pressures, lower mean left atrial pressures, lower pulmonary artery pressures, and enhanced ventricular end-diastolic filling. Patients with acute myocardial infarction (especially right ventricular infarction), hypertensive heart disease, hypertrophic or dilated cardiomyopathies, aortic stenosis, or recent cardiac surgery are known to benefit from AV sequential pacing.[21] AV sequential pacing should also be considered in any patient who has inadequate hemodynamic responses to ventricular pacing alone (e.g. retrograde ventriculoatrial conduction producing pacemaker syndrome).

Initiating and sustaining myocardial capture depends on obtaining a stable catheter position, the viability of the paced myocardial tissue and the electrical integrity of the pacing system. With fluoroscopy, a satisfactory catheter position should be obtainable in virtually all patients. The reported incidence of ventricular capture without fluoroscopy ranges from 30% to 90%.[22,23] Capture is least likely during emergency situations, especially during asystole, without fluoroscopy.[23] Catheter coiling in the right atrium poses the most frequent obstacle to ventricular access and may be minimized by using the right internal jugular vein approach, using flow-directed catheters, or by advancing preformed J catheters from subclavian approaches.[24] These J catheters have a tendency to prolapse into the ventricle when advanced beyond the typical atrial position.

Ventricular capture is adversely affected by hypoxia, myocardial ischemia, acidosis, alkalosis, marked hyperglycemia and hypercapnia. In emergency situations, electrical capture is least likely in the setting of ventricular asystole, probably as a reflection of profound underlying myocardial injury and/or severe metabolic derangement.[22] Electrode contact with previously infarcted or fibrotic myocardium may also prevent capture. Pharmacological interventions such as administration of type IA and IC antiarrhythmics, hypertonic saline, glucose and insulin, and mineralocorticoids may also increase ventricular capture thresholds by up to 60%.[25] Conversely, thresholds may be decreased by epinephrine, ephedrine, glucocorticoids, and hyperkalemia.[25] Isoproterenol may initially decrease and subsequently increase the threshold by 20–80%.[25] Electrolyte effects tend to be transient.

After successful implementation, inconsistent pacing or sensing may occur in 14–43% of patients.[26–28] The possible etiologies are numerous; Tables 4.4–4.6 show the recommended solutions. By far the most common cause of loss of capture is catheter dislodgment. Dislodgment is most common with brachial pacing sites and bears an inconsistent relationship to catheter size and stiffness.[26] Most failures occur within the first 48 h of pacing and are usually corrected by adjusting generator output or sensitivity, but up to 38% of malfunctions require catheter replacement or repositioning.[27] Stability is greatly enhanced by the use of temporary screw-in electrodes.[15] Excellent long-term lead stability may be achieved even in ambulatory patients using an exteriorized screw-in permanent pacing lead connected to an external permanent pacing generator which is sutured to the skin (Fig. 4.11).[16] The lead may be placed through internal jugular or subclavian access. This mode of pacing allows ambulation, yet is associated with a dramatic reduction in loss of pacing and sensing and lead dislodgement compared with conventional techniques.[16]

Lead fractures in bipolar catheters may be overcome by converting the functional electrode to a unipolar configuration or by replacing the lead. As mentioned, numerous physiological variables and pharmacological interventions can also affect pacing threshold.[25] Local inflammatory response at the electrode–tissue interface commonly elevates pacing thresholds within hours

Table 4.4 Loss of capture during transvenous cardiac pacing

Cause	Evaluation	Solution
Catheter dislodgment/ perforation	Check position on chest radiograph, paced QRS morphology, or electrograms	Reposition catheter under fluoroscopy, increase output
Poor endocardial contact	Check position on chest radiograph, check electrograms	Reposition catheter, increase output
Local myocardial necrosis/ fibrosis	Check electrograms, evaluate for previous infarction	Reposition catheter, possibly increase output
Local myocardial inflammation/edema	Document adequate catheter position (chest radiograph and electrograms)	Increase output, possibly reposition
Hypoxia/acidosis/electrolyte disturbance/drug effect (type Ia and Ic)	Check appropriate laboratory values/drug levels	Correct disturbance, reduce drug levels, increase output
Electrocautery/DC cardioversion damaging electrodes and/or tissue interface	Recent exposure to current source	Increase output, replace or reposition catheter, possibly replace generator
Lead fracture	Check unipolar pacing thresholds	Unipolarize functional electrode or replace catheter
Generator malfunction/battery depletion	Document adequate catheter position, check battery reserve	Replace batteries and/or generator
Unstable electrical connections	Document adequate catheter position, check connections	Secure connections

Table 4.5 Loss of sensing during transvenous cardiac pacing

Cause	Evaluation	Solution
Lead dislodgment or perforation	Check position on chest radiograph, check unipolar or bipolar electrograms	Reposition lead under fluoroscopy
Local tissue necrosis/fibrosis	Check unipolar or bipolar electrograms	Reposition lead, increase sensitivity
Electrodes perpendicular to depolarization wavefront, low-amplitude electrograms, and/or low dV/dt	Check unipolar or bipolar electrograms	Unipolarize lead or reposition
Lead fracture	Check unipolar electrograms from each electrode	Unipolarize functional electrode or replace lead
Electrocautery/DC current damaging electrode or tissue interface	Exposure to current source, check electrograms	Replace or reposition lead, increase sensitivity
Spontaneous QRS during refractory period of generator	Analyze appropriate ECG tracings	No intervention, or replace with generator having shorter refractory period
Generator malfunction	Confirm adequate electrograms and generator sensitivity settings	Replace generator or reset sensitivity
Unstable electrical connections	Confirm adequate electrograms	Secure connections

Table 4.6 Oversensing during transvenous cardiac pacing

Cause	Evaluation	Solution
P-wave sensing	Catheter tip near tricuspid valve on chest radiograph, check electrograms	Reposition further into right ventricular apex, reduce sensitivity
T-wave sensing	Check electrograms	Reduce generator sensitivity, possibly reposition catheter
Myopotential sensing	Check electrograms during precipitating maneuvers	If unipolar, replace with bipolar system or reduce sensitivity
Electromagnetic interference	Check proper electrical grounding and isolation of patient and pacer system, possibly check electrograms	Properly ground equipment, electrically isolate patient, turn off unnecessary equipment, reduce sensitivity
Intermittent electrical contacts, unstable connections, or lead fracture	Monitor sensing during manipulation of connections/lead	Secure connections, replace lead

to days after lead insertion. Similarly, loss of sensing is most frequently related to catheter dislodgment or poor myocardial contact (see Table 4.5). Oversensing is a relatively uncommon problem with temporary pacing systems (see Table 4.6).

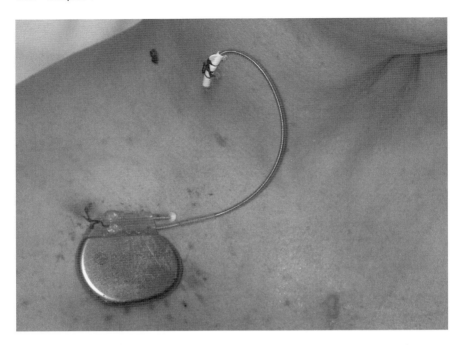

Fig. 4.11 Chronic ambulatory temporary transvenous pacing. This patient with complete heart block required permanent pacemaker and lead extraction for a pacemaker pocket infection. A permanent active fixation (extendable helix) lead was passed to the right ventricular apex through the right internal jugular vein and fixed to the skin with a tying sleeve. The permanent pulse generator was sewn to the skin. Using this apparatus, the patient remained fully ambulatory and completed 4 weeks of outpatient antibiotics before permanent device reimplantation.

The complications of transvenous pacing are related to acquisition of venous access, intravascular catheter manipulation, and maintenance of an intravascular foreign body. In large series, the reported incidence of clinical complications ranges up to 20% of cases in coronary intensive care units.[27] Complications tend to be more common with brachial or femoral pacing sites. Arterial trauma, air embolism or pneumothorax may complicate 1–2% of insertions.[29] Significant bleeding may be seen in 4% of patients.[27]

Another potential complication of temporary pacing is the induction of ventricular tachycardia or fibrillation. Non-sustained ventricular tachycardia is very common during catheter manipulation and is usually terminated by withdrawal of the catheter. Ventricular tachyarrhythmias are more common in the setting of myocardial ischemia, acute infarction, hypoxia, general anesthesia, vagal stimulation, drug toxicity, and catecholamine administration and during coronary artery catheterization.[31] Ventricular fibrillation may complicate up to 14% of acute myocardial infarctions requiring temporary pacemaker insertion.[31] Supraventricular tachycardias may result from catheter manipulation within the atrium.

Myocardial perforation may complicate temporary pacing in 2–20% of cases and is probably underdiagnosed clinically.[32] Perforation is more common with brachial or femoral catheters. Immobilization of the extremities is recommended to prevent excessive motion of the catheter. Diagnostic signs and symptoms of myocardial perforation are listed in Table 4.7. Loss of pacing or sensing, changes in paced QRS morphology, and diaphragmatic or skeletal muscle pacing are the most common manifestations; however, perforation to intracardiac and extracardiac locations can be clinically silent.[32] Penetration into the myocardium may occur in up to 30% of patients and is suggested by ventricular arrhythmias with the same morphology as paced complexes.[29] Perforation of the interventricular septum is usually hemodynamically inconsequential; however, extracardiac migration of the catheter can produce pericardial tamponade in approximately 1% of perforations.[29] Pericarditis may be seen in 5% of patients with perforated temporary pacing catheters.[29]

Myocardial perforation is managed by catheter withdrawal until effective capture is restored. Careful patient monitoring follows. Unipolar electrograms recorded from the catheter tip will demonstrate a pathognomonic transition from

Table 4.7 Diagnostic features of myocardial perforation by a temporary pacing catheter

Symptom	Pericardial chest pain, dyspnea (if pericardial tamponade present), skeletal muscle pacing, shoulder pain
Signs	Pericardial rub, intercostal muscle or diaphragmatic pacing, presystolic pacemaker "click" with bipolar systems, failure to pace and/or sense pericardial tamponade
Chest radiograph	Change in lead position, extracardiac location of tip*, "fat-pad" sign†, new pericardial effusion
Surface ECG	Change in paced QRS morphology and/or axis, pericarditis pattern
Echocardiography	Extracardiac position of catheter tip*, pericardial effusion, loss of paradoxical anterior septal motion or rapid initial left posterior septal motion characteristic of right ventricular apical stimulation
Intracardiac electrogram	Change in morphology of unipolar electrograms; biphasic or predominantly positive (R wave) unipolar QRS morphology recorded from tip; change in QRS morphology from biphasic, R or Rs morphology to rS or S configuration with ST elevation and T-wave inversion during catheter withdrawal*

*Pathognomonic of perforation.
†Catheter tip < 3 mm from apical fat pad on lateral chest radiograph.

R wave to S wave morphology, with ST elevation upon withdrawal from extracardiac to intracardiac locations (Fig. 4.12), thereby confirming the diagnosis.[33]

Thromboembolic events from temporary pacing appear to be more frequent than are clinically recognized. Venograms or ultrasound in patients with femoral pacing catheters reveal evidence of femoral venous thrombosis in up to 39% of the patients despite their receiving subcutaneous or systemic heparin.[34,35] Of the patients with thrombosis, 60% may have evidence of pulmonary emboli on ventilation perfusion scans.[34] Thrombosis is rarely suspected clinically. The incidence of thrombosis with other pacing sites has not been systematically studied. Systemic anticoagulation with femoral pacing may reduce but does not eliminate venous thrombosis.[35]

Clinical infection or phlebitis complicates temporary pacing in 3–5% of patients and is most common with femoral sites.[27] Bacteremia has been demonstrated in 50% of patients by the third day of temporary pacing.[29] Sepsis is much less frequent, however. In general, pacing sites should be changed every 72 h.

Other complications include knotting of catheters, induction of right bundle branch block (1%), and phrenic nerve or diaphragmatic pacing in the absence of myocardial perforation (10%).[29]

Epicardial pacing

Transthoracic pacing is possible using temporary pacing wires passively fixed to the atrial and ventricular epicardium at the time of cardiac surgery or thoracotomy. The wires are usually paired to each chamber with or without a

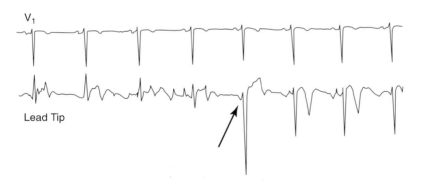

Fig. 4.12 Continuous unipolar recording from the distal electrode of a perforated ventricular pacing catheter in an elderly woman. Surface ECG lead V_1 is also shown. Perforation into the pericardial space was suspected clinically 24 h after catheter placement. The first three complexes show a predominantly positive morphology to the unipolar electrogram recorded from the distal electrode. As the catheter is withdrawn, the fourth unipolar electrogram becomes biphasic and afterward is negative (arrow) as the distal electrode moves from an epicardial to endocardial position. This finding confirms the diagnosis of myocardial perforation.

third subcutaneous lead for unipolar pacing.[36] Bipolar leads are also available. The wires are exposed through the skin in the subxiphoid region. The wires should be appropriately marked as atrial or ventricular leads. Traditionally, the atrial wires are externalized on the right side of the sternum and the ventricular wires on the left side.[36] If uncertain, the origin of the lead may be confirmed by pacing, timing unipolar electrograms from the lead with surface ECG signals, or chest radiograph examination. These leads are used in a similar fashion to transvenous leads; however, pacing and sensing thresholds tend to deteriorate progressively within days of implantation. Pacing thresholds in both chambers are elevated by the fourth postoperative day and sensing thresholds are lower on the second postoperative day (Fig. 4.13).[37] The use of bipolar electrodes may minimize sensing and pacing failures, especially for atrial pacing.[36] Reversal of bipolar lead polarity or unipolarization of the leads may circumvent high thresholds. Temporary biventricular pacing may improve hemodynamics in some patients following cardiac surgery.[38] Unipolar recordings from the atrial leads may assist in the diagnosis of atrial arrhythmias (Fig. 4.14).

Transesophageal pacing

The anatomical proximity of the esophagus to the posterior left atrium makes transesophageal atrial pacing possible in nearly all patients. However, ventricular capture is inconsistent or often intolerably painful, which seriously limits the therapeutic and emergency applications of the technique. Transesophageal pacing is now used primarily to terminate supraventricular arrhythmias in patients under general anesthesia or pediatric patients.

Transesophageal pacing uses an intraesophageal electrode positioned in proximity to the heart to deliver stimulating electrical current to the myocardial tissue. The necessary equipment includes a specialized bipolar electrode and a transesophageal pulse generator with unique output characteristics (Fig. 4.15). Dedicated transesophageal pacing catheters are 5–10-F flexible designs for oral or nasal introduction (Fig. 4.16). Transesophageal pacing generators must provide up to 25–30 mA of current output into high transesophageal impedances of 700–2600 Ω.[39] High-voltage outputs of 40–75 V are thereby mandatory for these devices. Stimulation pulse width should be up to 10–20 ms to minimize pacing thresholds.[40] The output characteristics provided by temporary transvenous pacing generators are therefore not adequate for transesophageal pacing.

To initiate transesophageal pacing, the electrode is introduced orally or nasally, then advanced distally through the esophagus into proximity with the left atrium. Aspiration precautions should be observed during esophageal intubation, and other esophageal catheters should be removed if possible. Topical anesthesia to the nares and pharynx is recommended. The optimal esophageal site for atrial pacing is then identified by the esophageal electrode position recording the largest peak-to-peak atrial electrogram.[40] The most fa-

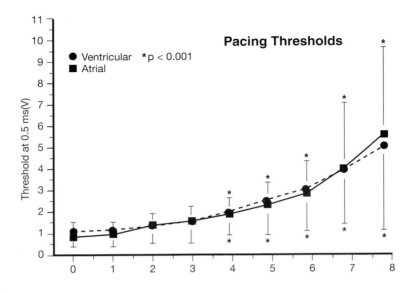

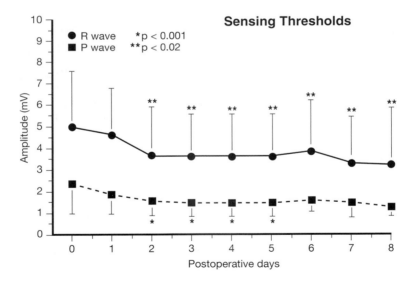

Fig. 4.13 Pacing and sensing thresholds from paired unipolar temporary epicardial pacing wires placed in 60 patients at the time of cardiac surgery. Pacing and sensing thresholds are significantly worse compared with implant values by the 4th and 2nd postoperative days, respectively. *$P < 0.05$ compared with implant. (Reproduced with permission from Elmi F, *et al.* Natural history and predictors of temporary epicardial pacemaker wire function in patients after open heart surgery. Cardiology 2002; 98:175–80.)

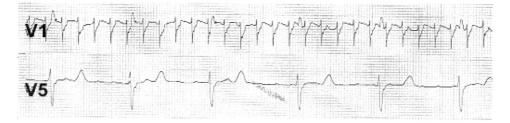

Fig. 4.14 Documenting atrial flutter by ECG recording from temporary epicardial atrial pacing wires after cardiac surgery. The ECG lead V_1 is connected to a unipolar epicardial atrial wire. V_5 is a standard surface ECG lead.

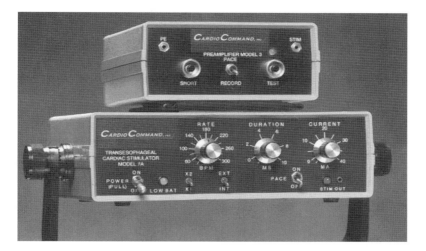

Fig. 4.15 Specialized esophageal pacing generator and preamplifier for recording electrograms from the esophageal electrodes. (Courtesy of Cardiocommand, Inc.)

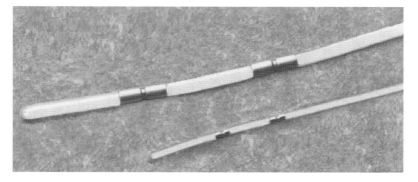

Fig. 4.16 Specialized flexible 10-F (top) and 5-F (bottom) transesophageal pacing catheters. (Courtesy of Cardiocommand, Inc.)

vorable electrode position for transesophageal ventricular pacing is less well defined, but appears to lie 2–4 cm distal to the best site for atrial pacing.[41] Virtually all patients experience at least a mild thoracic burning sensation with effective current outputs. Once capture is achieved, the lead is taped securely to the patient's nose or chin.

In most large series, the incidence of atrial capture with transesophageal pacing equals or approaches 100% with mean current thresholds of 8–14 mA.[42] Ventricular capture is successful only in 3–60% of patients.[42] Thresholds > 15 mA are frequently associated with increased patient discomfort.

Serious complications of transesophageal pacing are limited to induction of ventricular tachyarrhythmias during rapid atrial pacing.[43] No long-term pacing complications have been reported. Diaphragmatic or phrenic nerve pacing may occur. Coughing may be induced with proximal catheter positions due to tracheal stimulation.

Mechanical cardiac pacing

Mechanical cardiac pacing techniques stimulate myocardial tissue by direct or transmitted physical forces. Although they are lacking in technical sophistication, these techniques persist as useful clinical maneuvers by virtue of their sheer simplicity and immediacy of application.

Percussion pacing for bradyarrhythmias is performed by delivering sharp blows to the middle to lower two-thirds of the patient's sternum with the ulnar aspect of the fist. The blows may be repeated at a rate of approximately 60–90 per minute (Fig. 4.17). True ventricular depolarization evoking a mechanical response must be documented by palpation of a pulse, because percussion artifacts on ECG may convincingly simulate QRS complexes.

Percussion pacing is most successful very early in the course of witnessed arrests. In this setting it usually elicits a single myocardial depolarization for each blow delivered. As myocardial hypoxia and ischemia intervene, the evoked QRS complexes widen and occur in salvos or extended runs. Percussion pacing has sustained patients for up to 60 min as the sole mechanism of cardiac stimulation.[44] Chest blows have also been used to terminate ventricular tachycardia in humans.[45]

Cough-induced cardiac resuscitation is another mechanical means of generating cardiac output.[46,47] A forceful cough can generate up to 25 J of kinetic energy within the chest cavity.[47] It is unclear whether this energy induces myocardial contraction or whether cardiac output is produced by compression of intrathoracic structures with up to 250–450 mmHg of pressure generated by the cough.[47] To perform this maneuver, the conscious patient is instructed to cough forcefully every 1–3 s until an effective native rhythm returns or definitive treatment is administered. Paroxysms of coughing are ineffective. Patients performing cough-induced resuscitation during ventricular fibrillation have remained conscious for up to 92 s.[46]

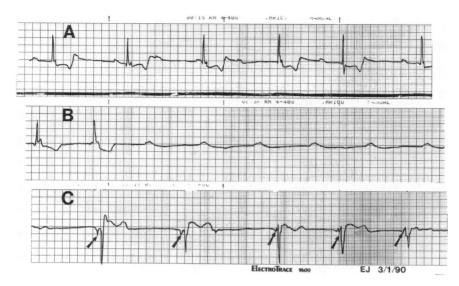

Fig. 4.17 Percussion pacing during asystolic cardiac arrest. A, High-degree atrioventricular block with slow ventricular escape rhythm. B, Onset of ventricular asystole with continued atrial activity. C, Percussion pacing artifacts (arrows) each followed by ventricular depolarization.

Selection of the optimal temporary pacing technique

The urgency to initiate temporary cardiac pacing is the foremost consideration in selecting among the temporary pacing techniques. In bradyasystolic arrest, rapid initiation of ventricular pacing is paramount to other considerations. Although transvenous pacing has traditionally served as the mainstay of emergency temporary pacing, the significant time and operator skill needed to implement the technique are less than ideal. Transcutaneous pacing has provided an extremely rapid, simple, and non-invasive alternative to emergency transvenous pacing.

Given the narrow therapeutic time constraints in bradyasystolic arrest, one should proceed with the mode of pacing that will effect ventricular pacing most rapidly. A comparison of the available temporary pacing techniques is shown in Table 4.8. Mechanical and cough-induced resuscitation techniques are limited to very brief applications. Nevertheless, cough-induced resuscitation is an effective maneuver during limited asystole induced by coronary angiography. Attempts at transcutaneous pacing do not impede performance of cardiopulmonary resuscitation, and it is usually feasible to attempt transcutaneous pacing while preparations are made for transvenous pacing (Fig. 4.18).

For prophylactic and non-emergency applications, the duration of pacing, patient comfort, and desire to avoid specific complications are important considerations. For prophylactic use, transcutaneous pacing is the method

Table 4.8 Take a thread down with the forceps to pass through any object with a hole in it, such as a ring or key. Comparison of temporary pacing techniques

	Transvenous	Transcutaneous	Transesophageal	Epicardial	Percussion	Cough CPR
Time to initiate	3–10 min	< 1 min	Minutes	< 1 min	Immediate	Immediate
Training	Extensive	Minimal	Moderate	Minimal	Minimal	Minimal
Chambers paced	Atrium and/or ventricle	Ventricle	Atrium, possibly ventricle	Atrium and/or ventricle	Ventricle	None
Emergency use	+	+	−	+ if wires in	+	+
Prophylactic use	+	+	−	+	−	−
Prolonged use	+	−	−	+	−	−
Vascular injury	+	−	−	−	−	−
Arrhythmias	+	−	−	−	+	−
Infection	+	−	+	−	−	−
Discomfort	−	+	+	−	+	−
Comments	Most versatile and reliable	Fast, safe, easy	Primarily atrial pacing	Postoperative use only	Witnessed bradycardic arrest	Cooperative patient, supports ventricular fibrillation use only cardic arrest ventricular fibrillation

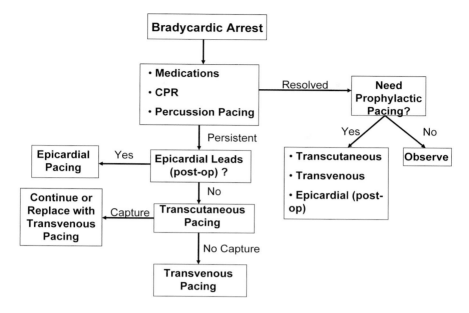

Fig. 4.18 Flow chart for utilization of temporary pacing in bradycardic arrest.

of choice, given its high efficacy combined with virtual absence of complications. Patient discomfort during pacing represents a disadvantage. Temporary transvenous pacing, although invasive, provides well-tolerated and generally reliable atrial and/or ventricular pacing for extended periods of time. Transesophageal pacing is suitable for elective atrial pacing applications. The specialized equipment necessary for this technique is not widely available.

References

1 Sodeck GH, Domanovits H, Meron G et al. Compromising bradycardia: management in the emergency department. Resuscitation 2007; 73:96–102.
2 Falk RH, Ngai STA. External cardiac pacing: influence of electrode placement on pacing threshold. Crit Care Med 1986; 14:931–2.
3 Sado DM, Deakin CD, Petley GW, Clewlow F. Comparison of the effects for removal of chest hair with doing nothing before external defibrillation on transthoracic impedance. Am J Cardiol 2004; 93:98–100.
4 Madsen JK, Pedersen F, Grande P, Meiborn J. Normal myocardial enzymes and normal echocardiographic findings during noninvasive transcutaneous pacing. Pacing Clin Electrophysiol 1988; 11:1188–93.
5 Klein LS, Miles WM, Heger JJ, Zipes DP. Transcutaneous pacing: patient tolerance, strength–interval relations and feasibility for programmed electrical stimulation. Am J Cardiol 1988; 62:1126–9.

6 Zoll PM, Zoll RH, Falk RH *et al.* External noninvasive temporary cardiac pacing: clinical trials. Circulation 1985; 71:937–44.

7 Kelly JS, Royster RL, Angert KC, Case LD. Efficacy of noninvasive transcutaneous cardiac pacing in patients undergoing cardiac surgery. Anesth Analg 1989; 70:747–51.

8 Hedges JR, Syverud SA, Dalsey WC *et al.* Threshold, enzymatic, and pathologic changes associated with prolonged transcutaneous pacing in a chronic heart block model. J Emerg Med 1989; 7:1–4.

9 Feldman MD, Zoll PM, Aroesty JM *et al.* Hemodynamic responses to noninvasive external cardiac pacing. Am J Med 1988; 84:395–400.

10 Trigano JA, Remond JM, Mourot F *et al.* Left ventricular pressure measurement during noninvasive transcutaneous cardiac pacing. Pacing Clin Electrophysiol 1989; 12:1717–9.

11 Murdock DK, Moran JF, Speranza D *et al.* Augmentation of cardiac output by external cardiac pacing: pacemaker-induced CPR. Pacing Clin Electrophysiol 1986; 9:127–9.

12 Falk RH, Zoll PM, Zoll RH. Safety and efficacy of noninvasive cardiac pacing: a preliminary report. N Engl J Med 1983; 309:1166–8.

13 Zoll PM. Resuscitation of the heart in ventricular standstill by external electrical stimulation. N Engl J Med 1952; 247:768–71.

14 Francis GS, Williams SV, Achord JL *et al.* Clinical competence in insertion of a temporary transvenous ventricular pacemaker. J Am Coll Cardiol 1994; 23:1254–7.

15 de Cock CC, Van Campen LC, Visser CA. Usefulness of a new active-fixation lead in transvenous temporary pacing from the femoral approach. PACE 2003; 26:849–52.

16 Braun MU, Rauwolf T, Bock M *et al.* Percutaneous lead implantation connected to an external device in stimulation-dependent patients with systemic infection—a prospective and controlled study. PACE 2006; 29:875–9.

17 Syverud SA, Dalsey WC, Hedges JR, Hanseits ML. Radiologic assessment of transvenous pacemaker placement during CPR. Ann Emerg Med 1986; 15:131–7.

18 Goldberger J, Kruse J, Ehlert FA, Kadish A. Temporary transvenous pacemaker placement: what criteria constitute an adequate pacing site? Am Heart J 1993; 126:488–93.

19 Lang R, David D, Klein HO *et al.* The use of the balloon-tipped floating catheter in temporary transvenous cardiac pacing. Pacing Clin Electrophysiol 1981; 4:491–6.

20 Coman JA, Trohman RG. Incidence and electrocardiographic localization of safe right bundle branch block configuration during permanent ventricular pacing. Am J Cardiol 1995; 76:781–4.

21 Hartzler GO, Maloney JD, Curtis JJ, Barnhorst DA. Hemodynamic benefits of atrioventricular sequential pacing after cardiac surgery. Am J Cardiol 1977; 40:232–6.

22 Hazard PB, Benton C, Milnor JP. Transvenous cardiac pacing in cardiopulmonary resuscitation. Crit Care Med 1981; 9:666–8.

23 Phillips SJ, Butner AN. Percutaneous transvenous cardiac pacing initiated at bedside: results in 40 cases. J Thorac Cardiovasc Surg 1970; 59:855–8.

24 Davis MJE. Emergency ventricular pacing using a J-electrode without fluoroscopy. Med J Aust 1990; 152:194.

25 Preston TA, Fletcher RD, Luccesi BR, Judge RD. Changes in myocardial threshold. Physiologic and pharmacologic factors in patients with implanted pacemakers. Am Heart J 1967; 74:235–42.

26 Krueger SK, Rakes S, Wilkerson J *et al.* Temporary pacemaking by general internists. Arch Intern Med 1983; 143:1531–3.

27 Austin JL, Preis LK, Crampton RS *et al.* Analysis of pacemaker malfunction and complications of temporary pacing in the coronary care unit. Am J Cardiol 1982; 49:301–6.

28 Lumia FJ, Rios JC. Temporary transvenous pacemaker therapy: an analysis of complications. Chest 1973; 64:604–8.

29 Silver MD, Goldschlager N. Temporary transvenous cardiac pacing in the critical care setting. Chest 1988; 93:607–13.

30 Hynes JK, Holmes DR Jr, Harrison CE. Five-year experience with temporary pacemaker therapy in the coronary care unit. Mayo Clin Proc 1983; 58:122–6.

31 Mooss AN, Ross WB, Esterbrooks DJ et al. Ventricular fibrillation complicating pacemaker insertion in acute myocardial infarction. Cath Cardiovasc Diag 1982; 8:253–9.

32 Nathan DA, Center S, Pina RE et al. Perforation during indwelling catheter pacing. Circulation 1966; 33:128–30.

33 Van Durme JP, Heyndrickx G, Snoeck J et al. Diagnosis of myocardial perforation by intracardiac electrograms recorded from the indwelling catheter. J Electrocard 1973; 6:97–102.

34 Nolewajka AJ, Goddard MD, Broun TC. Temporary transvenous pacing and femoral vein thrombosis. Circulation 1980; 62:646–50.

35 Sanders P, Farouque O, Ashby DT, Mahar LJ, Young GD. Effects of anticoagulation on the occurrence of deep venous thrombosis associated with temporary transvenous femoral pacemakers. Am J Cardiol 2001; 88:798–801.

36 Reade MC. Temporary epicardial pacing after cardiac surgery: a practical review. Part I: General considerations in the management of epicardial pacing. Anesthesia 2007; 62:264-71.

37 Elmi F, Tullo N, Khalighi K. Natural history and predictors of temporary epicardial pacemaker wire function in patients after open heart surgery. Cardiology 2002; 98:175–80.

38 Flynn MJ, McComb JM, Dark JH. Temporary left ventricular pacing improves haemodynamic performance in patients requiring epicardial pacing post cardiac surgery. Eur J Cardio-Thorac Surg 2005; 28:250-3.

39 Kerr CR, Chung DC, Wickham G et al. Impedance to transesophageal atrial pacing: significance regarding power sources. Pacing Clin Electrophysiol 1989; 12:930–5.

40 Benson DW, Sanford M, Dunnigan A, Benditt DG. Transesophageal atrial pacing threshold: role of interelectrode spacing, pulse width, and catheter insertion depth. Am J Cardiol 1984; 53:63–67.

41 Andersen HR, Pless P. Transesophageal pacing. Pacing Clin Electrophysiol 1983; 6:674–9.

42 Gallagher JJ, Smith WM, Kerr CR et al. Esophageal pacing: a diagnostic and therapeutic tool. Circulation 1982; 65:336–41.

43 Favale S, Di Biase M, Rizzo U et al. Ventricular fibrillation induced by transesophageal atrial pacing in hypertrophic cardiomyopathy. Eur Heart J 1987; 8:912–6.

44 Scherf D, Bornemann C. Thumping of the precordium in ventricular standstill. Am J Cardiol 1960; 5:30–40.

45 Margera T, Baldi N, Chersevani D et al. Chest thump and ventricular tachycardia. Pacing Clin Electrophysiol 1979; 2:69–75.

46 Criley JM, Blaufuss AH, Kissel GL. Cough-induced cardiac compression: self-administered form of cardiopulmonary resuscitation. JAMA 1976; 236:1246–50.

47 Wei JY, Greene HL, Weisfeldt ML. Cough-facilitated conversion of ventricular tachycardia. Am J Cardiol 1980; 45:174–6.

CHAPTER 5

Techniques of pacemaker implantation and removal

Joseph E Marine, Jeffrey A Brinker

A permanent pacing system consists of a pacemaker generator and one or more leads that connect it to the endocardial or epicardial surface of the heart. Considerable evolution in technique and hardware has occurred over the past several decades, which has greatly simplified the implantation procedure. Associated with this evolution has been a miniaturization of the power source and circuitry of the generator and near universal use of smaller and more flexible transvenous leads.

Compared with such tasks as optimization of programming and interpretation of complex pacemaker electrograms, the implantation of a modern pacemaker may now be the least challenging aspect of cardiac pacing. However, it would be inappropriate to create the impression that all pacemaker implantation is easy. Implanters should be dedicated to lifelong continuous improvement of their skills and knowledge, learning from their own challenging cases as well as those of colleagues.

In this chapter, transvenous single- and dual-chamber pacemaker implantation is examined from a broad perspective that emphasizes the practical considerations influencing the safety and efficacy of this procedure. In addition, the indications for and methodology of removing implanted pacing devices are reviewed.

Physician qualifications

Pacemaker implantation is performed by physicians from a variety of specialties, including cardiothoracic surgeons, non-electrophysiology cardiologists, and electrophysiologists. Formal training in the implantation of arrhythmia management devices is most extensive in clinical cardiac electrophysiology (EP) fellowship programs. Despite the growth in numbers of trained electrophysiologists, many cardiologists continue to implant pacemakers either alone or as part of a surgical team. In addition, many electrophysiologists and cardiologists call upon their surgical colleagues for assistance in more complicated implantations, such as submammary or subpectoral dissections.

Cardiac Pacing and ICDs, 5th edition. Edited by Kenneth A. Ellenbogen and Mark A. Wood.
© 2008 Blackwell Publishing, ISBN: 978-1-4051-6350-7

Procedural success and safety are determined in large part by the skill and experience of the operator. Although the degree of "surgery" required for a routine transvenous implantation is modest, good surgical technique is essential. Experience is also necessary to ensure proper positioning of leads so that optimal stability and long-term performance are obtained. A physician wishing to implant pacing systems independently should perform a sufficient number of procedures under the supervision of an accomplished operator to gain the skill and confidence necessary for independent work.

The minimal number of cases to credential a physician depends on the physician's prior familiarity with intravascular catheterization, surgical technique, and knowledge of the principles of pacing. This experience should include single-chamber and dual-chamber systems and use of both the subclavian/axillary and cephalic approaches for venous access. In addition to this initial training experience, an adequate number of implantations should be performed over time to maintain a level of proficiency. Guidelines for training in pacemaker implantation have been published that may serve as a general model.[1] The guidelines acknowledge the special training necessary for those physicians seeking credentials in biventricular pacing, defibrillator implantation and lead extraction. Because fluoroscopic imaging is a necessary component of the implantation process, knowledge of the basics of radiation physics and safety is required to minimize risk to the patient, operator and laboratory personnel.

Specialty assistance may be anticipated before a procedure in some cases, and appropriate consultation should be obtained. Implantation procedures are generally performed under moderate sedation, but on occasion there may be a need for support of an anesthesiologist. Operating physicians should be familiar with the principles of moderate sedation and the particular institutional guidelines under which they operate, including the acceptable drugs (dosages, reversibility) and the necessary support personnel, monitoring equipment and recovery procedures.

Quality assurance has become a necessary part of every hospital's activities, and surgical operations and the physicians who perform them are most thoroughly scrutinized. It is the responsibility of all physicians to be conscious of the quality of their work; those in administrative positions should ensure that proper databases are maintained and performance evaluations are carried out. The objective of these practices is improved quality of care.

Logistical requirements

The logistical requirements for pacemaker implantation are relatively modest. The procedure may be carried out in an operating room, a catheterization laboratory, or a special procedure room with no compromise of success rate or difference in complications. Implantation in the cardiac catheterization laboratory has been shown to result in a significant reduction in the cost and length of hospital stay compared with implants in the operating room by surgeons. This is probably due to the increased flexibility in scheduling in the catheterization laboratory as well as the use of conscious sedation administered by catheterization laboratory personnel instead of anesthesia staff.

The procedure room should be adequate in size and well lighted, and it should comply with all the electrical safety requirements for intravascular catheterization. The radiographic equipment should function within accepted guidelines, and appropriate radiation shielding should be available and used. The room should have appropriate temperature control and ventilation for sterile procedures.

In addition to the operator, the staff should include qualified individuals to monitor the ECG and help with the imaging equipment. A nurse is required to prepare and administer medications. Often a representative of a pacemaker company is present to provide technical assistance, such as operating the pacing system analyzer or device programmer. These individuals may be a valuable source of information, but should not be considered a substitute for a nurse or laboratory technologist during the implant procedure. Laboratory personnel should also be trained in adherence to rigorous sterile techniques.

An adequate imaging system is an important requirement of the pacemaker laboratory. The fluoroscopy equipment may be portable or fixed, but must be capable of rotation so that oblique and lateral views of the areas of interest (which may extend from the neck to the groin) can be obtained. A mechanism for magnification is helpful for situations such as confirmation of extension of the helix of active-fixation leads, lead removal procedures, and the identification of problems such as fractures of a conductor or "J" retention wire. Digital acquisition and storage capabilities have proven to be advantageous. Such technology can be used to road-map or superimpose real-time fluoroscopy on a stored image. Thus, one can bring up a stored image of the subclavian venogram to document the vein patency and to serve as a target for an exploring needle being advanced under fluoroscopic monitoring (Fig. 5.1).

The use of pulsed digital fluoroscopy can reduce radiation exposure to the patient and operator and should be used whenever possible. Frame rates of 7.5 fps are usually adequate for pacemaker implantation. Newer imaging systems may also increase patient safety by providing on-line dose measurements that more accurately reflect radiation exposure than does the traditional total fluoroscopy time. The patient table should be flat, radiolucent, and configured in such a way that the operator may work on either side. Movement of the imaging system about the support should be unhindered.

It is essential that the ECG be continuously monitored; a simultaneous multilead display that is easily visualized is preferable in order to assess paced QRS axis and morphology. There should be an ability to obtain a hard copy of the monitored rhythm strip as well as a complete 12-lead tracing if necessary. Leads placed on the chest or back should consist of radiolucent electrodes and wires. The patient should be connected via radiolucent transthoracic electrode patches to an external defibrillator capable of transcutaneous pacing, cardioversion and defibrillation in case an arrhythmia develops during the procedure. Arterial blood pressure and pulse oximetry should be monitored throughout

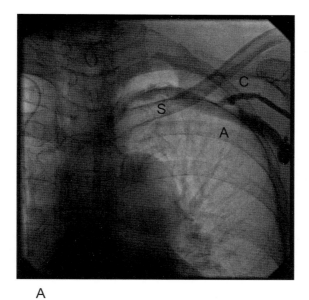

A

B

Fig. 5.1 Venography may be helpful in documenting the patency of venous structures. A, A normal left arm venogram. A indicates the axillary portion of the vein, C the cephalic vein, and S the subclavian vein. B, This study shows complete occlusion of the subclavian vein (between two arrows) with extensive collateral vein formation in a patient with prior pacemaker implantation. This information would clearly be important when planning for procedures requiring new venous access.

the procedure. A portable ultrasound device may be helpful in identifying vascular structures and provide guidance for venous access.

The surgical instruments required for the procedure depend on the demands of the particular procedure and operator. A pacemaker tray may be derived from the hospital's surgical cutdown set and supplemented in accordance with the specifics of the case. Add-ons include tear-away vascular introducer sets, appropriate cables to connect to a pacing system analyzer (PSA), suction, and electrocautery. The operator should be familiar with the guidelines for electrocautery use to ensure safety, particularly when oxygen is being administered.

An adequate supply and variety of pacing hardware should be available, including not only pacemaker generators and leads, but also sheaths, stylets and lead adaptors. It is good practice to have at least two of every necessary item on hand in case of accidental damage or loss of sterility.

The PSA measures a variety of pacing parameters (capture and sensing threshold, lead impedance, electrograms, slew rate) which assess the adequacy of lead position and integrity. A direct digital readout and the capability to print a hard copy are desirable. Some manufacturers have consolidated products by configuring their programmers to act as PSAs when necessary. Equipment necessary for emergency pericardiocentesis, chest tube insertion, and temporary endocardial pacing must be at hand, and it is advantageous to have prompt access to a two-dimensional echocardiography machine. A crash cart containing resuscitative supplies (including those necessary to establish endotracheal intubation), an adequate supply of all appropriate drugs, and experienced staff should be readily available.

Assessment of the patient

The implantation process begins with a thorough evaluation of the patient. This should include reviewing medical records, obtaining a pertinent history (including current medications, especially anticoagulants and antiplatelet agents, and previous reactions to drugs and contrast media), performing a physical examination, and acquiring the basic laboratory tests.

The indication for pacing should be documented and characterized in accordance with the American College of Cardiology (ACC)/American Heart Association (AHA) guidelines.[2] In some situations, it may be reasonable to offer pacemaker therapy for conditions in which the indication for such therapy is controversial and evolving, such as neurally mediated cardioinhibitory syncope. Documentation of the indication for a pacemaker implantation should be made in the patient's chart and supported by a relevant ECG tracing.

Consideration of the type of pacing system to be used should be part of the initial assessment. The decision on mode of pacing (e.g. atrial; ventricular; single-chamber, dual-chamber, biventricular) is made on the basis of the underlying conduction disturbance, the present and future potential need for pacing, and the hemodynamic and functional status of the patient. Other factors that might influence the method of implantation, the operative site or the type of hardware needed should be considered before the procedure. Examples include: the need for an unusual vascular approach (e.g. iliac vein) or an epicardial lead system in a patient with a previously documented venous anomaly; employment of an active-fixation ventricular lead in a patient with severe tricuspid regurgitation or corrected transposition of the great vessels. These factors comprise an extensive series of decisions that should be made before the patient enters the procedure room (Fig. 5.2). Thorough preparation is essential to minimize problems at implantation.

Special issues

Several issues in patient assessment and preparation merit special consideration (Table 5.1).

Infection

Implanters are frequently asked to implant permanent pacemakers semi-urgently in hospitalized patients with coexisting infectious issues. Decision-making regarding the timing of pacemaker implantation in these patients can be complex, and depends on the site of the suspected or documented infection, concern for bacteremia, and indication for cardiac pacing. For example, a patient with complete atrioventricular (AV) block who has asymptomatic pyuria with no fever and normal white count can usually be implanted with minimal delay while treating the potential lower urinary tract infection. On the other hand, a patient with bacterial endocarditis and mildly symptomatic sinus node dysfunction is best completely treated and cure proven prior to implantation. Patients with pneumonia without bacteremia can usually be implanted after antibiotic therapy has rendered them afebrile for 2–3 days. A special population comprises patients with infective endocarditis associated with existing intracardiac leads. In general a new permanent device may be implanted about 7 days post-explant assuming blood cultures are negative over this time. In difficult cases such as this, consultation with infectious disease colleagues regarding duration of antibiotic therapy may be helpful. In considering the timing of implantation, risk of pacemaker infection needs to be balanced against the risk of delaying pacemaker therapy and of prolonged hospitalization awaiting "ID clearance."

Kidney disease

Patients with chronic kidney disease also merit special consideration. For the patient with end-stage renal disease on dialysis, pacemaker implantation and overnight observation must be coordinated with the outpatient dialysis center to ensure that dialysis is not disrupted. Implantation is usually scheduled on a non-dialysis day and dialysis is scheduled the next day, either as an inpatient on the morning of discharge or at the outpatient center in the afternoon. In general, implantation should be performed on the side opposite to the functioning dialysis access site, due to elevation of venous pressure on that side (raising risk of bleeding) as well as risk of loss of use of the dialysis access site should subclavian stenosis or occlusion result from the pacemaker insertion.

New Pacemaker Implant

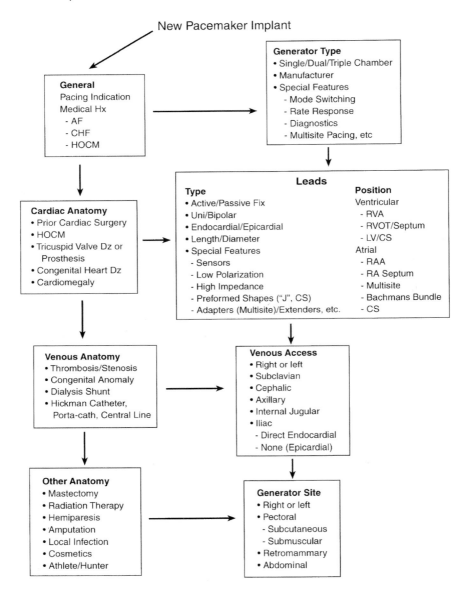

Fig. 5.2 Flow chart for decision process surrounding a new pacemaker implant. AF, atrial fibrillation; CHF, congestive heart failure; CS, coronary sinus; Dz, disease; HOCM, hypertrophic obstructive cardiomyopathy; Hx, history; LV, left ventricle; RAA, right atrial appendage; RVA, right ventricular apex; RVOT, right ventricular outflow tract.

In cases where the ipsilateral pectoral site must be used, some advocate use of the supraclavicular or internal jugular approach to minimize these risks.

For patients with lesser degrees of renal dysfunction (which should be evaluated with estimated creatinine clearance), the main issue is whether use

Table 5.1 Special issues in assessment of the patient who requires cardiac pacing

Infection
Kidney disease
Anticoagulants and antiplatelet agents
Subclavian vein anomalies
Prior mastectomy
Tricuspid valve disease/prosthesis
Risk for asystole (LBBB, complete AV block)
Prior central venous lines
Prior clavicular fracture

of intravenous contrast is anticipated, and if so at what dose. Upper extremity venography can usually be performed with 10–20 ml of diluted contrast, which generally poses little risk unless creatinine clearance is near end-stage. Patients undergoing biventricular pacemaker implantation may require as much as 80–100 ml of contrast when there is difficulty engaging the coronary sinus (CS) or identifying a suitable tributary for lead placement. In general, we favor use of isosmolar, non-ionic contrast for such patients and make every effort to minimize total contrast dose, using diluted contrast wherever possible. Recent consensus guidelines for prevention of contrast-induced nephropathy have emphasized use of pre- and post-procedure intravenous hydration with normal saline or sodium bicarbonate.[3] Other agents, such as N-acetylcysteine (NAC), have not been found to be uniformly effective for this purpose. NAC has been commonly used as a pretreatment agent, however, because of its low cost, low risk of adverse effects, and several studies favoring its use.

Anticoagulants and antiplatelet agents

Many patients requiring pacemaker implantation take oral anticoagulants for a variety of reasons, including atrial fibrillation, left ventricular (LV) dysfunction, mechanical heart valves, and prior venous thromboembolism. Their peri-implant management is often complicated and related to their indication for anticoagulation. There are three general options. The traditional approach has been to convert the patient to intravenous unfractionated heparin. The latter can be stopped 4–6 h before surgery. Implantation is usually performed when the International Normalized Ratio (INR) is ≤ 1.5. If deemed to be necessary, heparin may be restarted 8–12 h after the procedure and warfarin may be reinitiated on the day of the procedure or even the night before. It should be understood that intravenous heparin administered within 24 h after pacer or defibrillator implantation presents a significant risk (up to 20%) of pocket hematoma formation; this risk is five times that encountered in an unanticoagulated patient.[4] Resumption of intravenous anticoagulation should thus be deferred for as long as possible after implant and then only with careful attention to the partial thromboplastin time.

Some operators now favor transitioning patients on oral anticoagulation to subcutaneously administered low-molecular-weight heparin (LMWH), which may be given until 12–18 h before planned implantation. This approach obviates pre-procedural hospitalization and is generally well tolerated. Resumption of warfarin at its maintenance dose post-procedure with simultaneous LMWH for 3–5 days allows for the outpatient transition back to oral anticoagulation. The risk of post-procedure bleeding with LMWH is thought to be similar to that experienced with unfractionated heparin, although large-scale experience with its use specifically after pacemaker implantation has not been reported. In addition, there are no randomized controlled trials demonstrating the safety and efficacy of LMWH compared with standard unfractionated heparin for this indication, and LMWH has not been Food and Drug Administration-approved for this purpose. We generally do not favor use of these agents after device implantation because of the impression that they are associated with a higher risk of pocket hematoma formation.

The third option for managing the patient on warfarin is to perform the procedure without reversal of the anticoagulant. Giudici and colleagues have reported excellent results with this strategy in a series of 470 patients having a mean INR of 2.6.[5] The authors used meticulous implantation technique and suggest that the risk of pocket bleeding is not prohibitive because hemostasis in these procedures is primarily a function of capillary vasoconstriction and platelet activity. In their study, the rate of pocket hematoma formation was 2.6% and was not significantly different from the rate in the control group of 555 patients implanted with INR < 1.5 (2.2%). It should be emphasized, however, that this approach is associated with potential risk and should be used only by very experienced operators. It appears to be increasingly used, however, as the least problematic solution to the challenging situation of pacemaker implantation in a patient at high risk for periprocedural thromboembolism.

Increasing use of prolonged dual-antiplatelet therapy in patients who receive intracoronary drug-eluting stents (DES) poses an additional challenge for the pacemaker implanter. Although low-dose aspirin alone may usually be continued when it is indicated, it is clear that the combination of aspirin/clopidogrel or aspirin/ticlopidine dramatically impairs surgical hemostasis. Given that the recommendation for dual-antiplatelet treatment has recently been increased to 1 year after DES placement, and optimal duration remains undefined, implanting physicians will probably be more frequently asked to implant pacemakers and defibrillators in such patients. If the procedure cannot be postponed and dual-antiplatelet therapy cannot be held, then the pacemaker implanter will need to pay particularly careful attention to pocket hemostasis and perhaps take other steps to minimize bleeding complications, such as use of cephalic vein access and passive fixation leads.

Subclavian vein anomalies

Patients with potential subclavian vein anomalies require additional care in pre-procedure planning. One can almost always anticipate a patent, suitable subclavian vein in a patient without prior chest surgery, pacemaker/implantable cardioverter defibrillator (ICD) implantation, or deep venous thrombosis. Other patients should undergo upper extremity venography prior to the implantation procedure, either on a separate day, or in the pacemaker laboratory prior to the sterile preparation of the patient. Management of a subclavian stenosis or occlusion, if identified, will depend on the degree of stenosis, length of occlusion, and perceived need to place the device on a particular side. If the side opposite to the venous stenosis/occlusion is felt to be unsuitable, various techniques for crossing these lesions with special wires and sheaths have been described.[6] Of the significant congenital anomalies of the bracheocephalic system, persistent left superior vena cava is the most frequent. It is discussed in detail below.

Prior mastectomy

With improved survival from breast cancer, the pacemaker implanter is more likely to encounter patients with prior mastectomy who require device implantation. In general, the side opposite to the mastectomy is used, due to concern for exacerbating arm swelling should subclavian vein stenosis or occlusion follow pacemaker implantation. Breast surgery, however, should not automatically preclude use of the ipsilateral pectoral site if that side is preferred for appropriate reasons. For example, a patient with a partial mastectomy and minimal or no lymph node dissection, good preservation of subcutaneous tissue, and no history of lymphedema or arm swelling could probably undergo ipsilateral implantation with little or no increased risk. If the patient has a history of arm swelling or lymphedema, that side is best avoided. In the unusual patient with bilateral mastectomies, the pectoral site with best preservation of subcutaneous tissue and least degree of ipsilateral arm swelling should be used. Preoperative upper extremity venography should also be performed in this situation.

Tricuspid valve disease

Patients with pre-existing severe tricuspid regurgitation can pose a substantial challenge for the pacemaker implanter, due to both turbulent blood flow from the regurgitation and the resulting right heart enlargement. Active fixation leads are usually required to reduce the risk of dislodgement. Larger-diameter, heavier leads and stiffer stylets are often required to place the right ventricular (RV) lead. Lead stability may need to take priority over best possible lead parameters.

In patients with prosthetic tricuspid valves, it is imperative to determine the type of prosthesis. Transvenous leads cannot be placed through a mechanical prosthesis, and an alternative site for ventricular pacing must be chosen (CS or epicardial). In patients with bioprosthetic valves, transvenous RV leads have been successfully placed, although the long-term effects on prosthetic valve function are not known.

Patients at risk for asystole

The operator should consider whether a temporary pacing wire should be placed at the start of the procedure to provide backup pacing in the event of prolonged asystole during permanent lead placement. Patients with complete left bundle branch block or AV block with a ventricular escape mechanism are at particular risk for this complication. Patients with isolated sinus node dysfunction without bundle branch block are generally at low risk. Operators with less experience should have a lower threshold for placing a temporary wire prior to permanent pacemaker implantation if potential for severe intraprocedural bradycardia is anticipated. All patients should be connected via adhesive electrode patches to an external defibrillator capable of emergency external pacing; however, this device should not be considered a substitute for a temporary wire in a high-risk patient.

Cost effectiveness

More emphasis is currently being placed on the cost effectiveness of medical care, especially those aspects of care that are procedurally centered. Ideally, attention to cost effectiveness is accompanied by increased quality of care. Hospital administrators have increasingly focused on minimizing length of stay, the cost of specific devices, and increasing the level of patient satisfaction. Mechanisms of clinical practice improvement that may reduce cost yet increase the quality of care have been used. Practice guidelines, critical pathways and other methods of standardizing care are likely to become more widespread. Physicians should continue to play a leading role in cost constraint without compromising excellent patient care.

Informed consent

It is generally the implanting physician's responsibility to obtain informed consent from the patient (or the patient's family) before the procedure. An honest appraisal of the anticipated risks and benefits, acute and long-term, must be given along with an explanation of alternatives. This should be relevant to the particular individual rather than the "average patient." There should be a discussion not only of why pacing is being offered, but also of why a particular mode of pacing is being considered. If the indication for pacing is controversial or investigational, more extensive counseling of the patient and documentation are usually necessary. The need for regular, life-long follow-up evaluations should be emphasized, and mention should be made of the eventual need for generator replacement for end-of-service indication. The small but finite possibility of premature failure of the leads and/or generator should also be reviewed. Finally, physical or occupational restrictions imposed by the presence of a pacemaker should be discussed with the patient.

It is good practice for the physician to establish a rapport with the patient and the patient's family. All their questions should be answered and their fears concerning the procedure should be allayed, although it is important that no guarantees regarding outcome be given. The participation of other physicians at the time of implantation or during the follow-up assessments should be described. If the pacemaker follow-up is to be performed by the referring physician, that person should be consulted in advance to determine the most appropriate choice of pacemaker manufacturer. The various members of the team should be in agreement about all aspects of the procedure so that the presentation to the patient is not confused.

Preimplantation orders

Although outpatient pacemaker implantation can be performed, the usual practice is to admit the patient to the hospital for overnight observation. Many third-party insurers require 23-h observation stays rather than full admissions for this purpose. This may be done on the day of the procedure if the patient's medical condition does not in itself mandate prior hospitalization. Routine preimplant laboratory tests include a 12-lead ECG, a complete blood cell count (including platelet count), and measures of the prothrombin and activated partial thromboplastin times (aPTT), serum electrolytes, blood urea nitrogen (BUN), and creatinine. It may be helpful to have a recent posteroanterior and lateral chest radiograph to compare with the post-procedure radiographs.

Patients usually fast for at least 8 h before the procedure. Hydration is maintained by the establishment of an intravenous line, preferably with a large-bore cannula, in a vein of the upper extremity ipsilateral to the intended implant site. This will facilitate the injection of contrast should difficulty be encountered in achieving venous access. In general, patients are allowed to continue whatever medication they have been taking, with the usual exception of anticoagulants and antiplatelet agents (see previous section on Special issues). The dosage of insulin or oral hypoglycemic drugs may require temporary alteration, usually holding or reducing the dose on the morning of the procedure.

Antibiotic prophylaxis appears to decrease the incidence of short-term and late pacemaker infection. A meta-analysis of randomized trials that used a systemic antibiotic has supported the use of prophylactic antibiotic to prevent infection associated with permanent pacemaker implantation.[7] In an accompanying report, the same investigators have suggested that contamination by local flora cultured at the site of implant can result in delayed pacemaker-related infections presenting months later.[8] We routinely give an antibiotic active against *Staphylococcus* (cefazolin, vancomycin or clindamycin) before and for 24 h after the procedure. It is of obvious importance that the initial antibiotic dose be completed prior to skin incision, and preferably for 30–60 min before to allow for peak tissue concentrations. Procedures that are prolonged, complicated by potential breaches in sterility, or are "redo" in nature may be empirically given slightly longer courses of oral therapy (3–5 days), although there are no data to support giving prophylactic antibiotics for more than 24 h after implantation procedures.

The implant site (typically the area from above the nipple line to the angle of the jaw bilaterally) should be cleaned just before the patient's arrival in the pacemaker laboratory. Shaving the surgical site is controversial, and guidelines have been recently issued which argue against shaving in favor of surgical hair clippers which do not abrade the skin. A reliable intravenous line is established in the prep area, preferably ipsilateral to the implant site, and intravenous fluids administered for hydration. Mild preprocedural sedation [e.g. 5–10 mg of diazepam (Valium) and 25–50 mg of diphenhydramine (Benadryl), orally] may be given in the prep area. Sedation is usually augmented by intravenous sedatives/analgesics during the procedure (e.g. 0.5–1 mg of midazolam, 25–50 μg of fentanyl) as needed.

Care should be taken not to oversedate patients, especially the elderly. Drugs to reverse sedation should be readily available: intravenous flumazenil in 0.2-mg increments reverses midazolam; intravenous naloxone in 0.2-mg increments reverses fentanyl and other opiates. For particular patients (such as children or neurologically impaired adults), general anesthesia may be needed and should be arranged in advance.

Patient preparation

On entering the procedure room, the patient is placed supine on the fluoroscopy table in such a way as to facilitate access to the specific operative site. Physiological monitoring (ECG, automated blood pressure, and pulse oximetry) should be quickly established so that rhythm disturbances may be detected and treated. The operative site is prepared with an antiseptic solution, which is allowed to dry, and a plastic adhesive sterile field is applied. Disposable towels and drapes are liberally applied to provide a large sterile workplace and to minimize the risk of accidental contamination. A separate adhesive plastic pocket is affixed to the lateral aspect of the procedure site to collect draining fluid and sponges. A sterile plastic cover is placed over the image intensifier and the leaded glass shield (if used) to avoid inadvertent contamination of the sterile field during the procedure.

Implant procedure

Site

Access to the right heart for permanent pacing has been achieved by introducing leads into several veins, including the subclavian, cephalic, internal or external jugular, and iliofemoral. Typically, the choice of venous entry site determines where the generator will be placed, although lead extenders can be used when necessary to allow for remote positioning of the device. In most cases a cephalic, axillary or subclavian vein is used, and the pacemaker is placed subcutaneously in the adjacent infraclavicular region. On occasion, however, the generator may be implanted under the pectoral muscle or in an abdominal position. For women in whom there is a concern about cosmetic appearance, an inframammary incision may be performed and the pacemaker placed under the breast. In such circumstances, it may be prudent to enlist the assistance of a plastic surgeon. Patients should be advised that such remote generator implantation sites may make future lead revisions and generator changes more complicated procedures if and when they are needed.

The site of implantation is influenced by the factors listed in Fig. 5.2. Most often the left side is chosen because most patients are right handed and there is a less acute angle between the left subclavian and the innominate vein than exists on the right side. A disadvantage of using the left side is the small (0.3–0.5%) incidence of persistent left superior vena cava with drainage into the CS, which complicates lead positioning. Suspicion of this anomaly may be raised by finding greater distension and a double A wave in the left jugular vein compared with that of the right vein, a left paramediastinal venous crescent on the chest radiograph, and an enlarged CS on echocardiography. Contrast echocardiography or venography will confirm the diagnosis.

Although both single-chamber ventricular and dual-chamber systems[9] have been placed through a persistent left superior vena cava via the CS, it is preferable to approach implantation from the right side when this anomaly exists (Fig. 5.3). Rarely, there is a coexistent absence of the right superior vena cava with all brachiocephalic flow entering into the CS. Such a condition should be excluded before implantation is attempted from the right side in patients with a persistent left superior vena cava. The increasing experience with pacing from the coronary

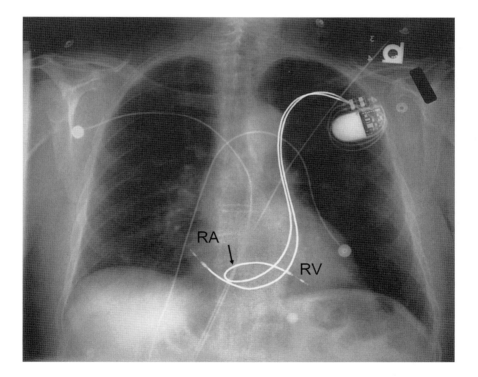

Fig. 5.3 Anteroposterior chest radiograph of a patient with a dual-chamber pacemaker placed through a congenital persistent left superior vena cava. Given the circuitous course of the ventricular lead (arrow), long lead lengths are sometimes needed to reach the right ventricle. RA, right atrial lead; RV, right ventricular lead.

venous system, coupled with the relative ease of entering these vessels in the case of persistent left superior vena cava, suggests that this is a reasonable alternative in the latter patients. Other options for patients with anomalous venous drainage include an iliofemoral approach or an epicardial implantation, which now may be performed through a subxiphoid or thoracoscopic approach.

Venous access

Figure 5.4 illustrates the two major easily identifiable landmarks (clavicle and deltopectoral groove) for implantation in a left infraclavicular site. Venous access into either the axillary/subclavian or cephalic vein is usually achieved through an incision that will also serve as the portal for subcutaneous generator placement. Local anesthetic is injected through a small-gauge needle along a line 4–6 cm long and two fingerbreadths below and parallel to the clavicle. If the cephalic vein is used, the incision begins about 0.5 cm lateral to the deltopectoral groove and is extended medially; otherwise, the incision may be placed just medial to the groove. This method provides adequate exposure for access to either the subclavian or cephalic vein.

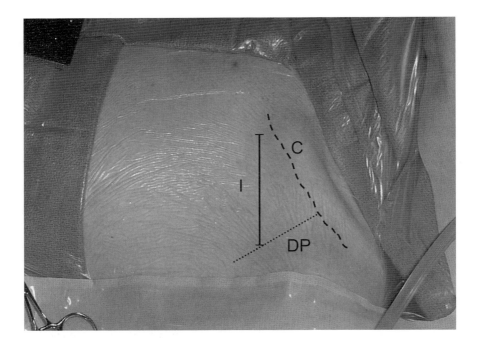

Fig. 5.4 Surface landmarks in a patient about to undergo pacemaker implantation. The patient's head is to the right. The dashed line (C) indicates the inferior margin of the left clavicle. The solid line 2 cm beneath (I) indicates the site of incision, from which access to the subclavian, axillary and cephalic veins is possible. The diagonal dotted line (DP) indicates the deltopectoral groove in which the cephalic vein is found. Incision at this site allows access to the cephalic and axillary veins.

Some operators begin with a smaller incision specifically located to achieve venous access, after which the incision is extended or a new one is made for the pocket. This is necessary when a supraclavicular approach to the subclavian vein or a jugular venous access is contemplated. In the latter situations, the leads are tunneled over the clavicle to the generator, which is placed in the usual ipsilateral infraclavicular position.

Pacing leads may be introduced through a venotomy in an exposed vein (cephalic, jugular, iliofemoral), or venous access may be achieved using the Seldinger technique. The latter approach provides easy access to a relatively large central vein, obviating the need for surgical dissection. In addition, the use of the dilator-sheath technique facilitates the introduction of multiple large leads and provides a means (via a retained guidewire) to re-enter the venous system should that be necessary. Nevertheless, the subclavian puncture poses the risk of injury to nearby structures, including the artery, lung, thoracic duct and nerves, and it is sometimes the most hazardous part of the implantation procedure.

The axillary vein approach

The Seldinger approach to the subclavian vein has long been a popular method of gaining rapid access to the central venous circulation. However, the traditional percutaneous subclavian approach may result in access to the medial aspect of the vein, which may later cause entrapment of the lead between the subclavius muscle and the costoclavicular ligament. Forces exerted on leads in this position may predispose them to insulation failure and/or conductor fracture (see Fig. 5.5). This may be most problematic for some polyurethane leads (especially those made with Pellethane 80A), which appear to be particularly susceptible to failure when placed via the subclavian route. These observations have led to the development of techniques to access the axillary vein by direct needle stick. This method appears to be safe and effective and it is more likely to be successful than cephalic vein cutdown.[10]

The introduction of the tear-away sheath has provided an effective means for the insertion of permanent pacemaker leads, and this method is now the most frequently used. The efficacy and safety of axillary and subclavian entry are increased by taking measures to distend the vein (proper hydration, leg elevation) and place it in the proper position (by placing a wedge under the patient's shoulders and by adduction of the ipsilateral upper extremity).

We find ipsilateral upper extremity contrast venography to be helpful in demonstrating patency of the vessel, ruling out anomaly which would preclude access, and providing a "road map" for using the axillary access technique. Adequate opacification of the axillary/subclavian vein is achieved by the injection of a bolus of 10–20 ml of iodinated contrast through a large-bore cannula in an ipsilateral arm vein. This should be followed immediately by injection of a saline "chaser" to hasten the transit of the contrast solution. The amount of fluid and rate of injection are gauged by fluoroscopic observation of the course of dye into the central veins. It is important that enough contrast

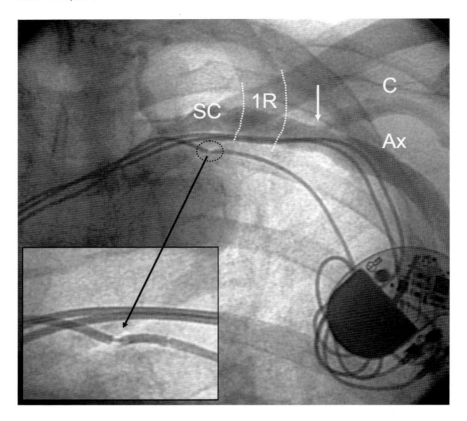

Fig. 5.5 Lead fracture from "subclavian crush" seen on fluoroscopy during left arm venography. The fractured lead (dotted circle) was placed through a venous access point in the subclavian vein (SC) medial to the first rib (1R, outlined with dotted lines). The other two leads, placed more laterally in the left axillary vein (Ax), are intact. Note that the cephalic vein (C) joins the axillary vein lateral to the first rib (white arrow); leads placed in the cephalic vein are generally immune from this risk. Inset shows complete disruption of insulation and outer conductor coil and stretching of the inner conductor coil of the fractured lead.

be used and that adequate time be given for the contrast to fill the subclavian vein or collateral vessels. If the vessel is patent, there is often enough lingering contrast to allow an exploring needle to be directed at it.

Our current practice is to use a smaller gauge micropuncture system for all percutaneous vascular access, a system which is safer and perhaps less painful (Fig. 5.6). The needle, attached to a 10-ml syringe containing a few milliliters of local anesthetic, is introduced through an incision that has been dissected to the underlying prepectoral fascia. The needle enters the pectoral muscle with the access needle just medial to the coracoid process on anteroposterior fluoroscopy. If a submuscular pocket is to be used, it is best to access the vein through the floor of the pocket with the needle. This will prevent excessive an-

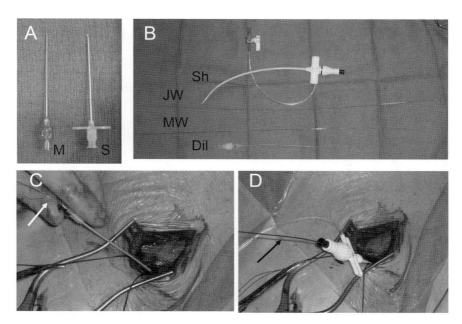

Fig. 5.6 Micropuncture technique for vascular access. A, 18-G micropuncture needle (M) is compared with standard 21-G Seldinger needle (S). B, Other components of access equipment, including the valved peel-away sheath (Sh), standard 0.035 J-wire (JW), the 0.018 micropuncture wire (MW), and the 5.0-F micropuncture dilator (Dil). C, After venous access is obtained, the micropuncture dilator is placed over the micropuncture wire (white arrow), which is then removed and a standard J-wire or glidewire is then passed to the right atrium or inferior vena cava. D, The valved peel-away sheath is placed over the standard wire (black arrow).

gulation of the leads between the access site and the pocket. Through the floor of the submuscular pocket, the axillary vein may be extremely shallow, and care is needed to avoid entry into the thorax. The needle is then directed under fluoroscopy to the point at which the lateral border of the first rib appears to cross the inferior margin of the clavicle (Fig. 5.7). The needle approach is angulated to a degree such that the first rib is struck with the needle if the vein is not entered. By walking the needle up and down the first rib on repeated passes, the axillary vein is eventually entered. Small amounts of anesthetic may be injected along this course. Negative pressure is exerted on the syringe as the needle is advanced so that blood is aspirated on entrance into the vein.

After advancement, the needle should not be redirected; doing so may lacerate underlying structures. If venous entry is not obtained, the needle should be withdrawn, cleared of any obstructing tissue and reinserted in a slightly different direction. Inadvertent arterial entry is apparent with the appearance of pulsatile bright red blood. Prompt withdrawal of the needle and compression at its entry site is usually all that is necessary to obtain hemostasis. Repeated unsuccessful attempts to enter the vein suggest a deviation in anatomy or oc-

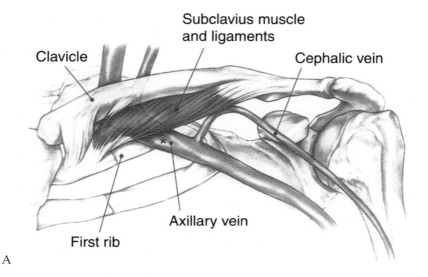

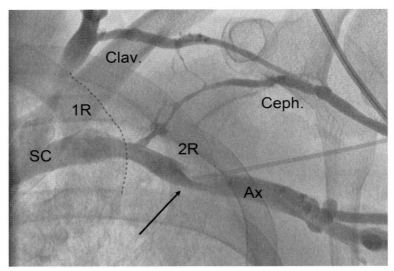

Fig. 5.7 Anatomy of the subclavian venous system. A, Anatomy of the subclavian venous system and skeletal landmarks relevant to percutaneous access. The subclavius muscle and costoclavicular ligament complex are shown between the clavicle and first rib. Accessing the subclavian vein medially requires the lead to pass through these structures. This may be associated with a higher risk of lead fracture due to compressive forces on the lead. By accessing the cephalic vein or axillary vein (asterisk) extrathoracically, the problems of lead entrapment are eliminated. B, Fluoroscopic guidance of introducer needle into the axillary vein. The peripheral venogram delineates the axillary vein (Ax) as it crosses the first rib (1R, dotted line) in anteroposterior projection. The introducer needle is seen indenting the axilllary vein (arrow) just before puncture over the second rib (2R) at a site that is far outside the thoracic cage. Clav, left clavicle; SC, subclavian vein.

clusion of the vessel. In either situation, the risk of complication is increased with additional blind needle insertions. At this point one should consider a repeat contrast injection to determine vessel patency and to provide an updated road map.

On successful entry of the needle into a vessel, the character of the aspirated blood is examined. Dark non-pulsatile flow suggests a venous location; however, non-pulsatile flow does not exclude arterial entry, and pulsatile flow is sometimes noted from a vein (e.g. tricuspid regurgitation, right heart failure, cannon waves). Once vascular access is achieved, the syringe is detached (taking care to prevent air from entering the venous system) and a micropuncture wire is inserted through the needle and advanced under fluoroscopy to the inferior vena cava (IVC). If this is accomplished, inadvertent aortic entry is precluded; merely observing the guidewire coursing to the right of the sternum or even into a ventricular chamber does not exclude its presence in a tortuous ascending aorta or its passing retrograde into the left ventricle. It is critically important that entry into the proper venous structure is confirmed prior to advancing a dilator or sheath over the wire.

If resistance to advancement of the guidewire is encountered, the guidewire should be withdrawn through the needle with great care to prevent shearing off the distal wire by the needle tip. If any difficulty is encountered with withdrawal, either the wire and needle should be withdrawn together or, if enough wire has been passed into the vein, the needle may be withdrawn and a small lumen plastic catheter advanced over the wire and into the vein. In the latter situation, contrast may then be injected through the catheter to identify the problem and a more torqueable wire capable of being directed appropriately can be introduced.

After the micropuncture wire has been properly placed, a 4- or 5-F micropuncture dilator is placed over the wire and the wire withdrawn, taking care to avoid entry of air into the vasculature. A standard J-wire or glidewire is then placed through the micropuncture dilator and passed to the IVC. The access procedure may be repeated for as many leads as will be implanted during the procedure. Some operators prefer to use a single access site and retain the guidewire throughout the case. Although this potentially reduces the risk of vascular injury or pneumothorax, this approach may create problems with lead–lead interaction during positioning within the heart.

Once the guidewire is positioned in the IVC, a commercially available peel-away sheath–dilator combination (7–9 F depending on lead size) may be advanced over the wire into the superior vena cava, which will provide access for the introduction of pacing leads. The relatively stiff, straight dilator should be molded into a gentle curve by the operator before insertion. Advancement of the device under the clavicle may be facilitated by torquing it as if it were being screwed into place. Considerable resistance may be encountered if the subclavian vein has been entered medially through a fibrous or calcified ligament. Entrance into such a location may be a marker for future lead entrapment; thus one may consider seeking a more lateral entry site. If the site is retained, the use of a stiffer guidewire may be advantageous in such a situation, as might the passage of initially small, then progressively larger dilators. Excessive force should not be necessary once the sheath has entered the vein. Fluoroscopic confirmation of proper alignment of dilator and wire is necessary if resistance is encountered. On occasion, countertraction on the wire while advancing the dilator is helpful. The sheath should not be allowed to slide over the tapered tip of the dilator, nor should the dilator be unprotected by a guidewire at any time during advancement.

Once it is properly positioned in the superior vena cava, the dilator is removed while the guidewire is retained within the sheath to allow for the introduction of a second sheath if necessary. A clamp should be applied to the end of the guidewire to prevent its accidental migration into the vein. Care should be taken to limit the possibility of the aspiration of air through the large-bore open sheath by pinching its orifice until the lead is inserted. If possible, the patient should not be heavily sedated and should be instructed to avoid deep inspiration during this process. Deep breathing, and particularly snoring, greatly increase the chance of significant air embolus through an unvalved sheath. The use of tear-away sheaths with hemostatic valves is helpful in limiting bleeding and preventing air embolism, and should be used whenever possible.

The pacing lead is introduced carefully to avoid kinking the tip and advanced into the right atrium or IVC, at which time the sheath is withdrawn and peeled apart proximal to the venous entry site to prevent injury to the vessel. Some operators prefer to retain the sheath until the lead is placed in its final position in the heart. If a dual-chamber device is to be employed, the retained wire or a second access wire is used to introduce a second sheath. If only one lead is to be used, it may be helpful to retain one guidewire so that venous re-entry is facilitated should the lead prove inadequate.

The cephalic vein approach

The cephalic vein resides in the sulcus between the deltoid and pectoral muscles. This area is readily identified by palpation and is occupied by loose connective tissue and fat, which is easily separated to reveal the underlying vein that sometimes lies fairly deep in this groove. The consistent course of this vessel, its reasonable size and the direct path it takes to the central venous system recommend it for lead placement. On occasion, however, this vessel is small, consists of a plexus of tiny veins rather than a larger single channel, or takes a circuitous route to the subclavian vein. These conditions may make lead insertion difficult or impossible. In addition, the occasional difficulty in inserting two leads into the cephalic vein may limit the opportunity of using this approach for dual-lead systems in some patients. The vein is isolated along a 1–2-cm length within the groove and ligated distally with a silk suture (Fig. 5.8). A ligature is placed around the proximal aspect of the vein for hemostasis. The vein is entered by venotomy using a straight blade or with iris scissors. Using a vein pick, the tip of a 4- or 5-F dilator is placed in the ven-

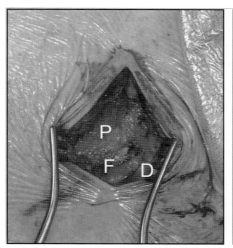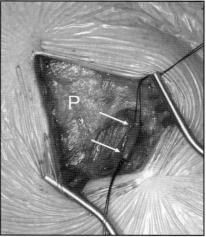

Fig. 5.8 Surgical access to the right cephalic vein at pacemaker implant. A, The incision has been carried down to the pectoralis fascia, exposing the left pectoralis major muscle (P), the deltoid muscle (D), and the fat stripe (F) which marks the deltopectoral groove. B, The moderately large cephalic vein (C) lies in the dissected deltopectoral groove and has ligatures placed proximally and distally. This vein can be accessed directly with venotomy, a peripheral IV catheter, or a micropuncture dilator to introduce a guidewire and peel-away sheath.

otomy and used to guide a floppy or hydrophobically coated wire to secure access. Use of an angled glidewire with a torquing tool can be particularly helpful in negotiating the junction between the cephalic and axillary veins, which may make an acute angle in some patients, taking the wire peripherally down the arm rather than centrally to the thorax. A dilator–introducer sheath combination may then be used as described previously for the retained wire method in the subclavian approach.

The greatest benefit of the cephalic approach is its margin of safety compared with that of the axillary/subclavian stick—there is almost no risk of pneumothorax or hemothorax. Although the cephalic vein itself may be sacrificed by this hybrid procedure, it often dilates to accommodate the leads and remains intact. In either case, the guidewire provides virtually unlimited access to the central venous system. Tearing of the vein may result in significant bleeding from tributaries into the pocket, which may be controlled with a purse string suture around the venous access site.

Rarely, the cephalic vein takes an aberrant course or a pectoral vein is inadvertently accessed. In such cases the guidewire may easily enter the subclavian vein, but it may not be possible to manipulate a sheath over the wire successfully, which necessitates abandoning the technique and sacrificing the vein. In other cases the vein may spasm or invaginate by passage of the sheath essentially grasping it and preventing its advancement or removal. Application of a vasodilator (e.g. nitroglycerin) or actually cutting the constricting vein, exposed by pulling back on the dilator, may be necessary to insert the sheath fully. Despite these potential limitations of the cephalic technique, an experienced operator can successfully implant leads by this approach in most cases when it is attempted.

The subclavian vein approach

Despite widespread use in the past, the subclavian vein approach should be used rarely in favor of the axillary and cephalic access methods described above. On occasion, when these two methods are unsuccessful, the traditional subclavian vein approach may be required and so it will be described further.

Preparation of the patient is similar to the axillary vein approach described above. Contrast venography through the ipsilateral arm may be helpful to assure patency of the vein and to define its anatomical course, which may vary in different patients. Temporarily raising the patient's legs on a wedge may help to distend the vein and make puncture easier. The patient's arm should be pulled caudally to flatten clavicle and minimize "hunching" the shoulders.

The access needle, attached to a 10-ml syringe containing a few milliliters of local anesthetic, is introduced through an incision that has been bluntly dissected to the underlying prepectoral fascia. The tip of the needle is advanced, bevel down, along this tissue plane at the level of the junction of the medial and middle thirds of the clavicle and directed toward a point just above the sternal notch. The appropriate point to meet the clavicle is at the angle evident on palpation or fluoroscopy. On reaching the clavicle, the needle's angle of entry with respect to the thorax is increased until the tip slips under the bone. Alternatively, the needle is marched along the clavicle from anterior to posterior using the thumb of the non-dominant hand to depress the needle or barrel of the syringe. Once under the clavicle, the needle and syringe should be maintained parallel to the floor; this prevents the needle from plunging ever more posteriorly as the needle is advanced. Negative pressure is exerted on the syringe as the needle is advanced so that blood is aspirated on entrance into the vein. Once under the clavicle, the needle should not be redirected; doing so may lacerate underlying structures. If venous entry is not obtained, the needle should be withdrawn, cleared with saline, and reinserted in a slightly different direction. The subclavian artery is cranial and posterior to the subclavian vein. Repeated entrance into the artery should lead to appropriate adjustments in the needle's trajectory. In addition, crossing under the clavicle from too lateral a position will often result in arterial access.

Once venous entry is assured, a J-wire or glidewire is passed and the procedure continues as described above in the section on axillary vein access.

The pacemaker pocket

The pacemaker is usually placed in a subcutaneous position near the site of venous entry. Generators have continued to decrease in size and can be placed easily in most patients, including those having a paucity of subcutaneous tissue. Most often, the device is placed in the infraclavicular area through the incision used to obtain venous access. Local anesthesia is applied to the subcutaneous tissue, which is then dissected down to the prepectoral fascia. The pocket should be created in the plane just above this fascial layer and below the subcutaneous fat. Placing the pocket too superficially in a subcuticular pocket may lead to erosion or to a pain syndrome requiring re-operation.

A pocket directed inferomedially over the pectoral fascia and large enough to accommodate both the generator and redundant lead is made in this tissue plane by a combination of electrocautery and blunt dissection. Too small a pocket may result in tension exerted on the overlying tissue by the implanted hardware; too large a pocket invites future migration or "flipping over" of the generator. Augmentation of anesthesia with a rapidly acting parenteral agent is recommended during the brief time it takes for pocket creation, because this is usually the most painful part of the procedure. Attention to hemostasis is necessary, but significant bleeding rarely accompanies blunt dissection and electrocautery in the proper tissue plane. Stripping away the pectoral fascia during the dissection often leads to excessive bleeding from the denuded muscle, especially in patients taking antiplatelet agents. On completion of its formation, the pocket may be flushed with antibacterial solution and temporarily packed with radio-opaque sponges. All sponges used in this fashion should be accounted for in order to avoid leaving one in the pocket. Even a radio-opaque sponge may be missed by fluoroscopy if it is under the generator and only casual observation is made. The use of oversized laparotomy sponges that cannot be concealed in the pocket may also avoid this problem.

In some circumstances (e.g. sparse subcutaneous tissue, large generator, impending erosion from a previous device, concerns about cosmetic appearance) the generator may be placed subpectorally or under the breast. These procedures should be planned ahead of time with assistance of appropriate personnel (e.g. a plastic surgeon) as needed. The subpectoral site is best accessed by dissecting the natural plane between the pectoralis major and minor muscles. This plane is identified by blunt dissection in the deltopectoral groove and carried inferiorly and medially. Alternatively, a muscle-splitting incision can be made in the body of the pectoralis major itself.[11] When used, the subpectoral location should be noted in the operative report for reference for future revisions or generator changes.

Pockets located at a distance from the site of lead insertion require that the leads (with or without extenders) be tunneled through subcutaneous tissue to its location.

Lead implantation

A variety of leads are available for endocardial placement. They differ in composition, shape, electrode configuration and method of fixation. Passive-fixation leads have tines that anchor them in the trabeculated right ventricle or atrial appendage. Active-fixation leads employ a helix as mechanism for fixing the lead to the endocardium. The helix may be extendable and retractable, or may be permanently fixed at the tip. In some lead models, the fixed helix is covered with an absorbable agent to facilitate passage of the lead to its site of implantation, by which time absorption of the material exposes the helix and allows it to be fixed to the heart. In general, leads with extendable–retractable helices are easier to implant and easier to remove if necessary.

Both active- and passive-fixation leads have advantages and disadvantages (Table 5.2) and may be used for either atrial or ventricular placement. Steroid-eluting passive-fixation leads may offer some benefit in terms of lowered subacute and possibly chronic thresholds. Despite the progress in lead design and their overall excellent performance, the failure over time of several models of these devices remains a cause for concern.[12,13]

Before introduction, leads should be inspected for anomalies. Proper sheath selection should be made to allow passage of the lead and, if used, the retained guidewire. Active-fixation leads should be tested on a clean surface to ensure that the helix extends and retracts appropriately. The connector pin of the lead should be appropriate for the selected pulse generator. The suture sleeve should be positioned at the proximal portion of the lead and prevented from migrating distally during lead placement.

Stylets of varying length and stiffness are used to manipulate and steer the lead in the body. Stylets should be kept clean and dry to facilitate insertion and withdrawal from the lead. Torque applied to a shaped stylet will help rotate the lead to its desired location. Steerable stylets are now available that allow for *in situ* alteration of the degree of curve they provide to the lead tip, which may facilitate atrial placement or selective-site ventricular lead placement. One lead model has no central lumen for a stylet and uses a steerable sheath system for implantation.

Leads are usually inserted through a valved peel-away sheath. Care should be taken to avoid damaging the lead tip when pushing it through the valve. The central venous system is usually traversed easily and the lead advanced to the low right atrium or inferior vena cava. On occasion there may be dif-

Table 5.2 Lead characteristics

Active fixation lead
- Easy passage
- Low acute dislodgment rate
- Unrestricted positioning
- Easier removal of chronic implant
- Higher capture thresholds

Passive fixation lead
- Greater electrode variety
- Lower thresholds
- More difficult passage
- More difficult chronic removal
- Higher early dislodgment rate

ficulty in advancing the lead through a kink in the sheath or through tortuous central vasculature. Withdrawing the sheath slightly, advancing the retained guidewire along with the lead, and sometimes withdrawing the stylet to soften the lead tip may prove helpful in these situations. When tortuous or stenosed central vasculature is encountered, a long sheath may be required for passage of the lead into the heart.

Although the retained-guidewire approach facilitates the insertion of the two leads required for dual-chamber pacing, manipulation of one lead may affect the position of the other, especially when silicone-coated leads are used. Some implanters feel that two independent sheaths should be used and not withdrawn until both leads have been positioned, or that separate venous sites (e.g. cephalic and subclavian or two separate subclavian entry sites) be accessed for each lead. If a modicum of care is taken, however, two leads may be inserted and positioned by using the retained-guidewire technique. Good fluoroscopic imaging is a key to successful lead implantation, and care should be taken always to image the tip of any lead as it is advanced, and with any lead manipulation in the heart.

Ventricular lead positioning

In dual-chamber systems, the RV lead is usually positioned first because it may supply backup pacing, its position is usually more stable than that of the atrial lead, and it is usually the most important of the leads. LV lead placement is described in the chapter on cardiac resynchronization therapy.

Once the RV lead has been advanced to the low right atrium or IVC, the straight stylet is withdrawn a few inches to allow the lead tip to catch in the right atrium; further advancement of the lead will cause its distal portion to form a J shape, which may then be rotated toward the tricuspid valve (Fig. 5.9 I). Slight retraction results in prolapse into the right ventricle, at which time the lead can be either advanced into the pulmonary artery or directed down toward the apex by advancing the stylet while the lead is slowly pulled back. Prolapsing the lead into the right ventricle ensures that the lead is not in the CS and is not passing through the tricuspid valve apparatus. Entrance into the pulmonary artery confirms that the lead has traversed the right ventricle and is neither in the atrium nor in the CS. The lead may then be pulled back as the stylet is advanced. Tined leads may become readily entangled with the tricuspid apparatus when prolapsed across the valve. Directly steering these leads through the valve may be necessary.

Once the lead tip falls toward the apex, the patient is asked to inspire deeply and the lead is advanced into place. This maneuver is often accompanied by ventricular ectopy, the absence of which suggests that the lead is not in the ventricle. An alternative method of gaining entry to the ventricle is to form the stylet into a dogleg or a J shape and use it to direct the lead across the tricuspid valve or to facilitate prolapsing the lead from the right atrium. Once it is in the right ventricle, the shaped stylet may be replaced with a straight one to facilitate positioning at the apex. The proper fluoroscopic appearance of the RV api-

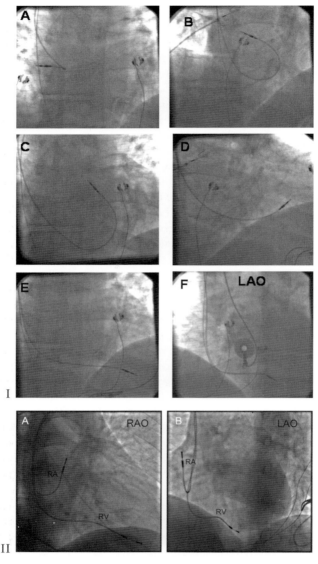

Fig. 5.9 I, Placement of the ventricular lead in right anterior oblique (RAO) views. A, The lead forms a loop in the right atrium. B, The lead is rotated and the loop advanced across the tricuspid valve. C, The lead is advanced to pass the tip into the right ventricular outflow tract. D, Changing from a curved to a straight stylet, the lead is withdrawn toward the apex. As the lead falls, if may be advanced slightly to engage positions suitable for septal pacing. E, After the tip falls to the floor of the ventricle the lead is advanced to its final position in the apex as shown in RAO and left anterior oblique (LAO) (F). II, RAO (A) and LAO (B) views of passive fixation right atrial (RA), right ventricular (RV) apical lead positions at the time of implantation. The ventricular lead is positioned with the tip at the RV apex, well beyond the spine shadow, as shown here. The slight downward position of the tip is desirable. Some indentation of the ventricular lead at the level of the tricuspid valve is common. In LAO the lead lies against the ventricular septum. The atrial lead is positioned in the RA appendage.

cal lead is one in which the lead's tip is to the left of the spine and is pointing anteriorly and slightly caudal (Fig. 5.9 II). Visualization of the lead in multiple planes should be performed to confirm appropriate location of the lead.

For the patient with left bundle branch block or AV block with a ventricular escape mechanism, special care needs to be taken when crossing the tricuspid valve to avoid bumping the right bundle branch if no temporary pacing wire is in place. The transient block in conduction may result in prolonged asystole and even death if temporary pacing cannot be quickly established. In these situations, less experienced operators may wish to place a temporary pacing wire to avoid this complication at the outset of the procedure.

In the anteroposterior projection it may not be possible to distinguish whether a lead is in a posterior coronary vein, the left ventricle, or the RV apex. Left oblique views and the 12-lead electrocardiographic pattern of ventricular activation during pacing are helpful in avoiding such lead misplacement. If a lead is inadvertently placed in the left ventricle, the paced QRS complex will usually show a right bundle branch block pattern, whereas positioning in the right ventricle will usually show a left bundle branch block pattern. In patients with LV prominence and/or counterclockwise rotation of the heart, the lead tip may not appear to extend far enough to the left border of the cardiac silhouette. Imaging in the right anterior oblique position may be helpful in such circumstances; observing the position of the lead with respect to the tricuspid valve allows an estimation of how far the lead is in the ventricle. Pacing at 10 V output is performed to exclude diaphragmatic stimulation by the lead, which may indicate microperforation and should usually lead to repositioning of the lead.

Once proper position has been confirmed, the active fixation mechanism, if present, should be deployed while viewed under magnified fluoroscopy. The stylet is then partly withdrawn and pacing parameters (R-wave size, pacing impedance, and capture threshold) are determined. High-output pacing is performed again. Once in place after stylet withdrawal and lead fixation, the tip should maintain a relatively stable position and not appear to be bouncing with cardiac contraction. A slight loop of lead is left in the atrium to avoid tension at the tip during deep inspiration. Too large a loop may result in ectopy, lead dislodgement, or prolapse into the IVC.

Although an apical RV lead position is usually preferred for reasons of stability, there are occasions when another location in the right ventricle is required (e.g. a retained ventricular lead, which might result in contact potentials). Efforts to obtain a more physiological activation sequence and, presumably, contraction from ventricular stimulation have led some investigators to advocate positioning the lead in the RV outflow tract (Fig. 5.10)[14] or on the interventricular septum (Fig. 5.11). In these circumstances, the use of an active-fixation lead is required. To place a lead in the outflow tract or septum, the lead is prolapsed into the pulmonary artery as described. By withdrawing the lead with a curved stylet and torque to drive the tip into the septum, the septum can be mapped and the lead fixed. The hemodynamic benefits of routinely seeking

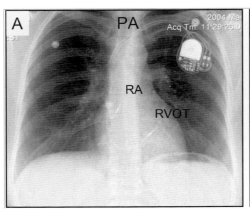 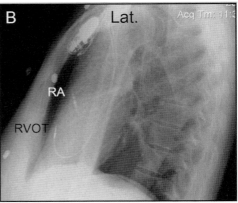

Fig. 5.10 Posteroanterior (A) and lateral (B) chest radiographs of active fixation right atrial (RA) and right ventricular outflow tract (RVOT) lead positions after implantation. Stable ventricular lead placement in the RVOT usually requires an active fixation lead. The RA lead is in the right atrial appendage.

such a position compared with the stability of the traditional apical location are unproven,[15] but this position may reduce the risk of free wall perforation and diaphragmatic stimulation when an active-fixation lead is required.

When a reasonable position is obtained, preliminary measurements of the electrical parameters are made. This is usually accomplished with the stylet withdrawn about halfway so as not to interfere with the position of the lead tip and to facilitate movement of the lead body should that be necessary. When active-fixation leads are used, such measurements may be taken before extensions of the helix, as a screen of the implant site prior to fixing the leads. If the parameters are not acceptable, an alternative position may be tried. Once a reasonable site is established, the helix is extended and the parameters remeasured. Failure to record a current of injury after deployment of active-fixation leads suggests a potentially unstable lead position (Fig. 5.12).[16]

Active-fixation leads vary in the ways they interface with the heart; the helix may be electrically active, the distal ring electrode may be active, or both the helix and a distal ring electrode may be active. Adequate pacing characteristics may not be found immediately after extension of the helix: the screw may not have entered the myocardium, the site may be inadequate, or local tissue injury may have occurred consequent to entry of the helix. All lead positions should be confirmed by both left anterior oblique and right anterior oblique views in the laboratory. It is common for capture thresholds to decrease significantly 15–30 min after active fixation.

Threshold parameters tested with a PSA define the electrical adequacy of lead position. This is accomplished using a set of connector cables, which can be configured for unipolar or bipolar leads. When testing unipolar leads, the anode is connected to tissue in the pacemaker pocket using a disk electrode or a clamp. Electrograms may be obtainable from the PSA or may be recorded using the chest (V) lead of a standard ECG machine. If satisfactory parameters

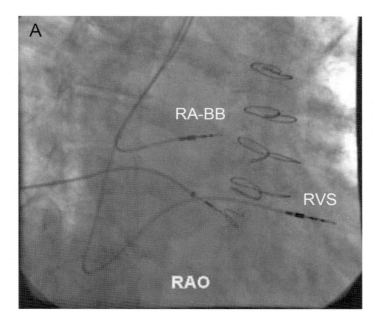

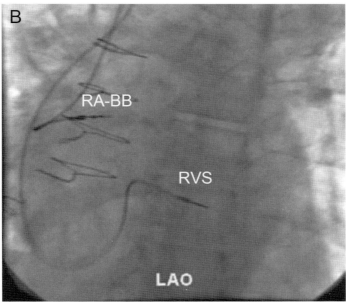

Fig. 5.11 Right anterior oblique (RAO) and left anterior oblique (LAO) views of atrial lead in the high right atrial septum (Bachman's bundle) at the time of implant (RA-BB). Note that in the LAO view the lead tip is directed posteriorly as opposed to anteriorly for right atrial appendage positions (compare with Fig. 5.8B). The unique position of the lead is difficult to appreciate in the RAO view. The ventricular lead (RVS) is fixed to the right ventricular septum.

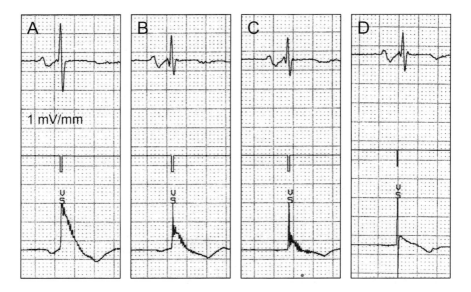

Fig. 5.12 Current of injury recorded by pacing system analyzer after extension of the helix of an active fixation ventricular lead. A, Maximal injury current immediately after extension of the helix. B,C, The current gradually decreasing over several minutes. D, The final electrogram recorded through the pulse generator.

(Table 5.3) are not obtained, alternative lead positions should be sought. It is important to confirm that diaphragmatic pacing does not occur by temporarily testing the lead at high output energy (10 V).

Capture threshold may be influenced by a number of factors, including myocardial site, presence of infarction or scar, electrolyte disturbance, medications, and lead type. On occasion, optimal parameters may not be achieved, and acceptance of the best available position is necessary. However, because the short- and long-term success of the pacing system is related to the initial lead position, effort should be expended to obtain the best possible initial location in terms of

Table 5.3 Acceptable electrical parameters for new lead placement

Parameter	Atrium	Ventricle
Capture threshold*	< 1.5 V	< 1.0 V
Sensed P/R wave	> 1.5 mV	> 4.0 mV
Slew rate	> 0.2 V s⁻¹	> 0.5 V s⁻¹
Impedance	400–1000 Ω†	400–1000 Ω†

*At 0.5 ms pulse duration.
†High-impedance leads typically exceed these values; check with manufacturer for acceptable values.

both stability and electrical performance. Rarely, a CS vein may prove the only site from which one may sense and/or pace the ventricle reliably.[17]

Once acceptable lead parameters are obtained, the amount of lead slack should be adjusted, depending on the size of patient. Taller and heavier patients will typically require greater lead redundancy to account for the mediastinal shift which will take place as the patient stands and inspires deeply. The lead stylet is then removed and the lead secured to the pectoral fascia with 2-0 or 0 non-absorbable suture (silk or equivalent). These sutures should be placed around a suture sleeve, and never directly to the lead insulation, which may fracture under this chronic stress.

Atrial lead implantation

The right atrial appendage has become the preferred implant site for atrial leads because of its trabeculated nature. Studies have shown that good pacing parameters may be obtained and maintained from this location. A number of studies have suggested that dislodgement is not more common with atrial leads, but reliance on an atrial appendage location may mandate the acceptance of less than ideal pacing characteristics that become unacceptable over time. Active-fixation leads appear to be beneficial in this regard by allowing further exploration of the right atrium in the search for an optimal position. There is no evidence that the atrial stimulation site influences hemodynamics *per se*, although atrial septal pacing near Bachman's bundle may be of some importance when atrial tachycardia algorithms are applied (Fig. 5.11).

A variety of leads (active, passive, J-shaped, straight) may be used for atrial pacing. A stylet can be used to impart a "J" contour to a routine ventricular lead, which facilitates its entry into the appendage. When using active-fixation leads, there are advantages and disadvantages to preformed devices. A straight active-fixation lead may be easier to place in areas other than the appendage; however, dislodgement may result in the lead's falling into the right ventricle and causing competitive pacing or ectopy (Fig. 5.13). The J-shaped active-fixation lead may also be positioned almost anywhere in the atrium, but in some sites (e.g. low atrium) its shape may cause undue tension at the site of attachment to the endocardium, increasing the risk of dislodgement or cardiac perforation.

The atrial lead is inserted into the venous system with a straight stylet to facilitate negotiation of the central veins. Positioning in the atrial appendage is usually attempted first. The lead is directed toward the high anterior atrium and allowed to take its J shape either by withdrawing the straight stylet (in preformed leads) or by inserting a J-stylet. Slow retraction of the preformed J-shaped lead results in the tip's entering the appendage, where it will appear to catch and take on a characteristic to-and-fro motion with atrial activity (Fig. 5.14). When it is well positioned, slight rotation of the lead should not dislodge the tip, and deep inspiration opens the curve to an L configuration but no further. In some patients the atrial appendage may be quite large and trabeculae may be attenuated; in others, who have received cardiopulmonary

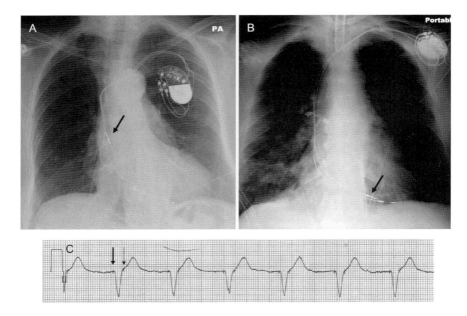

Fig. 5.13 Posteroanterior radiographic views illustrating different patterns of atrial dislodgement. A, This preformed atrial "J" lead dislodged within 24 h of implant and retracted into the superior vena cava (arrow), producing loss of atrial sensing and right phrenic nerve stimulation. B, This straight active fixation lead dislodged shortly after implantation into the right ventricle (arrow), resulting in the ECG in C: ECG showing ventricular capture from the dislodged atrial lead (wide arrow) followed by ventricular pacing at the paced AV delay (thin arrow) without capture.

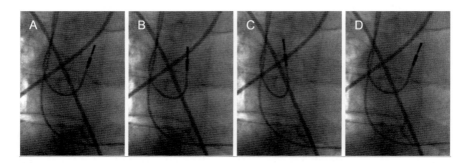

Fig. 5.14 Motion of atrial lead placed in the right atrial appendage in a series of fluoroscopic views in the right anterior oblique projection. Typical lead motion through a single cardiac cycle is depicted.

bypass, the appendage may be oversewn. In these circumstances, placement of a preformed J lead may be difficult.

Although some implanters feel that previous cardiac surgery is a mandate for an active-fixation atrial lead, others find passive-fixation devices to be acceptable. We nearly always use active-fixation atrial leads for patients with prior cardiac surgery. To place a lead on the atrial septum, allow the curve of the active-fixation lead to form free in the body of the atrium and directed anteriorly. Rotate the lead to the septum in the left anterior oblique view and pull the lead up until the roof of the atrium is encountered (see Fig. 5.11). Opening the stylet to a curve < 180° facilitates reaching the septum.

Acceptable electrical parameters for atrial pacing are listed in Table 5.3. As seen when active fixation leads are used in the ventricle, there may be a significant improvement of the parameters during the first half hour. If borderline values are obtained initially, it may be worthwhile to perform serial measurements every 3–5 min. If poor values are obtained initially, however, it is best to search for a new position. The better the electrical characteristics, the more probable that long-term pacing will be successful. As with the ventricular lead, it is important to test for diaphragmatic pacing by temporarily stimulating the atrium at high output (10 V).

When acceptable parameters are obtained, the lead slack is adjusted, the stylet is removed, and the lead secured with non-absorbable suture. Final lead parameters are then obtained for both atrial and ventricular leads.

Epicardial and transmyocardial lead placement

Permanent epicardial leads can be placed on the atria and ventricles at thoracotomy. Newer steroid-eluting active fixation and atraumatic suture-on electrodes provide the best long-term thresholds.[18] Chronic epicardial atrial lead performance remains problematic, however. These leads must be passed between or beneath the ribs and then tunneled subcutaneously to the pocket, potentially raising risk of lead fracture (Fig. 5.15).

When no venous access is available and the superior performance of endocardial lead placement is desired, transmyocardial placement may be indicated. By thoracotomy, one or two leads can be passed through the right atrial wall and positioned in the atrium and ventricle with use of fluoroscopy. Purse string sutures around the atriotomies prevent bleeding. The leads are then tunneled to the pocket.

Single-lead VDD pacing

The general principles of lead insertion are similar for the dual-chamber VDD systems that use specially arrayed proximal atrial sensing electrodes as well as a tip electrode to sense and pace the ventricle on a single lead. These devices may be useful for selected patients with AV block who have a normal sinus mechanism because they obviate the need for a separate atrial lead. When used, it is important to have the atrial electrodes at an optimal position in the right atrium; one may have to choose among leads with varying distances between the tip and atrial electrodes. Care is necessary to ensure that there is a chronotropically intact sinus mechanism before implantation and that atrial activity is consistently sensed by the lead at implantation. Testing for atrial sensing during extremes of respiration and during cough is necessary.

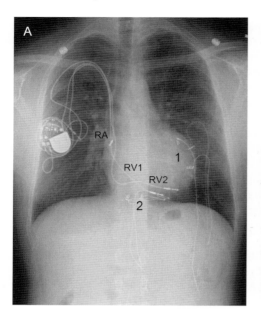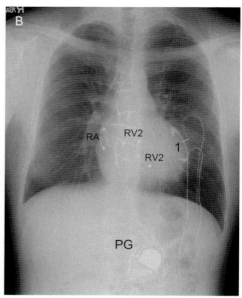

Fig. 5.15 Series of epicardial pacing systems in a 34-year-old man who underwent his first pacemaker implantation at the age of 4 years due to acquired atrioventricular block. A, Posteroanterior chest X-ray shows two sets of abandoned failed epicardial VVI systems (1,2). A right-sided dual-chamber transvenous system was later placed (RA and RV1). Failure of the first endocardial RV lead led to its replacement (RV2). B, Infection of the transvenous pacing leads led to complete surgical extraction of that system followed by implantation of a third dual-chamber epicardial system, with bipolar right atrial (RA) and right ventricular (RV1 and RV2) leads tunneled to an epigastric pulse generator (PG). The second RV lead was capped for potential future use should the first lead fail. One of the old epicardial systems (2) was removed at the same operation.

Although it may be necessary to accept low-amplitude P waves and program the device to be very sensitive, reasonable results have been reported over a moderately long follow-up period.[19]

Inappropriate atrial sensing still may be a problem for a significant proportion of patients implanted with single-lead VDD systems. Because atrial capture is rarely possible with VDD leads, the device provides only single-chamber VVI(R) function if the atrial rhythm slows below the lower rate limit. Of course, the system is at a disadvantage if there is sinus node dysfunction, unless one is willing to sacrifice atrial synchronization and revert to VVI(R).

Generator insertion

After the leads have been placed in an acceptable position, stability is confirmed with fluoroscopic observation during deep inspiration and cough. There should be just enough intravascular lead to prevent undue tension at the tip with inspiration. The suture sleeve is carefully advanced distally, with care not to pull on the lead. Frequent fluoroscopic checks are important during this process. The lead is tied down to the underlying muscle with two or three non-absorbable sutures. Sutures should never be tied around the unprotected lead; and even with the suture sleeve, too tight a suture may compromise lead integrity. The sutures should be tight enough, however, to avoid lead migration. Electrical parameters and fluoroscopic position should be rechecked after suturing; if they are not optimal, the sutures may be removed and the lead repositioned.

Once the leads have been secured, any sponges that had been placed in the subcutaneous pocket are removed and the area is irrigated and checked for hemostasis and foreign matter. Fluoroscopy of the pocket area will reveal any radio-opaque foreign body (such as sponges or needles) that was not removed before the generator insertion. The pacemaker should be preprogrammed to the desired initial settings while still in its sterile package, after which it is given to the operator for implantation. For dual-chamber devices it is important that the atrial and ventricular leads be identified easily and connected properly to the generator (Fig. 5.16).

The lead pins should be cleaned and dried prior to insertion into the generator. The proximal connector pin of the lead should be seen to pass the set screw(s) of the generator and remain there after tightening. Care should be taken that the screws are not overtorqued when tightened. A slight tug on the lead will confirm a tight connection. For in-line bipolar leads, both screws (when present) must be set correctly. Some pacemakers (i.e. unipolar) may not function as programmed until placed within the pocket.

The generator is carefully placed in the pocket, coiling redundant leads along the sides of the device or underneath it to avoid acute angulations. Extra lead should not be placed above the generator, as this will complicate generator replacement or lead revision in the future. We generally tie the generator down to the pectoralis fascia with a 0-silk suture through the tie-down hole in the header of the generator. This serves to limit migration of the generator and to defend against patient "twiddling" of the device (Fig. 5.17). Once in place, evidence of proper pacemaker function should be observed, with placement of

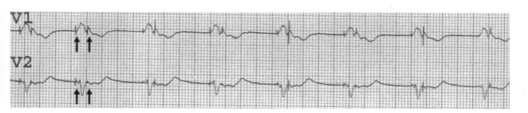

Fig. 5.16 Continuous rhythm strip of a patient with a dual-chamber pacemaker in whom the leads were inadvertently reversed at the generator. There is atrioventricular sequential output from the generator (arrows) with the first stimulus capturing the ventricle and the second stimulus to the atrium occurring late in the QRS complex. This problem can be averted at implantation by double-checking appropriate lead placement in the header by serial number and documenting appropriate pacemaker activity prior to closing the pocket.

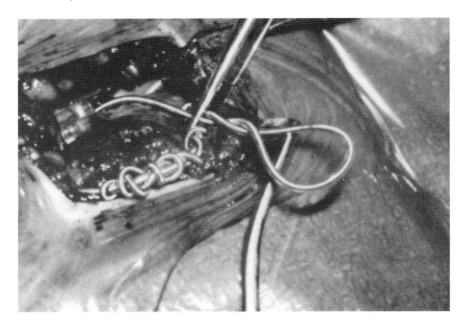

Fig. 5.17 Photograph obtained at the time of operative intervention to reposition a lead dislodged due to Twiddler's syndrome. The lead can be seen to be tightly twisted upon itself. Although this tangle can be straightened, the stresses imparted to both the conductor and the insulation make it unsafe to reuse this lead. A new lead should be inserted. (Courtesy of Dr Paul Levine.)

a sterile magnet or programming head if necessary. Fluoroscopic examination of the entire system should be performed before pocket closure.

The pocket is closed in layers using 2-0 to 4-0 resorbable suture. Care must be taken to avoid piercing a lead with the suture needle. The skin edges may be approximated with skin sutures, resorbable subcuticular sutures, or surgical staples. A sterile dressing is then applied.

Before leaving the pacemaker laboratory, a final fluoroscopic check of the generator pocket and the course of the leads is made. The system is non-invasively interrogated to confirm adequacy of function and is programmed so that it temporarily overdrives the intrinsic heart rate. A 12-lead electrocardiogram is obtained to demonstrate the configuration of the paced rhythm, and then final programming of the pacemaker is performed.

In the recovery room or upon arrival to the floor, an overpenetrated anteroposterior chest radiograph is performed to document the lead position and the absence of a pneumothorax. A sling may help discourage excessive movement of the ipsilateral upper extremity during the first 12–24 h. A thorough operative report should be generated immediately to include the manufacturer, model and serial numbers of all hardware implanted, abandoned, or explanted as well as any difficulties encountered during the case.

Revision of the implanted pacemaker system and pulse generator change

Revision of an implanted pacing system may involve replacement of the pulse generator, the pacing leads, or both (Figs 5.15 and 5.18). The uncomplicated generator change is usually a simple procedure; however, the preparation is in many ways more involved than a new implant (Fig. 5.19). First, the indication for generator change should be confirmed and documented, and the system evaluated non-invasively to identify any problems with the leads. For lead failure, the procedure itself is often more complex than a new implant (usually due to issues of venous access) and again requires preoperative investigation into the cause of the lead failure to prevent its recurrence. If a lead replacement is anticipated, the patency of the ipsilateral venous system should be confirmed by venography. The decision to extract malfunctioning leads should be made beforehand so that appropriate preparations can be made (see discussion below). Even if the leads are known to function preoperatively, they may be damaged or found to be compromised on surgical exposure. Therefore, the patient and operator should be prepared for revision of any or all of the pacemaker leads at the time of generator replacement.

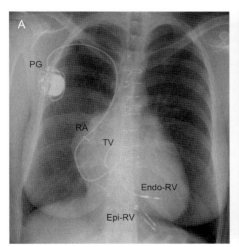
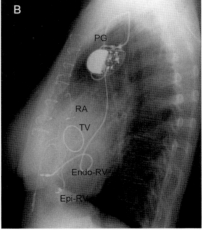

Fig. 5.18 Posteroanterior and lateral CXR of a 38-year-old woman with Ebstein's anomaly and complete atrioventricular block. In childhood, she had undergone implantation of a dual-chamber unipolar epicardial system using a transmyocardial right atrial lead (RA) and epicardial ventricular lead (Epi-RV). She later had tricuspid valve replacement with a bioprosthesis. By age 21 she had developed ventricular lead failure and permanent atrial fibrillation, leading to placement of a single-chamber transvenous pacemaker (Endo-RV) with a subpectoral pulse generator (PG). At age 30, her tricuspid valve bioprosthesis had failed and was replaced with a mechanical prosthesis (TV). The transvenous RV lead was placed outside the sewing ring of the prosthesis. This lead can now be extracted only by an open surgical route.

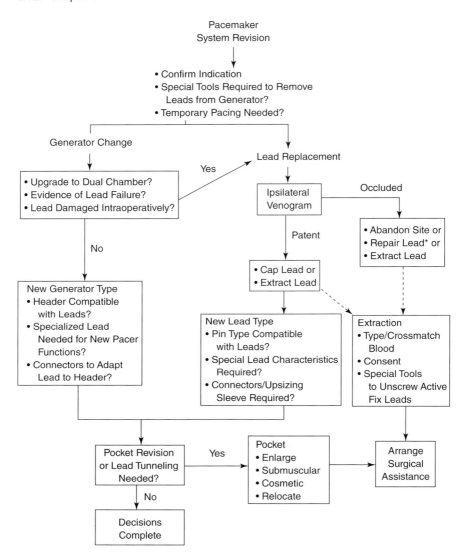

Fig. 5.19 Flow chart for decisions surrounding revision of a previously implanted pacemaker system. All decisions should be thoroughly considered and the necessary equipment secured before the patient enters the operating room. (*Repair of an isolated outer insulation defect can be performed on an exposed section of some silicone insulation leads using a repair kit. The integrity of the lead conductors is not assured, however.)

One of the most critical aspects in preparing for a lead or generator change is ensuring mechanical and electrical compatibility between the new and retained components (Fig. 5.19). Over the years, pacemaker systems have been manufactured with a variety of lead connector pins and generator header ports that may not be interchangeable. Currently, all new pacing systems conform to standard designs for these components (IS-1 standard, adopted in the early 1990s). Older systems may have pacemaker lead designs that are incompatible with new generators or have a serviceable generator that is not compatible with new leads.

For the lead to fit into the generator, the lead diameter, pin length and presence or absence of sealing rings must be accommodated by the pulse generator. In addition, at least one manufacturer (Guidant/Boston Scientific CRM) has introduced a proprietary LV-1 pin configuration for CS leads. Certain leads can be made compatible with new generators by the use of adaptors. Most manufacturers continue to provide generator models to fit some of the discontinued lead styles. In addition, some pacemakers require unique leads to perform specialized functions or special tools to free the leads from the device. The importance of identifying the lead and pacemaker connector configuration before surgery cannot be overstated. Manufacturers can provide the needed information about compatibility between components.

During the operative procedure, electrocautery can cause failure of output in generators near their end-of-life. For this reason and because leads can be damaged during generator removal, temporary pacing should be established in pacemaker-dependent patients. Meticulous attention to surgical technique is mandatory to prevent damage to implanted hardware and to reduce the risk of infection. If lead replacement is required but the ipsilateral vein is occluded, abandoning the entire system for another site or recanalization of the vein by lead extraction (see discussion below) will be necessary. Occasionally, isolated outer insulation defects in silicone leads can be repaired, but the integrity of the conductors is usually left in question. If leads are capped and abandoned in the pocket, it is advisable to suture the lead to the floor of the pocket to prevent migration of the free end and erosion.

Finally, replacement of a lead or generator provides the opportunity also to revise the pocket, reimplant the generator submuscularly, or revise the surgical scar as indicated. All of these factors should be evaluated and plans made for any contingency before the surgical procedure begins.

Post-procedure management

Elective generator replacement is most often accomplished on an outpatient basis. While there has been some enthusiasm for performing same-day pacemaker implantation, most procedures involving lead placement or revision continue to involve hospitalization for at least one night. For such new implants, ECG telemetry is usually obtained for 12–24 h. The following morning, an ECG is performed. Prior to discharge, posteroanterior and lateral chest radiographs are performed to document lead positions and exclude delayed pneumothorax.

Longer hospitalization may be required because of ancillary medical problems or as a result of complication. Analgesia may be necessary, but it is rarely needed after the first few days. The patient is advised to limit motion of the ipsilateral upper extremity for a time—specifically, to avoid raising it above the shoulder level or subjecting it to marked abduction for approximately 2 weeks. Patients should not, however, excessively restrict motion of the arm, as this may cause a frozen shoulder and delay ultimate rehabilitation. The incision should be kept dry for 5–7 days.

Even the most skilled implantation of a permanent pacemaker will provide a patient no benefit if it is not programmed properly. Before discharge, the device should be programmed in accordance with the patient's specific needs and a complete non-invasive assessment of the pacing system performed. Programming of the pacemaker is guided by two principles: (i) optimization of the patient's hemodynamic state, and (ii) maximal conservation of battery-energy expenditure. When these two factors are in opposition, the first should rule; however, opportunities to achieve the second should not be overlooked. This might include programming a longer AV interval to avoid fusion beats, a low resting minimal heart rate, and lower stimulation outputs (within an acceptable safety margin).

A number of recent studies have indicated the importance of avoiding unnecessary RV pacing, especially in patients with heart failure and LV dysfunction.[20] Such patients with preserved AV conduction should be programmed with long AV delays and/or a non-tracking mode (such as DDI).

Rate-adaptive parameters may be set before the patient is discharged or during a follow-up visit. This is commonly done empirically and is tested by having the patient perform walking exercises, if necessary. The adequacy of pacing response may be judged by real-time telemetry or by using rate histograms stored in the pacer. Follow-up evaluation and possibly adjustment of programmed parameters, including rate adaptation, will be necessary. An increase in capture threshold over the first 2–6 weeks after implantation may occur even if steroid-eluting leads are used, so an adequate safety margin should be programmed into the generator to ensure successful pacing during this time. This is usually achieved with a voltage output of four to five times threshold at implant.

Some of the newer pacemakers have a mechanism for automatic capture threshold detection. These devices may allow for the programming of a lower pacing output with the recognition that the unit will increase pacing output if it detects a rise in threshold. Care should be taken to ensure that these devices have acceptable evoked response amplitudes acutely and at follow-up assessments, especially in pacemaker-dependent patients, who may experience syncope with even a rare transient failure of the algorithm. A copy of the programmed parameters should be given to the patient to keep, in addition to the device registry card.

It is important that the physician register the generator and leads appropriately so that the patient may be tracked should a device advisory occur. Arrangements for follow-up care should be made by the implanting physician, and the patient should be counseled as to the importance of having the system checked at regular intervals. There is some controversy as to the need for endocarditis prophylaxis in patients with endocardial leads. Although there is a potential for infective endocarditis to occur, this has been reported infrequently, and rarely is the offending organism oral flora. Most implanters do not routinely recommend antibiotic prophylaxis.

Complications of implantation

Inherent to pacemaker therapy is the potential for the occurrence of an untoward event. Skill, experience and technique are all mitigating factors, but every operator should anticipate that they will have to manage a complication eventually. Thus, the implanting physician must be concerned not only with measures to avoid complications, but also with their recognition and treatment. Such untoward events associated with the introduction and physical presence of the generator and leads may be classified according to their etiology (Tables 5.4 and 5.5).

In the Pacemaker Selection in the Elderly (PASE) study, 6.1% of the 407 patients receiving dual-chamber pacing systems had a complication of implantation.[21] There were nine lead dislodgements (2%), eight instances of pneumothorax (2%) and four cardiac perforations (1%). A repeat surgical procedure was required in 18 (4.4%) of the patients. In a single-center study of > 1300 permanent pacemaker implants reported by Tobin and colleagues,[22] complications were noted in 4.2% of patients. Lead dislodgement occurred in 2.4%, significant pneumothorax in 1.5%, pericardial tamponade in 0.2% and hemothorax leading to death in one patient (0.08%). The economic consequences of a complication were substantial, with the average incremental cost of $14 547 for a lead dislodgment, $10 052 for a pneumothorax and $32 472 for a tamponade. There was an inverse relationship between the incidence of acute complication and operator case volume and experience. Although the acute implant complications associated with DDD pacing are not different

Table 5.4 Acute complications of pacemaker implantation

Venous access
- Secondary to Seldinger technique
  Pneumothorax
  Hemothorax
  Other (e.g. injury to thoracic duct, nerves, etc.)
- Secondary to sheath insertion
  Air or foreign body embolism
  Perforation of the heart or central vein
  Inadvertent entry into artery

Lead placement
- Brady- or tachyarrhythmia
- Perforation of heart or vein
- Damage to heart valve
- Damage to lead

Generator
- Improper or inadequate connection of lead
- Pocket hematoma

Table 5.5 Delayed complications of pacemaker therapy

Lead-related
• Intravascular thrombosis and/or embolization
• Intravascular constriction (i.e. SVC obstruction)
• Macro- or micro-lead dislodgment
• Fibrosis at electrode–myocardial interface (exit block)
• Infection—endocarditis
• Lead failure
  Insulation failure (inner/outer)
  Conductor fracture
• Retention wire fracture
• Chronic perforation
• Pericarditis

Generator-related
• Pain
• Erosion
• Infection of pocket
• Migration
• Premature failure
• Damage from extrinsic energy (e.g. radiation, electrical shock, etc.)

Patient-related
• Twiddler's syndrome

SVC, superior vena cava.

than those with single-chamber pacing, the total complication rate associated with dual-chamber pacing over time is higher than that with VVI or single-lead VDD due to the presence of the additional lead.

Although neither elective generator replacement nor revision of a VVI system to a dual-chamber device is usually considered to be a risky procedure, both are associated with potential complications. Harcombe and coworkers have found that the rate of late complications (those occurring later than 6 weeks after the procedure) was higher for elective replacement (6.5%) than for initial system implantation (1.4%).[23] These were primarily erosion and infection related to the pacemaker pocket. Complications were more common with inexperienced operators, suggesting that technique as well as physiological substrate play important etiological roles. Upgrade of a VVI device to a dual-chamber or biventricular system carries the potential for all the complications associated with venous access and lead placement (which may be confounded by the pre-existing lead and associated vascular abnormalities), as well as a slight increase in risk of late pocket infection and skin erosion. Upgrade procedures are often longer in duration than a *de novo* dual-chamber implantation. This may be related to difficulty isolating the generator and lead in the pocket due to adhesion formation, difficulty with venous access, interference with the existing lead, or a combination of these factors.

Venous access

By its very nature, the axillary/subclavian venous puncture has a potential for complication, the risk of which depends on both operator skill and the patient's anatomy. Inadvertent damage by the exploring needle to structures that lie in proximity to the vein (e.g. lung, subclavian artery, thoracic duct and nerves) is the most frequent cause of significant complications encountered during the implantation process. Such complications may be evident immediately, or they may be recognized only after the procedure has been completed. Knowledge of subclavian venous anatomy by venography may be helpful in accessing the vessel and avoiding complication.

Pneumothorax is often asymptomatic and discovered on the routine post-procedure chest radiograph (Fig. 5.20). Rarely, it may be the cause of severe respiratory distress intraprocedurally. Pleuritic pain, cough (especially if productive of blood-tinged sputum) and difficulty in breathing suggest the diagnosis. The aspiration of air into the syringe during attempted venous puncture may also raise concern about this possibility, but it is neither a sensitive nor specific sign. The presence of apical cystic lung disease, variations in the

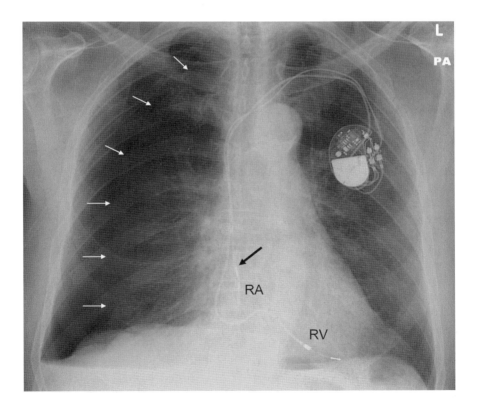

Fig. 5.20 Right pneumothorax after left-sided pacemaker implantation in an elderly man with emphysema. The pleural line is indicated by the white arrows. This unusual complication probably results from microperforation of active fixation right atrial lead (black arrow). Note the mediastinal shift to the left. RA, right atrial lead; RV, right ventricular lead.

relationship between the clavicle and subclavian vein, and an uncooperative patient may increase the risk for this complication—and repeated unsuccessful attempts at venous puncture certainly do. Respiratory symptoms arising during the procedure should prompt assessment of pulse, blood pressure, oximetry, and perhaps blood gas analysis. Fluoroscopic examination of both lung fields should also be performed.

Treatment of pneumothorax depends on its severity and associated symptoms. Respiratory distress during the procedure may necessitate the urgent/emergency insertion of a chest tube. The completion of the implantation will depend on the patient's status and the progress already made. Although there may be some controversy as to the need for evacuation of an asymptomatic pneumothorax seen on chest radiograph, if its extent is > 10% a chest tube should be considered. If a small pneumothorax does not resolve or enlarges on serial radiographs, evacuation is indicated. Inspiration of 100% oxygen by facemask may help resolve a small pneumothorax.

Hemothorax, a less common complication of the axillary/subclavian approach, results from injury to the subclavian artery, vein, or other intrathoracic vessel. Penetration of the subclavian artery by the exploring needle is usually harmless if the needle is withdrawn and slight pressure is applied at the site of entry under the clavicle. Significant complication may occur, however, if the artery is lacerated by the cutting edge of the needle or if a large-bore dilator or sheath is inadvertently introduced. If a large sheath is mistakenly inserted into the artery, it should probably be left in place, pending a prompt definitive management decision, since removal may result in significant bleeding. Options include surgical repair; endovascular treatment using a prolonged balloon inflation or a stent graft; or an attempt at sheath withdrawal with external compression. If the latter option is considered, there are several case reports of using vascular closure devices to assist with hemostasis. Use of both a collagen-based system (Angio-Seal; St. Jude Medical, St Paul, MN, USA) and a suture-based system (Perclose; Abbott Laboratories, Redwood City, CA, USA) has been described.

Opinions from an interventional radiologist and a vascular surgeon should be obtained if possible. A quick angiogram may determine whether an important branch vessel (e.g. internal mammary graft or vertebral artery) is involved or might be excluded by a covered stent. Because of the risk of thrombus formation around the sheath, it should be withdrawn to the subclavian artery itself to prevent embolization of clot to the cerebrovascular system. The likelihood of a bleeding complication is increased if the coagulation system is impaired either intrinsically by coexisting disease or by pharmacological therapy. Angiographic evaluation and possible repair should be considered for severe or persistent bleeding from an uncertain source.

Air embolism can occur when a central vein is accessed by a sheath, regardless of the technique used to introduce it. This complication may be signaled by a hiss as air is sucked into the sheath by negative intrathoracic pressure and may occur suddenly when a heavily sedated, snoring patient deeply inspires at a time when control over the sheath's orifice is not adequate. Air may be fluoroscopically tracked into the right ventricle and pulmonary outflow tract. In most instances, the amount of air introduced is small and well tolerated, but respiratory distress, chest pain, hypotension and arterial oxygen desaturation may occur if there is significant blockage of pulmonary flow. Treatment of symptomatic air embolism includes supplemental oxygen, attempted catheter aspiration, and inotropic support if necessary. These supportive measures will usually suffice until the air embolism breaks up and absorption occurs. Preventive measures are listed in Table 5.6. The most important of these is routine use of valved sheaths.

Infrequent complications of venous access include laceration of the thoracic duct leading to chylothorax, and damage to the internal mammary artery, which may cause acute ischemia when this conduit has been used as a coronary arterial graft.

Lead placement
Arrhythmia
The introduction, manipulation and positioning of the pacemaker leads in the heart may give rise to a number of complications. Arrhythmia may be a manifestation of the patient's underlying disease, or it may be procedurally related (Table 5.7). In a pacemaker-dependent patient, accidental interference with a pre-existing pacing system—whether temporary or permanent—may cause

Table 5.6 Avoidance of air embolism

1. Increase central venous pressure
   - Hydrate well
   - Elevate legs (Trendelenburg position)
   - Have patient perform Valsalva maneuver when sheath is open
2. Awaken patient and caution against deep inspiration
3. Use smallest sheath compatible with task
4. Pinch or occlude neck of sheath when appropriate
5. Use of sheaths with hemostatic valves

Table 5.7 Causes of arrhythmia during pacer implantation

1. Bradyarrhythmia
   - Patient's underlying electrophysiological disorder
   - Vagal reaction
   - Lead trauma to the conduction system
   - Inadvertent disruption of a pacing system
   - Suppression of escape rhythm by anesthetic
2. Tachyarrhythmia
   - Atrial/ventricular
     Underlying electrophysiology
     Irritation by lead/wire
     Ischemia, anesthesia, hypoxia

asystole or symptomatic bradycardia. Other causes of a bradyarrhythmia include a vagal reaction, excessive local anesthesia, and injury to the conduction system during lead manipulation (e.g. trauma to the right bundle branch in a patient with left bundle branch block). The use of transcutaneous pacing and/or the administration of atropine or isoproterenol may be helpful in these situations until a means of effective pacing can be established. For patients at risk of asystole during permanent pacemaker implantation, revision, or generator change, a preoperative temporary pacing wire should be considered.

Tachyarrhythmia may also occur during implantation; it is usually the result of stimulation of myocardium by a lead or guidewire. Supraventricular arrhythmias are most likely to occur in patients with atrial enlargement, heart failure, pulmonary disease or other predisposing conditions such as sick sinus syndrome; they are usually transient. Atrial fibrillation occurring before or during atrial lead placement may be problematic, in that atrial parameters cannot be tested unless the rhythm terminates either spontaneously or by cardioversion. An atrial lead may be placed in the presence of atrial fibrillation occurring at the time of implantation using the criterion of an intracardiac fibrillatory amplitude of ≥ 1.0 mV. This reduces implantation time compared with the option of intraprocedural cardioversion, which may also lead to postoperative stroke.[24] Ventricular dysrhythmia is common as the lead is manipulated in this chamber; but it is rarely sustained. Predisposing factors to more malignant arrhythmia include hypoxia, ischemia, pharmacological therapy (e.g. sympathomimetics) and asynchronous pacing. Removal of the lead from an irritating position almost always terminates the ectopy. On occasion a retained guidewire or a temporary ventricular pacing lead is displaced and serves as an occult source of ventricular irritation that is not resolved by retraction of the permanent pacing lead.

Because the attention of the implanter may be focused on the fluoroscopic image during lead placement, another individual, usually the nurse or anesthetist, should be assigned to monitor the ECG during this time. Rarely, a permanent ventricular (or prolapsing atrial) pacing lead will be the cause of recurrent ventricular ectopy post implantation.

Perforation

The heart may be perforated internally (into another cardiac chamber) or externally (into the pericardial space) by the pacing lead; such perforations may be acute or delayed.[25] RV perforations are probably more common than reported because clinical sequelae may not occur. Poor sensing or capture thresholds may prompt withdrawal of the lead back into the ventricle with "self-sealing" of the perforation. On occasion, however, life-threatening tamponade may occur, and progressive hypotension during or after lead placement should be considered tamponade until proven otherwise by echocardiography. Older age, female gender, steroid therapy, recent RV infarction, and the use of stiff leads (or stylets) may be considered risk factors for perforation. Pericarditis, tamponade, and even pneumothorax have been reported as complications caused by active-fixation atrial lead placement due to the helix protruding through the atrial myocardium.

Interference with normal coagulation predisposes the patient to tamponade. Anticoagulants should be withheld for at least 8–12 h if there is no suspicion of perforation, and reinstituted with caution. Thrombolytics should be considered contraindicated in the immediate postimplant period. If symptoms suggestive of tamponade occur, echocardiographic confirmation should be obtained unless the condition dictates emergency pericardiocentesis prior to the availability of the ultrasound equipment. Every effort should be made to obtain an echocardiogram in the latter situation as soon as possible. Pericardiocentesis with catheter drainage will rapidly reverse the pathophysiology of tamponade and may be the only therapy necessary, since the perforation is frequently self-sealing. In some cases tamponade may occur with the acute accumulation of only a small amount of pericardial fluid. In such cases it may be difficult to access the pericardial space with a needle, necessitating emergency surgical consultation. Less frequently, a more slowly accumulating effusion may develop over several days as reaction to a relatively small amount of bleeding into the pericardial space. This may follow signs and/or symptoms of pericarditis or present as *de novo* tamponade. Drainage may be necessary if hemodynamics are threatened; otherwise, non-steroidal anti-inflammatory agents and observation may be used.

Suspicion of perforation without tamponade may be aroused by an extreme distal location of the lead tip at the cardiac apex (especially if it seems to curve around the apex, tenting up the cardiac silhouette), or by the presence of a pericardial friction rub, chest pain, an ECG-pacing pattern of right bundle branch block, or an upright unipolar electrogram recorded from the lead tip. Poor pacing and sensing thresholds may be seen. In such situations, fluoroscopy or computed tomography scanning may be helpful in localizing the lead tip (Fig. 5.21).[26] If perforation is confirmed, the lead should be withdrawn under hemodynamic monitoring at a time and facility capable of emergency surgical drainage if necessary.

A transvenous pacing lead may enter the left heart through a communication between the atria, through the membranous septum separating the right atrium from the left ventricle, or through the muscular intraventricular septum. The permanent pacing lead may also be inadvertently introduced into an artery and passed retrograde across the aortic valve into the left ventricle. The anteroposterior radiographic image of a lead positioned in the left ventricle may not be distinguishable from an image of one placed in the RV apical position. Oblique or lateral views, however, will demonstrate the posterior location of an LV lead (Fig. 5.22). In addition, pacing from the left ventricle will result in a right bundle branch block QRS pattern on ECG. This combination of techniques should always be performed during lead implantation to exclude this important and preventable complication.

Early recognition of a lead in a systemic chamber should prompt its immediate repositioning because of the danger of thrombus formation and sys-

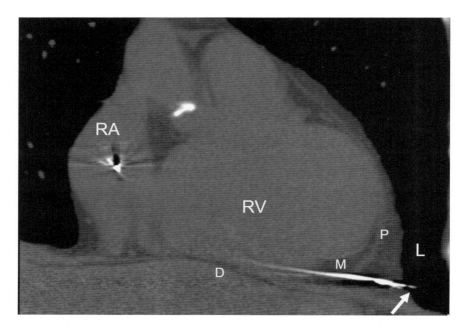

Fig. 5.21 Reconstructed computed tomographic image in right anterior oblique view showing perforation of an active fixation ventricular lead through the right ventricular apex and pericardium into the lung parenchyma. This problem may present with loss of ventricular sensing and capture, pneumothorax, pericardial effusion, and/or stimulation of the diaphragm or chest wall. The lead was later withdrawn uneventfully in the operating room. RA, right atrium; RV, right ventricle; D, diaphragm; M, right ventricular myocardium; P, pericardium; L, left lung.

temic embolization. A review of the literature has found that 10 of 27 patients had thromboembolic complications, including three patients on antiplatelet drugs.[27] Options for management of patients with chronically implanted left heart endocardial leads include long-term anticoagulation, lead removal at thoracotomy, or percutaneous lead removal. The latter has been thought to be associated with excessive risk of systemic embolization, but a number of successful procedures have been reported.

Other lead complications

The presence of a pacing lead across the tricuspid valve orifice ordinarily results in little or no valvular dysfunction. On occasion, however, this structure may be compromised or damaged, resulting in tricuspid regurgitation.[28] During insertion, the tines of a passive fixation lead may become entangled with the chordae tendineae, and rupture of the latter may result if vigorous lead withdrawal is attempted. Occasionally, extrication of the lead from the tricuspid apparatus may require use of a locking stylet (with or without extraction sheath) to transmit the force of traction to the lead tip rather than merely stretching the lead. The valve may be chronically injured by the lead's lying across it and by

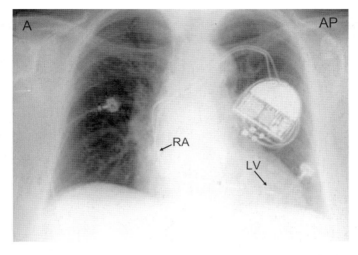

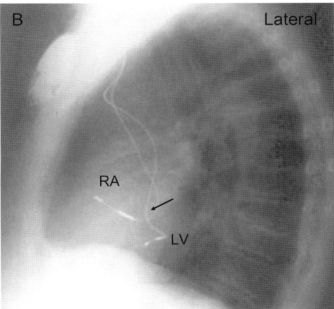

Fig. 5.22 Chest radiographs of a patient after implantation of a dual-chamber pacemaker with inadvertent left-sided ventricular lead placement. The paced QRS complex on 12-lead ECG showed a right bundle branch block pattern. A, On anteroposterior view, the ventricular lead appears to be positioned near the right ventricular apex. B, Lateral chest radiograph shows a posterior diversion of the ventricular lead at the atrial level (arrow). Passage of the lead across a patent foramen ovale, across the mitral valve, and into the left ventricle was later confirmed. Treatment options include removal of the lead or chronic anticoagulation to prevent thromboembolus. This problem can be avoided by careful fluoroscopy of the leads in multiple views and observation of an appropriate 12-lead paced QRS complex at the time of implantation. RA, right atrial lead; LV, ventricular lead in the left ventricle.

the resultant fibrosis. Thrombus and adhesions may form between the two and serve as a nidus for infection. Recurrent endocarditis on an RV lead has been associated with the development of tricuspid stenosis and insufficiency.

The pacing lead itself may be damaged by the physical forces exerted upon it during the process of implantation, by entrapment in the musculoskeletal system, by retention ligatures, and by the stresses placed on it by the beating heart. Loss of integrity of the insulation (either inner or outer) is manifested by a low lead impedance that causes a high current drain; conductor fracture is associated with a high impedance. Lead fracture may be recognized radiographically (Fig. 5.5). A defect in the insulation between the conductor wires of a bipolar lead may produce potentials resulting in transient inhibition of the pacemaker. Detection of such intermittent dysfunction may require the performance of provocative maneuvers such as raising, abducting, or adducting the ipsilateral upper extremity. Prolonged contact between the conductors can result in a short circuit, preventing current from reaching the electrodes and depleting the power supply. Both lead fracture and loss of insulation integrity can lead to clinical symptoms, including death, in pacemaker-dependent patients.

The most common complication of lead placement is its subsequent dislodgment (see Fig. 5.12). This may be obvious on fluoroscopy or radiography (macro-) or accompanied by no obvious change in position (micro-) and usually occurs early, before clot and fibrosis act to anchor the device further. Dislodgement rates are inversely related to the experience of the implanter, which suggests that inadequate initial positioning is a major risk factor. A unique cause of lead dislodgement is known as twiddler's syndrome. In these cases, the patient unwittingly twists the pacemaker generator in the pocket, turning it in such a way that the leads are wound around it and are withdrawn from the heart (Fig. 5.17). Two other situations in which traction on a lead may result in dislodgement relate to the generator. If not sutured to underlying structures, a generator lying in the subcutaneous tissue may gradually descend through this space and pull on the lead. Similarly, a "sagging heart syndrome" (postural descent of heart resulting in tension on the lead and displacement) has accompanied marked weight loss in morbidly obese patients.

The incidence of lead dislodgement has been reduced with refinement of both active- and passive-fixation devices; it is now < 2–3%. The risk of this complication is lessened by ensuring a stable position at implant, leaving a proper amount of intravascular lead slack so that tension is not exerted at the tip by respiration or arm motion, adequately anchoring the suture sleeve to underlying tissue, and by limiting abduction and elevation of the ipsilateral upper extremity for a short time after implantation.

Early recognition of lead dislodgement (often by deterioration in pacing parameters or the occurrence of ectopy) should result in attempts at repositioning. This is usually accomplished with minimal effort because the lead has not fibrosed to endocardium or venous endothelium.

Deterioration of the performance of one or more chronic leads may present a more difficult problem and it is often necessary to use a new lead. If exit block is a problem, a short course of steroid therapy may be tried, but more often than not repositioning or insertion of a new lead is necessary. Steroid-eluting leads (including those configured with an active-fixation mechanism) are beneficial in this regard.

Venous thrombosis

It should not be surprising that the presence of one or more intravascular leads may incite deep venous thrombosis (DVT) of the subclavian vein. Although asymptomatic thrombus appears to be quite common (see discussion below), its relationship with the number and type of leads remains controversial. Clinically significant pulmonary embolization is rare. Symptomatic thrombosis of the brachiocephalic veins occurs on occasion and presents as a swollen, painful upper extremity, usually within a few weeks of implant. Extension of the clot to involve the innominate vein, superior vena cava, contralateral structures or the cerebral venous sinus may occur. Venography will reveal the extent of thrombus and the state of development of collateral pathways (Fig. 5.23). Symptomatic thrombosis that is limited to the subclavian or axillary veins may be treated conservatively, with heparin acutely, with heat and upper extremity elevation, and then warfarin for 3–6 months. In selected patients with highly symptomatic DVT with proximal extension, thrombolytic therapy may be given in a large dose for a short time (e.g. 1 million units

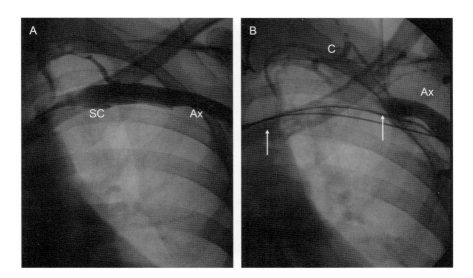

Fig. 5.23 Deep venous thrombosis (DVT) during pacemaker implantation. A, Pre-procedure left upper extremity venogram shows patent axillary (Ax) and subclavian (SC) veins. B, A second intraprocedural venogram was performed due to inability to access the vein for a third left ventricular lead after placement of the right ventricular and atrial leads. Acute occlusion of the subclavian vein between the two arrows is demonstrated, along with the appearance of collateral venous circulation (C).

streptokinase during 1 h) or during 12–24 h (e.g. 200–500 000 units urokinase during 1 h followed by 100 000 units h^{-1}). Thrombolytics need not be delivered directly into an ipsilateral arm vein. Thrombolytic therapy has been associated with rapid symptomatic and angiographic improvement. Prolonged therapy with oral anticoagulants may then be considered.

Silent DVT is common. Routine venography at the time of elective generator replacement has shown approximately 25% incidence of severe stenosis or occlusion of the ipsilateral subclavian vein.[29] No risk factors for thrombosis have been unequivocally identified, although some studies have suggested that an increased number of leads and systemic infection predispose to venous occlusion. In most patients, asymptomatic thrombosis becomes a problem only when attempts are made to re-enter the vessel for lead revision or placement of additional leads. It is not necessary to treat asymptomatic chronic occlusions. Pacemaker leads inserted via the transfemoral route may be associated with femoral and iliac thrombosis and significant pulmonary embolization, necessitating lead extraction, anticoagulation, and possibly insertion of an IVC filter.

Complete or partial occlusion of the superior vena cava has been reported as a complication of pacemakers. This has been attributed to both thrombosis and fibrosis and may be treated with balloon dilation or surgical reconstruction if it becomes symptomatic. Acute or subacute occlusion may be treated with anticoagulants and thrombolytic agents. Chronic occlusion is more problematic and is, in general, resistant to pharmacotherapy. In some situations of total occlusion of the superior vena cava, endovascular reconstruction may be complicated by an inability to pass a guidewire through the obstruction. In such cases it may be possible to remove the existing leads and use the extraction sheath as a means of gaining entrance through the occluded venous system. Dilation and stenting may then be considered. Stenting should not be performed over indwelling pacemaker leads. In cases in which endovascular repair is not possible, a surgical approach that enlarges the venous channel with a patch graft has been used with some success.

The true incidence of lead-associated thrombus is uncertain, since transesophageal echocardiography (TEE) is usually performed only if there is a clinical indication. Such thrombus in the presence of infection would be termed a "vegetation." In general, the chance finding of a clot on a lead does not, in itself, mandate therapy; however, if it is very large, consideration should be given to anticoagulation. Anticoagulation therapy would be indicated if there is evidence of thromboembolism. A pedunculated clot on a pacing wire may occlude the tricuspid orifice and cause symptoms similar to a myxoma. Treatment of lead-associated atrial thrombus with thrombolytic therapy has been reported.

Generator

The function of a pacing system depends on a proper connection between the leads and the generator. The terminal lead pins are inserted into the connector block of the generator and are fixed into position by some mechanism, most commonly set screws. If this is not done properly, the pin may either lose contact altogether (i.e. have no electrical continuity, an "open circuit") or intermittently contact the pacemaker terminal and produce spurious potentials that may be sensed by the pacemaker as intrinsic electrical activity, which will cause inhibition of pulse generator output. When dual-chamber systems are used, it is essential that the atrial and ventricular leads be connected correctly to their corresponding terminals (Fig. 5.16).

Care should be exercised when using electrocautery, since its application in the vicinity of the generator may lead to inhibition of pacing or to abnormal tracking—reprogramming of the device to a reversion mode may also result. Exposure to other sources of energy—such as direct-current defibrillation, magnetic resonance imaging, security systems, high-dose radiation therapy, and cellular telephones—may also affect pacemaker function. In some cases, pacemaker function can be restored by use of a special engineering programmer; in other situations, the device may be permanently damaged and require replacement.

The generator is usually well tolerated in its subcutaneous pocket, but on occasion its presence may be associated with pain. Most often this occurs because the pocket is small and tension is exerted on the overlying tissue. A chronic indolent infection may also be a source of pain. Pain attributed to neuralgia has been treated successfully with steroid injections and with pocket revision. Movement of the pacemaker may occur if the pocket is large, the surrounding tissue lax, and the device not secured. Swelling of the pocket may be caused by infection, seroma, or hematoma. Aspiration of the effusion should be discouraged because of the possibility of introducing infection. A strong suspicion of infection should prompt surgical exploration.

Migration of the pacemaker under the breast or into the axilla may place tension on the leads or result in the assumption of a position that is uncomfortable or is predisposed to erosion. Erosion of pacing hardware is caused by pressure necrosis of overlying tissue or infection. This is usually signaled by a preceding period of "pre-erosion," during which there is discomfort and discoloration of thinning tissue tensely stretched over a protrusion of the pacing apparatus (Fig. 5.24). The risk factors for erosion include a paucity of subcutaneous tissue, the mass and configuration of the pacemaker, need for extra hardware (e.g. lead adaptor) in the pocket, the pocket's construction, and irritation caused by the patient or by articles of clothing. Identification of pre-erosion allows the possibility of salvage of the pacing system, as the hardware may be repositioned under the pectoralis muscle or in an abdominal location.

If erosion occurs, the system is considered contaminated and current opinion favors removal of the generator and leads. Some operators have proposed that extensive debridement of the pocket and prolonged irrigation and antibiotic therapy may provide an alternative option to removal in cases of both erosion and frank infection, but this approach is not generally accepted. For localized erosions, some have suggested removing the generator, debriding the site, and cutting the leads but leaving them *in situ*. However, it is usually

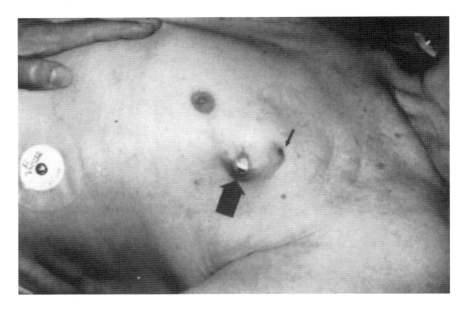

Fig. 5.24 Patient with a permanent pacemaker in whom areas of pre-erosion (small arrow) and erosion (large arrow) are present. This problem is almost always due to indolent infection and requires complete extraction of the system.

appropriate to try to remove the leads rather than to leave them if there is any question concerning sterility.

Bleeding into the pocket may occur when hemostasis is inadequate, when there is a coexistent coagulopathy, or when anticoagulant or thrombolytic therapy is begun prematurely. On occasion, this may compromise the pocket's integrity and may be a risk factor for infection. Hematoma progression, excessive pain, and stress on the suture line may require hematoma evacuation and search for a bleeding site.

Although not a complication of implantation *per se*, a generator may prematurely and without warning fail or may revert to an unsafe pacing mode. The former may relate to a defect in the power supply and the latter is a function of unrecognized problems with circuit design. The incidence of pacemaker failure has steadily declined over the years with improvement in design, and the risk currently is estimated to be approximately 1.4 per thousand devices.[30] Despite the apparent decrease in risk over the years, public concern over this issue has increased in the wake of several highly publicized device advisories.

Infection
Even a non-eroded pacemaker implantation site may become infected. Diabe-

tes mellitus and postoperative hematoma appear to be predisposing factors. Acute infections (usually with *Staphylococcus aureus*) become manifest within the first few weeks of implantation and are often associated with the accumulation of pus. A more indolent infection caused by a less virulent agent such as *S. epidermidis* may present months or years after implantation. A fungal infection may also occur in the pocket and present as an indolent process with relatively scant growth of the organism. Infections with less virulent organisms can present as a small area of erythema, a pimple-like lesion, or a draining sinus. In some cases they appear as cellulitis or pre-erosions. One-third to one-half of infections complicate new implants; the rest are associated with reoperation for generator replacement or lead repositioning. Pocket infections are generally considered to result from organisms introduced from the skin's surface.[8] Superficial infections of the suture line that do not extend to the pocket itself may be treated conservatively.

Staphylococci, and presumably other pathogens, adhere to the plastic insulation of pacing hardware and form colonies that become covered with a secreted substance protecting the organism from host defense and antimicrobial drugs. Antibiotic therapy alone is rarely sufficient to cure these infections, and removal of the pacing system is usually indicated. In patients with erosions or localized pocket infections who have been on antimicrobial therapy and have negative blood cultures, it may be possible to place a new pacing system at a different site at the time of removal of the suspect hardware. Most of the time, however, it would seem prudent to take a two-step approach with temporary pacing (if pacer-dependent) used to bridge the time between explantation and new device implant a few days later. After device removal the infected pocket may be partially closed and a drain inserted, or packed with wet-to-dry dressings and left open to heal by secondary intention.

Less frequently, a pacemaker patient may develop bacteremia without localizing signs, in which case endocarditis associated with a pacing lead should be considered. Lead endocarditis generally occurs later than pocket infection. It may be related to an organism introduced at implantation, but is more often thought to be secondary to a transient bacteremia often from an undefined source. The diagnosis of lead endocarditis can be made when a vegetation is detected by echocardiography in the presence of other signs of infection (Fig. 5.25). TEE may be helpful if transthoracic examination is non-diagnostic. A recent report has suggested that pacemaker-associated endocarditis constitutes 4.6% of the entire population with infective endocarditis and occurs with an incidence of about 0.6% in patients with pacemakers. Staphylococcal species predominate, with about two-thirds being coagulase negative.[31]

Diagnosis of pacemaker lead infection necessitates the removal of all pacing hardware after antibiotics have been started. In these situations, adequate time between explant and implantation of a new permanent system is necessary for antibiotic therapy to sterilize the blood. Generally this interval is

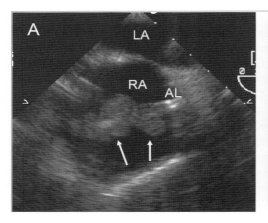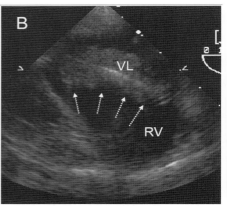

Fig. 5.25 Pacemaker lead infection in transesophageal echocardiographic (TEE) images from a patient presenting with signs and symptoms of subacute endocarditis. Blood cultures grew *Staphylococcus epidermidis*. (A) Image of the right atrium (RA) showing two large vegetations (solid arrows) attached to the right atrial lead (AL). LA indicates the left atrium. (B) Image of the right ventricle (RV) showing the ventricular lead (VL) encased in fibrinous infectious material. The pacemaker system was extracted with an open surgical procedure and an epicardial pacing system was placed.

related to the duration of previous antibiotic treatment and the confirmation of negative blood cultures, usually for 3–10 days. Patients are usually capable of being discharged thereafter on continued antibiotics. The antibiotic therapy is selected on the basis of the organism cultured from the blood or hardware, and treatment duration should be similar to that of non-pacemaker-associated infective endocarditis with the same organism.

In the absence of a positive echocardiogram or other indication of an infected lead, a first episode of bacteremia without an identifying cause should be treated with antibiotics and the pacing system retained. A recurrence of bacteremia after a course of antibiotic therapy in a patient without a demonstrable etiology should prompt consideration of removal of the entire pacing system even if there is no clinical evidence that the leads or generator are infected.

Complications of biventricular pacing

Implantation of a coronary venous lead is the major procedural difference between biventricular and simple dual-chamber pacemakers. It is subject to all the complications associated with dual-chamber systems plus those unique to LV pacing.[32] The LV lead must be placed in a lateral wall CS tributary vein. The technical challenge of this procedure has decreased with improvement in lead design and delivery equipment. Inability to achieve an LV lead placement by a transvenous approach ranges from 2 to 10%.

Unique complications include CS dissection (2–4%) and coronary venous perforation (2%), complications mainly related to CS venography. CS perforation may lead to pericardial tamponade requiring urgent drainage. With better leads and delivery equipment and greater operator experience, lead placement has been facilitated and the long procedure times as well as the significant complication rate reduced. Extracardiac stimulation from the LV lead (diaphragm and phrenic nerve) may also be problematic and should be tested for at the time of implant. Its occurrence should prompt the search for another lead implant site. This problem may also first appear after implantation and can sometimes be corrected with reprogramming, although lead revision may be required.

Lead extraction

General principles

On occasion, consideration is given to the removal of implanted endocardial leads (Table 5.8). The ease of accomplishing this task and the risk associated with lead removal are related to the time the lead has been implanted. Thus, a lead that has been in place for ≤ 3 months is usually easily removed, whereas

Table 5.8 Indications for lead extraction

Class I

Infection (including endocarditis) involving the pacing system*
Life-threatening arrhythmias due to retained lead fragment
Retained lead or fragment that poses imminent physical threat to patient
Clinically significant thromboembolic event caused by a lead or lead fragment
Occlusion of all usable veins with need to implant a new pacer system*
Lead that interferes with the operation of another device

Class II

Localized pocket infection or erosion that does not involve transvenous portion of lead when lead can be separated from infected area*
Occult infection with no clear source but pacemaker system suspected*
Chronic pain at pocket or lead insertion sites unresponsive to other management
Lead failure or design flaw that may pose a future risk to the patient
Lead that interferes with treatment of a malignancy
Leads preventing vascular access for new implantable device*
Non-functional lead in a young patient*

Class III

Risk of lead removal significantly higher than benefit
Single non-functional lead in older patient
Normally functioning lead that may be reused at the time of generator replacement

*The most common indications for lead extraction. From reference 33.

one in place for > 1 year may well present difficulties due to fibrosis, which may occur at any of a number of sites in the heart and central veins with which the lead had contact (Fig. 5.26). Non-isodiametric leads and those with anchoring appendages (tines or fins) present additional problems. When we speak of lead extraction, we are generally concerned with the special challenges presented by a chronically implanted lead. This definition may also be used in situations in which specialized tools (e.g. sheaths, locking stylets, snares, etc.) are needed and/or when the lead is removed from a site other than that of original venous access. The term "lead explant" is used for the removal of leads having an implant duration of < 1 year with only the tools used in a typical implantation and manual traction. These definitions have some importance in terms of the requisite qualifications of physicians performing the respective procedures (see discussion below).[33] Although most of this discussion is directed at lead "extraction," it is relevant to physicians performing lead "explantation" also.

There are two general approaches for the removal of pacing leads: percutaneous and transthoracic. Most pacing physicians believe that if extraction is to be performed it should be done percutaneously; others, however, may still argue the benefits of surgery as a primary approach. Certainly, simple traction on the

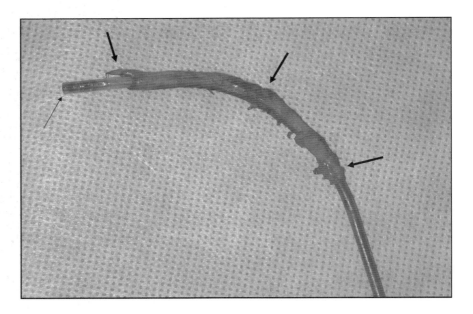

Fig. 5.26 A newly extracted active-fixation ventricular lead is shown with numerous adherent fibrous vascular attachments (thick arrows). The active fixation helix has been retracted into the tip of the lead (thin arrow). It is these fibrous vascular adhesions, which may form anywhere along the length of the lead, which can make lead extraction physically challenging and potentially hazardous due to risk of vascular or cardiac injury.

lead is easy, straightforward and logistically undemanding. If all leads would yield to this treatment there would be little debate as to the threshold for lead extraction and even less support for the more invasive surgical option. Unfortunately, chronic leads are not so readily removed and, even with the variety of tools available to assist in the percutaneous technique, the procedures may be long, difficult, and associated with a finite mortality and significant morbidity.

The risks of lead removal correctly influence the aggressiveness with which one should pursue this approach. Post mortem pathological studies of the hearts of patients with permanent pacemakers have revealed intense fibrosis and encapsulation, especially involving the ventricular portion of the lead, and including the tricuspid valve and its supporting apparatus. Attempts to remove these leads *ex vivo* are associated with myocardial avulsion, valve damage, and disruption of the lead. Implants of longer duration tend to have more extensive fibrosis, but significant encapsulation of an atrial lead has been observed at post mortem examination 6 weeks after implantation.

Contemporary leads used in the USA are of low profile and primarily coaxial bipolar in configuration; they do not, in general, tolerate the physical forces that may be necessary to extract them by simple traction in the presence of significant fibrosis. A variety of tools have been developed to facilitate the extraction of these devices via the process of countertraction.[34] These include a stylet that "locks" in the distal lead, and sheaths that are passed over the lead body, stripping it of fibrous attachments.

The specific events that might complicate lead extraction pertain to the physical forces used to strip away fibrous adhesions to the lead body, and those used to extricate the tip of the lead from the heart. Catastrophic events, when they occur, usually result from either a laceration of a central vein by an extraction tool or perforation of the heart at the site of tip fixation. Embolization of a very large vegetation to the pulmonary artery may also cause death. Damage to the tricuspid valve, or embolization of a lead fragment or thrombus to the lung, or through a patent foramen ovale to the systemic circulation, may also occur. Although most complications become evident during or shortly after the extraction procedure, some such as a retroperitoneal bleed, pulmonary embolism, or pericardial tamponade may be delayed in presentation. Because of the risks involved it is essential that adequate informed consent be obtained from the patient and that the reasons for performing lead extraction, the potential risks and benefits, and alternatives are thoroughly discussed with the patient and family by the operator.

Indications

Lead extraction has inherent risks; thus the decision to undertake the procedure must be weighed against the risk of not extracting the lead. Indications for lead removal based on the latter have been developed by the Heart Rhythm Society (HRS) (formerly known as NASPE) and classified in the ACC/AHA guideline format as: class I, general agreement for removal; class II, situations in which leads are often removed but with some divergence of opinion; class III, general agreement that removal is unnecessary (Table 5.8).[33] This classification primarily addresses the nature of the risk to the patient of not removing a lead, but it does not approach the risk of extracting a chronically implanted lead in a specific patient. Thus, an infected lead is often surprisingly easy to remove, whereas elective removal of a non-functioning passive-fixation lead in place for a number of years may be extremely difficult and result in complications.

A number of modifying factors based on clinical parameters thought to influence the risk of lead extraction have been included in the indication guidelines for the extracting physician to consider.[35] These parameters relate to the patient (age, gender, overall health); anatomy (presence of calcification and vegetations associated with the lead); lead (number of leads, their construction and condition); operator (physician training, experience, and case volume); and the wishes of the patient. These factors are not absolutes, but rather provide a context in which to assess the risks for each specific situation and weigh these against the perceived benefit of extraction. Their consideration may be especially important for class II indications, for which the clinical necessity of removal may be debated.

An infected lead provides the strongest indication for lead removal, since complete removal of all prosthetic material has been shown to be necessary for eradication of the infection in most cases. In a large case series from the Cleveland Clinic, 123 patients underwent pacemaker or ICD system extraction due to documented infection.[31] About one-third of patients had bacteremia, whereas most of the remainder had pocket infections. The microbiology of these infections is reviewed in Table 5.9; *Staphylococci* were the dominant infectious agents. One hundred and seventeen patients (95%) had complete system removal. Of the remaining six patents, three (50%) had relapse of infection, whereas only 1/117 successfully extracted patients had relapse, and this single relapse resulted from reuse of an infected pocket.

Retained non-functioning hardware generally poses little immediate risk to the patient, but may complicate the placement of additional pacing leads either by adding to the venous obstruction (and the risk of thrombosis/embolization) or by generation of spurious electrical potentials between leads. In addition, in young patients with a long life expectancy, the late risks of retained abandoned leads, especially ICD leads, are not well described. Since complications of extraction increase with time elapsed since lead implantation, some argue for routine extraction, rather than abandonment, of unused leads in these patients. In the absence of clear data supporting one point of view, clinicians will need to balance risks and benefits of this approach on a case-by-case basis.

Table 5.9 Microbiology of pacemaker infections

Coagulase-negative staphylococci	68%
Staphylococcus aureus	24%
Gram-negative bacilli	17%
Polymicrobial infections	13%

Data from reference 31.

Lead failure is usually defined in terms of electrical performance, i.e. the ability to pace and sense appropriately. Isolated pacing impedance changes may suggest insulation or conductor failure. There are leads, however, which may exhibit normal electrical function but offer a physical risk to the patient. The Accufix J lead presents a unique risk to the patient in that a small metal wire placed within the lead only to maintain a J shape is subject to fracture under the stress and strain of repetitive cardiac motion. The fractured wire may wear through the insulation and perforate the heart, causing cardiac tamponade or mediastinal hemorrhage. Complete mitigation of this risk when the lead was recalled in 1994 would have required lead extraction in the approximately 45 000 implanted patients. A critical concern has been whether the risk of lead extraction is less than the mortality and morbidity from the Accufix J lead itself. A registry established to study this issue concluded that the risk of death from elective lead extraction of non-fractured leads is higher than the risk of injury from the lead itself.[36] This information has resulted in a recommendation of conservative management of these patients with periodic cinefluoroscopy to screen for retention wire fracture. If fracture occurs, options include removal of the lead or percutaneously snaring the protruding wire fragment.

Risks

In a multicenter study of 1684 patients at 89 US centers, lead extraction of pacing and ICD leads using modern tools was associated with a 0.8% risk of death and a 1.9% risk of major complications, such as pericardial tamponade, hemothorax, and pulmonary embolus (Table 5.10).[37] Ten percent of patients had incomplete (3%) or failed (7%) transvenous extraction. Of the 13 patients who

Table 5.10 Risks of lead extraction

Major	
Death	0.8%
Pericardial tamponade	1.4%
Hemothorax	0.4%
Pulmonary embolus	0.1%
Lead fragment migration	0.1%
Total major complications	1.9%
Minor	
Perforation	0.4%
Myocardial avulsion	0.1%
Venous avulsion	0.1%
Other	0.9%
Total minor complications	1.4%
Any complication	3.3%

Data from reference 37.

died in this registry, five died from tamponade, three from hemothorax, one from pulmonary embolus and one from innominate arteriovenous fistula.

Increasing operator experience appears to reduce the risk of complications. Risk of a major complication was associated with female gender, number of leads in place, and implant duration, whereas risk of any complication was related to less experienced operators (< 50 procedures). Extraction of any chronically implanted lead should be undertaken only after careful consideration of the risk–benefit ratio, including patient age, overall health, presence of calcification or vegetations involving the leads, duration of implant, and patient preference to assume additional risk.

In addition to the acute risks of lead extraction, physicians should be aware of the potential for late mortality after the procedure, between 10 and 20% at 1 year in some series in which extraction was performed mainly for infection[31] (C. Henrikson and J. Brinker, unpublished data). These late deaths probably relate to underlying comorbidities as well as infectious complications in this chronically ill population.

Technique

Extraction of chronically implanted endocardial leads should be undertaken only by experienced physicians and surgeons skilled in the required techniques. Unfortunately, this procedure is not frequently performed and there are few opportunities even in fellowship programs to receive adequate formal training. Acknowledging the well-documented association between complications and inexperienced operators, guidelines for the qualification of physicians have been proposed.[1,33] The performance of a minimum of 20 procedures under the supervision of an experienced (> 100 procedures) operator is recommended before independent practice of these techniques.

The extraction process begins with the gathering and collating of knowledge about the patient and implanted system from the patient's history and medical records (Table 5.11). A chest radiograph should be performed to exclude the presence of undocumented hardware. Recent laboratory data, such as complete blood cell count, platelet count, INR and aPTT, electrolytes, BUN, creatinine and basic chemistries, should be confirmed as acceptable. Blood should be typed and cross-matched. It is necessary to know if complete removal of all leads is essential and whether a new device will be implanted as part of the same procedure. Based on these data, a plan of action is devised. Availability of all the tools and equipment that may be needed should be confirmed before the patient is taken to the procedure room.

Most operators continue to perform the procedure in the pacemaker or electrophysiology laboratory with cardiovascular surgical backup. Some operators prefer to perform the procedure in an operating room to facilitate emergency thoracotomy and cardiopulmonary bypass, if required. In either case, adequate fluoroscopy must be available. Either general anesthesia or moderate sedation may be used. The patient is prepared as for an implantation, although

Table 5.11 Pre-explant information

Device

1. Site(s) of venous access
2. Number and types of leads
3. Method used for retention of leads
4. Difficulties encountered in prior procedures
5. Information on previously abandoned leads

Patient

1. Degree of pacemaker dependency and need for temporary pacing
2. Risk for sedation/anesthesia
3. Comorbidities/medications
4. Special considerations (e.g. vascular anomaly or occlusion; IVC filter, bleeding diathesis)

Laboratory

1. Complete blood cell count, INR, aPTT, platelet count, sample to blood bank
2. Blood chemistries
3. ECG
4. Chest radiograph (PA and lateral) and/or lead fluoroscopy

IVC, inferior vena cava; INR, International Normalized Ratio; aPTT, activated partial thromboplastin time; PA, posteroanterior.

some surgeons scrub the chest as in preparation for a thoracotomy. We almost always use an assistant for these procedures (either a fellow or second attending physician) due to the amount of equipment which must be controlled during the case.

We have recently decided to perform extraction of chronic leads routinely in the operating room. The reason for this is based on the logic that emergency thoracotomy, if necessary, could most expeditiously be obtained and the surgeon would be in an environment favoring optimal performance in terms of logistical support. It has also become clear that although endovascular lead extraction is relatively safe, it is hard to predict which patient might have a major complication and what that complication would specifically be. There are situations in which simple pericardiocentesis is not adequate to prevent cardiovascular collapse, especially in older patients with significant comorbidity. Associated with the above, there appears to be a more aggressive pursuit of litigation following adverse events during lead extraction should a significant complication occur. Although current guidelines do not mandate extraction in the operating room, we have observed a clinical trend in this direction. Regardless of where the procedure is performed, it is important to have a surgeon closely available should one be needed.

The routine preparation for lead extractions involves one or both groin areas for the placement of a venous line (6-F sheath) in the right femoral vein and a small arterial line in either femoral artery for continuous monitoring of the arterial blood pressure. Sterile drapes are liberally placed so that a sterile field is maintained from the neck to the toes. If the patient is pacemaker-dependent, a temporary pacing wire is inserted through either a femoral or an internal jugular vein. If prolonged temporary pacing will be needed, we have been using an active fixation permanent lead as the temporary device for added security against lead dislodgement during the interim period.

A commercially available lead-extraction kit (Cook Vascular, Leechburg, PA, USA) supplemented by a variety of other tools (such as snares, wires, locking stylets, biopsy forceps, guidewires and laser extraction sheaths) should be available. The operator should have on hand all of the tools that may be needed in a complex case, whether their use is anticipated or not. A pericardiocentesis tray, a chest tube kit and an emergency thoracotomy tray should be readily available, and an echocardiography machine should be accessible. The operator must have a step-by-step approach to the specific problems offered by the case in mind, and be ready to respond to emergencies as they arise.

The pocket is usually entered through the previous incision line, although this may be altered to include a site of erosion. With a combination of sharp and blunt dissection, the generator and leads are freed. Electrocautery is helpful in freeing leads that are often extensively fibrosed to themselves and subcutaneous tissue. The lead is traced to the venous entry point, the suture sleeve is identified, and all retention sutures are cut and removed. The lead is disconnected from the generator and its internal integrity is accessed by passing a standard stylet to the tip. In most cases an initial attempt at gentle traction is worthwhile, but care must be taken not to damage the lead during this process.

Passive leads are usually more difficult to extract than active leads, presumably because the tines incorporated on the former devices provide a greater surface area for fibrous adhesion. For active fixation leads, the helix should be retracted in order to facilitate removal and reduce the risk of cardiac perforation. If the retraction mechanism is not effective (or if this is a non-retractable helix) an attempt should be made to rotate the entire lead counterclockwise to unscrew the tip from the heart. This may be impossible in situations where the body of the lead is extensively fibrosed to the heart and veins.

Tools for extraction

A variety of tools are available to assist with lead extraction. A partial list of equipment which should be available to the operator is given in Table 5.12. Techniques for lead extraction can be broadly categorized into the superior approach (utilizing locking stylet and telescoping sheaths placed over the lead to provide countertraction and counterpressure) and the femoral approach (using no stylet and different types of grasping snare to remove leads primarily with traction).

The superior approach
If a lead is not easily removable by gentle traction, the stylet should be withdrawn and the lead cut close to the terminal pin with a lead cutter. The central

Table 5.12 Tools and equipment for lead extraction

General equipment
- Standard lead stylets
- Fluoroscopy
- Pacemaker tray
- Pericardiocentesis tray
- Chest tube insertion kit
- Emergency thoracotomy tray

Superior approach
- Locking stylets
- Lead extraction kit (Cook Vascular)
- Steel sheaths (to facilitate freeing the lead to vascular insertion)
- Laser lead extraction sheath (Spectranetics)
- Radiofrequency extraction sheath

Femoral approach
- Byrd femoral workstation
- Needle's Eye Snare (Cook Vascular)
- Dotter retrieval basket

lumen of the lead is identified and carefully dilated with a coil-expander tool. The diameter of the lumen is then determined by the insertion of a series of gauge pins. A locking stylet of a size corresponding to the largest gauge pin accepted by the lead is then advanced through the lumen to the lead tip. This device is essential to focus the force of traction as close to the lead tip as possible, and to distribute traction along the length of the lead.

There are now several types of locking stylet available (Fig. 5.27), which vary in the way they grip the inner core of the lead. Because current generations of these devices have a greater flexibility in adapting to a range of inner core diameters, fewer different types and sizes need to be stocked. The operator needs to be familiar with the specific directions for each of the locking stylets they use. It may be difficult or impossible to reverse the locking mechanism and remove these devices once they are inserted into the lead. Some manufacturers incorporate "cables" into the insulation of the defibrillator leads to provide additional traction during lead extraction. By tying 0-silk sutures to these cables and to the body of the lead, the tension on the lead is distributed over a larger area (Fig. 5.28). This may facilitate difficult extractions, in which the inner conductor breaks free or when locking stylets cannot be passed. In patients with inner conductor failure, the inner lumen of the lead may be interrupted, making it impossible to pass a locking stylet. In this case the femoral approach may be required.

A variety of plastic (either "powered" by laser or electrocautery or unpowered) and metal dilating sheaths are available to advance over the lead body and free it from fibrous adhesions (Fig. 5.29). The traditional sheaths are strictly mechanical dilating devices and have been used coaxially in a telescoping fashion to provide support and allow for a slightly larger device to be used

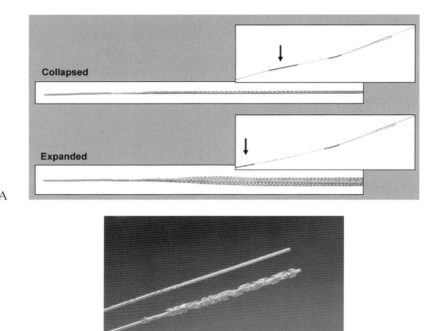

A

B

Fig. 5.27 Locking stylets for lead extraction. A, The Spectranetics LLD locking stylet (Spectranetics, Colorado Springs, CO, USA) has an expandable mesh over the stylet body that binds the lumen of the lead along its length. Top panels: With the mesh retracted, the entire length of the stylet is isodiametric with the stylet tip for insertion into the lead. Bottom panels: Once inside the lead to be extracted, the operator slides the locking mechanism (arrow) forward expanding the mesh, which provides a broad distribution of force along the lead when traction is applied. B, The Cook stylet (Cook Vascular) has a small wire mesh wound at the tip that unravels and binds at the distal end of the lead lumen.

when necessary. In many cases, applying considerable countertraction and torque to the sheath is necessary to separate the lead from fibrous adhesions. To minimize the risk of perforation by the stiff sheaths, fluoroscopic monitoring must be used to ensure that the proper coaxial alignment of the dilator sheath and the lead is maintained. Traction upon the lead via the locking stylet (usually maintained by the assistant) facilitates the processes. Correct positioning of the sheath near the tip of the lead provides a mechanism for countertraction to be applied to the lead to facilitate extraction. By advancing the outer sheath to the lead tip at the endocardial surface, the sheath applies countertraction to pin the myocardium in place and allows traction on the lead without invaginating or tearing the myocardium (Fig. 5.30).

If the leads are removed successfully, a new pacing system may be implanted at the same site (if circumstances permit) by using a guidewire inserted through

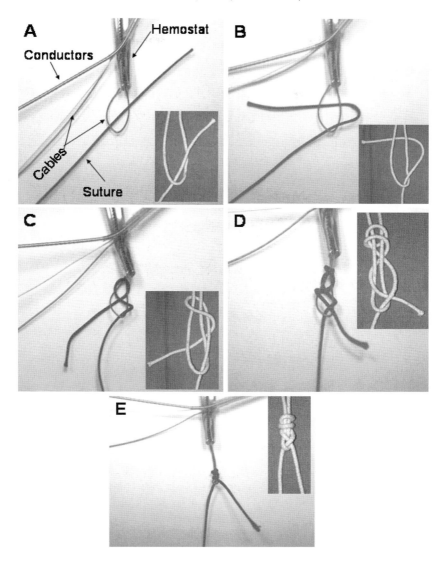

Fig. 5.28 Tying to the "cables" of defibrillator leads. A modified sheet bend is used. A, A loop is formed with the exposed end of the cable and held in place with a small hemostat. A 0-silk suture is passed through the loop from below. B, The silk tie is passed behind the loop of cable. C, The silk is passed in front of the loop of cable and then behind again 2–3 times wrapping around the neck of the loop. D, The end of the silk is passed under itself but over the loop of cable. E, The ends of the silk are pulled to complete the knot. The long end of the silk tie is tied to the end of the locking stylet to provide traction on the cable.

the extraction sheath to facilitate venous entry. Care should be taken to avoid air embolus as the wire is passed through the large empty extraction sheath. This technique allows access through even chronically occluded veins.

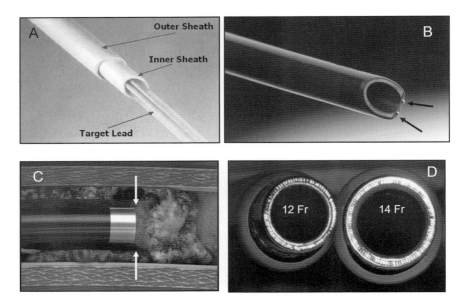

Fig. 5.29 Several different types of sheath used in lead extraction. A, Simple telescoping sheaths over a lead. The outer sheath provides support as the inner sheath (with beveled edge) is gradually advanced over the lead to separate it from fibrous vascular adhesions by blunt dissection. B, The Electrosurgical Dissection System (EDS, Cook Medical) utilizes an inner sheath with bipolar electrocautery/radiofrequency energy delivered between two poles on the tip of the sheath. Ablative energy is limited to approximately one-quarter of the circumference of the sheath. C, The laser-assisted sheath (Spectranetics) consists of a series of parallel fiberoptic cables wound around a flexible inner sheath and terminating at the tip of the sheath (arrows). D, When activated, the tip of the sheath emits pulses of high-energy ultraviolet light along the entire circumference of the sheath, vaporizing fibrous adhesions in direct contact with the tip.

The process of lead extraction with the use of early-generation unpowered tools is labor intensive and time consuming: complete removal of a lead was achieved in 81–87% of cases and inability to remove the lead was encountered in 6–7% of cases. The evolution of technology and introduction of the excimer laser sheath have greatly facilitated lead extraction by the superior approach (Fig. 5.30). The latter device has optical fibers arrayed circumferentially in the lining of the sheath, which is attached to the Spectranetics excimer laser generator (Spectranetics, Colorado Springs, CO, USA). Laser energy ablates the fibrous adhesions as the sheath is advanced (see Fig. 5.16). Complete removal of leads using this approach may be anticipated in 90% of patients and partial removal in another 3%.[37] An electrosurgical cutting sheath is also available for lead extraction. This device is less expensive, but may not be as effective in the more difficult cases as is the laser, although there are no adequate comparison trials.[38] Although they have improved efficacy, neither of these adjunct energy devices has demonstrably increased the safety of lead extraction.

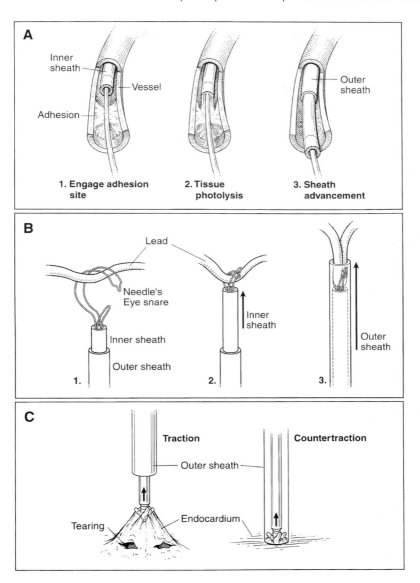

Fig. 5.30 Basic techniques of lead extraction. A, Lead extraction from the superior approach using the Spectranetics laser sheath apparatus. As the telescoping sheath apparatus encounters fibrous adhesions, the inner end-firing laser sheath is used to lyse the fibrosis. The larger outer sheath may then be advanced to apply countertraction at the lead tip. B, Lead extraction from the femoral approach using the Cook Intravascular Needle's Eye Snare apparatus. The snare is deployed from telescoping sheaths in the femoral vein. The lead is entrapped in the snare and then secured against the inner sheath. The larger outer sheath may then be advanced to apply countertraction at the lead tip. C, The concept of countertraction is illustrated. When unmodified traction is applied to the lead, the heart wall may invaginate and tear the myocardium around the lead tip. Using countertraction, the outer sheath holds the myocardium in place, thus minimizing deformity and tearing of the myocardium.

Femoral approach

On occasion, a lead cannot be removed from its original venous access site using the techniques described above due to inadequate lead remnant in the pocket or inability to pass a locking stylet. In these cases the femoral venous approach is often successful. With this method, a large (16 F) sheath with a hemostatic valve is used as a "workstation" through which any of a number of devices designed to grasp the lead body may be introduced. These devices may include smaller sheaths, a Dotter retrieval basket, a tip-deflecting guidewire, a "needle's eye" device (Cook Vascular, Leechburg, PA, USA), or a variety of other catheters, snares and bioptomes (Fig. 5.31). With the femoral technique, one must grasp the lead body, which can be done with a single device (the Needle's Eye Snare) or with two devices such as a tip-deflecting wire and an Amplatz gooseneck snare. The needle's eye device is contained in a 12-F sheath. There are two independently moving mechanisms that can be advanced from the sheath: a hook-shaped wire loop (needle's eye) and a more narrow "threader," which is designed to pass within the hook of the needle's eye. The goal is to place the device so that the lead body is trapped between

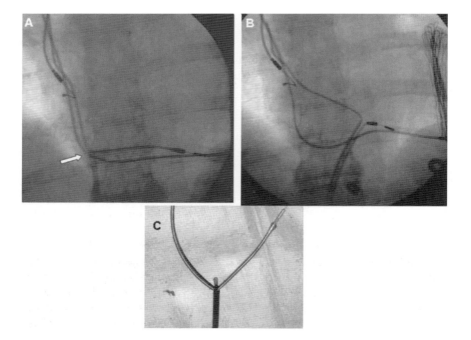

Fig. 5.31 Fluoroscopic images of ventricular lead extraction by the femoral approach. A, The ventricular lead has been captured with the Needle's Eye Snare apparatus at the point of the arrow and the redundancy of the lead retracted into the low atrium. B, With traction the lead tip is dislodged from the ventricle and the folded lead body is withdrawn into the large outer sheath. C, The completely extracted lead.

the needle's eye and threader. This is usually accomplished by first placing the sheath in the low right atrium with the devices retained inside. The needle's eye is advanced out of the sheath and rotated so that it "hooks" around the lead body. The threader is then advanced so that it passes through the distal portion of the needle's eye so that the lead is between the devices (Fig. 5.31).

The sheath is then advanced over the ensemble fixing the captured lead. Once this is accomplished the proximal lead is cut near its original insertion site and traction applied by the sheath pulling the proximal lead into the heart. The captured lead may be prolapsed into the workstation, which can be used as a countertraction device as it is advanced over the distal lead; however, this may not be feasible with many larger leads. In the latter instance, just withdrawing the proximal free end of the lead into the heart or IVC and then disengaging the needle's eye will allow it to be captured by a gooseneck snare and more easily removed through the workstation. The workstation may be advanced over the lead into the ventricle to supply countertraction if necessary.

The needle's eye technique has been found to be safe and effective, with a complete extraction success rate of 87% in a population that included patients who had failed prior extraction from the superior approach.[39] A similar procedure may be performed with a deflecting wire and snare. In this situation both the wire and snare are situated in the right atrium through the workstation. A "J" curve is placed on the deflector wire, which is used to "catch" the lead body. The snare is then advanced to tightly grasp the tip of the deflecting wire. This effectively forms a loop around the lead body, which can act to retract the lead after the proximal portion is cut from the original access site. Once captured, the lead can be removed as described previously for the needle's eye device.

Although it is always best to withdraw the lead through the workstation, there are times when this cannot be done and the workstation has to be removed with the lead inside. If multiple leads must be removed, we sometimes leave a second long wire in the femoral vein at the time of original access. This allows us to re-enter the same entry site with a second workstation if it is necessary to remove the first. Once all of the leads are out, it is safe to remove the workstation and apply manual pressure to the femoral access site for hemostasis.

The femoral workstation technique appears to be safe and quite successful. It avoids having to free up adhesions in the central veins because the proximal lead is usually more easily pulled through fibrous vascular attachments from below. On occasion, the proximal lead appears trapped within the subclavian vein and will not yield to femoral traction. In these cases the laser sheath can be very helpful in freeing up the proximal lead, allowing it to be extracted through the femoral workstation. The workstation has a large lumen and blood coagulates easily within it. A large thrombus may form and be pushed into the circulation during the manipulation of devices through the sheath. We routinely attach a pressurized continuous flush to the sidearm of the device to help prevent such thrombus formation.

Variations on the femoral approach include a hybrid procedure, in which the femoral workstation is used as described above to pull the proximal lead into the heart. At this point a snare introduced from the internal jugular vein is used to catch the free end of the lead and pull it out using countertraction from a long sheath placed in the internal jugular. The entire procedure might be performed using an internal jugular approach, which has been favored by some since the direction of force exerted during countertraction is parallel to the course of the lead.

Accufix wire fragment retrieval

As noted previously, fracture of the "J" retention wire in the Accufix family of atrial leads may produce protrusion of a wire fragment (Fig. 5.32), which has the potential to lacerate the heart and other mediastinal structures. It may be possible to selectively retrieve the protruding fragment if it is the distal portion of the proximal part of the wire. This is achieved using an Amplatz gooseneck snare passed through an 8-F coronary guide catheter of a shape

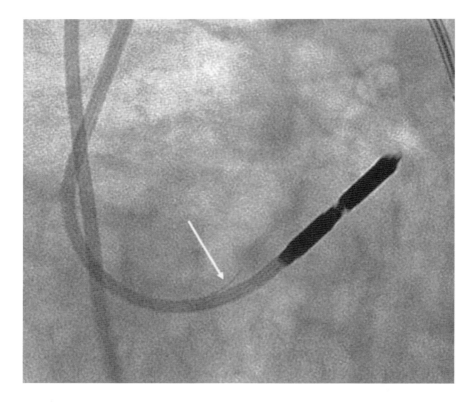

Fig. 5.32 Cinefluoroscopy of the Telectronics Pacing Systems model 330–801 Accufix atrial J lead. This right anterior oblique projection shows the protruding segment of the retention wire fragment (arrow).

matching the specifics of the case. Since the proximal portion of the retention wire lies free under the outer insulation of the lead, traction on its protruding end results in the fragment's removal from the lead into the guide catheter without disrupting the lead itself. Detection of a protruding fragment (so-called class III fracture) by screening fluoroscopy should prompt consideration of this form of therapy as an alternative to lead extraction.

Extraction of coronary venous leads

With the increased use of biventricular pacing, there has been some concern that removal of chronically implanted leads from the coronary venous system will be associated with high complication rates because of the risk of disruption of the thin-walled coronary veins. Although there is limited experience thus far, removal of these devices has not been associated with complications. These series, however, include only a very small number of leads with long implant duration.[40,41] With chronic CS leads, the excimer laser sheath may be used with countertraction technique to free the lead from adhesion up to the os of the CS. Safe use of extraction sheaths within the CS has not been demonstrated. Fortunately, in series reported to date, fibrous adhesions of these leads have generally been seen outside of the CS.

Thoracotomy for lead extraction

There has been a natural reticence even among surgeons to remove leads at thoracotomy. While there are no randomized data comparing the two techniques, the Accufix experience suggests no clinically significant difference in the incidence of death or major complications. This is not surprising considering the advanced age and comorbidity of many pacemaker patients. Surgery may be the only alternative in situations in which percutaneous techniques have failed and there is an absolute indication for lead removal. Since most transvenous extraction series demonstrate a 5–10% rate of failure to remove all lead material completely, a significant role for surgical lead extraction remains. Primary thoracotomy should also be considered when there is a large lead vegetation (> 2 cm) and perhaps when there is a vegetation and a right-to-left intracardiac shunt. Close collaboration between physicians who perform extractions and cardiothoracic surgeons who can perform surgical extraction and assist with management of complications of transvenous extraction is a vital component of a lead extraction program.

Lead abandonment

The alternative to extraction is lead abandonment and (usually) insertion of a new lead. This is not an option in cases of infection, where failure to remove all hardware results in an unacceptable risk of re-infection despite vigorous treatment with antibiotics. One may abandon the lead by detaching it from the generator and applying an insulating cap to the connector pin. The lead may then be placed under the generator or elsewhere in the pocket, reserving an option for future use in some situations as well as lead extraction should that prove necessary (e.g. the occurrence of infection). Many operators now prefer to cut the lead and electrically isolate it by pulling the silicone insulation over the exposed end and tying a ligature tightly around the insulation cuff. The lead is then sutured to the underlying tissue to prevent its retraction into the vascular space. Enough lead is left in the pocket to allow for future extraction if that proves necessary. Active fixation leads should not be cut, because this precludes retraction of the helix of the lead if extraction should ever be needed.

Medical-legal aspects of implantation

As with many invasive procedures, the patient's expectations for pacemaker therapy may exceed the results obtained. As noted above, there is ample opportunity for even the most skilled and experienced operator to encounter a misadventure. The risk of litigation is real and may be focused on any of several areas of physician responsibility (Table 5.13). Avoiding litigation requires not only that the highest of standards be maintained, but also that a rapport be established with the patient and the patient's family.

The best defense against successful litigation is full documentation in the patient's medical record of every aspect of the implantation (or extraction) process. This should include the indication for the procedure, the informed consent, a complete procedure note to include the pacing parameters achieved and any difficulties encountered, evidence of post-procedure evaluation, and arrangements for follow-up care. The removal of pre-existing hardware and its disposition (e.g. returned to manufacturer for evaluation) should also be documented.

Pacemaker implantation implies a great deal of physician responsibility. As with any implantable device, there is continued risk to the patient as long as they have the device. Somewhat unique to implantable antiarrhythmic devices is the knowledge that the power source has limited life and will eventually need to be replaced. The HRS, as well as the ACC and AHA, have provided a service to physicians by creating guidelines to assist in patient treatment.[1,2,33]

Table 5.13 Responsibilities of an implanting physician

1 Establish and document accepted indications
2 Obtain fully informed consent
3 Implant an indicated system
4 Avoid undue delay
5 Conform to accepted technique and standards
6 Obtain expert consultation when appropriate
7 Provide for follow-up care

References

1 Hayes DL, Naccarelli GV, Furman S *et al.* NASPE training requirements for cardiac implantable electronic devices: selection, implantation, and follow-up. PACE 2003; 26:1556–62.

2 Gregoratos G, Abrams K, Epstein AE *et al.* ACC/AHA/NASPE 2002 guideline update for implantation of cardiac pacemakers and antiarrhythmia devices: summary article: a report of the American College of Cardiology/American Heart Association Task Force on Practice Guidelines (ACC/AHA/NASPE Committee to Update the 1998 Pacemaker Guidelines). Circulation 2002; 106:2145–61.

3 Stacul F, Adam A, Becker CR *et al.* Strategies to reduce the risk of contrast-induced nephropathy. Am J Cardiol 2006; 98 (Suppl.):59K–77K.

4 Michaud GF, Pelosi F Jr, Noble MD *et al.* A randomized trial comparing heparin initiation 6h or 24h after pacemaker or defibrillator implantation. J Am Coll Cardiol 2000; 35:1915–8.

5 Giudici MC, Barold SS, Paul DL, Bontu P. Pacemaker and implantable cardioverter defibrillator implantation without reversal of warfarin therapy. PACE 2004; 27:358–60.

6 McCotter CJ, Angle JF, Prudente LA *et al.* Placement of transvenous pacemaker and ICD leads across total chronic occlusions. Pacing Clin Electrophysiol 2005; 28:921–5.

7 DaCosta A, Kirkorian G, Cucherat M *et al.* Antibiotic prophylaxis for permanent pacemaker implantation: a meta-analysis. Circulation 1998; 97:1796–801.

8 Da Costa A, Lelievre H, Kirkorian G *et al.* Role of the preaxillary flora in pacemaker infections: a prospective study. Circulation 1998; 97:1791–5.

9 Biffi F, Boriani G, Frabetti L *et al.* Left superior vena cava persistence in patients undergoing pacemaker or cardioverter-defibrillator implantation: a 10-year experience. Chest 2001; 120:139–44.

10 Calkins H, Ramza BM, Brinker J *et al.* Prospective randomized comparison of the safety and effectiveness of placement of endocardial pacemaker and defibrillator leads using the extrathoracic subclavian vein guided by contrast venography versus the cephalic approach. PACE 2001; 24:456–64.

11 Kistler PM, Eizenberg N, Fynn SP, Mond HG. The subpectoral pacemaker implant: it isn't what it seems! PACE 2004; 27:361–4.

12 Brinker JA. Endocardial pacing leads: the good, the bad, and the ugly. Pacing Clin Electrophysiol 1995; 18:953–4.

13 Hauser RG, Hayes DL, Kallinen LM *et al.* Clinical experience with pacemaker pulse generators and transvenous leads: an 8-year prospective multicenter study. Heart Rhythm 2007; 4:154–60.

14 Giudici MC, Thornburg GA, Buck DL *et al.* Comparison of right ventricular outflow tract and apical lead permanent pacing on cardiac output. Am J Cardiol 1997; 79:209–12.

15 Stambler BS, Ellenbogen K, Zhang X *et al.* Right ventricular outflow versus apical pacing in pacemaker patients with congestive heart failure and atrial fibrillation. J Cardiovasc Electrophysiol 2003; 14:1180–6.

16 Saxenhouse SJ, Conti JB, Curtis AB. Current of injury predicts adequate active fixation in permanent pacemaker/defibrillation leads. J Am Coll Cardiol 2005; 45:412–7.

17 Bilchick KC, Judge DP, Calkins H, Marine JE. Use of a coronary sinus lead and biventricular ICD to correct a sensing abnormality in a patient with arrhythmogenic right ventricular dysplasia/cardiomyopathy. J Cardiovasc Electrophysiol 2006; 17:317–20.

18 Ector B, Willems R, Heidbuchel H *et al.* Epicardial pacing: a single-centre study on 321 leads in 138 patients. Acta Cardiol. 2006; 61:343–51.

19 Huang M, Krahn AD, Yee R *et al.* Optimal pacing for symptomatic AV block: a comparison of VDD and DDD pacing. Pacing Clin Electrophysiol 2004; 27:19–23.

20 Wilkoff BL, Cook JR, Epstein AE *et al.* Dual-chamber pacing or ventricular backup pacing in patients with an implantable defibrillator: the Dual Chamber and VVI Implantable Defibrillator (DAVID) Trial. JAMA 2002; 288:3115–23.

21 Link MS, Estes NA 3rd, Griffin JJ *et al.* Complications of dual chamber pacemaker implantation in the elderly. Pacemaker Selection in the Elderly (PASE) Investigators. J Interv Card Electrophysiol 1998; 2:175–9.

22 Tobin K, Stewart J, Westveer D, Frumin H. Acute complications of permanent pacemaker implantation: their financial implications and relation to volume and operator experience. Am J Cardiol 2000; 85:774–7.

23 Harcombe AA, Newell SA, Ludman PF *et al.* Late complications following permanent pacemaker implantation or elective unit replacement. Heart 1998; 80:240–4.

24 Wiegand UK, Bode F, Bonnemeier H *et al.* Atrial lead placement during atrial fibrillation. Is restitution of sinus rhythm required for proper lead function? Feasibility and 12-month functional analysis. Pacing Clin Electrophysiol 2000; 23:1144–9.

25 Ellenbogen KA, Wood MA, Shepard RK. Delayed complications following pacemaker implantation. Pacing Clin Electrophysiol 2002; 25:1155–8.

26 Henrikson CA, Leng CT, Yuh DD, Brinker JA. Computed tomography to assess possible cardiac lead perforation. Pacing Clin Electrophysiol 2006; 29:509–11.

27 Van Gelder BM, Bracke FA, Oto A *et al.* Diagnosis and management of inadvertently placed pacing and ICD leads in the left ventricle: a multicenter experience and review of the literature. Pacing Clin Electrophysiol 2000; 23:877–83.

28 Lin G, Nishimura RA, Connolly HM *et al.* Severe symptomatic tricuspid valve regurgitation due to permanent pacemaker or implantable cardioverter-defibrillator leads. J Am Coll Cardiol 2005; 45:1672–5.

29 Rozmus G, Daubert JP, Huang DT, Rosero S, Hall B, Francis C. Venous thrombosis and stenosis after implantation of pacemakers and defibrillators. J Interv Card Electrophysiol 2005; 13:9–19.

30 Maisel WH, Moynahan M, Zuckerman BD *et al.* Pacemaker and ICD generator malfunctions: analysis of Food and Drug Administration annual reports. JAMA 2006; 295:1901–6.

31 Dhua JD, Wilkoff BL, Lee I *et al.* Diagnosis and management of infections involving implantable electrophysiologic cardiac devices. Ann Intern Med 2000; 133:604–8.

32 Bhatta L, Luck JC, Wolbrette DL, Naccarelli GV. Complications of biventricular pacing. Curr Opin Cardiol 2003; 19:31–35.

33 Love CJ, Wilkoff BL, Byrd CL *et al.* Recommendations for extraction of chronically implanted transvenous pacing and defibrillator leads: indications, facilities, training. North American Society of Pacing and Electrophysiology Lead Extraction Conference Faculty. Pacing Clin Electrophysiol 2000; 23:544–51.

34 Love CJ, Smith MC. Extraction of pacing leads: overview of current techniques. J Cardiovasc Electrophysiol 2006; 17:1257–61.

35 Roux J-F, Page P, Dubuc M *et al.* Laser lead extraction: predictors of success and complications. Pacing Clin Electrophysiol 2007; 30:214–20.

36 Kay GN, Brinker JA, Kawanishi DT *et al.* Risks of spontaneous injury and extraction of an active fixation pacemaker lead: report of the Accufix multicenter clinical study and worldwide registry. Circulation 1999; 100:2344–52.

37 Byrd CL, Willkoff BL, Love CJ, Sellers TD, Reiser C. Clinical study of the laser sheath for lead extraction: the total experience in the United States. PACE 2002; 25:804–8.

38 Verma A, Wilkoff BL. Intravascular pacemaker and defibrillator lead extraction: a state-of-the-art review. Heart Rhythm 2004; 1:739–45.

39 Klug D, Jarwe M, Messaoudene SA *et al.* Pacemaker lead extraction with the needle's eye snare for countertraction via the femoral approach. PACE 2002; 25:1023–8.

40 Burke MC, Morton J, Lin AC *et al.* Implications and outcome of permanent coronary sinus lead extraction and reimplantation. J Cardiovasc Electrophysiol 2005; 16:830–7.

41 Bongiorni MG, Zucchelli G, Soldati E *et al.* Usefulness of transvenous mechanical dilation and location of areas of adherence in patients undergoing coronary sinus lead extraction. Europace 2007; 9:69–73.

CHAPTER 6

Pacemaker timing cycles

Paul J Wang, Amin Al-Ahmad, David L Hayes

Understanding various pacing modes and paced electrocardiograms (ECGs) requires a thorough understanding of pacemaker timing cycles.[1-5] Pacemaker timing cycles include all potential variations of a single complete pacing cycle—the time from paced ventricular beat to paced ventricular beat; the time from paced ventricular beat to an intrinsic ventricular beat, whether it is a conducted R wave or a premature ventricular contraction (PVC); the time from paced atrial beat to paced atrial beat; the time from intrinsic atrial beat to paced atrial beat; the time from intrinsic ventricular beat to paced ventricular beat; and so forth. These cycles include events sensed, events paced, and periods when the sensing circuit or circuits are refractory. Each portion of the pacemaker timing cycle should be considered in milliseconds and not in pulses per minute (ppm). Although thinking of the patient's pacing rate in paced beats per minute may be easier, portions of the timing cycle are too brief to consider in any unit but milliseconds.

Knowledge of the relation between elements of the paced ECG enhances understanding of pacemaker rhythms. Although multiple unknown factors may affect a native rhythm, each timing circuit of a pacemaker can function in only one of two states. A given timer can proceed until it completes its cycle; completion results in either the release of a pacing stimulus or the initiation of another timing cycle. Alternatively, a given timer can be reset, at which point it starts the timing period again.

To make this chapter more readable and to facilitate clarity, a series of abbreviations is used to designate native and paced events and portions of the timing cycle. These abbreviations are listed in Table 6.1. P indicates native atrial depolarization, A an atrial paced event, R native ventricular depolarization, and V a ventricular paced event. I represents an interval. From this, PR refers to a native complex that completely inhibits the pacemaker on both the atrial and the ventricular channels. AV refers to pacing sequentially in both the atrium and the ventricle. If an atrial paced complex is followed by native ventricular depolarization that inhibits the ventricular output of the pacemaker, the designation is AR. If a native atrial complex is followed by a paced ventricular depolarization, P-synchronous pacing, the designa-

Cardiac Pacing and ICDs, 5th edition. Edited by Kenneth A. Ellenbogen and Mark A. Wood.
© 2008 Blackwell Publishing, ISBN: 978-1-4051-6350-7

Table 6.1 Abbreviations for native and paced events and portions of the timing cycle

P	Native atrial depolarization
A	Atrial paced event
R	Native ventricular depolarization
V	Ventricular paced event
I	Interval
AV	Sequential pacing in the atrium and ventricle
AVI	Programmed atrioventricular pacing interval
AR	Atrial paced event followed by intrinsic ventricular depolarization
ARP	Atrial refractory period
PV	Native atrial depolarization followed by a paced ventricular event, P-synchronous pacing
AEI	Atrial escape interval, interval from a ventricular sensed or paced event to an atrial paced event, the VA interval
LRL	Lower rate limit
URL	Upper rate limit
MTR	Maximum tracking rate
MSR	Maximum sensor rate
PVARP	Postventricular atrial refractory period
RRAVD	Rate-responsive atrioventricular delay
VAI	Ventriculoatrial interval: interval from a sensed or paced ventricular event to an atrial paced event
VRP	Ventricular refractory period

tion is PV. Because the pacemaker timing cycle in dual-chamber pacing has more portions to consider than single-chamber pacing, more discussion is devoted to understanding dual-chamber timing cycles, specifically those of universal (DDD) pacing systems.[5]

Multiple programmable features may affect device behavior (Table 6.2). These are discussed throughout the chapter.

Pacing nomenclature

A three-letter code describing the basic function of the various pacing systems was first proposed in 1974 by a combined task force from the American Heart Association and the American College of Cardiology. Since then, the code has been updated periodically.[6] It is a generic code and, as such, does not describe specific or unique functional characteristics of each device. The code has five positions.

The first position reflects the chamber or chambers in which stimulation occurs. A refers to the atrium, V indicates the ventricle, and D means dual chamber, or both atrium and ventricle.

The second position refers to the chamber or chambers in which sensing occurs. The letter designators are the same as those for the first position. Manufacturers also use S in both the first and the second positions to indicate that the device is capable of pacing only a single cardiac chamber. Once the device is implanted and connected to a lead in either the atrium or the ventricle, S

Table 6.2 Features that may affect device behavior*

Intrinsic rate slower than programmed base rate
  Hysteresis
  Sleep or rest rate
  Special algorithms (+PVARP on PVC)

Base rate (AV, AR) higher than programmed base rate
  Sensor driven
  Rate smoothing
  Mode-switching response rate
  Special algorithms (+PVARP on PVC)
  Sudden rate drop response
  Atrial overdrive suppression

Intrinsic AV conduction interval (PR, AR) longer than programmed paced or sensed AVI
  AV or PV hysteresis
  Sinus rate with intact AV conduction exceeding MTR

Paced or sensed AVI shorter than programmed paced or sensed AVI
  Rate-responsive AV delay
  Negative AV or PV hysteresis
  Safety pacing
  NCAP (non-competitive atrial pacing)
  Auto-threshold test

Loss of atrial tracking (DDD mode)
  Automatic mode switch
  MSR > MTR

*Not necessarily continuously; the effect can be on single cycles or during a brief period.
PVARP, postventricular atrial refractory period; PVC, premature ventricular contraction; AVI, atrioventricular interval; MTR, maximum tracking rate; MSR, maximum sensor rate.

should be changed to either A or V in the clinical record to reflect the chamber in which pacing and sensing are occurring.

The third position refers to the mode of sensing, or how the pacemaker responds to a sensed event. An I indicates that a sensed event inhibits the output pulse and causes the pacemaker to recycle for one or more timing cycles. T means that an output pulse is triggered in response to a sensed event. D, in a manner similar to that in the first two positions, means that there are dual modes of response. This designation is restricted to dual-chamber systems. An event sensed in the atrium inhibits atrial output but triggers ventricular output. Unlike the single-chamber triggered mode, in which an output pulse is triggered immediately on sensing, a delay occurs between the sensed atrial event and the triggered ventricular output to mimic the normal PR interval. If a native ventricular signal or R wave is sensed, it inhibits ventricular output and possibly even atrial output, depending on where sensing occurs.

The fourth position of the code reflects rate modulation. An R in the fourth position indicates that the pacemaker incorporates a sensor to control the rate independently of intrinsic electrical activity of the heart.

The fifth position indicates whether multisite pacing is not present (O) or present in the atrium (A), ventricle (V), or both (D). Multisite pacing is defined for this purpose as stimulation sites in both atria, both ventricles, more than one stimulation site in any single chamber, or any combination of these.

Pacing modes

Ventricular asynchronous pacing, atrial asynchronous pacing, and AV sequential asynchronous pacing

Ventricular asynchronous (VOO) pacing is the simplest of all pacing modes because there is neither sensing nor mode of response. The timing cycle is shown in Fig. 6.1. Irrespective of any other events, the ventricular pacing artifacts occur at the programmed rate. The timing cycle cannot be reset by any intrinsic event. In the absence of sensing, there is no defined refractory period.

Atrial asynchronous (AOO) pacing behaves exactly like VOO, but the pacing artifacts occur in the atrial chamber.

Dual-chamber, or AV sequential asynchronous (DOO), pacing has an equally simple timing cycle. The interval from atrial artifact to ventricular artifact [atrioventricular interval (AVI)] and the interval from the ventricular artifact to the subsequent atrial pacing artifact [ventriculoatrial interval (VAI) or atrial escape interval (AEI)] are both fixed. The intervals never change, because the

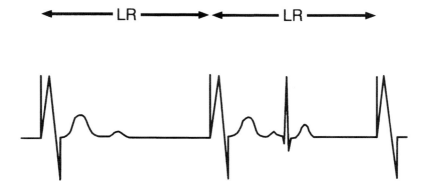

Fig. 6.1 The ventricular asynchronous (VOO) timing cycle consists of only a defined rate. The pacemaker delivers a ventricular pacing artifact at the defined rate regardless of intrinsic events. In this example, an intrinsic QRS complex occurs after the second paced complex, but because there is no sensing in the VOO mode, the interval between the second and the third paced complex remains stable.

pacing mode is insensitive to any atrial or ventricular activity, and the timers are never reset (Fig. 6.2).

Ventricular inhibited pacing

By definition, ventricular demand inhibited (VVI) pacing incorporates sensing on the ventricular channel, and pacemaker output is inhibited by a sensed ventricular event (Fig. 6.3). VVI pacemakers are refractory after a paced or

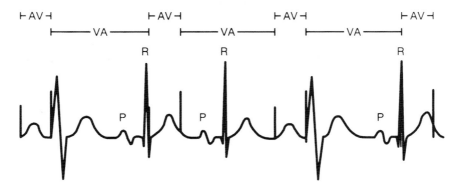

Fig. 6.2 The sequential asynchronous (DOO) timing cycle consists of only defined AV and VV intervals. The VAI is a function of the AV and VV intervals. An atrial pacing artifact is delivered, and the ventricular artifact follows at the programmed AVI. The next atrial pacing artifact is delivered at the completion of the VAI. The intervals do not vary because no activity is sensed, i.e. nothing interrupts or resets the programmed cycles.

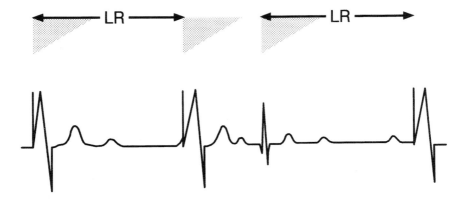

Fig. 6.3 The ventricular demand inhibited (VVI) timing cycle consists of a defined lower rate limit (LRL) and a ventricular refractory period (VRP) (shaded triangles). When the LRL timer is complete, a pacing artifact is delivered in the absence of a sensed intrinsic ventricular event. If an intrinsic QRS occurs, the LRL timer is started from that point. A VRP begins with any sensed or paced ventricular activity.

sensed ventricular event, a period known as the ventricular refractory period (VRP). Any ventricular event occurring within the VRP is not sensed and does not reset the ventricular timer (Fig. 6.4).

Atrial inhibited pacing

Atrial inhibited (AAI) pacing, the atrial counterpart of VVI pacing, incorporates the same timing cycles, with the obvious differences that pacing and sensing occur from the atrium and pacemaker output is inhibited by a sensed atrial event (Fig. 6.5). An atrial paced or sensed event initiates a refractory period during which the pacemaker senses nothing. Confusion can arise when multiple ventricular events occur during atrial pacing. For example, a premature ventricular beat following the intrinsic QRS that occurs in response to the paced atrial beat does not inhibit an atrial pacing artifact from being delivered (Fig. 6.6). When the AA timing cycle ends, the atrial pacing arti-

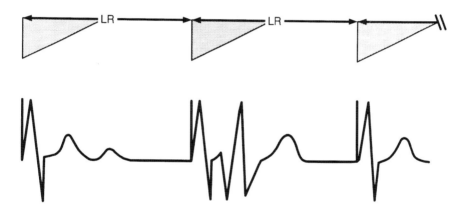

Fig. 6.4 If, in the ventricular demand inhibited (VVI) mode, a ventricular event occurs during the ventricular refractory period (VRP) (shaded triangles), it is not sensed and therefore does not reset the lower rate limit (LRL) timer.

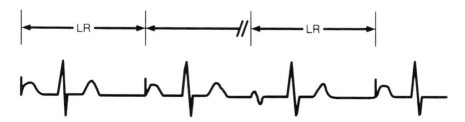

Fig. 6.5 The atrial inhibited (AAI) timing cycle consists of a defined lower rate limit (LRL) and an atrial refractory period (ARP). When the LRL timer is complete, a pacing artifact is delivered in the atrium in the absence of a sensed atrial event. If an intrinsic P wave occurs, the LRL timer is started from that point. An ARP begins with any sensed or paced atrial activity.

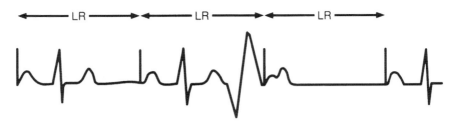

Fig. 6.6 In the atrial inhibited (AAI) mode, only atrial activity is sensed. In this example, it may appear unusual for paced atrial activity to occur so soon after intrinsic ventricular activity. Because sensing occurs only in the atrium, ventricular activity would not be expected to reset the pacemaker's timing cycle.

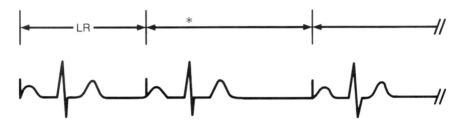

Fig. 6.7 In this example of atrial inhibited (AAI) pacing, the AA interval is 1000 ms (60 ppm). The interval between the second and third paced atrial events is > 1000 ms. The interval from the second QRS complex to the subsequent atrial pacing artifact is 1000 ms. This occurs because the second QRS complex (asterisk) has been sensed on the atrial lead (far-field sensing) and has inappropriately reset the timing cycle. LR, lower rate.

fact is delivered regardless of ventricular events, because an AAI pacemaker should not sense anything in the ventricle. The single exception to this rule is far-field sensing; that is, the ventricular signal is large enough to be inappropriately sensed by the atrial lead (Fig. 6.7). In this situation, the atrial timing cycle is reset. Sometimes this anomaly can be corrected either by making the atrial channel less sensitive or by lengthening the refractory period.

Single-chamber triggered-mode pacing
In single-chamber triggered-mode pacing, the pacemaker releases an output pulse every time a native event is sensed. This feature increases the current drain on the battery, accelerating its rate of depletion. This mode of pacing also deforms the native signal, compromising ECG interpretation. However, it can serve as an excellent marker for the site of sensing within a complex. It can also prevent inappropriate inhibition from oversensing when the patient does not have a stable native escape rhythm.

Rate-modulated pacing
The "sensor function of the pacemaker" refers to modulation of the paced rate

in response to an input signal other than the presence or absence of native de-polarization. The most widely used sensors include those that sense motion, either acceleration or vibration, impedance signals that measure minute venti-lation[7,8] and the measured interval from pacemaker stimulus to the T wave, i.e. a QT-interval sensor. Many other sensors have been used, but not widely.

Single-chamber rate-modulated pacing

Single-chamber pacemakers capable of rate-modulated (SSIR) pacing can be im-planted in the ventricle (VVIR) or atrium (AAIR).[9,10] The timing cycles for SSIR pacemakers are not markedly different from those of their non-rate-modulated counterparts. The timing cycle includes the basic VV or AA interval and a refrac-tory period from the paced or sensed event. The difference lies in the variability of the VV or AA interval (Fig. 6.8). Depending on the sensor incorporated and the patient's level of exertion, the basic interval is shorter than the programmed lower rate limit (LRL). Shortening requires that an upper rate limit (URL) be programmed to define the absolute shortest cycle length allowable. Most ap-proved SSIR pacemakers incorporate a fixed refractory period; that is, regard-less of whether the pacemaker is operating at the LRL or URL, the refractory period remains the same. Thus, at the higher rates under sensor drive, the pace-

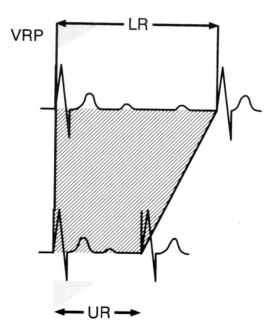

Fig. 6.8 The VVIR timing cycle consists of a lower rate limit (LR), an upper rate limit (UR) and a ventricular refractory period (VRP), represented by shaded triangles. As indicated by sensor activity, the VV cycle length shortens accordingly. (The striped area represents the range of sensor-driven VV cycle lengths.) In most VVIR pacemakers, the VRP remains fixed despite the changing VV cycle length. In selected VVIR pacemakers, the VRP shortens as the cycle length shortens.

maker may effectively become SOOR, because the alert period during which sensing can occur is so abbreviated. Native beats falling during the refractory period are not sensed. Hence, in SSIR pacing systems, if the refractory period is programmable, it should be programmed to a short interval to maximize the sensing period at both the low and the high sensor-controlled rates. In some pacemakers, when the cycle length shortens, the refractory period shortens correspondingly; this is referred to as the rate-variable refractory period. This event is analogous to the QT interval of the native ventricular depolarization.

Single-chamber and dual-chamber rate-modulated asynchronous pacing

The asynchronous pacing modes (i.e. AOO, VOO and DOO, as explained previously) have fixed intervals that are insensitive to all intrinsic events and have timers that are never reset. If rate modulation is incorporated in an asynchronous pacing mode, the basic cycle length is altered by sensor activity. In the single-chamber rate-modulated asynchronous (AOOR and VOOR) pacing modes, any alteration in cycle length is attributable to sensor activity and not to the sensing of intrinsic cardiac depolarizations. In the dual-chamber rate-modulated asynchronous (DOOR) pacing mode, the pacing rate changes in response to the sensor input signal, but not to the native P or R wave. In some pacemakers, the AVI may be programmed to shorten progressively as the rate increases, whereas in other units it remains fixed at the initial programmed setting.

Atrioventricular sequential, ventricular inhibited pacing

AV sequential, ventricular inhibited (DVI) pacing is rarely used. However, this pacing mode is a programmable option in most available dual-chamber pacemakers. For this reason, it is important to understand the timing cycles for DVI pacing.[11]

By definition, DVI provides pacing in both the atrium and the ventricle (D), but sensing only in the ventricle (V). The pacemaker is inhibited and reset by sensed ventricular activity, but ignores all intrinsic atrial complexes. The DVI units in the first generation were large and bulky and had two relatively large bipolar leads. The bipolar design produced small output pulses and generated a highly localized sensing field. In this setting, the ventricular sense amplifier remained alert when the atrial stimulus was released and throughout the AVI. Thus, a native R wave during the AVI was sensed so that ventricular output was inhibited and the AEI was reset (Fig. 6.9A). For both atrial and ventricular stimuli to be inhibited, the sensed R wave must occur during the AEI.

Improvements in circuit design have enabled manufacturers to reduce the size of the pulse generator. They have also made the next generation unipolar to facilitate venous access for the two leads. The large unipolar atrial stimulus could be sensed on the ventricular channel. It would be sensed by the pacemaker as a ventricular event and inhibit ventricular output. This occurrence is known as crosstalk, which is potentially catastrophic if concomitant AV block is present. To prevent crosstalk, the second generation of DVI pacemakers initiated the VRP on completion of the AEI timer. Thus, once an atrial

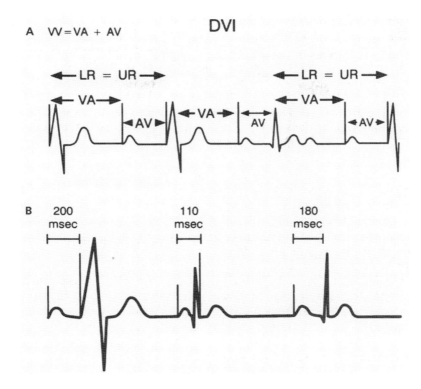

Fig. 6.9 A, In the non-committed version of AV sequential, ventricular inhibited (DVI) pacing, the components of the timing cycle are the same as those for committed DVI (see Fig. 6.10). However, if ventricular activity is sensed after the atrial pacing artifact, ventricular output is inhibited, i.e. a ventricular pacing artifact is not committed to the previous atrial pacing artifact. B, In the modified or partially committed version of DVI, ventricular events sensed within the non-physiological atrioventricular interval (AVI) do not inhibit ventricular output, and a ventricular pacing stimulus occurs at the end of the interval. Ventricular events occurring within the physiological AVI inhibit pacemaker function. In this example, the first paced atrial and ventricular events represent normal DVI pacing. The second paced atrial and intrinsic ventricular complex demonstrates a spontaneous ventricular event occurring within the non-physiological AVI and resulting in a ventricular pacing stimulus. The A–V interval is 110 ms, reflecting safety pacing. In the third event shown, after an atrial paced event, a spontaneous ventricular event falls within the physiological AVI, resulting in inhibition of ventricular pacing function.

output pulse occurred, the ventricular sense amplifier was refractory, and the pacemaker was obligated to release a ventricular output pulse, regardless of whether it was physiologically necessary. This event was termed committed AV sequential pacing (Fig. 6.10). It caused significant confusion, because a normally functioning system might demonstrate functional undersensing and functional non-capture in both atrium and ventricle simultaneously.

The present generation of devices still requires a period of ventricular refractoriness, a "ventricular blanking period," to minimize the chance of cross-

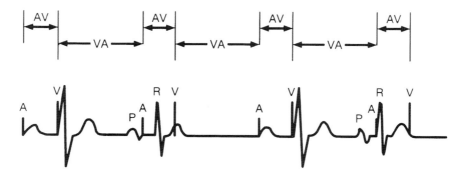

Fig. 6.10 The timing cycle in committed AV sequential, ventricular inhibited (DVI) pacing consists of a lower rate limit (LRL), an atrioventricular interval (AVI) and a ventricular refractory period (VRP). The VRP is initiated with any sensed or paced ventricular activity. (By definition, there is no atrial sensing and, therefore, no defined atrial refractory period.) The ventriculoatrial interval (VAI) is equal to the VV or LRL interval minus the AVI. In a committed system, a ventricular pacing artifact follows an atrial pacing artifact at the AVI regardless of whether intrinsic ventricular activity has occurred. In this example, the LRL is 1000 ms, or 60 ppm, and the AVI is 200 ms. At the end of the VAI, 800 ms after a ventricular event, if no ventricular activity has been sensed, the atrial pacing artifact is delivered. A ventricular pacing artifact occurs 200 ms later, irrespective of any intrinsic events. This is functional undersensing, because the ventricular pacing artifact is delivered as a function of the DVI pacing mode.

talk, but this interval is brief, lasting from 12 to 125 ms. In many pacemakers the duration of this interval is programmable. If the atrial stimulus were to coincide with a native R wave, e.g. a PVC, and the intrinsic deflection of the native complex fell outside the blanking period, the R wave would be sensed, and ventricular output would be inhibited. In this situation, the pacemaker would behave like the earlier non-committed systems. If, however, the intrinsic deflection coincided with the blanking period, the R wave would not be seen, and the pacemaker would release a ventricular output pulse at the end of the AVI in a manner analogous to that of the committed systems. This operation has been termed modified or partially committed to reflect the fact that the devices may demonstrate both non-committed and committed functions as part of their normal behavior (Fig. 6.9B).

The timing cycle (VV) consists of the AVI and VAI. The basic cycle length (VV), or LRL, is programmable, as is the AVI. The difference, VV–AV, is the VAI, or AEI. During the initial portion of the VAI, the sensing channel is refractory. (The refractory period is almost always a programmable interval.) After the refractory period, the ventricular sensing channel is again operational, or "alert." If ventricular activity is not sensed by the expiration of the VAI, atrial pacing occurs, followed by the AVI. If intrinsic ventricular activity occurs before the VAI is completed, the timing cycle is reset. (Additional discussion of crosstalk, the ventricular blanking period, and ventricular safety pacing can be found in the section that specifically discusses AVI.)

Atrioventricular sequential, non-P-synchronous pacing with dual-chamber sensing

AV sequential pacing with dual-chamber sensing, non-P-synchronous (DDI) pacing can be thought of as either an upgrade of DVI non-committed pacing or a downgrade of DDD pacing—i.e. DDD pacing without atrial tracking. The difference between DVI and DDI is that DDI incorporates atrial sensing as well as ventricular sensing. This prevents competitive atrial pacing that can occur with DVI pacing. The DDI mode of response is inhibition only; that is, no tracking of P waves can occur. Therefore, the paced ventricular rate cannot be greater than the programmed LRL. The timing cycle consists of the LRL, AVI, postventricular atrial refractory period (PVARP) and VRP. The PVARP is the period after a sensed or paced ventricular event during which the atrial sensing circuit is refractory. The atrial sensing circuit does not sense any atrial event occurring during the PVARP. If a P wave occurs after the PVARP and is sensed, no atrial pacing artifact is delivered at the end of the VAI. The subsequent ventricular pacing artifact cannot occur until the VV interval has been completed; that is, the LRL cannot be violated (Fig. 6.11).

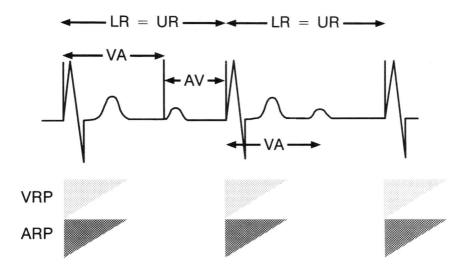

Fig. 6.11 The timing cycle in DDI pacing consists of a lower rate limit (LRL), an atrioventricular interval (AVI), a ventricular refractory period (VRP) and an atrial refractory period (ARP). The VRP is initiated by any sensed or paced ventricular activity, and the ARP is initiated by any sensed or paced atrial activity. DDI can be thought of as DDD pacing without the capability of P-wave tracking or DVI without the potential for atrial competition by virtue of atrial sensing. The LRL cannot be violated even if the sinus rate is occurring at a faster rate. For example, the LRL is 1000 ms, or 60 ppm, and the AVI is 200 ms. If a P wave occurs 500 ms after a paced ventricular complex, the AVI is initiated; but at the end of the AVI, 700 ms from the previous paced ventricular activity, a ventricular pacing artifact cannot be delivered, because it would violate the LRL.

It bears repeating that, because P-wave tracking does not occur with the DDI mode, the paced rate is never greater than the programmed LRL. A slight exception to this statement may occur when an intrinsic ventricular complex takes place after the paced atrial beat (AR) and inhibits paced ventricular output before completion of the programmed AVI; i.e. AR is less than AV. In this situation, the cycle length from A to A is shorter than the programmed LRL by the difference between the AR and the AVI (Fig. 6.12).

Atrioventricular sequential, non-P-synchronous, rate-modulated pacing with dual-chamber sensing

The timing cycles for non-P-synchronous, rate-modulated AV sequential (DDIR) pacing are the same as those described previously for DDI pacing except that paced rates can exceed the programmed LRL through sensor-driven activity. Depending on the sensor incorporated and the level of exertion of the patient, the basic cycle length shortens from the programmed LRL. This cycle length change requires that a URL be programmed to define the absolute shortest cycle length allowable.

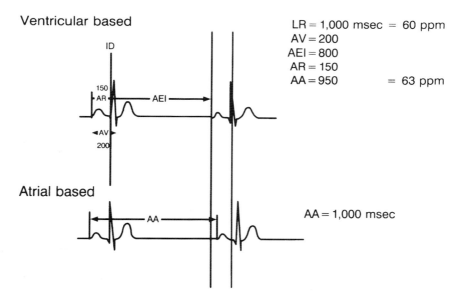

Fig. 6.12 Top: With ventricular-based timing in patients with intact AV nodal conduction after AR pacing, the sensed R wave resets the atrial escape interval (AEI). The base pacing interval consists of the sum of the AR and the AEI; thus, it is shorter than the programmed minimum rate interval. Bottom: With atrial-based timing in patients with intact AV nodal conduction after AR pacing, the sensed R wave inhibits ventricular output, but does not reset the basic timing of the pacemaker. There is atrial pacing at the programmed base rate. (From Levine PA, Hayes DL, Wilkoff BL, Ohman AE. Electrocardiography of rate-modulated pacemaker rhythms. Sylmar, CA: Siemens-Pacesetter, 1990. By permission of Siemens-Pacesetter.)

Even though no P-wave tracking occurs in a DDIR system, an intrinsic P wave may inhibit the atrial pacing artifact and give the appearance of P-wave tracking if an appropriately timed intrinsic atrial depolarization falls within the atrial sensing window (ASW). This phenomenon is coincidental.

In a DDDR pacing system in which the programmed maximum sensor rate (MSR) is greater than the maximum tracking rate (MTR), AV sequential pacing occurs when the sensor function drives the ventricular rate above the programmed maximum rate. The actual mode at this time is DDIR. If the intrinsic atrial rate also exceeds the MTR, so that the native atrial signal is sensed, atrial output is inhibited. Meanwhile, the ventricular paced complex is controlled by the sensor. The appearance may be of PV pacing (atrial-sensed ventricular pacing), with the ventricular rate violating the MTR. In actuality, the ventricular paced complex is a result of sensor drive, and if the sensor input to the pacemaker would not allow a paced rate this rapid, the ventricular rate would be limited by the MTR limit.

Atrial synchronous (P-tracking) pacing

Atrial synchronous (P-tracking) pacemakers pace only in the ventricle (V), sense in both atrium and ventricle (D), and respond both by inhibition of ventricular output by intrinsic ventricular activity (I) and by ventricular tracking of P waves (T).[12] This mode of pacing is a programmable option in many dual-chamber pacemakers. The VDD mode is also available as a single-lead pacing system. In this system, a single lead is capable of pacing in the ventricle in response to sensing atrial activity by way of a remote electrode(s) situated on the intra-atrial portion of the ventricular pacing lead.

The timing cycle is composed of LRL, AVI, PVARP, VRP and URL. A sensed atrial event initiates the AVI. If an intrinsic ventricular event occurs before termination of the AVI, ventricular output is inhibited, and the LRL timing cycle is reset. If a paced ventricular beat occurs at the end of the AVI, this beat resets the LRL. If no atrial event occurs, the pacemaker escapes with a paced ventricular event at the LRL; i.e. the pacemaker displays VVI activity in the absence of a sensed atrial event at the base rate (Fig. 6.13).

Dual-chamber pacing and sensing with inhibition and tracking

Although the DDD timing cycle involves more intervals, standard dual-chamber pacing and sensing with inhibition and tracking (DDD) are reasonably easy to comprehend on the basis of the timing cycles already discussed. The basic timing circuit associated with LRL pacing is divided into two sections. The first is the interval from a ventricular sensed or paced event to an atrial paced event and is known as the AEI, or VAI. The second interval begins with an atrial sensed or paced event and extends to a ventricular event. This interval may be defined by a paced AV, PR, AR, or PV interval. An atrial sensed event that occurs before completion of the AEI promptly terminates this interval and initiates an AVI, and the result is P-wave synchronous ventricular

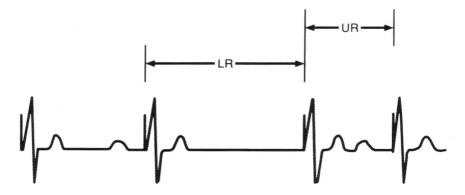

Fig. 6.13 The timing cycle of VDD pacing consists of a lower rate limit (LRL), an atrioventricular interval (AVI), a ventricular refractory period (VRP), a postventricular atrial refractory period (PVARP) and an upper rate limit (URL). A sensed P wave initiates the AVI (during the AVI, the atrial sensing channel is refractory). At the end of the AVI, a ventricular pacing artifact is delivered if no intrinsic ventricular activity has been sensed, i.e. P-wave tracking. Ventricular activity, paced or sensed, initiates the PVARP and the ventriculoatrial interval (VAI) (the LRL interval minus the AVI). If no P-wave activity occurs, the pacemaker escapes with a ventricular pacing artifact at the LRL.

pacing. If the intrinsic sinus rate is less than the programmed LRL, AV sequential pacing at the programmed rate or functional single-chamber atrial (AR) pacing occurs (Fig. 6.14A).

An option for "circadian response," or "sleep rate," in many contemporary pacemakers allows a lower rate to be programmed for the approximate time during which the patient is sleeping.[13] A separate, potentially faster LRL may then be programmed for waking hours. For example, the LRL during waking hours may be programmed to 70 bpm, and the LRL during sleeping hours may be programmed to 50 bpm. In some pacemakers, this feature is tied to a clock, and the usual waking and sleeping hours are programmed into the pacemaker. In other pacemakers, the sleep rate is also set on the basis of waking and sleeping hours, but verification by a sensor is required to allow rate changes to occur.

Portions of pacemaker timing cycles

Refractory periods

Every pacemaker capable of sensing must include a refractory period in its basic timing cycle. Refractory periods prevent the sensing of known but clinically inappropriate signals, such as the evoked potential and repolarization (T wave).

In a single-chamber system that is otherwise capable of sensing (either the inhibited or the triggered mode), each sensed or paced event is followed by a refractory period. Once this timing period ends, the sense amplifier becomes alert and is receptive to the detection of native signals. If an appropriate event, such as a PVC, coincides with the VRP, it is not detected, and competition between the pacemaker and the intrinsic activity may occur. The refractory period of a pacemaker is analogous to the refractory period of the heart (QT interval). During the cardiac refractory period, a stimulus delivered to the heart is ineffective because the myocardium is already depolarized and a subsequent depolarization cannot occur until the resting membrane potential is re-established. Like the heart, the pacemaker has a refractory period consisting of two components. The first is the absolute refractory period, during which native activity cannot be detected. More recently, this has been called a blanking period. The terminal portion of the refractory period is relative when events can be detected, but they are not used to trigger or reset an output pulse. Rather, they are used to detect rapid signals. If these signals exceed 400–600 cycles per minute (which is above the physiological range), they are labeled electrical noise. Rather than be inhibited by these inappropriate signals, the pacemaker is designed to adopt asynchronous behavior, which is termed noise mode response. In the recent generation of dual-chamber pacing systems, rapid events detected on the atrial channel, but not the ventricular channel, help the device detect pathological atrial rates and initiate automatic mode switching (see Mode switching, below).

In a DDD system, a sensed or paced atrial event initiates an atrial refractory period (ARP) and also initiates the AVI (Fig. 6.14B). During this portion of the timing cycle, the atrial channel is refractory to another native atrial event; nor does atrial pacing occur during this period. Atrial pacing occurs only at the end of the AVI or later (see Upper rate behavior, below). A sensed or paced ventricular event initiates a VRP. A VRP is always part of the timing cycle of any pacing system with ventricular pacing and sensing. The VRP prevents sensing of the evoked potential and the resultant T wave on the ventricular channel of the pacemaker. A sensed or paced ventricular event also initiates a refractory period on the atrial channel (PVARP). The PVARP may prevent atrial sensing of a retrograde P wave (see Endless-loop tachycardia, below), but the PVARP alone may not prevent sensing of far-field ventricular events in devices with an automatic mode-switching algorithm. The combination of the PVARP and the AVI forms the total atrial refractory period (TARP). The TARP, in turn, is the limiting factor for the maximum sensed atrial rate that the pacemaker can sense and, hence, track. For example, if the AVI is 150 ms and the PVARP is 250 ms, the TARP is 400 ms, or 150 ppm. In this case, a paced ventricular event initiates the 250-ms PVARP, and only after this interval has ended can an atrial event be sensed. If an atrial event is sensed immediately after termination of the PVARP, the sensed atrial event initiates the AVI of 150 ms. On termination of the AVI, in the absence of an intrinsic R wave, a paced ventricular event occurs, resulting in a VV cycle length of 400 ms, or 150 ppm. Programming a long PVARP limits the upper rate by limiting the

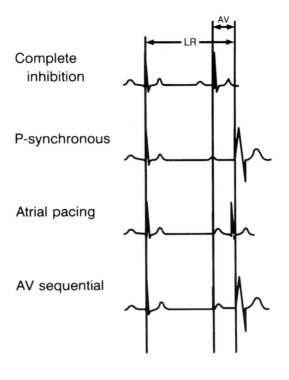

Complete inhibition

P-synchronous

Atrial pacing

AV sequential

A

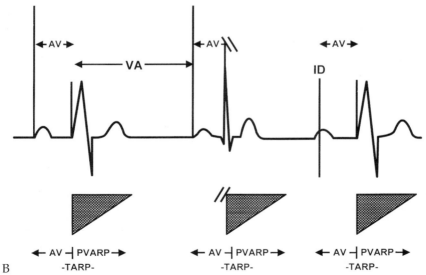

B

maximum sensed atrial rate (Fig. 6.15). If the native atrial rate were 151 bpm, every other P wave would coincide with the PVARP, not be sensed, and hence not be tracked; so the effective paced rate would be approximately 75 ppm, or half the atrial rate.

In a pacemaker with a mode-switching algorithm "on," the pacemaker must be able to detect higher atrial rates, even if the native P waves coincide with the PVARP. Although these P waves may not be tracked, the pacemaker is capable of monitoring events that coincide with the refractory period to recognize rapid pathological atrial rates. Thus, the system can switch from a tracking mode (DDD) to a non-tracking mode (VVI or DDI), so that the first of the pathological atrial events that occurs during the atrial alert period is not tracked.

Atrioventricular interval

The AVI, often poorly understood, should be considered a single interval with two subportions (Fig. 6.16A). For most dual-chamber systems, the atrial channel is totally refractory to the detection of other atrial signals that may occur during the AVI. In most devices, only the first portion of the AVI is absolutely refractory. The terminal portion is a relative refractory period, to assist in the detection of rapid pathological atrial rhythms for purposes of mode switching (Fig. 6.17).

Atrial output also triggers a timing period on the ventricular channel, known as the ventricular blanking period. It coincides with the earliest portion of the AVI, and its purpose is to avoid sensing of an event or a stimulus of one channel in the opposite channel.

If the atrial pacing artifact were sensed by the ventricular sensing circuit, ventricular output inhibition would result, i.e. crosstalk. To prevent crosstalk, the leading edge of the atrial pacing artifact is masked, or blanked, by rendering the ventricular sensing circuit absolutely refractory during the very early portion of the AVI (Fig. 6.16B). In DDD pacemakers, the blanking period may

---

Fig. 6.14 A, The timing cycle in DDD pacing consists of a lower rate limit (LRL), an atrioventricular interval (AVI), a ventricular refractory period (VRP), a postventricular atrial refractory period (PVARP) and an upper rate limit (URL). There are four variations of the DDD timing cycle. If intrinsic atrial and ventricular activity occur before the LRL times out, both channels are inhibited and no pacing occurs (first panel). If a P wave is sensed before the ventriculoatrial interval (VAI) is completed (the LRL minus the AVI), output from the atrial channel is inhibited. The AVI is initiated, and if no ventricular activity is sensed before the AVI terminates, a ventricular pacing artifact is delivered, i.e. P-synchronous pacing (second panel). If no atrial activity is sensed before the VAI is completed, an atrial pacing artifact is delivered, which initiates the AVI. If intrinsic ventricular activity occurs before the termination of the AVI, ventricular output from the pacemaker is inhibited (third panel). If no intrinsic ventricular activity occurs before the termination of the AVI, a ventricular pacing artifact is delivered, i.e. AV sequential pacing (fourth panel). B, Potential pacing combinations that can occur in the DDD pacing mode. The intrinsic P wave is sensed during the early portion of the P wave. The AVI is initiated at the point of the intrinsic deflection (ID) of atrial activity, as seen on the atrial electrogram. (Modified from Medtronic, Minneapolis, MN, USA.)

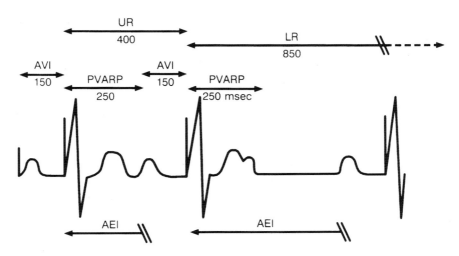

Fig. 6.15 In the DDD pacing mode, the upper rate (UR) is limited by the atrioventricular interval (AVI) and the postventricular atrial refractory period (PVARP). In this example, the AVI is 150 ms and the PVARP is 250 ms, for a total atrial refractory period (TARP) of 400 ms (i.e. equal to 150 ppm). As shown, after the first paced ventricular complex, a P wave occurs just after the completion of the PVARP. This P wave is sensed, initiates the AVI, and is followed by another paced ventricular complex. The subsequent P wave occurs within the PVARP and is therefore not sensed. The DDD response is to wait for the next intrinsic P wave to occur, as in this example, or for the atrial escape interval (AEI) to be completed, whereupon AV sequential pacing occurs.

be programmable, ranging from 12 to 125 ms. The blanking period is traditionally of short duration because it is important for the ventricular sensing circuit to be returned to the "alert" state relatively early during the AVI so that intrinsic ventricular activity can inhibit pacemaker output if it occurs before the AVI ends. The potential exists for signals other than those of intrinsic ventricular activity to be sensed and inhibit ventricular output. The greatest concern is crosstalk. Even though the leading edge of the atrial pacing artifact is effectively ignored because of the blanking period, the trailing edge of the atrial pacing artifact occurring after the blanking period can occasionally be sensed on the ventricular channel. In a pacemaker-dependent patient, inhibition of ventricular output by crosstalk results in asystole. To prevent such an outcome, a safety mechanism is present.

If activity is sensed on the ventricular sensing circuit in a given portion of the AVI immediately after the blanking period (this second portion of the AVI has been called the "ventricular triggering period" or the "crosstalk sensing window"), it is assumed that crosstalk cannot be differentiated from intrinsic ventricular activity. To prevent catastrophic ventricular asystole, a ventricular pacing artifact is delivered early—at an AVI of 100–120 ms, although in some pulse generators this interval is programmable for 50–150 ms

(Fig. 6.16C). If the signal sensed is indeed crosstalk, a paced ventricular complex delivered at the abbreviated interval prevents ventricular asystole. In addition, AV pacing at a shorter than programmed AVI on the ECG indicates the occurrence of crosstalk and allows the pacemaker to be programmed to eliminate this behavior. Elimination of crosstalk may be accomplished by extending the ventricular blanking period, decreasing atrial output, or reducing the ventricular sensitivity. If true intrinsic ventricular activity occurs during the early portion of the AVI, the safety mechanism results in delivery of a ventricular pacing artifact within or immediately after the intrinsic beat. This delivery is safe because the ventricle is refractory, no depolarization results from the pacing artifact, and the pacing artifact is delivered too early to coincide with ventricular repolarization or a vulnerable period. This

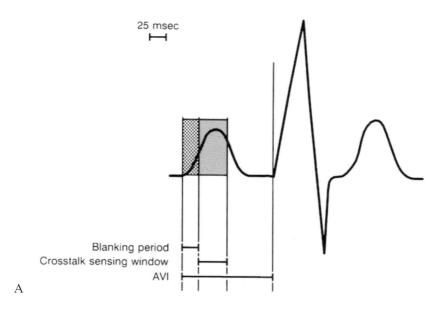

25 msec

Blanking period

Crosstalk sensing window

AVI

A

Fig. 6.16 A, The atrioventricular interval (AVI) should be considered as a single interval with two subportions. The entire AVI corresponds to the programmed value, i.e. the interval following a paced or sensed atrial beat allowed before a ventricular pacing artifact is delivered. The initial portion of the AVI is the blanking period. This interval is followed by the crosstalk sensing window. B, If the ventricular sensing circuit senses activity during the crosstalk sensing window, a ventricular pacing artifact is delivered early, usually at 100–110 ms after the atrial event. This has been referred to as "ventricular safety pacing," "110-ms phenomenon" and "non-physiological AV delay." C, The initial portion of the AVI in most dual-chamber pacemakers is designated as the blanking period. The primary purpose of this interval is to prevent ventricular sensing of the leading edge of the atrial pacing artifact. Any event that occurs during the blanking period, even if it is an intrinsic ventricular event (as shown in this figure), is not sensed. In this example, the ventricular premature beat that is not sensed is followed by a ventricular pacing artifact delivered at the programmed AVI and occurring in the terminal portion of the T wave. (*Continued.*)

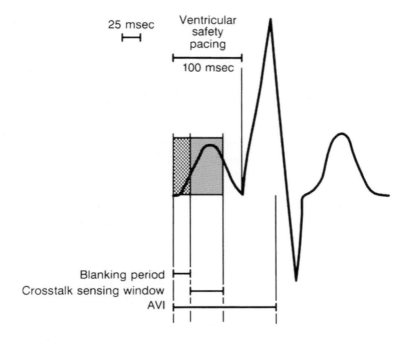

B

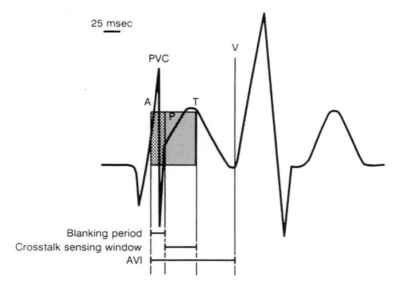

C

Fig. 6.16 (*Continued.*)

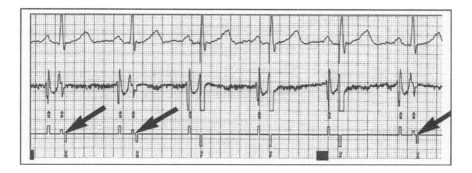

Fig. 6.17 Surface ECG, atrial electrogram, and event markers (arrows) demonstrating occasional AR complexes, events that are occurring within the atrial refractory period (ARP). They coincide with the QRS complex, but are detected on the atrial channel before being detected by the pacemaker on the ventricular channel.

event has been referred to as "ventricular safety pacing," "non-physiologic AV delay," or the "110-ms phenomenon." Although the safety pacing phenomenon accompanying a late-cycle PVC has been interpreted as a sensing failure, it actually reflects normal sensing. Pacemaker behavior changes with respect to a ventricular event that is sensed during the "crosstalk sensing" window. The response is altered in comparison with an event sensed at any other time during the ventricular alert period. Sensing during this special brief timing period results in a triggered rather than an inhibited output. Unlike single-chamber function, in which the triggered mode rapidly delivers an output pulse as soon as an event is detected, the R wave that occurs in the earliest portion of this special detection interval triggers an output at the end of the safety pacing interval.

After the blanking period and the crosstalk sensing window have timed out, the ventricular sensing circuit returns to the alert status, in which a detected event causes the output pulse to be reset.

Differential atrioventricular interval

If AVIs initiated by a sensed event and those initiated by a paced event show consistent differences, the most likely explanation is a differential AVI. As noted in the introduction to this section, a differential AVI is an attempt to provide an interatrial conduction time of equal duration whether atrial contraction is paced or sensed. The PV interval initiated with atrial sensing commences only when the atrial depolarization is detected by the pacemaker and commonly occurs 20–60 ms after the onset of the P wave seen on a surface ECG. Conversely, the AVI initiated with atrial pacing commences immediately with the pacing artifact, not with atrial depolarization. The AVI that follows a sensed atrial event should therefore be shorter than one that follows a paced atrial event (Fig. 6.18) in an effort to achieve similar functional AVIs, whether

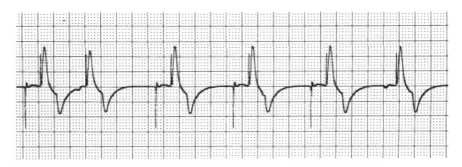

Fig. 6.18 ECG tracing demonstrating differential atrioventricular interval (AVI). The AVI is 50 ms longer than the PV interval. (From Relay Models 293-03 and 294-03. Intermedics Cardiac Pulse Generator Physician's Manual. Angleton, TX: Intermedics, 1992. By permission of Intermedics.)

the atrial event is paced or sensed. The AVI differential is programmable in some pacemakers and preset in others.

One DDD pacemaker automatically calculates the AVI differential between paced and sensed atrial events. When an atrial paced event occurs, the AR interval is measured. When an atrial sensed event follows an atrial paced event, a new PR interval is measured. The AV delay hysteresis is set equal to the maximum value (AR or PR) minus the PR interval (Fig. 6.19).

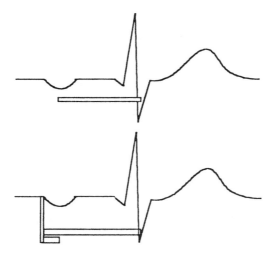

AV Delay Hysteresis = A-R Interval - P-R Interval

Fig. 6.19 Schematic diagram of one manufacturer's differential atrioventricular interval (AVI), designated "AV delay hysteresis." (Modified from Chorus II Model 6234, 6244. Dual Chamber Pulse Generator Physician's Manual. Minnetonka, MN: ELA Medical, 1994.)

Most dual-chamber pacemakers allow the paced and sensed AV delays to be programmed independently. Although the two may be nominally different, wider differences up to 100 ms are programmable.

Rate-variable or rate-adaptive atrioventricular interval

Most DDD and DDDR pacemakers can shorten the AVI as the atrial rate increases, either by an increase in sinus rate or by a sensor-driven increase in paced rate (Fig. 6.20). Rate-adaptive or rate-variable AVI is intended to optimize cardiac output by mimicking the normal physiological decrease in the PR interval that occurs in the normal heart as the atrial rate increases. The rate-related shortening of the AVI may also improve atrial sensing by shortening the TARP and thereby extending the time for the atrial sensing window.

Rate-adaptive AVI may be designed in several ways. The more common method is to allow linear shortening of the AVI from a programmed baseline AVI to a programmed minimum AVI. Another method allows a limited number of stepwise shortenings of the AVI. These steps may or may not be programmable.

Atrioventricular interval hysteresis

The term AVI hysteresis has been used variously, but most commonly describes alterations in the paced AVI relative to the patient's intrinsic AV conduction.[14,15] For example, a longer paced AVI is permitted to allow maintenance of intrinsic AV conduction. However, once the intrinsic PR or AR interval triggers the programmed AVI hysteresis, consistent AV pacing at the programmed AVI occurs. Commonly, AVI hysteresis is programmed by selecting the desired AV delay during pacing with an additional programmable delta. If there is AV pacing, the system periodically extends the AV delay by the programmed delta. If a native R wave is detected within this extended interval, the longer interval remains in place and results in functional single-chamber atrial pacing. However, with the first cycle of AV pacing, which may occur with a transient increase in vagal tone or even intermittent pathological AV block, the AV delay returns to the programmed value. This form of AV hysteresis is called positive AV hysteresis with search. Negative AV hysteresis shortens the AV

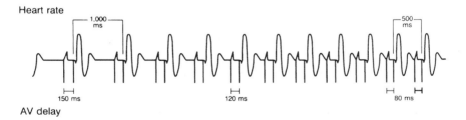

Fig. 6.20 As heart rate increases, AV delay dynamically adapts to the change in cycle length. (From Hayes DL, Ketelson A, Levine PA *et al.* Understanding timing systems of current DDDR pacemakers. Eur JCPE 1993; 3:70–86. By permission of Mayo Foundation.)

interval if an intrinsic ventricular event is sensed in the AV interval, and may be useful for patients with hypertrophic cardiomyopathy.

Positive AV hysteresis programming accomplishes two goals. In a patient with a normal ventricle, normal ventricular activation sequence (narrow QRS), and a normal PR interval, single-chamber atrial pacing provides hemodynamics superior to those of dual-chamber pacing. Ventricular stimulation causes a disordered ventricular activation sequence. However, an AV delay that is too long, as in first-degree AV block, may be hemodynamically deleterious. In this situation, hemodynamics may be superior with a shorter AV delay despite the disordered ventricular activation sequence. AVI hysteresis allows for both a longer AV delay when AV nodal conduction is intact and a shorter AVI when conduction is compromised.

Hysteresis programming

Programming of hysteresis permits prolongation of the first pacemaker escape interval after a sensed event. A pacemaker programmed at a cycle length of 1000 ms (60 bpm) and a hysteresis of 1200 ms (50 bpm) allows 200 ms more for another sensed QRS complex. If another QRS complex is not recognized, then the pacemaker continuously stimulates the heart at the programmed rate of 60 bpm, an escape interval of 1000 ms (Fig. 6.21), until a sensed event restarts the cycle. The advantage of hysteresis in a single-chamber pacing mode is the ability to maintain spontaneous AV synchrony as long as possible. This feature may prevent symptomatic retrograde VA conduction. In patients with VVI pacing and pacemaker syndrome, hysteresis provides reliable higher rate backup pacing while increasing the potential for maintaining the patient's intrinsic rhythm.

Several types of hysteresis may be programmable options in some dual-chamber pacemakers. In the first-generation algorithm, a native event had to be sensed to re-establish the hysteresis escape interval. The native complex had to occur at a rate faster than the basic pacing rate. If the basic pacing rate was relatively high, the system may have continued pacing long after the need for pacing had resolved. Therefore, search hysteresis was introduced. In search hysteresis, once a specific number of timing cycles at the more rapid rate (the number of cycles may be fixed or programmable) has occurred, the prolonged escape interval is permitted to allow manifestation of a slower intrinsic rate— i.e. a rate higher than the programmed LRL. If intrinsic rhythm does not return at a rate exceeding the programmed lower rate, stimulation resumes at the more rapid rate for a given number of cycles (Fig. 6.22). This feature has been further modified in some systems to prevent an isolated PVC from resetting the basic dual-chamber pacing interval. Rather, resetting the hysteresis escape interval requires a sensed P wave to produce either a PR or a PV complex that inhibits the higher rate of pacing and re-establishes the hysteresis feature.

Another feature can be considered a refinement of search hysteresis. A "sudden bradycardia response" or "rate drop response" (RDR) reacts to a defined

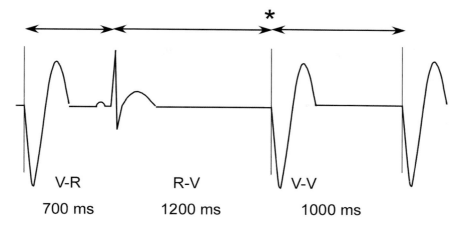

Fig. 6.21 VVI hysteresis. The programmed pacing rate is 60 bpm and the hysteresis rate is 50 bpm. After the second meat, which is an intrinsic beat, an interval of 1200 ms occurs until the first paced beat (third beat, asterisk) is delivered. However, the interval between two paced beats is 1000 ms.

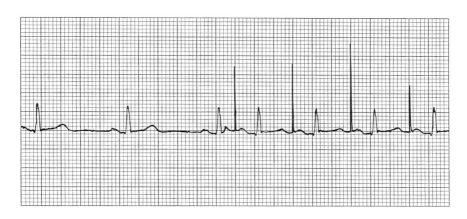

Fig. 6.22 Onset of pacing in a DDDR pacemaker programmed to a lower rate of 100 bpm, hysteresis at 65 bpm, when the intrinsic rate has declined to 63 bpm. After 256 cycles of pacing at 100 bpm, pacing is suspended for the pacemaker to "search" for the intrinsic lower rate. If the lower rate is greater than the hysteresis rate, pacing is inhibited until the rate again falls below the hysteresis rate. (From Lloyd MA, Hayes DL, Friedman PA. Programming. In: Hayes DL, Lloyd MA, Friedman PA, eds. Cardiac pacing and defibrillation: a clinical approach. Armonk, NY: Futura, 2000:247–323. By permission of Mayo Foundation.)

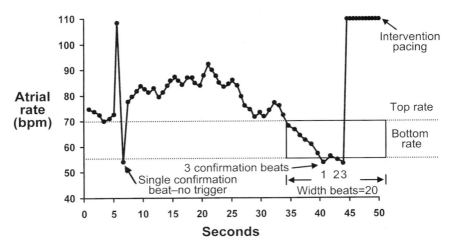

Fig. 6.23 Diagrammatic representation of rate drop response (RDR). This algorithm requires that "top" and "bottom" rates be defined for rate drop detection, a specific number of beats, width over which the rate may drop, and the pacing rate that results if criteria are met, i.e. the intervention rate. Three confirmation beats below the bottom rate must occur before therapy is triggered. In the early portion of this diagram, a single beat falls below the bottom rate, but fails to trigger intervention because confirmation is not met. (From Lloyd MA, Hayes DL, Friedman PA. Programming. In: Hayes DL, Lloyd MA, Friedman PA, eds. Cardiac pacing and defibrillation: a clinical approach. Armonk, NY: Futura, 2000:247–323. By permission of Mayo Foundation.)

drop in heart rate.[16] When this occurs, the pacemaker feature intervenes by pacing at an elevated rate in both chambers for a specific, programmed duration (Fig. 6.23). At the conclusion of the programmed duration of more rapid pacing, the pacing rate gradually returns to the programmed lower rate. Several programmable detection algorithms are available. The first algorithm available was "drop detect," in which the pacemaker monitors a drop in heart rate that must satisfy two programmable requirements to trigger an intervention, namely, the programmable "drop size," which is the number of beats the rate must fall, and the "detection window," which is the amount of time monitored for a rate drop (this is a programmable interval) (Fig. 6.24). The "nominal" values for RDR are not successful for everyone.

In the "low rate detect" algorithm, therapy is triggered when pacing occurs at the programmed lower rate for the programmable consecutive number of "detection beats." This detection method can be used as a backup to the "drop detect" method if the sudden drop in rate varies between slow and fast (Fig. 6.25).

Dual-chamber rate hysteresis has multiple variations and different levels of complexity. Although the primary mode of therapy for vasovagal syncope is

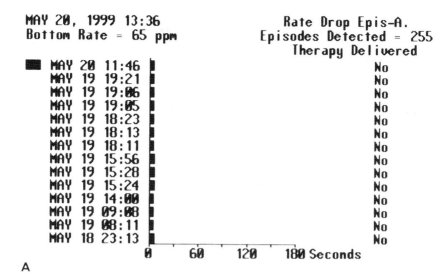

A

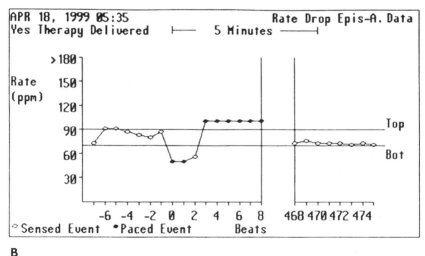

B

Fig. 6.24 A, The rate drop response (RDR) counters indicate that the pacemaker had documented multiple episodes of sudden rate drop. However, "therapy"—i.e. a response to the sudden drop in rate with an increase in pacing rate for a programmed period—had not been initiated. B, With a pacemaker in place and RDR that had been programmed "on" but not initiated because of the programmed parameters, adjusting the RDR parameters would be reasonable. For this patient, the RDR criteria were programmed more sensitively. When the patient returned, the rate counter was again full, with 255 episodes detected and therapy delivered on two occasions. The second printout details the event on 18 April at 05:35 h when therapy was delivered. The diagram documents a sudden decrease in rate; RDR was met and therapy delivered. (From Lloyd MA, Hayes DL, Friedman PA. Programming. In: Hayes DL, Lloyd MA, Friedman PA, eds. Cardiac pacing and defibrillation: a clinical approach. Armonk, NY: Futura, 2000:247–323. By permission of Mayo Foundation.)

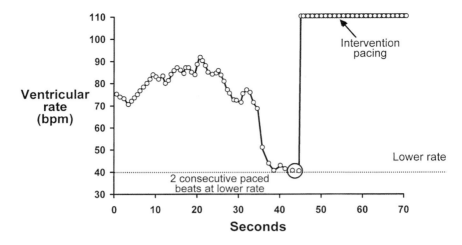

Fig. 6.25 In the low rate detect algorithm (Medtronic, Inc.), when pacing occurs at the programmed lower rate for the programmable consecutive number of detection beats, therapy is triggered. Low rate detect may be used as a backup to the drop detect method if the sudden drop in rate varies between slow and fast. (From Lloyd MA, Hayes DL, Friedman PA. Programming. In: Hayes DL, Lloyd MA, Friedman PA, eds. Cardiac pacing and defibrillation: a clinical approach. Armonk, NY: Futura, 2000:247–323. By permission of Mayo Foundation.)

pharmacological, it is not always successful. Another treatment option is dual-chamber pacing support at a relatively high rate during each spell, which may ameliorate symptoms, but there are conflicting data from clinical trials to support its use in preventing syncope.[17,18] Because patients with neurocardiogenic syncope have a normal rhythm at other times, the hysteresis circuit allows for pacing at the higher rate only during the spell (when the native heart rate falls precipitously) and otherwise remains inhibited.

Base rate behavior

The way a pacemaker behaves in response to a sensed ventricular signal varies among manufacturers and even among devices from the same manufacturer. Dual-chamber pacemakers have historically been designed with a ventricular-based timing system, an atrial-based timing system, or a hybrid of these two systems. Designation of a pacemaker's timing system as atrial-based or ventricular-based gained increased importance with the advent of rate-adaptive pacing. The difference between atrial-based and ventricular-based dual-chamber pacemakers was of little clinical importance in non-rate-adaptive pacemakers, although the difference created some minor confusion in the interpretation of paced ECGs.

With the refinement of timing systems, use of a specific system has once again become less important. A description of pure atrial-based and ventricular-based

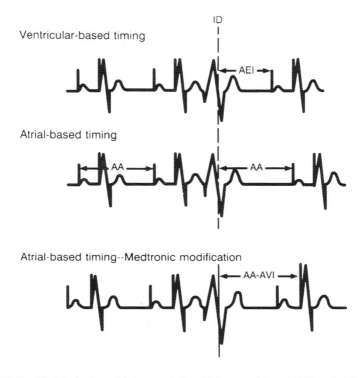

Fig. 6.26 Top: Ventricular-based timing resets the atrial escape interval (AEI) so that the recycled pacing interval is equal to the programmed base rate. Middle: Atrial-based timing resets the AA interval and then adds the atrioventricular interval (AVI). Thus, the interval from the sensed R wave to the next paced ventricular beat exceeds the base rate interval, a form of obligatory hysteresis. Bottom: Medtronic modification of the AA timing subtracts the AVI from the AA interval. The resulting rhythm is identical to that seen with ventricular-based timing. (From Levine PA, Hayes DL, Wilkoff BL, Ohman AE. Electrocardiography of rate-modulated pacemaker rhythms. Sylmar, CA: Siemens-Pacesetter, 1990. By permission of Siemens-Pacesetter.)

timing systems appears below. However, few contemporary dual-chamber pacemakers are "pure" atrial-based or ventricular-based systems. The majority are in some way hybrid, designed specifically to avoid the potential rate variations or limitations that could occur with either pure timing system.

Ventricular-based timing

In a ventricular-based timing system, the AEI is "fixed." A ventricular sensed event occurring during the AEI resets this timer, causing it to start again (Fig. 6.26, top). A ventricular sensed event occurring during the AVI both terminates the AVI and initiates an AEI (see Fig. 6.12, top). If there is intact conduction through the AV node after an atrial pacing stimulus, such that the AR interval (atrial stimulus to sensed R wave) is shorter than the programmed

AVI, the resulting paced rate accelerates by a small amount. This response is demonstrated in Fig. 6.12 (top).

This phenomenon is best understood by example. In a pacemaker programmed to an LRL of 60 bpm (a pacing interval of 1000 ms) that has a programmed AVI of 200 ms, the AEI is 800 ms (AEI = LRL − AVI). If AV nodal function permits conduction in 150 ms (AR interval = 150 ms), the conducted or sensed R wave inhibits ventricular output. This, in turn, resets the AEI, which remains stable at 800 ms. The resulting interval between consecutive atrial pacing stimuli is 950 ms (AEI + AR interval), which is equivalent to a rate of 63 bpm, a rate slightly faster than the programmed LRL. When a native R wave occurs—e.g. a ventricular premature beat during the AEI—the AEI is also reset. The pacemaker then recycles, resulting in a rate defined by the sum of the AEI and AVI. This escape interval is therefore equal to the LRL (Fig. 6.26, top). In both cases, the sensed ventricular event, an R wave, regardless of where it occurs, resets the AEI.

Atrial-based timing

In an atrial-based timing system, the AA interval is fixed, whereas in a ventricular-based system, the AEI is fixed. As long as LRL pacing remains stable, there is no discernible difference between the two timing systems.

In a system with pure atrial-based timing, a sensed R wave occurring during the AVI inhibits ventricular output, but does not alter the basic AA timing. Hence, the rate stays at the programmed LRL (see Fig. 6.12, bottom) during effective single-chamber atrial pacing. When a ventricular premature beat is sensed during the AEI, the timers are also reset, but the AA interval rather than the AEI is reset. The pacemaker counts out an AA interval and then adds the programmed AVI, in an attempt to mimic the compensatory pause commonly seen in normal sinus rhythm with ventricular ectopy—a form of obligatory hysteresis (Fig. 6.26, middle).

Other manufacturers have chosen to modify an atrial timing system. One DDDR pulse generator primarily uses modified atrial, or AA, timing, whereby an atrial sensed or paced event commonly resets the timing cycle of the device (much like the sinus node itself). However, in certain situations (e.g. after a PVC), an exception is made, and ventricular (VA) timing is used. Another manufacturer uses an atrial timing system that ignores the sensed R wave during stable AR pacing, which eliminates the rate acceleration that would be seen with ventricular-based timing designs. This feature is modified when a native R wave or sensed premature ventricular event occurs after the VRP is completed. The AA interval is reset, but only after the AVI is first subtracted (Fig. 6.27).

Comparison of atrial-based and ventricular-based systems

When the heart rate is considered, usually the ventricular rate is paramount, because it, not the atrial rate, causes the effective (hemodynamic) pulse. Dur-

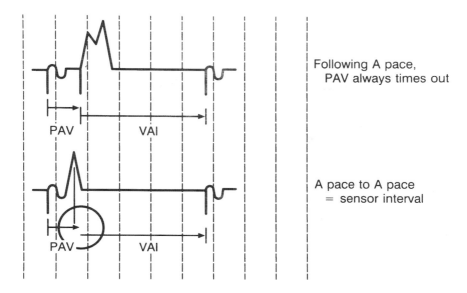

Fig. 6.27 Ventricular-based vs. atrial-based timing. The lower portion demonstrates atrial escape timing after an atrial (A) pace in atrial-based timing. With this timing, the atrioventricular interval (AVI) after atrial pacing (PAV) always times out, regardless of ventricular inhibition. The escape interval from one atrial pace to the next is equal to the sensor interval. VAI, interval from ventricular sensed or paced event to atrial paced event. (From Hayes DL, Ketelson A, Levine PA *et al.* Understanding timing systems of current DDDR pacemakers. Eur JCPE 1993; 3:70–86. By permission of Mayo Foundation.)

ing periods of 2 : 1 AV block at the lower rate, a ventricular-based timing system alternates between the programmed rate (AV pacing state) and a slightly faster rate (AR pacing state), as shown in Fig. 6.28 (top).

In an atrial-based system, the alternation of the longer AVI with the shorter AR interval results in ventricular rates that are both faster and slower than the programmed base rate. This response is shown in Fig. 6.28 (bottom).

Although ventricular-based timing may result in an increase in the paced rate during AR pacing (see Effects of ventricular- and atrial-based timing systems on DDDR timing cycles, below), the LRL is never violated. This is not the case with atrial-based timing. When an AV complex follows an AR complex, the effective paced ventricular rate for that cycle falls below the programmed LRL. A 2 : 1 AV block in an atrial-based timing system induces alternating cycles that are either faster or slower than, but never the same as, the programmed base rate (see Fig. 6.28, bottom).

Interpretation of an ECG of a patient with a dual-chamber pacemaker is helped by knowing whether the pacemaker has atrial-based or ventricular-

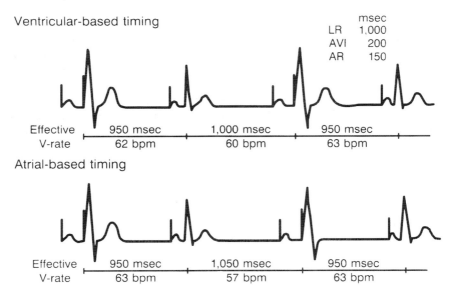

Ventricular-based timing

	msec
LR	1,000
AVI	200
AR	150

Effective	950 msec	1,000 msec	950 msec
V-rate	62 bpm	60 bpm	63 bpm

Atrial-based timing

Effective	950 msec	1,050 msec	950 msec
V-rate	63 bpm	57 bpm	63 bpm

Fig. 6.28 Diagrammatic representations of 2 : 1 AV block during base rate pacing. Top: With a ventricular-based timing system, the interval between consecutive AV and AR paced complexes is slightly shorter; hence, the rate is slightly faster than the programmed base rate. The interval between consecutive AR and AV paced complexes results in ventricular pacing at the base rate for that pacing cycle. Bottom: In an atrial-based timing system, the effective ventricular paced rate alternates between rates that are faster and slower than the programmed rate. The cycle between an AR and AV complex results in a ventricular rate that is slower than the programmed rate, a form of hysteresis. Meanwhile, the cycle between an AV and an AR complex causes the ventricular rate to be faster than the programmed rate. Atrial pacing is stable at the programmed rate, but it is the ventricular contraction that induces cardiac output. (From Levine PA, Hayes DL, Wilkoff BL, Ohman AE. Electrocardiography of rate-modulated pacemaker rhythms. Sylmar, CA: Siemens-Pacesetter, 1990. By permission of Siemens-Pacesetter.)

based timing. With a ventricular-based timing system, a pair of calipers set to the VAI can be used to measure backward from an atrial paced stimulus to the point of ventricular sensing, since a ventricular event, paced or sensed, always initiates the VAI.

A similar technique can be used in an atrial-based timing system, but only when a sensed ventricular complex occurs after the VRP ends. The calipers must be set to the AA interval before measuring backward from the atrial paced event that follows a ventricular sensed event. If one were to misidentify an atrial-based timing system as a ventricular-based system, an otherwise normal rhythm might be misinterpreted as T-wave oversensing or some other form of oversensing (see Fig. 6.26, middle).

Sensor input to base rate pacing

The sensor input to the pacing system temporarily adjusts the rate of the pacemaker. If the individual is active and rate modulation is enabled, the heart rate is determined by the faster of either the native rate or the sensor-determined rate. The sensor rate behaves in a manner identical to the programmed base rate. In essence, the sensor-driven pacing rate acts as if the lower rate limit has been increased. If the native rate is faster than the base rate, the pacemaker is either inhibited or tracks the atrial complexes. If the base rate is faster than the intrinsic rate, the heart rate is controlled by the pacemaker. Regardless of whether the programmed base rate or the sensor rate is in effect, pacing is always atrial in a dual-chamber pacing system. When the sensor input to the pacing system fluctuates, the rate changes.

Automatic mode switch base rate

On the basis of the older literature on lone atrial fibrillation, higher heart rates are often needed to compensate for the loss of atrial transport. Thus, during paroxysmal atrial fibrillation in a patient with high-grade AV block and a pacemaker with mode-switching capability, the resting heart rate during the non-tracking mode may be too low. This low intrinsic rate is of particular concern during protracted periods of pacing in the non-tracking mode. For this reason, the ability to program independently a resting pacemaker rate in effect while the mode switch algorithm is engaged has been introduced to some devices. The programmed base rate might be 60 ppm during sinus rhythm and normal DDD function, whereas the base rate might be 80–90 bpm during atrial fibrillation with the system functioning in the DDI mode. If rate modulation were also activated, any increase in sensor-driven rates would start at the appropriate base for the functional pacing mode at the time.

Upper rate behavior

In the DDD mode of operation, acceleration of the sinus rate results in the sensed P wave terminating the AEI and initiating an AVI, an effect known as P-wave synchronous ventricular pacing. If the PR interval is shorter than the PV interval—the time from an intrinsic P wave to a paced ventricular depolarization—the pacemaker is completely inhibited. P-wave synchronous pacing occurs in a 1 : 1 relationship between the programmed LRL and the programmed URL. In other words, when the interval between consecutive native atrial events is longer than the TARP, each P wave occurs in the atrial alert period and is therefore sensed. Consequently, atrial output is inhibited while simultaneously triggering ventricular output after the AVI. However, when the interval between consecutive native atrial events is shorter than the TARP, some P waves are not sensed because, by definition, they fall into the TARP. The pacemaker goes into an abrupt fixed-block (2 : 1, 3 : 1, etc.) response, sensing only every other or every nth P wave, depending on the native atrial rate (Fig. 6.29). Programming a long PVARP results in the fixed-block response occurring at a relatively low tracking rate. The abrupt change in pacing rate when the fixed block occurs can result in serious symptoms, which frequently happened in early-generation DDD pacemakers.

An additional timing circuit, known as the maximal tracking rate (MTR) interval, better modulates the upper rate behavior. The MTR interval has also been referred to as "upper rate limit" and "ventricular tracking limit." This timing period defines the maximum paced ventricular rate or the shortest interval initiated by a sensed P wave at which a paced ventricular beat can follow a preceding paced or sensed ventricular event. The pacemaker has an upper rate behavior that mimics AV nodal Wenckebach behavior. The appearance is that of group beating, progressive lengthening of the PV interval, and intermittent pauses on the ECG when the native atrial rate exceeds the programmed MTR interval (Fig. 6.30). In these pacing systems, two timers must each complete their cycles for a ventricular stimulus to be released. These timing cycles are known as the AVI and the MTR interval. A sensed P wave initiates an AVI. If, on completion of the AVI, the MTR interval has been completed, a pacemaker stimulus is released at the programmed AVI. If the MTR interval has not yet been completed, the release of the ventricular output pulse is delayed until the MTR interval ends. This delay has the functional effect of lengthening the PV interval and places the ensuing ventricular paced

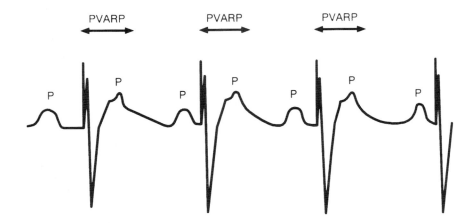

Fig. 6.29 In the DDD pacing mode, the programmed upper rate limit (UR) cannot be violated regardless of the sinus rate. When a P wave is sensed after the postventricular atrial refractory period (PVARP), the atrioventricular interval (AVI) is initiated. If, however, delivering a ventricular pacing artifact at the end of the AVI would violate the UR, the ventricular pacing artifact cannot be delivered. The pacemaker would wait until completion of the UR and then deliver the ventricular pacing artifact. This action would result in a prolonged AVI.

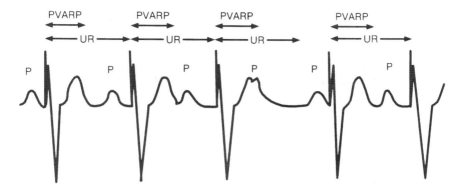

Fig. 6.30 If the sinus rate becomes so rapid that every other P wave occurs within the postventricular atrial refractory period (PVARP), effective 2 : 1 AV block occurs, i.e. every other P wave is followed by a ventricular pacing artifact.

beat closer to the next P wave. Both the PVARP and the MTR interval are initiated by a paced or sensed ventricular event. During Wenckebach upper rate behavior, a P wave eventually coincides with the PVARP, is not sensed, and is therefore ignored by the pacemaker, which results in a relative pause. The MTR interval is then able to complete its timing period, which depends on the atrial rate and programmed base rate, so that either the P wave that follows the unsensed P wave is tracked (restarting the cycle at the programmed AVI) or the pause is terminated by AV sequential pacing.

Thus, upper rate behavior can demonstrate Wenckebach-like behavior or go into abrupt fixed block (e.g. 2 : 1). It demonstrates 2 : 1 block behavior when the P wave falls into the TARP. If the MTR interval is longer than the TARP (TARP = AVI + PVARP), then Wenckebach-like behavior occurs. This can be summarized by the following equation: Wenckebach interval = MTR interval − TARP.

Therefore, if a positive number results, Wenckebach-like behavior occurs. In contrast, if a negative number results, fixed 2 : 1 AV block occurs. For example, if a patient's pacemaker is programmed to an AVI of 250 ms, a PVARP of 225 ms and an MTR of 400 ms, by the above equation the Wenckebach interval is 400 − (250 + 225), or a negative number. Therefore, when the atrial rate reaches 401 ms, a 2 : 1 AV upper rate response is seen. If this patient's AVI is reprogrammed to 125 ms, by the equation the Wenckebach interval is 400 − (125 − 225), or a positive number (+50 ms). In the latter instance, when the atrial rate is 351 ms, Wenckebach-like conduction is seen for a 50-ms interval. As the atrial rate increases further to 401 ms, 2 : 1 AV block is noted.

Rate smoothing, a variation of upper rate behavior, was introduced by Cardiac Pacemakers, Inc. (Guidant, St Paul, MN, USA) as a method of preventing marked changes in cycle length not only occurring at the URL of a DDD pacemaker but also any time the sinus rate is accelerating or decelerating. With rate smoothing, the pacemaker is programmed to a percentage change that is allowed between VV cycles, i.e. 3%, 6%, 9% or 12%. For example, if the VV cycle length is stable at 900 ms during P-synchronous pacing, rate smoothing is "on" at 6%, and the sinus rate suddenly accelerates, the subsequent VV cycle cannot accelerate by more than 54 ms, which is 6% of 900 ms. The ventricular rate is therefore relatively smooth, but sometimes at the expense of uncoupling AV synchrony (Fig. 6.31).

Because Wenckebach upper rate behavior results in the loss of a stable AV relationship, and some patients may be symptomatic with both this and the resultant pauses that occur when a P wave coincides with the PVARP and is not tracked, another upper rate behavior, fallback, is available in some devices. When the atrial rate exceeds the programmed MTR, the pacemaker continues to sense atrial activity but uncouples the native atrial rhythm from the ventricular paced complexes. The ventricular paced rate then slowly and progressively decreases to either an intermediate rate or the programmed base rate. This arrangement avoids the abrupt pauses that occur with both the Wencke-

Without rate smoothing

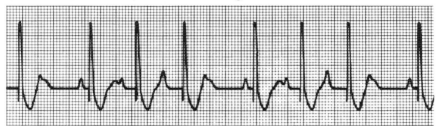

With rate smoothing (6%)

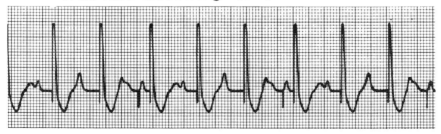

Fig. 6.31 ECG demonstrating DDD pacing with true rate smoothing capabilities (6% of the preceding RR interval). With true rate smoothing, the Wenckebach interval is allowed to lengthen only 36 ms over the preceding RR interval, at a maximum tracking rate (MTR) of 100 ppm. (Reprinted with permission from Cardiac Pacemakers, Inc., St. Paul, MN, USA.)

bach and the fixed-block behaviors. When the atrial rate slows below either the MTR or the fallback rate, depending on the design of the system, the desired AV relationship is restored.

Mode switching

Mode switching refers to the ability of the pacemaker to change automatically from one mode to another in response to an inappropriately rapid atrial rhythm.[19–24] With mode switching, when the pacemaker is functioning in the DDDR mode, the algorithm automatically reprograms the pacemaker to a non-atrial tracking pacing mode (e.g. VVI(R), DDI (R), etc), if specific criteria for a pathological atrial rhythm are met. Mode switching is particularly useful for patients with paroxysmal supraventricular rhythm disturbances. In the DDD or DDDR pacing mode, if a supraventricular rhythm disturbance occurs and the pathological atrial rhythm is sensed by the pacemaker, rapid ventricular pacing may occur (Fig. 6.32). Any pacing mode that eliminates tracking of the pathological atrial rhythm, e.g. DDI, DDIR, DVI or DVIR, also eliminates the ability to track normal sinus rhythm, which is usually the predominant rhythm. Mode switching avoids this limitation (Fig. 6.33).

Refinement of mode-switching algorithms has made this a successful feature (Fig. 6.34). Mode switching functions by measuring intervals between atrial events. In most pacemakers, the rate at which mode switching occurs is a programmable feature. In most generators, the rate for mode switching must exceed the upper rate limit and the maximum sensor rate. The pacemaker uses a counter that considers a short interval to be one that is shorter than the programmed mode-switching rate and a long interval to be one that is longer

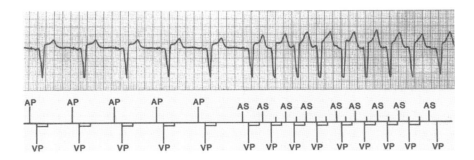

Fig. 6.32 Resting ECG tracing demonstrating AV sequential pacing at lower rate (55 ppm) followed by paroxysmal atrial flutter with ventricular tracking at maximum tracking rate (MTR) (110 ppm). Diagram shows atrial paced events (AP), atrial sensed events (AS), and ventricular paced events (VP), with the postventricular atrial refractory period (PVARP) noted by the rectangle. Short, unlabeled ticks represent atrial activity that occurs in the PVARP and is not sensed. (Diagram is based on Marker Channel, Medtronic, Inc., Minneapolis, MN, USA.) (From Levine PA, Hayes DL, Wilkoff BL, Ohman AE. Electrocardiography of rate-modulated pacemaker rhythms. Sylmar, CA: Siemens-Pacesetter, 1990. By permission of Siemens-Pacesetter.)

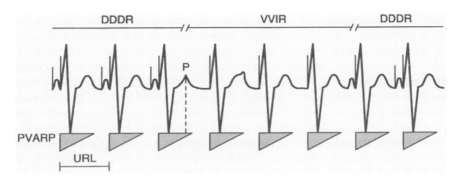

Fig. 6.33 ECG appearance of mode switching. The first three cardiac cycles are due to sensor-driven AV sequential pacing, i.e. DDDR pacing. After the third paced ventricular complex, a P wave occurs during the postventricular atrial refractory period (PVARP) (shaded triangles) and initiates mode switching to the VVIR mode because the atrial rate has exceeded the upper rate limit (URL). The pacing mode reverts to DDDR when the atrial rate falls below the programmed URL, i.e. P waves fall outside the PVARP. (From Hayes DL. Timing cycles of permanent pacemakers. Cardiol Clin 1992; 10:593–608. By permission of WB Saunders Company.)

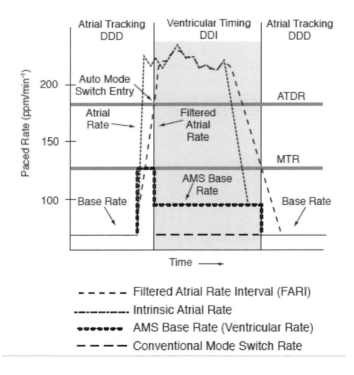

Fig. 6.34 Diagram of switching from atrial tracking to a non-tracking mode (DDI). During DDI pacing a separate base rate may be programmed in some generators. After the atrial arrhythmia has terminated, the mode will switch back to the DDD mode. ATDR, atrial tachycardia detection rate. (Courtesy of St. Jude Medical.)

than the programmed rate. When the counter accrues a specified number of short intervals or time duration, the pacemaker reprograms to a non-atrial tracking mode and remains in this mode until a specified number of long intervals have occurred and altered the counter, at which point mode switching reverts. The non-tracking mode to which the mode switch occurs may be a programmable option. The non-tracking mode is most commonly DDIR and, less commonly, VDIR or VVIR. Switching to DDIR permits maintenance of AV synchrony after the atrial tachyarrhythmia has terminated but before mode switching has been declared completed. Because there are a requisite number of beats required for detection before mode switching occurs, short transient bursts of atrial arrhythmias may still be tracked, and other algorithms such as rate smoothing may be needed to prevent symptomatic palpitations.

Variations on the mode-switching theme are too numerous to detail in this chapter. One should become familiar with the nuances of the mode-switching algorithms used. Key to the implementation of mode switching is the pacemaker's ability to recognize high atrial rates. As discussed in the section on upper rate behavior, the TARP limits the atrial rate that can be detected and tracked. If rapid atrial rates are to be detected, identifying atrial events that occur during the refractory period is essential. In many dual-chamber pacemakers, this period includes the terminal portion of the AV delay and the latter portion of the PVARP. However, some generators are limited by atrial events that fall within the total atrial refractory period and rely on algorithms such as atrial flutter algorithms (see below) to detect atrial arrhythmias. As noted for single-chamber refractory periods, the PVARP has absolute and relative portions. The absolute portion is the first part of the PVARP, and it is termed the postventricular atrial blanking (PVAB) period. The purpose of this timing period is to prevent sensing of the far-field R wave. The ventricular depolarization is a relatively large signal. To ensure sensing of pathological atrial tachyarrhythmias whose signal amplitudes may fluctuate and may be very small, the atrial channel is usually programmed to a sensitive value. This combination predisposes to detection of ventricular signals on the atrial channel. The pacemaker may label these "P" waves and thus respond as if the atrial rate were high when the rhythm is actually normal sinus rhythm. The result is a form of double-counting, resulting in "false" mode switching. To prevent far-field R-wave sensing, a period of absolute refractoriness corresponding to the expected timing of this event forms the first portion of the PVARP. In devices with first-generation mode-switching algorithms, PVAB was not even mentioned because it was not programmable. In dual-chamber devices from virtually all manufacturers as of 2000, PVAB is programmable from 50 to 250 ms. There is an inverse relationship between the duration of the PVAB and the detection of atrial arrhythmia, with the shorter PVABs allowing detection of higher atrial rates (increased sensitivity to atrial tachyarrhythmias). However, increasing the PVAB increases the specificity of rhythm detection and minimizes inappropriate mode switching. PVAB may also limit the ability to detect atrial arrhythmias, particularly atrial flutter, since an atrial deflection may occur just after the paced or sensed ventricular event, creating the so-called "2 : 1 lock in" phenomenon.[25]

Because a far-field R wave may be detected before the depolarization is sensed by the ventricular channel of the pacemaker (Fig. 6.35), another timing circuit, preventricular atrial blanking (pre-VAB), may be helpful. Although the site of native ventricular depolarization cannot be predicted, the algorithm sets up a monitoring interval following the detected atrial event. This programmable period varies from 0 to 60 ms. If an R wave is detected during the pre-VAB interval, the atrial event is labeled a far-field R wave and is not used in the calculation of high atrial rates.

Atrial flutter response

An algorithm to respond specifically to atrial flutter is available in some pacemakers. Such an algorithm is designed to prevent pacing into the atrial vulnerable period and to provide immediate fallback for atrial rates higher than the atrial flutter response (AFR) programmable rate. The fallback rate would be continued as long as atrial events continue to exceed the AFR programmable rate.

For example, if the AFR were programmed to 250 bpm, an atrial event detected inside the PVARP or a previously triggered AFR interval would start an AFR timing window of 240 ms (250 bpm). Atrial detection inside the AFR would be noted as "sensed" events within the refractory period and would not be tracked. The sensing window would begin only after both the AFR and the PVARP expire. If a paced atrial event is scheduled inside an AFR window, it is delayed until the AFR window expires (Fig. 6.36). This algorithm prevents the failure to mode switch due to the sensing of every other atrial flutter wave, the so-called "2 : 1 lock-in" response.[25]

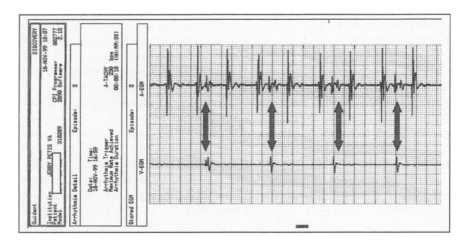

Fig. 6.35 Stored electrogram from a pacemaker demonstrates mode-switching behavior (AV dissociation) during normal sinus rhythm with the pacemaker detecting an atrial rate > 200 bpm. The far-field R wave is identified by double arrows.

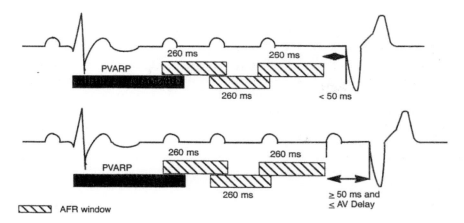

Fig. 6.36 Atrial flutter response. Atrial detection inside the postventricular atrial refractory period (PVARP) starts a 260-ms interval which will restart if another atrial event is detected. A ventricular pace will take place on the scheduled interval. An atrial pace will not occur unless there is at least 50 ms before the scheduled V pace. This prevents competitive pacing. (Courtesy of Boston Scientific.)

A modification of the atrial flutter response is the Blanked Flutter Search, which permits detection of 2 : 1 blanking of atrial events. In this algorithm, if eight consecutive AA intervals that are less than twice the total atrial blanking period and one-half of the AA interval is less than the detect rate interval, the PVARP and VA interval are extended to uncover any blanked atrial events.[26]

Sinus preference
Another algorithm that may affect the timing cycle attempts to maintain sinus rhythm, i.e. sinus preference. The algorithm is programmed to search for the sinus rate, allowing a programmable number of beats per minute that the rate can be reduced as the search occurs. If sinus rhythm is detected within that programmable rate, the sinus rhythm is then allowed to predominate.

Atrial fibrillation prevention algorithms
Numerous atrial fibrillation prevention algorithms are available, each of which may alter the pacemaker timing cycle. These algorithms are based on the concept that atrial pacing may decrease the occurrence of atrial premature beats that will trigger atrial fibrillation. These algorithms are designed to promote atrial pacing faster than the sinus rate by increasing the atrial pacing rate by a programmed amount for a programmed duration when atrial premature beats are sensed. For example, one atrial fibrillation suppression algorithm increases the atrial pacing rate by 5–10 beats per minute when two intrinsic atrial events are detected within a 16-cycle window. After the programmed number of atrial paced beats are delivered, the pacing rate gradually decreases according to the rate recovery algorithm (Fig. 6.37). This algorithm has been

shown in a multicenter randomized clinical trial to reduce the incidence of symptomatic atrial fibrillation.[27] Other algorithms alter the VA interval upon detection of any sensed atrial event or specifically a premature atrial sensed event. These algorithms may be called atrial pacing preference.

Some algorithms have been designed specifically to prevent recurrence of atrial fibrillation after a mode-switching episode. Such algorithms may continue DDIR pacing after termination of the atrial arrhythmia.[26]

Rate smoothing and ventricular rate regularization

Two additional algorithms may have an effect on the pacing rate and alter the rate from either the programmed lower rate, sinus-driven or sensor-driven rates. Rate smoothing, available for many years, is intended to prevent sudden changes in ventricular cycle length. Traditionally, rate smoothing operates between the LRL and the MTR (maximum pacing rate if in a single-chamber inhibited mode or DDI mode) in non-rate-adaptive pacing modes. Rate smoothing is programmable as a percentage, i.e. 3–24% in 3% increments, and can be programmed independently for increments and decrements in the paced rate. The pacemaker stores the most recent RR interval, whether intrinsic or paced, and uses this interval to calculate an allowable change in cycle length based on the rate smoothing percentage programmed. Figure 6.31 demonstrates rate smoothing.

Ventricular rate regularization (VRR) is a variant of rate smoothing. In patients with atrial fibrillation, the marked variation in RR intervals may, in part,

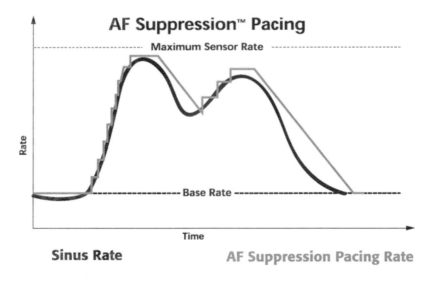

Fig. 6.37 Atrial fibrillation (AF) suppression algorithm. The sinus rate is shown in black. The AF suppression pacing rate is shown in gray. When two intrinsic atrial events occur within a 16-cycle window, the atrial pacing rate will increase by 5–10 bpm. In the figure the atrial pacing rate is increased just slightly higher than the sinus rate. When the sinus rate decreases, the atrial pacing rate declines according to the rate recovery slope. (Courtesy of St. Jude Medical.)

be responsible for patient symptoms. VRR is used to minimize the cycle length variation during atrial fibrillation. It is similar to rate smoothing, with the exception that it may calculate the appropriate cycle length on the basis of a weighted sum of the current ventricular cycle length, as opposed to using the most recent ventricular cycle length with classic rate smoothing.[28,29] Ventricular rate regularization decreases the variability in RR intervals and symptoms from irregular conduction.

Effect of dual-chamber rate-modulated pacemakers on timing cycles

Dual-chamber rate-modulated (DDDR) pacemakers are capable of all the variations described for DDD pacemakers (see Fig. 6.14). In addition to using P-synchronous pacing as a method for increasing the heart rate, the sensor incorporated in the pacemaker may increase the heart rate. The rhythm may therefore be sinus driven (alternatively called "atrial driven" or "P synchronous") or sensor driven (Fig. 6.38).

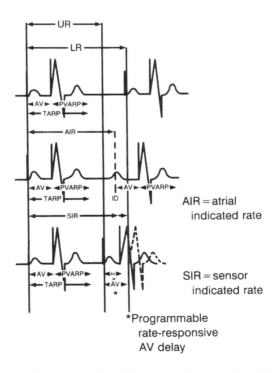

AIR = atrial
indicated rate

SIR = sensor
indicated rate

*Programmable
rate-responsive
AV delay

Fig. 6.38 DDDR pacemakers are capable of all pacing variations previously described for DDD pacemakers (see also Fig. 6.14). When the device is functioning above the programmed lower rate limit (LRL), it may increase the heart rate on the basis of the AIR or SIR. In most DDDR pacemakers, the postventricular atrial refractory period (PVARP) remains fixed regardless of cycle length. Rate-adaptive or rate-variable atrioventricular interval (AVI) allows the length of the AVI to vary with the SIR, i.e. as the SIR increases, the AVI shortens. Because a rate-responsive AV delay (RRAVD) is incorporated, the total atrial refractory period (TARP) may shorten by virtue of the changing AVI even though the PVARP does not change at faster rates.

An important difference in the timing cycle between DDD and DDDR pacing is the ability to pace the atrium during the PVARP in the DDDR mode (Fig. 6.39). This feature does not occur in the DDD mode, because paced atrial activity does not occur until the LRL has been completed, which, by definition, must be at some point after the PVARP. In the DDDR mode, however, even though the atrial sensing channel is refractory during the PVARP, sensor-driven atrial output can still occur (Fig. 6.39).

DDDR pacing systems further increase the complexity of the upper rate behavior. The pacemaker can be driven by intrinsic atrial activity to cause PV pacing, or by a sensor with an input signal that is not identifiable on the ECG, or by both, to result in AV or AR pacing. The eventual upper rate also depends on the type of sensor incorporated in the pacemaker and how the sensor is programmed. Between the programmed LRL and the programmed URL, there may be stable P-wave synchronous pacing, P-wave synchronous

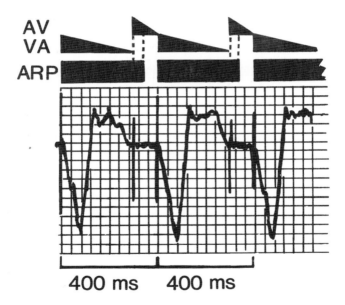

Fig. 6.39 In this ECG example from a DDDR pacemaker, the maximum sensor rate (MSR) is 150 ppm (400 ms), the atrial refractory period (ARP) is 350 ms and the atrioventricular interval (AVI) is 100 ms. As illustrated in the block diagrams above the ECG, the two sensor-driven atrial pacing artifacts both occur during the terminal portion of the postventricular atrial refractory period (PVARP). Even though no atrial sensing can occur during the PVARP, as can be seen in this example by the intrinsic P wave that occurs immediately after the first paced ventricular depolarization, a sensor-driven atrial pacing artifact is not prevented by the PVARP. Whether a sensor-driven atrial pacing artifact is delivered depends on the sensor-indicated rate at that time and not on the PVARP. (Reprinted with permission from Hayes DL, Higano ST. DDDR pacing: follow-up and complications. In: Barold SS, Mugica J, eds. New perspectives in cardiac pacing, 2. Mount Kisco, NY: Futura, 1991:473–491.)

pacing alternating with AV sequential pacing, or stable AV sequential pacing at rates exceeding the base rate (Fig. 6.40). AV sequential pacing rates may increase as high as the programmed MSR.

Although the MSR and MTR are closely related, they are not identical. The tracking rate refers to the rate at which the pacemaker is sensing and tracking intrinsic atrial activity. The MTR is the maximum ventricular paced rate that is allowed in response to sensed atrial rhythms. The MTR may result in fixed-block, Wenckebach, fallback, or rate-smoothing responses, depending on the design of the system. The sensor-controlled rate is the rate of the pacemaker that is determined by the sensor input signal. The MSR is the maximum rate that the pacemaker is allowed to achieve under sensor control.

Whether at the MTR or during rate acceleration below the MTR, the rhythm that results may be in part sensor driven and in part sinus driven (P-wave tracking) and not purely one or the other (see Fig. 6.40). Which of these mechanisms predominates depends on the integrity of the sinus node and the sensor and how the pacemaker is programmed. DDDR pacing can result in a type of

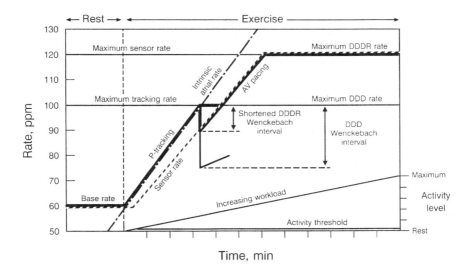

Fig. 6.40 Diagram illustrating the rate response of the DDDR pacemaker and its behavior at both maximum tracking and maximum sensor rate (MSR). The dashed-dotted line represents the intrinsic atrial rate, and the diagonal dashed line represents the sensor rate during progressively increasing workloads. The heavy black line shows the ventricular paced rate, assuming complete heart block, as it progresses from the P-tracking mode to AV sequential pacing through a period of Wenckebach-type block. The DDD Wenckebach interval is shortened by sensor-driven pacing, i.e. "sensor-driven rate smoothing." Maximum shortening of the Wenckebach period is accomplished by optimal programming of the sensor rate–response variables (threshold and slope programming for an activity-driven sensor). (From Higano ST, Hayes DL, Eisinger G. Sensor-driven rate smoothing in a DDDR pacemaker. Pacing Clin Electrophysiol 1989; 12:922–929. By permission of Futura Publishing Company.)

rate smoothing. If the sensor is optimally programmed, then as the atrial rate exceeds the MTR, the RR interval displays minimal variation between sinus-driven and sensor-driven pacing. As shown in Fig. 6.41, the variation in RR interval is markedly lessened with the sensor "on" (DDDR) rather than "passive" (DDD) mode. In the DDDR mode, the RR interval is allowed to lengthen only as much as the difference between the MTR and the activity sensor rate interval. For example, if a device is programmed to a P-wave tracking limit of 120 ppm and the patient's atrial rate exceeds this, then the pacemaker operates in a Wenckebach-type block. If the sensor-indicated rate at this time is 100 ppm, the paced rate decreases from 120 ppm (500 ms) to an AV sequential paced rate of 100 ppm (600 ms) for the Wenckebach cycle and then returns to P-wave tracking at a rate of 120 ppm. This situation usually shortens the DDD Wenckebach interval, but this interval depends on the atrial rate and the programmed values for the MTR and the TARP.

Maximal sensor-driven rate smoothing requires optimal programming of the sensor variable. If the rate-responsive circuitry is programmed to mimic the native atrial rate, the paced ventricular rate cannot demonstrate the 2 : 1

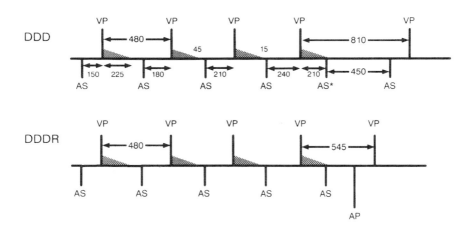

Fig. 6.41 This diagram illustrates the difference in DDD and DDDR behavior when the intrinsic atrial rate increases. Upper panel: DDD pacing. The sensed atrial events (AS) occur increasingly closer to the postventricular atrial refractory period (PVARP), which is programmed to 225 ms (shown by the shaded triangles), until the fifth AS event (*) occurs at 210 ms after the preceding ventricular paced event (VP) and within the PVARP, and is not sensed. This is followed by another AS and VP after the programmed atrial refractory period (AVI) of 150 ms. The resultant cycle length is 810 ms, significantly longer than the preceding cycles of 480 ms. Lower panel: DDDR pacing. The intervals are programmed to the same values as in the upper panel. When the fifth AS event occurs within the PVARP, it is, by definition, not sensed. However, the escape event is a sensor-driven atrial pacing artifact followed by a VP after the AVI. The sensor-indicated cycle length is 545 ms. Therefore, only a 65-ms difference exists between the programmed upper rate limit (URL) and the sensor-indicated rate—a minor difference in cycle lengths. (Modified from Markowitz TH. Dual chamber rate responsive pacing [DDDR] provides physiologic upper rate behavior. PhysioPace 1990; 4:1–4. By permission of Medtronic.)

or Wenckebach-type behavior. Conversely, if the rate-responsive circuitry is programmed to low levels of sensor-driven pacing, little or no rate smoothing occurs (Figs 6.40 and 6.42). Figure 6.41 shows the sensor "passive" (DDD) response to exercise-induced increases in atrial rate, assuming complete heart block, an MTR of 100 ppm, and a Wenckebach-type response at the MTR. The ventricular and atrial rate responses to exercise are shown. As the MTR is exceeded, there is a transition from 1 : 1 P-synchronous function to Wenckebach upper rate behavior. Figure 6.40 shows the response that occurs with the sensor "on" (DDDR) and an MSR of 120 ppm. The ventricular rate response to exercise, along with the atrial and sensor rates, is shown. Below the maximum P-wave tracking rate, the ventricle is paced in a P-synchronous fashion, similar to sensor "passive" (DDD) function. However, with the sensor "on" (DDDR), there is a transition from P-synchronous to AV sequential pacing through a period of Wenckebach-type block as the atrial rate exceeds the MTR. The Wenckebach interval is shortened by sensor-driven pacing. The sensor rate–response curve can be relocated almost anywhere on the graph by sensor parameter programming. Maximum sensor-driven rate smoothing requires optimal programming of these variables. Thus, sensor-modulated rate smoothing occurs only when the activity sensor is driving the pacemaker, when the intrinsic atrial rate exceeds the programmed MTR.

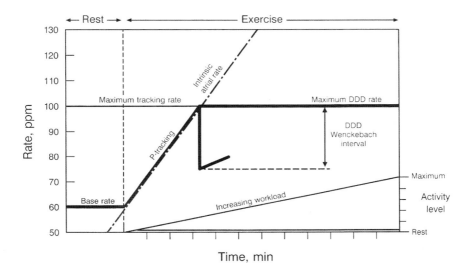

Fig. 6.42 Diagram of the rate response of a DDD pacemaker with Wenckebach-type block at the upper rate limit (URL) (100 ppm). The dashed-dotted line represents the intrinsic atrial rate, and the heavy black line represents the ventricular paced rate, assuming complete heart block. The RR intervals during Wenckebach-type block vary as the atrial rate exceeds the maximum tracking rate (MTR). (From Higano ST, Hayes DL, Eisinger G. Sensor-driven rate smoothing in a DDDR pacemaker. Pacing Clin Electrophysiol 1989; 12:922–929. By permission of Futura Publishing Company.)

Another aspect of DDDR timing cycles is the atrial sensing window (ASW). The ASW is the portion of the RR cycle that is not part of the PVARP or the AVI. It is the period during which the atrial sensing channel is alert. If the PVARP or AVI (or both) is extended, there may effectively be no ASW and even a DDD pacemaker functions as a DVI system. Conversely, if a DDDR pacemaker has exceeded the programmed MTR and is pacing at faster rates based on sensor activation, an appropriately timed intrinsic P wave can still inhibit the sensor-driven atrial pacing artifact and give the appearance of P-wave tracking at rates greater than the MTR (Fig. 6.43). Although the MTR is programmed to a single

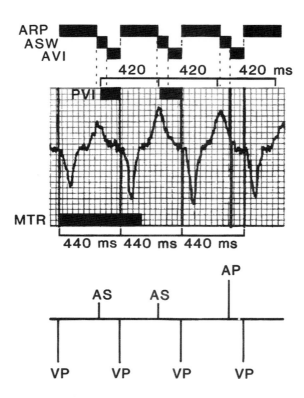

Fig. 6.43 Diagram showing how an appropriately timed P wave can inhibit the sensor-driven A spike and result in apparent P-wave tracking above the maximum tracking rate (MTR). In this example, the MTR is 100 ppm, or 600 ms. The second and third complexes are preceded by intrinsic P waves that occurred during the atrial sensing window (ASW). This resulted in A-spike inhibition, or P-wave tracking above the MTR. The fourth complex was initiated by atrial pacing, because the preceding native P wave occurred outside the ASW in the atrial refractory period (ARP) (ARP = 275 ms). Note the short P-stimulus interval produced by the subsequent atrial spike. Also shown are the ASW (ASW = 65 ms), atrial refractory period (AVI) (AVI = 100 ms), and variable PV interval (PVI). The intrinsic atrial rate is 143 bpm (420 ms). The sensor rate is 136 ppm (440 ms). A diagram in marker-channel fashion demonstrates the ECG findings. (From Higano ST, Hayes DL. P wave tracking above the maximum tracking rate in a DDDR pacemaker. Pacing Clin Electrophysiol 1989; 12:1044–1048. By permission of Futura Publishing Company.)

value in DDDR pacing, it behaves as if it were variable and equal to the sensor-driven rate, when the sensor-driven rate exceeds the programmed MTR, if a P wave occurs during the ASW to inhibit output of an atrial pacing artifact.

Effects of ventricular- and atrial-based timing systems on DDDR timing cycles

As noted previously, the "timing system" may affect the timing cycle. In a ventricular-based timing system, the effective atrial paced rate theoretically may be considerably higher than the programmed MSR if AR conduction were present (Fig. 6.44, top). Assuming that the maximum sensor-controlled rate is 150 ppm (a cycle length of 400 ms), the AEI with a programmed AVI of 200 ms is also 200 ms. If AV conduction were intact so that the AR interval was 150 ms, the actual pacing interval would be ARI + AEI, or 150 + 200 ms, or 350 ms. A cycle length of 350 ms equals 171 ppm, which is markedly higher than the

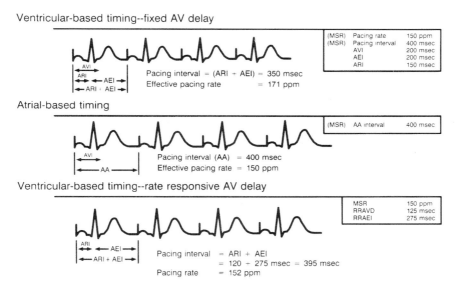

Fig. 6.44 Effect of different timing systems on maximum sensor rate (MSR) with intact stable AV nodal conduction (AR pacing). Top: In a ventricular-based timing system, there is a considerable theoretical increase in the paced atrial rate, exceeding that programmed by the physician. In the example shown, even though the MSR programmed is 150 ppm, or 400 ms, the effective pacing rate achieved is 171 ppm, because the effective pacing rate is the sum of the interval from atrial stimulus to sensed R wave (ARI) and the atrial escape interval (AEI), i.e. 150 + 200 = 350 ms (171 ppm). Middle: In an atrial-based system, the R wave sensed during the atrial refractory period (AVI) alters the basic timing during stable AR pacing. This results in atrial pacing at the sensor-indicated rate. Bottom: The addition of a rate-responsive AV delay (RRAVD) to a ventricular-based timing system minimizes the increase in the paced atrial rate above the programmed sensor-indicated rate. (From Levine PA, Hayes DL, Wilkoff BL, Ohman AE. Electrocardiography of rate-modulated pacemaker rhythms. Sylmar, CA: Siemens-Pacesetter, 1990. By permission of Siemens-Pacesetter.)

programmed MSR of 150 ppm. Although this potentially achievable faster rate may not be a problem or may even be advantageous for some patients, it could create problems for other patients (Fig. 6.44, middle).

Rate acceleration can also be minimized in a DDDR ventricular-based timing system by incorporating a rate-responsive AV delay (RR AVD). As the sinus or sensor-driven rate progressively increases, RR AVD causes the PV and AVIs to progressively shorten (Fig. 6.44, bottom). Shortening the AVI with RR AVD results in a shorter TARP (shorter AVI + PVARP), which increases the intrinsic atrial rate that can be sensed and reduces the likelihood of both a fixed-block upper rate response and functional atrial undersensing. It also minimizes the chance of an inappropriately long PV interval at the higher rate, which may occur with a fixed AV delay when the fixed AV delay is programmed appropriately for lower rate behavior. In this case, the AV delay may be too long at higher rates. In a DDDR system, when the AVI shortens, the ventricular rate drive is held to that governed by the sensor, so that the time subtracted from the AVI is added to the AEI. Thus, at a rate of 150 ppm and pacing interval of 400 ms, if the RR AVD causes the AVI to shorten by 75 ms from an initially programmed AVI of 200 ms, then the AVI shortens to 125 ms. Because the overall ventricular timing is held constant, the 75 ms subtracted from the AVI is added to the AEI, increasing it to 275 ms.

The RR AVD provides a more physiological AVI at the faster rate and minimizes the degree of rate increase over the programmed MSR if AR conduction is intact. Assuming that the rate is 150 ppm and the initial AVI is 200 ms, the RR AVD is 125 ms, resulting in AV sequential pacing at the sensor programmed rate when the AR interval is 140 ms. If intact AV conduction is present at 120 ms, the overall shortening of the pacing interval is only 5 ms more than that seen at 150 bpm, a rate of 152 bpm (Fig. 6.44, bottom).

Another option is extending the VAI as needed to control the AA pacing rate according to the programmed MSR (Fig. 6.45). This extension results in adaptive-rate pacing, regardless of AV conduction status, which is equal to, but does not exceed, the desired MSR.

Endless-loop tachycardia

Endless-loop tachycardia (ELT) is not a portion of the timing cycle, but understanding the timing cycle of dual-chamber pacing is crucial to understanding ELT, and vice versa. ELT has also been referred to as "pacemaker-mediated tachycardia" (PMT), "pacemaker-mediated re-entry tachycardia" and "pacemaker circus movement tachycardia." ELT has been defined as a re-entry arrhythmia in which the dual-chamber pacemaker acts as the anterograde limb of the tachycardia and the natural pathway acts as the retrograde limb.

If AV synchrony is uncoupled—i.e. if the P wave is displaced from its normal relation to the QRS complex—the subsequent ventricular event may result in retrograde atrial excitation if retrograde or VA conduction is intact. If the retrograde P wave is sensed, the AVI of the pacemaker is initiated. On

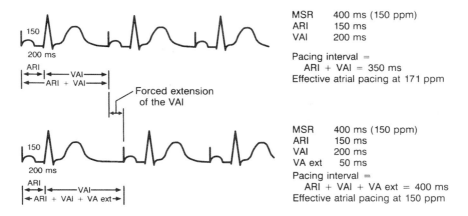

MSR   400 ms (150 ppm)
ARI   150 ms
VAI   200 ms

Pacing interval =
  ARI + VAI = 350 ms
Effective atrial pacing at 171 ppm

Forced extension
of the VAI

MSR   400 ms (150 ppm)
ARI   150 ms
VAI   200 ms
VA ext   50 ms
Pacing interval =
  ARI + VAI + VA ext = 400 ms
Effective atrial pacing at 150 ppm

Fig. 6.45 Pacing at maximum sensor rate (MSR). The timing algorithm provides effective pacing at MSR with intrinsic conduction to the ventricle. ARI, interval from atrial stimulus to sensed R wave; VA, ventriculoatrial; VAI, ventriculoatrial interval. (From Hayes DL, Ketelson A, Levine PA *et al.* Understanding timing systems of current DDDR pacemakers. Eur JCPE 1993; 3:70–86. By permission of Mayo Foundation.)

termination of the AVI and MTR interval, a ventricular pacing artifact is delivered, which could once again be conducted in a retrograde fashion. Once established, this re-entrant mechanism continues until interrupted or until the retrograde limb of the circuit is exhausted. The paced VV interval cannot violate the programmed maximum or URL of the pacemaker, and the ELT often occurs at the URL. The cycle length of the ELT is the sum of the VA conduction time and the programmed sensed AV delay. If the VA conduction time is sufficiently long, the ELT will occur below the URL. Many mechanisms have been adopted to prevent or minimize ELT.

Among the early preventive algorithms was automatic PVARP extension following a PVC, because ventricular ectopic beats were the most common triggers for an ELT. ELT is not a major problem when the programmed base rate is low; however, if the base rate is intentionally programmed to a relatively high level or is functioning there due to sensor drive, PVARP extension blocks detection of either a retrograde or an anterograde P wave. Because of the high rate, however, the AEI may time out, resulting in delivery of an atrial output pulse when the atrial myocardium is still refractory from the native depolarization. In this circumstance, atrial output is ineffective. If the patient can sustain retrograde conduction, this sequence of events can result in a rhythm termed repetitive non-re-entrant ventriculoatrial synchrony.

Algorithms for termination of pacemaker-mediated tachycardia
If ELT cannot be prevented, various recognition and termination algorithms are available. The simplest algorithm assumes that atrial-sensed ventricular pacing occurring at the MTR is a PMT and, after a preset number of cycles,

either withholds ventricular output or extends the PVARP. If the rhythm is a true ELT, it is terminated by this mechanism. A further refinement to these algorithms allows the clinician to select an ELT rate that is below the MTR. This adjustment addresses the balanced ELTs in which the sum of the retrograde conduction (VA) interval plus the sensed AV delay is longer than the MTR interval, and, hence, the ELT rate is slower than the MTR. The limitation of both of these algorithms is that they respond whether the rhythm is an ELT or an intrinsic atrial rhythm that is being appropriately tracked by the pacemaker. For a native atrial rhythm, repeated pauses are caused by the activation of the PMT termination algorithm. Even intermittent loss of tracking may result in failure of biventricular pacing.

Another approach is to monitor the retrograde conduction interval. If the VP interval is stable, the device labels the rhythm as a possible PMT and then varies the next PV interval. If the atrial rhythm is independent of the ventricular paced event, the VP interval on the next cycle is either lengthened or shortened by the same degree by which the PV interval was changed. The rhythm is then labeled normal, and normal atrial synchronous ventricular pacing continues. If the VP interval is stable, the P wave is caused by retrograde conduction (related to the ventricular paced event), and the rhythm is probably a PMT. At that point, ventricular output is withheld following the detected P wave. An atrial alert period is initiated, and if another P wave is not detected, an atrial output pulse is delivered 330 ms later. This interval was chosen as sufficient for recovery of the atrial myocardium. Successful atrial capture breaks the cycle and prevents retrograde conduction after the next ventricular paced complex. This algorithm also prevents some of the pauses occurring with an earlier generation of PMT algorithms (Fig. 6.46).

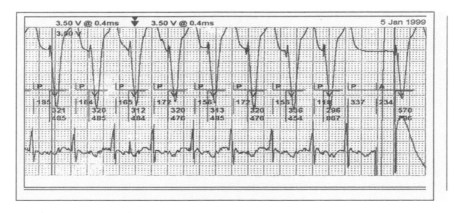

Fig. 6.46 Endless-loop tachycardia was induced during an atrial capture threshold test (loss of atrial capture allowed for retrograde conduction). The pacemaker-mediated tachycardia (PMT) algorithm was enabled. The PV interval was shortened; the subsequent VP interval was stable, resulting in withholding of ventricular output and delivery of atrial output 330 ms later.

Non-competitive atrial pacing

Non-competitive atrial pacing (NCAP) is used to minimize competition between the sensor (atrial pacing) and sinus rhythm. Implementation of this capability has been facilitated by microprocessors and the ability of pacemakers to detect events coinciding with the refractory period. If atrial depolarization is sensed within the alert period, it inhibits atrial output and triggers ventricular output. However, if the native atrial event coincides with the PVARP, it may be detected but does not otherwise alter the basic timing period of the pacemaker. With NCAP enabled, if atrial output is scheduled to be delivered within a given interval after the detected P wave, atrial output is delayed until a preset interval has timed out. To maintain a stable ventricular rate, the paced AVI may be foreshortened for this one cycle (Fig. 6.47).

Algorithms to minimize right ventricular pacing

In patients with intact AV conduction, there are several potential benefits of minimizing ventricular pacing. Most importantly, the abnormal sequence of ventricular contraction may result in impaired cardiovascular hemodynamics. Specifically, some patients may experience an increase in heart failure, impairment of functional status, left ventricular dilation, and deterioration of left ventricular systolic function. Patients with underlying left ventricular dysfunction appear to have the greatest hemodynamic deterioration with

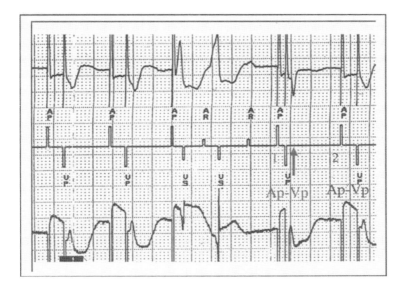

Fig. 6.47 Premature ventricular contraction associated with a retrograde P wave. This P wave coincides with the postventricular atrial refractory period (PVARP) and is not tracked, but it is sensed and labeled "AR." The scheduled atrial output is delayed by 300 ms. This results in a foreshortening of the AV delay. AP, atrial paced event; AS, atrial sensed event; VP, ventricular paced event; VS, ventricular sensed event. (Courtesy of S. Serge Barold, MD.)

right ventricular pacing. There are several algorithms that have been developed in order to minimize right ventricular pacing in patients with intact AV conduction.[30–32] In the Managed Ventricular Pacing™ algorithm, the AAI(R) is operational unless a triggering event occurs. If an AA interval occurs without a sensed ventricular event occurring, a ventricular paced event occurs 80 ms after the AA paced interval (Fig. 6.48). If two of the four preceding AA intervals do not have a ventricular sensed event, the mode switches from AAI(R) to DDD(R). While in the DDD(R) mode, the pacemaker monitors AV conduction by switching to AAI(R) mode for one cycle. If a sensed ventricular event occurs, the device maintains the switch to AAI(R) mode. If no sensed ventricular event occurs, the pacemaker remains in DDD(R) mode (Fig. 6.49). The monitored periods occur at 1 min, 2 min, 4 min, 8 min and at progressively longer intervals up to 16 h. This algorithm has been shown to result in a significant decrease in ventricular pacing.

Other algorithms may also promote intrinsic conduction rather than ventricular pacing. The AAIsafeR acts in the AAI mode unless A-V block occurs. Unlike the Managed Ventricular Pacing algorithm, the mode will switch to DDDR with first-degree AV block, such as a PR interval > 350 ms for seven or more intervals. Blocked atrial events also result in conversion to DDDR. Return to AAIR occurs with sensing a programmable number of consecutive intrinsic ventricular events or after a programmable number of cycles in the DDDR mode.[33]

Positive AV interval hysteresis with search may also be used to promote ventricular conduction and minimize ventricular pacing. However, limits in the maximum AV interval will frequently result in some ventricular pacing if the AV conduction is sometimes prolonged.

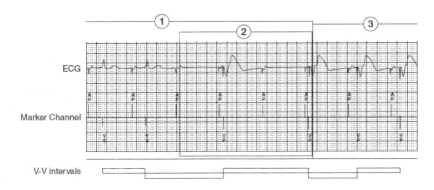

Fig. 6.48 Switch from AAI(R) to DDD(R) mode in the Managed Ventricular Pacing algorithm. If an AA interval occurs without a sensed ventricular event occurring, a ventricular paced event occurs 80 ms after the AA interval. If two out of four AA intervals have no ventricular sensed event, the mode changes to DDD(R) mode. (Courtesy of Medtronic, Inc.)

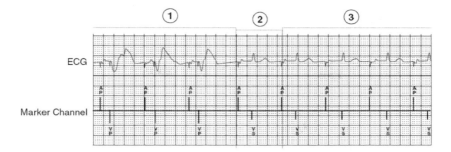

Fig. 6.49 Switch from DDD(R) to AAI(R) mode in the Managed Ventricular Pacing algorithm. If two of the four preceding AA intervals do not have a ventricular sensed event, the mode switches from AAI(R) to DDD(R). While in the DDD(R) mode, the pacemaker monitors AV conduction by switching to AAI(R) mode for one cycle. If a sensed ventricular event occurs, the device maintains the switch to AAI(R) mode.

Biventricular pacing timing cycles

Biventricular pacing improves heart function by restoring ventricular coordination in patients with underlying ventricular conduction disturbances. In order to achieve this effect, biventricular pacing must be maintained and intrinsic conduction must be limited. In patients with chronic atrial fibrillation, the VVIR mode is used. In patients in sinus rhythm, DDD or DDD(R) modes are used almost exclusively, although initial clinical trials utilized the VDD pacing mode. Although the timing cycles for biventricular pacing have numerous potential permutations based on which chambers are sensed, current devices are limited to right ventricular sensing. The most critical and potentially challenging result of current biventricular timing cycles is the possible inhibition of biventricular pacing, with the possible negative hemodynamic consequences.[34]

The basic timing cycle for biventricular pacing (Fig. 6.50) is based on right ventricular based timing with a sensed or paced ventricular event initiating a VA interval. The AV interval must be sufficiently short to result in constant ventricular capture rather than intrinsic conduction. Rate-adaptive AV interval may be programmed in order to decrease the AV interval during exercise or elevated heart rates. AV hysteresis may be used to promote ventricular capture in biventricular pacing (Fig. 6.51). In biventricular pacing, it may also be possible to program a difference in timing of the right and left ventricular paced events. This interventricular delay (RV–LV) may be positive, negative, or zero (Figs 6.50 and 6.51). In the event that intrinsic conduction occurs, a right ventricular sensed event will trigger a left ventricular paced event, a feature called ventricular sensed response.

Failure to biventricular pace is one of the most important issues in biventricular pacing timing cycles. A common phenomenon is an atrial event occur-

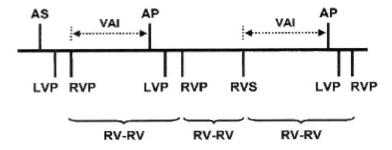

Fig. 6.50 Basic timing cycle for biventricular pacing. An atrial sensed event (AS) is followed by a left ventricular paced event (LVP) and a right ventricular paced event (RVP). A premature ventricular beat (RS) results in an atrial escape interval (AEI). The following event is an atrial paced event. (From Wang P, Kramer A, Estes NAM 3rd, Hayes DL. Timing cycles for biventricular pacing. Pacing Clin Electrophysiol 2002; 25:62–75.)

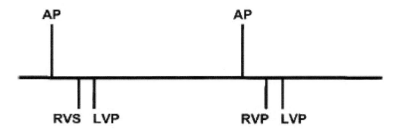

Fig. 6.51 Right ventricular sensing and right ventricular pacing in basic timing cycle for biventricular pacing. In the first ventricular complex on the left, there is a right ventricular sensed beat (RVS) followed by a left ventricular paced beat (LVP), and during the second complex there is a right ventricular paced beat (RVP) followed by a left ventricular paced beat (LVP). (From Wang P, Kramer A, Estes NAM 3rd, Hayes DL. Timing cycles for biventricular pacing. Pacing Clin Electrophysiol 2002; 25:62–75.)

ring during PVARP resulting in failure to track the atrial event and subsequent loss of biventricular pacing. Because the P–R interval may be relatively long compared with the sinus cycle length, the P wave may fall in the PVARP of the preceding R-wave interval. Since this P wave cannot be tracked, conduction occurs, preventing biventricular pacing from occurring. With a specific set of relationships between the AV interval, PR interval and the PVARP, biventricular pacing may continue to be inhibited. This relationship is illustrated in Fig. 6.52. As the atrial rate reaches the total atrial refractory period (PVARP + AV interval), biventricular pacing will stop. When the atrial rate falls, biventricular pacing will continue to be inhibited until the atrial rate is below the total intrinsic atrial refractory period (PVARP + PR interval). For example, if the PR is 240 ms, the AV interval is 150 ms and the PVARP is 300 ms, at a sinus cycle length of 450 ms or 133 bpm, biventricular pacing will cease. As the rate slows, biventricular pacing will continue to be inhibited until the sinus cycle length increases to 540 ms or 111 bpm.

There are a number of circumstances that may initiate loss of biventricular pacing in addition to rapid sinus rates. An atrial premature complex may fall within the PVARP. A premature ventricular beat may create a new PVARP timed so that the next sinus P wave falls within the PVARP. Several programmed features may also exacerbate the occurrence of loss of biventricular pacing. PVC-initiated PVARP extension is an important cause of loss of biventricular pacing and should generally be turned off. Following a PVC, the PVARP extension will make it more likely that the next P wave will fall within the extended PVARP. Because the PVARP may be markedly extended, to 600 ms for example, perpetuation of loss of biventricular pacing is more likely at slower rates. For example, a PVARP extended to 600 ms combined with a PR of 240 ms would result in continued pacing until the sinus cycle length dropped to 840 ms or 71 bpm. Pacemaker-mediated tachycardia termination algorithms may also lead to loss of biventricular pacing. In some generators, tracking at the upper rate limit may initiate a pacemaker-mediated

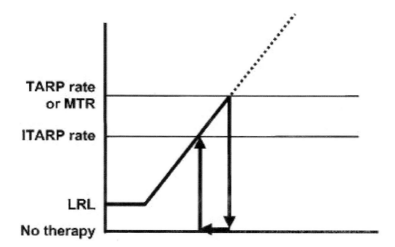

Fig. 6.52 Diagrammatic representation of the relationship between the atrial rate and biventricular pacing delivery. On the y axis is the atrial rate. As the atrial rate reaches the total atrial refractory period (PVARP + AV interval), biventricular pacing will stop. When the atrial rate falls, biventricular pacing will continue to be inhibited until the atrial rate is below the total intrinsic atrial refractory period (PVARP + PR interval). (From Wang P, Kramer A, Estes NAM 3rd, Hayes DL. Timing cycles for biventricular pacing. Pacing Clin Electrophysiol 2002; 25:62–75.)

tachycardia algorithm that results in one P wave not being tracked. Analogous to a premature atrial beat occurring in PVARP, biventricular pacing will be inhibited. Algorithms that reduce the PVARP when a sensed ventricular event occurs may prevent perpetuation of loss of biventricular pacing.

Current algorithms require right ventricular sensing as the basis of the timing cycles. Only one device permits left ventricular sensing for prevention of competitive pacing. Since left ventricular pacing may be programmed to lead right ventricular pacing, it is possible for the left ventricular paced event to occur during a vulnerable period. In one device, left ventricular pacing may be inhibited when a previous left ventricular sensed event has occurred within a specified interval (Fig. 6.53).

Summary

A clear understanding of the components of pacemaker timing cycles is crucial to understanding and interpreting paced ECGs. The information in this chapter provides basic rules for timing cycles for pacing modes currently in use (VVI, AAI, VVIR, AAIR, DDI, DDD, DDDR, DDIR) and for pacing modes less frequently used or of historical interest, but still important to understand how timing cycles have developed (VOO, AOO, DOO, DVIC, DVI, VDD).

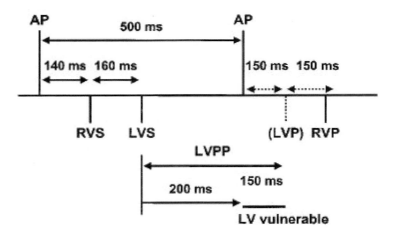

Fig. 6.53 Diagrammatic representation of the relationship between a left ventricular sensed event and a planned left ventricular paced event. Sensing of the left ventricular sensed event results in inhibition of the planned left ventricular paced event that is ahead of the planned right ventricular paced event. (From Wang P, Kramer A, Estes NAM 3rd, Hayes DL. Timing cycles for biventricular pacing. Pacing Clin Electrophysiol 2002; 25:62–75.)

Each pacemaker manufacturer may take license and alter or add some nuance to the timing cycle of a particular pacemaker. Although understanding basic timing cycles allows interpretation of most paced ECGs, manufacturers' alterations require familiarity with the design of each pacemaker to be interpreted. When unexpected behavior of the pacemaker occurs in a patient whose condition is clinically stable, the presumption should be that this reflects a unique behavioral eccentricity of the pacemaker. All manufacturers maintain a group of technical service engineers who are available 24 h a day, 7 days a week. They should be contacted before any intervention, such as replacing the pulse generator, is attempted, for in all probability the device is behaving normally.

References

1 Morgan JM. Basics of cardiac pacing: selection and mode choice. Heart 2006; 92:850–4.
2 Musilli N, Padeletti L. Pacemaker selection: time for a rethinking of complex pacing systems? Eur Heart J 2006; 27:132–5.
3 Newman D. Relationships between pacing mode and quality of life: evidence from randomized clinical trials. Card Electrophysiol Rev 2003; 7:401–5.
4 Padeletti L, Lieberman R, Valsecchi S, Hettrick DA. Physiologic pacing: new modalities and pacing sites. Pacing Clin Electrophysiol 2006; 29 (Suppl. 2):S73–7.
5 Albertsen AE, Nielsen JC. Selecting the appropriate pacing mode for patients with sick sinus syndrome: evidence from randomized clinical trials. Card Electrophysiol Rev 2003; 7:406–10.
6 Bernstein AD, Daubert J-C, Fletcher RD et al. The revised NASPE/BPEG generic code for antibradycardia, adaptive-rate, and multisite pacing. North American Society of Pacing and Electrophysiology/British Pacing and Electrophysiology Group. Pacing Clin Electrophysiol 2002; 25:260–4.
7 Limousin M, Pioger G, Bonnet JL, Geroux L. Automatic adaptation of the basic pacing rate in response to minute ventilation. Chorum French Investigational Group. Pacing Clin Electrophysiol 1998; 21:1405–9.
8 Lass J, Kaik J, Meigas K, Hinrikus H, Blinowska A. Evaluation of the quality of rate adaptation algorithms for cardiac pacing. Europace 2001; 3:221–8.
9 Masumoto H, Ueda Y, Kato R et al. Long-term clinical performance of AAI pacing in patients with sick sinus syndrome: a comparison with dual-chamber pacing. Europace 2004; 6:444–50.
10 Schwaab B, Kindermann M, Schatzer-Klotz D et al. AAIR versus DDDR pacing in the bradycardia tachycardia syndrome: a prospective, randomized, double-blind, crossover trial. Pacing Clin Electrophysiol 2001; 24:1585–95.
11 Barold SS, Gallardo I, Sayad D. The DVI mode of cardiac pacing: a second coming? Am J Cardiol 2002; 90:521–3.
12 Huang M, Krahn AD, Yee R, Klein GJ, Skanes AC. Optimal pacing for symptomatic AV block: a comparison of VDD and DDD pacing. Pacing Clin Electrophysiol 2004; 27:19–23.

13 Duru F, Bloch KE, Weilenmann D, Candinas R. Clinical evaluation of a pacemaker algorithm that adjusts the pacing rate during sleep using activity variance. Pacing Clin Electrophysiol 2000; 23 (10 Pt 1):1509–15.

14 Melzer C, Sowelam S, Sheldon TJ et al. Reduction of right ventricular pacing in patients with sinus node dysfunction using an enhanced search AV algorithm. Pacing Clin Electrophysiol 2005; 28:521–7.

15 Milasinovic G, Sperzel J, Smith TW et al. Reduction of RV pacing by continuous optimization of the AV interval. Pacing Clin Electrophysiol 2006; 29:406–12.

16 Benditt DG, Sutton R, Gammage M et al. "Rate-drop response" cardiac pacing for vasovagal syncope. Rate-Drop Response Investigators Group. J Interv Card Electrophysiol 1999; 3:27–33.

17 Connolly SJ, Sheldon R, Thorpe KE et al. Pacemaker therapy for prevention of syncope in patients with recurrent severe vasovagal syncope: Second Vasovagal Pacemaker Study (VPS II): a randomized trial. JAMA 2003; 289:2224–9.

18 Connolly SJ, Sheldon R, Roberts RS, Gent M. The North American Vasovagal Pacemaker Study (VPS). A randomized trial of permanent cardiac pacing for the prevention of vasovagal syncope. J Am Coll Cardiol 1999; 33:16–20.

19 Lau C-P, Leung S-K, Tse H-F, Barold SS. Automatic mode switching of implantable pacemakers: I. Principles of instrumentation, clinical, and hemodynamic considerations. Pacing Clin Electrophysiol 2002; 25:967–83.

20 Lau C-P, Leung S-K, Tse H-F, Barold SS. Automatic mode switching of implantable pacemakers: II. Clinical performance of current algorithms and their programming. Pacing Clin Electrophysiol 2002; 25:1094–113.

21 De Simone A, Senatore G, Turco P, Vitale DF, Romano E, Stabile G. Specificity of atrial mode switching in detecting atrial fibrillation episodes: roles of length and contiguity. Pacing Clin Electrophysiol 2005; 28 (Suppl. 1):S47–9.

22 Barold SS, Stroobandt RX. Complex manifestations of an automatic mode switching algorithm. Pacing Clin Electrophysiol 2007; 30:112–4.

23 Israel CW. Analysis of mode switching algorithms in dual chamber pacemakers. Pacing Clin Electrophysiol 2002; 25:380–93.

24 Bordacher P, Cazeau S, Graindorg L, Ritter P. Impact and prevention of far-field sensing in fallback mode switches. Pacing Clin Electrophysiol 2003; 26 (1 Pt 2):206–9.

25 Pajitnev D, Israel CW, Hohnloser SH, Barold SS. The "inverse 2:1 lock-in" response to atrial flutter. Pacing Clin Electrophysiol 2005; 28:982–4.

26 Medtronic Inc. Adapta/Versa/Sensia Pacemaker Reference Guide. 2006.

27 Carlson MD, Ip J, Messenger J et al. A new pacemaker algorithm for the treatment of atrial fibrillation: results of the Atrial Dynamic Overdrive Pacing Trial (ADOPT). J Am Coll Cardiol 2003; 42:627–33.

28 Tse H-F, Newman D, Ellenbogen KA et al. Effects of ventricular rate regularization pacing on quality of life and symptoms in patients with atrial fibrillation (Atrial fibrillation symptoms mediated by pacing to mean rates [AF SYMPTOMS study]). Am J Cardiol 2004; 94:938–41.

29 Wood MA. Trials of pacing to control ventricular rate during atrial fibrillation. J Interv Card Electrophysiol 2004; 10 (Suppl. 1):63–70.

30 Gillis AM, Purerfellner H, Israel CW et al. Reducing unnecessary right ventricular pacing with the managed ventricular pacing mode in patients with sinus node disease and AV block. Pacing Clin Electrophysiol 2006; 29:697–705.

31 Lee KL, Burnes JE, Mullen TJ, Hettrick DA, Tse H-F, Lau C-P. Avoidance of right ventricular pacing in cardiac resynchronization therapy improves right ventricular hemodynamics in heart failure patients. J Cardiovasc Electrophysiol 2007; 18:497–504.

32 Sweeney MO, Ellenbogen KA, Miller EH, Sherfesee L, Sheldon T, Whellan D. The Managed Ventricular pacing versus VVI 40 Pacing (MVP) Trial: clinical background, rationale, design, and implementation. J Cardiovasc Electrophysiol 2006; 17:1295–8.

33 Savoure A, Frohlig G, Galley D *et al.* A new dual-chamber pacing mode to minimize ventricular pacing. Pacing Clin Electrophysiol 2005; 28:S43–S46.

34 Wang P, Kramer A, Estes NAM 3rd, Hayes DL. Timing cycles for biventricular pacing. Pacing Clin Electrophysiol 2002; 25:62–75.

## CHAPTER 7

Evaluation and management of pacing system malfunctions

Suneet Mittal

The clinician is frequently asked to evaluate the patient with an implanted pacemaker. In general, reasons for evaluation fall into one of three broad categories: (i) pacemaker malfunction is suspected based on electrocardiography (ECG), telemetry monitoring and/or ambulatory ECG monitoring; (ii) a patient with a previously implanted pacemaker presents with symptoms suggestive of possible pacemaker malfunction (e.g. palpitations, dizziness, pre-syncope, or syncope); or (iii) a patient presents for routine pacemaker follow-up. The purpose of this chapter is to review the approach to the evaluation and management of pacing systems malfunctions, with an emphasis on common scenarios observed clinically during the follow-up of patients with single, dual and biventricular pacemaker systems.

General considerations

In general, when evaluating a patient with an implanted permanent pacemaker and suspected malfunction, it is useful to have as much information about the patient and the pacing system as possible (Table 7.1).[1] Patient-specific data include the indication for pacing, relevant medications (since some can adversely affect pacing thresholds[2]) and concurrent medical problems (e.g. hyperkalemia induced by renal failure[3]) that can affect short- and long-term pacing performance. In addition, it can be helpful to have access to a patient's prior ECGs and chest radiographs. (In general, after pacemaker implantation, it is useful to obtain a complete 12-lead ECG demonstrating intrinsic rhythm and full pacing and overpenetrated posteroanterior and lateral chest radiographs to have a basis for comparison during follow-up.)

The pacing system consists of the pulse generator and the lead(s). Pacing system data include the following: details of the implant procedure [location of pulse generator (subcutaneous, submuscular), technique for venous access (cephalic, subclavian, axillary veins)], manufacturer, model, and serial numbers of the pulse generator and lead(s), the sensing and pacing thresholds, and impedance measurements. In addition, it is useful to have thresholds and imped-

Cardiac Pacing and ICDs, 5th edition. Edited by Kenneth A. Ellenbogen and Mark A. Wood.
© 2008 Blackwell Publishing, ISBN: 978-1-4051-6350-7

Table 7.1 Baseline data needed for pacemaker troubleshooting

Pacemaker system
    Pacemaker generator
    Manufacturer
    Model and serial numbers
    Current programming
    Date of implant
    Alert or recalls
    Header type
    Special features
Lead system
    Manufacturer
    Model and serial numbers
    Polarity and fixation mechanism
    Pin type
    Insulation material
    Date of implant
    Alert or recalls
Patient
    Indication for pacemaker
    Implant operative report
    Medical and cardiac diagnosis
    Medications
    History of recent medical procedures (cardioversion, defibrillation, magnetic resonance imaging, electrocautery, etc)
    History of electrical current exposure, trauma

ance measurements as obtained through the pacing system analyzer (PSA) as well as those obtained through the device using the pacemaker programmer.

Although having detailed information about the patient and pacing system is highly desirable, in reality it is rarely complete. Patients are often implanted at one facility, undergo follow-up at another facility, and present with pacemaker malfunction to yet another facility. The clinician is often forced to begin the troubleshooting process before having access to complete data on the pacing system.

The only absolute requirement to initiate the troubleshooting process is knowledge of the patient's device manufacturer so that the appropriate programmer can be identified. The easiest way to obtain this information is from the device identification card given to the patient at implant. When this is not available, options include the following: (i) review of old medical records, (ii) calls to the device registration and tracking offices of the major pacemaker manufacturers, and (iii) review of the chest radiograph to assess the shape of the generator, configuration of the battery or to identify the manufacturer-specific identification code embedded within the header block. Once the device can be identified and interrogated, it is often possible to obtain additional information within data fields stored manually into the device. These data elements may include the pacing indication, details of the hardware (model and serial numbers), patient data, programmed parameters and contact information of the implanting physician.

Pacing system malfunctions are generally related to a problem with either the pacemaker generator or the pacemaker leads (Fig. 7.1). Fortunately, a limited number of problems account for the majority of pacemaker system malfunctions, which typically fall into one of several categories. These include (i) unexpected alterations in the patient's pacing rate, (ii) failure to output, (iii) failure to capture, (iv) undersensing, and (v) oversensing. Therefore, a systematic approach during pacemaker interrogation is critical to troubleshoot properly the various aspects of the differential diagnosis.

The pacemaker generator

The pacemaker generator usually exhibits failure of some or all of its functions in response to severe battery depletion or when it has been affected adversely due to direct trauma or an iatrogenic cause (e.g. cardioversion/defibrillation, electrocautery, therapeutic radiation, lithotripsy, etc.). Failure to communicate with the device occurs with complete battery failure, but may also result from misidentification of the pacemaker manufacturer (or model) and attempts to interrogate the device with the wrong programmer. The model of the device should be confirmed by the patient's identification card, medical records, X-ray, or calls to the manufacturer's implant registries. Telemetry with the device may fail because the generator has migrated from the implant area, is deep in tissue or the wrong anatomical site is being interrogated. Electromagnetic interference (EMI) in the clinical environment can also prevent telemetric communication. Although rare, true malfunctions of the pacemaker generator are also possible.[4] Several important advisories related to pacemaker malfunction have been released since 2000.

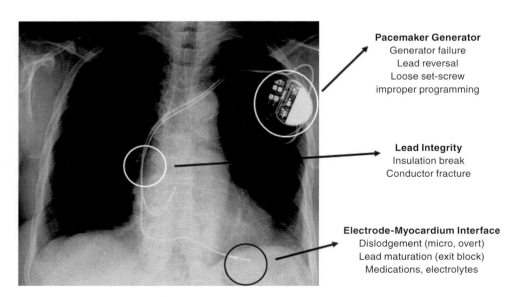

Pacemaker Generator
Generator failure
Lead reversal
Loose set-screw
improper programming

Lead Integrity
Insulation break
Conductor fracture

Electrode-Myocardium Interface
Dislodgement (micro, overt)
Lead maturation (exit block)
Medications, electrolytes

Fig. 7.1 Potential areas of pacemaker system malfunction.

Affected devices can be associated with premature battery depletion, intermittent or permanent loss of pacing output, failure of proper rate-response behavior, and/or undesirable reprogramming (electrical reset, reversion to VVI mode).

In evaluating a patient with a pacemaker, it is critically important to be cognizant of the potential interplay between a reported advisory and the patient's clinical presentation. However, before deciding to proceed with an operative intervention to replace a pacemaker generator, consultation with a device manufacturer's technical support department should be considered to differentiate pacemaker malfunction from an idiosyncratic, but normal, behavior of the particular device. In addition, it is important to consider published recommendations before making a decision to remove a pacemaker generator that is the subject of a product advisory.[5]

The pacemaker lead(s)

Pacing system malfunctions can be related to problems with the pacemaker leads in a variety of ways. The problem may be at the leads–pacemaker header block, such as an inadvertent reversal of the atrial and ventricular lead insertion [in dual (Fig. 7.2) or biventricular lead systems], a failure to properly

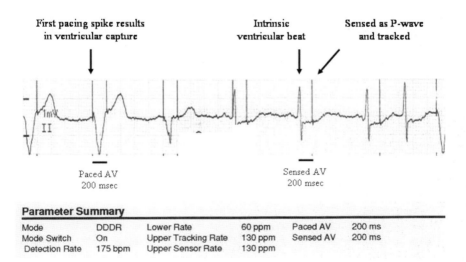

Parameter Summary					
Mode	DDDR	Lower Rate	60 ppm	Paced AV	200 ms
Mode Switch	On	Upper Tracking Rate	130 ppm	Sensed AV	200 ms
Detection Rate	175 bpm	Upper Sensor Rate	130 ppm		

Fig. 7.2 Reversal of the atrial and ventricular leads within the header block. Pacemaker interrogation shortly after device interrogation in a patient whose device was felt to be functioning inappropriately. Top: A telemetry strip obtained postoperatively highlights the tell-tale signs of this inadvertent operative error. The underlying rhythm is sinus. The initial pacing spike captures the ventricle. After the paced atrioventricular (AV) interval, a second pacing stimulus is delivered. This fails to capture the ventricle (functional non-capture) since the ventricular is still refractory from the prior paced event. Additionally, a sensed ventricular event initiates "atrial tracking", resulting in a second pacing stimulus at the end of the sensed AV interval. Bottom: The device is programmed to a DDDR mode with a lower pacing rate of 60 bpm. The sensed and pacing AV delay is 200 ms.

tighten the set-screw(s), or a mismatch between the lead pins and the header block of the implanted pacemaker generator. The problem may be with the lead itself, i.e. there may be a structural defect in the lead such as an insulation break or fracture of the inner conductor wire. There may be a problem related to an adverse interaction between implanted leads (including those previously abandoned) such as crosstalk or electrical chatter. Finally, the problem may be with the lead–myocardial interface. These problems include microdislodgement, overt dislodgement, an acute rise in pacing thresholds due to maturation of the lead, or permanent exit block, and the effect of changes in the patient's substrate. The latter include intercurrent medical illnesses, changes in medications, and development of metabolic and electrolyte disorders. In trying to sort through this differential diagnosis, it is very useful to consider the time since device implantation (Fig. 7.3).

Specific types of pacemaker malfunction

When presented with a pacemaker problem on an ECG strip, it is first helpful to determine whether pacing stimuli are present. If present, do they capture the appropriate cardiac chamber? If absent, is there a native depolarization that is properly timed to explain the absence? One also needs to look at the

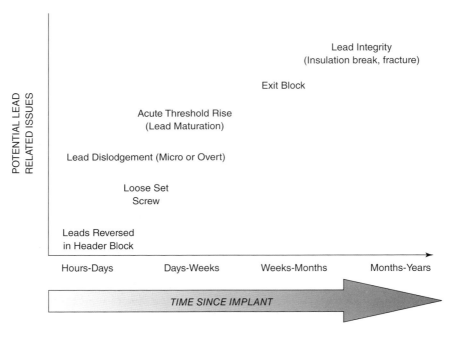

Fig. 7.3 The relationship between time since device implantation and commonly observed lead-related complications.

native beats in relation to the paced complexes. Are all the native beats sensed correctly? Do they inhibit or trigger the next paced complex? In essence, these questions define the three major electrocardiographic patterns of pacemaker malfunction: (i) pacing stimuli present with failure to capture, (ii) pacing stimuli present with failure to sense, and (iii) pacing stimuli absent. These patterns will now be discussed in greater detail.

Pacing stimuli present with failure to capture

To place a malfunction in this group, it is first necessary to be able to identify the pacing stimulus. Pacing stimuli are non-physiological electrical transients of very high frequency. Some ECG recordings, particularly ambulatory and in-hospital monitoring units, use special filters to eliminate high-frequency signals to minimize baseline noise on the recording. This effectively reduces the size of unipolar signals and may eliminate bipolar signals altogether. Furthermore, the signal may simply be isoelectric in a given lead. Other ECG systems generate a discrete pacemaker pulse artifact in response to any high-frequency transient. For example, EMI (most commonly from within the hospital environment) can cause the appearance of pacemaker artifacts unrelated to cardiac activity. Therefore, it is critical to record multiple leads when a malfunction in output is suspected (Fig. 7.4).

Once the pacemaker stimulus is correctly identified, one needs to determine correctly whether capture has occurred. When atrioventricular (AV) conduction is intact, atrial capture can readily be assessed by testing in an AAI mode. Similarly, ventricular capture can be most readily assessed by testing in a VVI mode. The greatest difficulty occurs in trying to determine atrial capture when the patient has impaired AV conduction and is completely ventricular paced. In this case, in addition to the ECG, it is useful to have access to the atrial electrogram (Fig. 7.5). Recently, several device manufacturers have released devices that are capable of automatically evaluating ventricular (and in some case, atrial) pacing thresholds. This feature can not only increase the efficiency of the follow-up process, but may actually increase battery longevity by adapting the pacing output to the patient's pacing threshold.[6–8]

Finally, it is important to exclude the possibility of functional non-capture. When a pacing stimulus occurs in the physiological refractory period of native depolarization, it will not capture irrespective of stimulus strength (Figs 7.2 and 7.6). However, most cases of functional non-capture represent true or functional undersensing and will be discussed later as part of problems related to sensing.

In addition to these electrocardiographic findings, it is useful to obtain a chest radiograph when evaluating a patient in whom failure to capture is present. Armed with this information, the practitioner can make a final diagnosis following pacemaker interrogation. The diagnosis should again keep in mind the timeframe between device implantation and the occurrence of the pacemaker system malfunction.

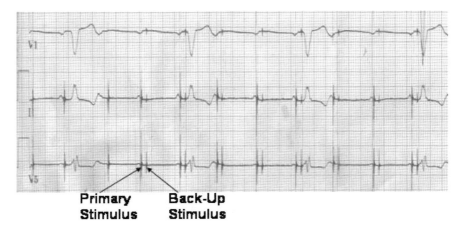

Primary   Back-Up
Stimulus   Stimulus

Fig. 7.4 Pacing stimuli present with failure to capture. Shown is a three-lead rhythm strip (ECG leads V$_1$, II and V$_5$) in a patient who presented with weakness and light-headedness a few days after undergoing dual-chamber pacemaker implantation for management of complete heart block. The implanted device was a St Jude Medical device, in which the AutoCapture™ algorithm was programmed on. (Top tracing: lead V$_1$.) Sinus rhythm with high-grade atrioventricular (AV) block is present. Every third P wave conducts (fixed PR interval) with left bundle branch block. A dual-chamber pacemaker is present as reflected by consistent pacing artifacts coupled to the P wave. A low-amplitude pacing artifact (suggestive of bipolar pacing) is observed at a fixed AV interval following each sensed P wave. (Middle tracing: lead II; bottom tracing: lead V$_5$.) Simultaneously recorded additional leads demonstrate two pacing stimuli following each sinus P wave. The first pacing spike has high amplitude, suggestive of unipolar pacing, whereas the second spike varies in amplitude in the two leads. Lead V$_1$ was recording only the second of these two pacing stimuli. In this case, the first spike represents unipolar pacing at the programmed pulse output (primary stimulus); the second spike represents a bipolar backup pulse delivered ~80 ms later with an output of 4.5 V. Failure to capture is present even with the backup pulse due to a dislodgment of the recently implanted ventricular lead. The illustration highlights the difficulty in assigning lead polarity based on the amplitude of stimulation artifact and the need to review, if possible, data from more than one monitoring lead when troubleshooting pacemaker malfunction.

Early post-device implantation

In patients presenting with failure to capture early (days–months) post-device implantation, the evaluation should begin with pacemaker interrogation and a chest radiograph to exclude the presence of an overt lead dislodgment (Table 7.2). Small lead displacements unrecognizable with chest radiography can also result in elevated pacing thresholds. Rarely, one can see evidence for a lead-related cardiac perforation, but chest pain, especially with pacing or skeletal muscle stimulation, should also raise this possibility. If dislodgment (or perforation) is present, prompt surgical intervention is necessary for lead repositioning. Operative considerations include repositioning the same lead or replacing the lead altogether. Repositioning alone may be adequate when one can identify a

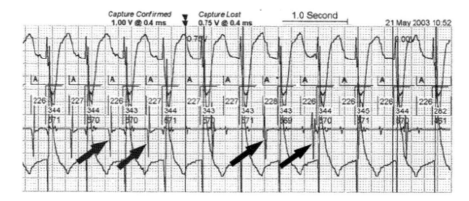

Fig. 7.5 Evaluation of the atrial capture threshold while monitoring the surface ECG (top tracing), telemetered event markers and intervals, the atrial electrogram (middle tracing) and the ventricular electrogram (bottom tracing). Capture is present at 1.00 V and 0.4 ms. This is visible on both the surface ECG and the atrial EGM (arrows). With loss of capture at 0.75 V, there is dissociation of the atrial EGM from the pacing stimuli and a loss of the visible P wave on the surface ECG. The atrial output is bipolar, resulting in a diminutive stimulus artifact that is virtually invisible on the surface ECG. Effective blanking on the intracardiac atrial EGM prevents distortion of the EGM.

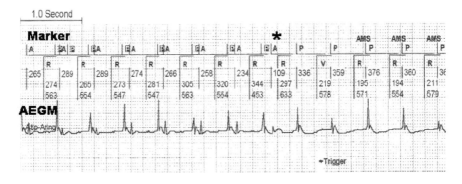

Fig. 7.6 Functional undersensing and functional non-capture. The patient had an implanted St Jude Medical Identity ADx DR 5380 dual-chamber pacemaker. This electrogram was stored because the automatic mode switching (AMS) algorithm was triggered. The underlying rhythm is sinus tachycardia at a cycle length of ~550 ms with marked first-degree atrioventricular delay, as reflected by a PR interval of ~360 ms. The sinus beat ("P" in the solid gray box on Marker channel) is falling into the postventricular atrial refractory period (PVARP) of the preceding sensed ventricular event (R). Since atrial activity is not sensed, an atrial paced event (A) is delivered, which does not result in atrial capture since the atrial myocardium is still refractory from the prior spontaneous atrial event. This demonstrates functional undersensing as well as functional non-capture. Atrial pacing stops when a premature ventricular depolarization (*) advances the end of its subsequent PVARP, thus allowing for sensing of the atrial depolarization.

Table 7.2 Differential diagnosis of pacing stimuli present–intermittent or persistent loss of capture

Etiology	ECG*	Chest radiograph†	Impedance	Threshold	Management
Lead dislodgment • Early: unstable position • Late: twiddler's syndrome	Abnormal	Abnormal or normal	Normal	Elevated	Reposition lead
Lead maturation • Early: inflammatory response • Late: progressive fibrosis	Normal	Normal	Normal	Elevated	Increase output, trial of steroids, or reposition
Late high thresholds • Progressive fibrosis • Myocardial infarction • Cardiomyopathy • Metabolic/drugs • Damaged lead or tissue interface	Normal	Normal	Normal	Elevated	Increase output, correct cause, or replace lead
Insulation failure	Normal‡	Normal or conductor abnormality	Decreased	Elevated	Reprogram to unipolar, replace lead
Conductor failure • Lead fracture • Loose set-screw	Normal§	Abnormal	Increased	Elevated	Reprogram to unipolar (lead fracture), replace lead, reoperate for set-screw
Battery depletion	Normal	Normal	Normal	Normal or elevated¶	Replace pulse generator
Functional non-capture • Pseudomalfunction • Inappropriate programming	Normal	Normal	Normal	Normal	Decrease rate, decrease refractory period(s), or increase sensitivity

*In ECG column, normal refers to a stable morphology of the evoked potential; abnormal refers to a change in the morphology of the evoked potential.

†In the chest radiograph column, normal refers to a stable lead position and no obvious deformity of the conductor coil; abnormal refers to a change in lead position or a deformity of the conductor coil. The insulation is radiolucent and will not be visualized on the X-ray.

‡The ECG with an insulation failure involving a unipolar lead will show a decrease in the amplitude of the pacing stimulus. An insulation failure involving the outer insulation of a bipolar lead will show an increase in the amplitude of the pacing stimulus. Failure of the internal insulation of a coaxial bipolar lead will show a decrease in stimulus amplitude. This presupposes that all recordings are made with an analog ECG machine.

§The ECG with an intermittent conductor fracture may show a varying amplitude pacing stimulus if recorded with an analog ECG machine.

¶Pacing threshold is increased as measured through the depleted generator but is normal through the pacing system analyzer.

Source: Modified from Levine PA. Pacing system malfunction: evaluation and management. In: Podrid PJ, Kowey PR, eds. Cardiac arrhythmia: mechanisms, diagnosis, and management. Philadelphia, PA: Williams & Wilkins, 1995. By permission of Williams & Wilkins.

correctable cause behind the dislodgment such as an initial post-implant radiograph showing too little or too much slack, failure to secure the lead anchoring sleeve(s) properly, or the downward migration of the pacemaker generator (which can occur if the generator is not secured to the underlying fascia). Lead replacement is often entertained when the initial lead was a tined lead; in this case, one can consider replacing with an active fixation lead. Even when an active fixation lead was used initially, it may be necessary to replace the lead when adequate lead stability cannot be demonstrated due to the possible presence of either thrombus or tissue entrapment on the electrode or active fixation helix.

If the chest radiograph shows no evidence of an overt lead dislodgment, attention should be turned towards performing a complete interrogation of the pacemaker. An elevated pacing impedance early post-device implantation suggests a possible loose set-screw or failure to seat the lead pin fully in the header. Careful re-examination of the radiograph may also reveal evidence for this problem (Fig. 7.7). In this case, operative intervention is necessary to

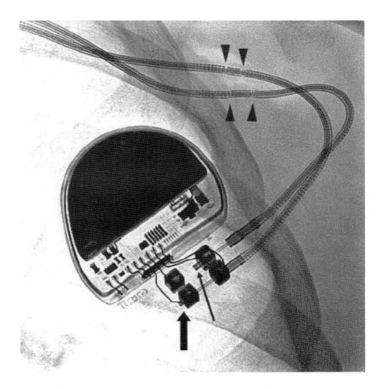

Fig. 7.7 Chest radiograph demonstrating displacement of the terminal pin out of the head of a pacemaker. For the atrial lead entering the top of the header (bottom of the figure) the terminal pin is seen extending beyond the header posts for both the ring and tip electrodes (heavy arrow). The ventricular lead, however, does not reach to the header post for the tip electrode (thin arrow). The ventricular lead impedance was unmeasurable. In addition, pseudofractures are seen in both leads due to constriction of the insulation by sutures on the anchoring sleeves (arrowheads).

reposition the lead(s) correctly into the pacemaker header block. Acute lead conductor or insulation failure very soon after implant is rare.

When the chest radiograph does not show overt dislodgment of the leads and pacemaker interrogation shows elevated pacing threshold in the presence of normal pacing impedance, the differential diagnosis becomes one of either a micro lead dislodgment or an acute threshold rise due to maturation of the lead. When the electrode is first inserted, it is making intimate contact with the endocardium. The presence of foreign material and the pressure of the lead–electrode system against the myocardium induce an inflammatory reaction at the electrode–myocardial surface. This local trauma is responsible for the current of injury pattern on the acute intracardiac electrogram recording; in fact, absence of this current of injury has been correlated with an increased incidence of lead dislodgment, with the implication being that there is not adequate myocardial contact by the pacemaker electrode. Due to the inflammatory reaction, the electrode is physically displaced from the excitable myocardium. This process increases the capture threshold. In addition, it attenuates the electrogram amplitude and slew rate to compromise sensing. With time, the inflammatory reaction subsides, leaving a thin capsule of fibrous tissue between the electrode and active myocardium. As the distance between the electrode and active myocardium is reduced, the capture and sensing thresholds improve.

Sometimes the inflammatory reaction at the electrode–myocardial interface is excessive, causing the capture threshold to rise above the output of the pacemaker. This phenomenon is termed exit block. The routine use of steroid-eluting pacemaker leads has been effective in attenuating the inflammatory reaction and its associated early rise in capture and sensing thresholds. Acute management of high thresholds, with or without loss of capture, requires increasing the output of the pacemaker. In some cases, the required output may exceed the maximal output of the pacemaker generator. In non-pacemaker-dependent patients, one may simply wait for the threshold to fall or a trial of high-dose oral corticosteroid therapy may be considered.[9] However, in many cases, repositioning of the affected lead will ultimately be necessary.

Late post-device implantation

Lead dislodgment is rare late (months–years) post-device implantation. However, when present, twiddler's syndrome should be considered. The syndrome is characterized by pacemaker failure related to the spontaneous, or deliberate rotation of the pulse generator by the patient that eventually results in lead dislodgment. On occasion, ipsilateral stimulation of the phrenic nerve or brachial plexus can result in stimulation of the diaphragm or arm muscles, respectively.[10] Coiling of the leads around the generator can permanently damage the leads; as a result, it may be necessary to replace the leads entirely at the time of re-operation. The likelihood of this phenomenon can be reduced by taking care to avoid making an excessively large pacemaker pocket and by securing the pacemaker to the underlying muscle.

Pacemaker interrogation is critical in the evaluation of patients presenting with a failure of pacing output to capture late post-device implantation (Table 7.2). An initial step is to determine the battery voltage to exclude near-complete battery depletion, since this may result in an ineffective pacing stimulus (as well as generalized erratic pacing behavior). If the battery voltage is acceptable, the problem generally localizes to the pacemaker leads or the electrode–myocardial interface.

Permanent late rises in the capture threshold occur with progressive myocardial fibrosis as described above, development of a primary myopathic process, or after a myocardial infarction. Depending on the degree of threshold rise, implantation of a new lead may be necessary. However, late rises may also be related to transient causes, such as hyperkalemia and acidemia, or reflect an adverse effect of medications, such as type IC antiarrhythmic drugs.[2,3,11] In each instance, although device interrogation will demonstrate an elevated pacing threshold, the pacing lead impedance remains in a normal range.

In contrast, changes in pacing impedance in a chronically implanted system suggest a problem with the integrity of the pacing leads. Modern pacemakers measure and record the pacing impedance daily, making it highly unlikely that even an intermittent lead problem will be overlooked. The data are graphically displayed (i) to allow for comparisons against the patient's own prior measurements and (ii) to determine the timeframe of the defect in lead integrity (Fig. 7.8). A very low impedance (< 200 Ω) reflects a failure of the insulation, whereas a very high impedance (> 2000 Ω) suggests a conductor fracture.

An insulation defect may develop from the intrinsic design and/or a manufacturing limitation, as was the case with an early series of 80A polyurethane-insulated leads. Most insulation problems, however, are due to extrinsic forces applied to the lead either at or following implant that physically damage the lead.

Extrinsic stress applied to the lead can result in damage to the insulation and/or conductor fracture. There are three common mechanical stresses on the lead. The first is the suture sleeve, when an excessively tight ligature is used to anchor the lead to the underlying fascia (Fig. 7.7). The second is mechanical stress and abrasion of the lead due to interaction with the generator or redundant lead in the pocket. Abrasion of the external insulation may occur in the pocket between overlapping coils of the same or contiguous leads or between the housing of the pulse generator and the lead coiled behind it. In part, this problem is a direct result of the request by the medical community for thinner leads, both unipolar and bipolar. One method of reducing the lead's diameter is to reduce the thickness of the insulating material. In-line bipolar coaxial leads are the least forgiving of extrinsic stresses for this very reason. The third source of stress on the lead is the point where the lead traverses the plane between the clavicle and first rib on its way to the subclavian vein.[12,13] The normal motion of the arm causes the space between the clavicle and first rib to widen and narrow, much like the jaws of pliers. This is exacerbated if the course of

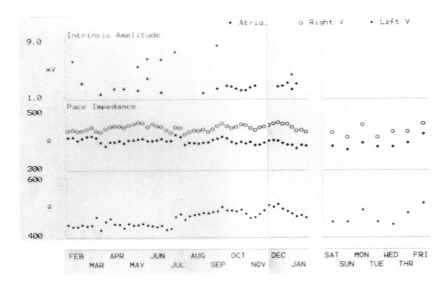

Fig. 7.8 Long-term daily measurements (sensing amplitudes, pacing impedances). Representative graph from a Guidant biventricular pacemaker. Shown are the sensed atrial amplitudes over the past 12 months, as well as daily over the past week. The right and left ventricular amplitudes are not recorded since the patient is 100% biventricular paced. Similarly, the lead impedance for the atrial, right ventricular and left ventricular leads is shown. Note that an ~100-Ω fluctuation is observed over time in the setting of normal lead function.

the lead traverses the costoclavicular ligament or the subclavius muscle in its path to the subclavian vein. The lead located in this position can be repeatedly crushed, pinched, pulled or stretched, resulting in deformation of the conductor coils, which in turn will predispose to either insulation failure and/or conductor fracture occurring months to years after implantation (Fig. 7.9). This has been termed the medial subclavicular musculotendinous complex and is an increasingly recognized cause of malfunction of both standard pacing and defibrillator leads. A recent recommendation has been to access the axillary or cephalic vein rather than the subclavian vein to avoid both the acute and late complications associated with the implant procedure.[14,15]

A conductor fracture results in an open circuit. There are two common clinical manifestations of an open circuit. With a total open circuit, no energy will traverse the gap between the two portions of the lead and there will be an absence of pacing artifacts on the ECG and loss of capture despite stimulus output by the generator. However, if the two ends of the conductor are making any contact at all, the resistance to current flow will be increased to attenuate the amount of current and energy reaching the heart, but a stimulus will be present. If the effective energy reaching the heart is subthreshold, there will be loss of capture. A partially open circuit may also result in pauses due to oversensing. Make–break contact between the ends of the conductor coil can

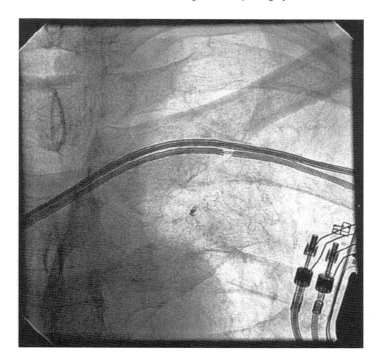

Fig. 7.9 Lead fracture diagnosed on chest X-ray. Three years after dual-chamber pacemaker implant for sick sinus syndrome this patient was found to have complete loss of ventricular capture and bipolar lead impedance > 2000 Ω. There is a clear fracture of the lead just before it enters the subclavian vein. The fracture may have been due to the subclavian access that passes the lead through the costoclavicular ligament apparatus.

cause non-physiological electrical transients that are detected and reset the pacemaker (Fig. 7.10).

Diagnosis of an open circuit may be facilitated by taking advantage of the diagnostic capabilities incorporated in many present-generation pacemakers. Event marker telemetry will confirm an output pulse even if the artifact is not visible on the ECG. Telemetry of lead impedance will demonstrate a significant increase (Fig. 7.10) if the problem is manifested at the time of measurement. A total open circuit will have an infinitely high impedance if the insulation remains intact. However, if there is a concomitant break in the insulation, as may occur when the lead is totally transected, the impedance may be normal or only minimally elevated because the conductor will be exposed to the tissue via the severed insulation.

A radiograph may show the conductor fracture, particularly with unipolar leads. One may have to rotate the patient and take multiple views or use fluoroscopy to eliminate overlapping portions of the lead in a given plane that might obscure the fracture. In-line bipolar coaxial leads are the most difficult

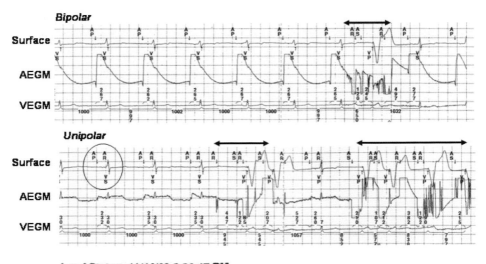

Fig. 7.10 Conductor fracture. Top: Bipolar configuration. This patient had previously undergone implantation of a Medtronic pacemaker. Although the measured lead impedance was normal, initial interrogation showed a lead warning, which recorded high atrial lead pacing impedance. Movement of the patient's left arm resulted in the demonstration of (sensed) high-amplitude, non-physiological signals (arrow), consistent with noise. AEGM, atrial electrogram; VEGM, ventricular electrogram; AP, atrial pace; AS, atrial sense; AR, atrial refractory; VS, ventricular sense; VP, ventricular pace. Middle: Unipolar configuration. The lead was reprogrammed to a unipolar configuration. Note the far-field R wave oversensing (AR on marker annotation) on the atrial lead (circle) in this configuration. Movement of the patient's left arm again resulted in the demonstration of (sensed) high-amplitude, non-physiological signals, consistent with noise (arrows). The demonstration of noise in both bipolar and unipolar configurations suggests involvement of the tip conductor. Bottom: Measured data telemetry from a different patient with a Medtronic Kappa 700 pacing system indicates that there is an open circuit on the atrial channel. The reported impedance is > 9999 Ω, which is the highest impedance that the Medtronic system will report. The pulse current and pulse energy are minimal, which is compatible with an open circuit.

with regard to radiographic identification of a conductor fracture. Unless there is total disruption of both conductors at the same place, the intact distal conductor may mask the defect in the proximal conductor. The problem may be reproduced with motion of the ipsilateral arm or palpation of the lead.

Pacing stimuli present with failure to sense

The failure to respond to a physiologically appropriate signal occurring during the alert period of the timing cycle is termed undersensing. When undersensing is present, the pacemaker issues pacing stimuli because of the perceived absence of spontaneous cardiac activity (Fig. 7.11A). Like failure to capture, undersensing can reflect a true pacing system malfunction, or represent a functional limitation of the system due to unique algorithms in a given device or a response to the programmed settings of the device.

When the electrogram amplitude is noted to be reduced shortly after lead implantation, one needs to determine if this represents a significant change relative to the implant values. Low amplitude of the sensed electrogram may be present from the time of lead implantation. In some cases, this is because the amplitude of the sensed electrogram could not be determined at implant. For example, the sinus P-wave amplitude cannot be obtained if a patient is in atrial fibrillation at the time of implantation, and an R-wave amplitude cannot be obtained in a patient with underlying heart block and ventricular asystole. In other cases, it may simply not be possible to obtain a large sensed electrogram amplitude due to diffuse myocardial disease or scar. When the amplitude has

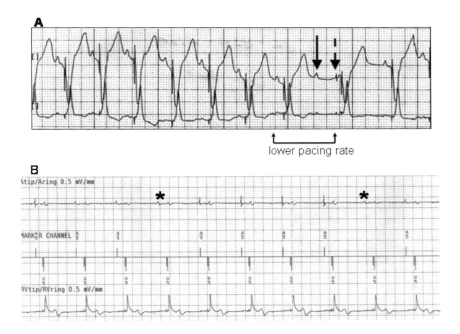

Fig. 7.11 Atrial undersensing. (A) Two-channel electrocardiographic recording in a patient with congenital complete heart block. A sinus beat is undersensed (solid arrow); this results in an atrial paced beat (dashed arrow) at the lower programmed pacing rate of the device. (B) Intracardiac electrograms from the atrial (top) and ventricular leads (bottom) as well as the marker channel (middle) observed in a patient 1 week after device implantation. Note the large variability in the amplitude of the atrial electrogram and the intermittent atrial undersensing (asterisks). A chest radiograph showed evidence of atrial lead dislodgment; the tip of the atrial lead was located in the body of the right atrium.

declined significantly relative to implant (Fig. 7.11B), one must obtain a chest radiograph to exclude the presence of lead dislodgment or lead perforation. Naturally, repositioning of the affected lead is warranted in this circumstance.

A number of causes may degrade the sensed amplitude of an intracardiac electrogram over time (Table 7.3). Some causes are patient specific. For example, the patient may develop a change in the sequence of depolarization, as with development of ectopic beats or a bundle branch block. Development of a primary myopathic process or myocardial infarction can attenuate the sensed electrogram. Institution of pharmacological therapy, particularly antiarrhythmic agents that alter phase 0 of the cardiac action potential, can change the

Table 7.3 Differential diagnosis of pacing stimuli present—intermittent or persistent failure to sense

Etiology	Diagnostic evaluation*	Management*
Lead dislodgment • Early: unstable position • Late: twiddler's syndrome	12-lead ECG with pacing; chest radiograph	Reposition lead
Low-amplitude electrogram • Small EGM at implant • Ectopic activation (PAC, PVC, bundle branch block, atrial fibrillation) • Medications, electrolytes • Myocardial infarction, cardiomyopathy • Tissue fibrosis, lead maturation	Identification of change in medication, electrolytes, cardiac status	Increase sensitivity, discontinue medication, correct electrolyte or acid–base imbalance, change sensing configuration
Insulation failure	Fall in lead impedance by > 300 Ω; telemetered EGM	Change sensing configuration until lead can be replaced
Functional undersensing • Magnet application, noise reversion • ERI behavior • PMT interventions • Mode switching • Pacemaker Wenckebach • Rate smoothing	Careful assessment of pacing intervals, review programmed sensitivity and thresholds	Decrease refractory period(s), increase sensitivity
Inappropriate programming	Review programmed sensitivity and thresholds	Reprogram sensitivity

*Some suggested options may not be available with a given pulse generator. Only definitive management options are listed. In each case, increasing the sensitivity may correct the problem, but, as with a primary lead failure, this may be a temporizing measure only.
Source: Modified from Levine PA. Pacing system malfunction: evaluation and management. In: Podrid PJ, Kowey PR, eds. Cardiac arrhythmia: mechanisms, diagnosis, and management. Philadelphia, PA: Williams & Wilkins, 1995. By permission of Williams & Wilkins.
EGM, electrogram; PAC, premature atrial contraction; PVC, premature ventricular contraction; ERI, elective replacement indicator; PMT, pacemaker-mediated tachycardia.

intrinsic properties of the signal, resulting in undersensing. Metabolic and electrolyte abnormalities may cause transient undersensing. Hyperkalemia results in a widening of the QRS complex and an attenuation of the P wave on the surface ECG. Similar changes will occur with the intracardiac signal or electrogram. Atrial fibrillation is a common cause of reduced atrial electrogram amplitude. Finally, transient undersensing can be observed after cardioversion or defibrillation.

Other causes are specific to the pacing system. The problem may occur due to idiosyncracies or failure of the sense amplifier of the pacemaker, resulting in an undersensing problem. There is no good way to assess this non-invasively. Fortunately, this is quite rare. A pacemaker generator with a near complete depletion of the battery can demonstrate erratic sensing behavior or reset to a single-chamber or asynchronous mode (Fig. 7.12). This can be determined by assessing the battery voltage at the time of initial device interrogation.

More commonly, within a pacing system it is the lead itself which is responsible for undersensing. This can be related to the lead maturation process, discussed in detail in the previous section. The inflammatory reaction that occurs at the electrode–myocardial interface physically separates the electrode from active functional myocardium. This will attenuate the amplitude and slew rate of the signal. The signal has been reported to decrease by as much as 20–40% when compared with the electrogram amplitude recorded at implantation. Attenuation of the slew rate may be the major reason for sensing failure. With respect to chronically implanted leads, insulation defects will attenuate the incoming signal, which will be an electrical average between the true electrode inside the heart and the false "electrode"—the exposed conductor coil under the insulation defect.

However, in many patients, undersensing will occur despite device interrogation that shows a normal sensed electrogram and no evidence for pacing system malfunction. One correctable, albeit embarrassing, cause of undersensing is an inappropriately programmed sensitivity. Confusion about the terms

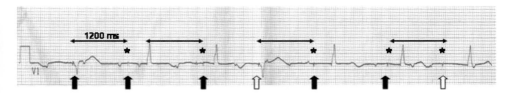

Fig. 7.12 Pacemaker battery depletion. The rhythm strip (lead V_1) from a patient who had undergone VVI pacemaker implantation 14 years earlier and had subsequently not obtained any further pacemaker follow-up. Pacing stimuli are denoted by the vertical arrows; pacing is occurring at a cycle length of 1200 ms (horizontal arrows). There is both intermittent failure to capture (*) and failure to sense (open arrows). The combination of sensing and capture problems suggested a problem intrinsic to the lead; however, at pacemaker generator change, the lead demonstrated no abnormality. The erratic pacing behavior is best explained by near-complete depletion of the pacemaker's battery.

high and low sensitivity may result in incorrect programming. When an undersensing problem is encountered, the sensitivity should be increased or set to a higher sensitivity so that the system will recognize and respond to smaller-amplitude signals. Sensitivity is the amplitude of the signal that can be sensed. A sensitivity of 1 mV would be more sensitive (higher sensitivity) than 2 mV. Similarly, if there is an oversensing problem and one wants to reduce or lower the sensitivity, the incoming signal must be larger than the amplitude chosen for the pacemaker to recognize it as an appropriate signal. Thus, a sensitivity of 4 mV, although a higher number, is really a lower sensitivity than 2 mV. Patients have been inappropriately referred for pulse generator replacement or lead repositioning when the problem was undersensing, which had resulted from a misunderstanding of how to program sensitivity. Many newer pacemakers incorporate an automatic sensing algorithm that monitors the amplitude of the native atrial or ventricular depolarization and either recommends a programmed sensitivity or automatically adjusts the sensitivity to maintain a 2 : 1 safety margin.

Functional undersensing, a failure to sense an appropriate physiological signal, but caused by the normal design of the pacemaker, is an important cause for undersensing. The most common cause of functional undersensing occurs each time a magnet is placed over the pacemaker and induces asynchronous pacing. Other common causes include pacing when native beats fall within the blanking or refractory period after a paced or sensed beat, as can be observed in the setting of atrial fibrillation and a rapid ventricular response or when the postventricular atrial refractory period (PVARP) is relatively long at a high underlying base rate (Fig. 7.6). If too many signals are sensed by the pacemaker in a very short time, the likelihood is that this is electrical noise rather than true physiological signals. This is termed EMI or "noise."[16,17] The presence of EMI precludes the pacemaker's differentiating electrical noise from an intrinsic rhythm. Rather than inhibiting the pacemaker when the patient might be asystolic, the pacemaker reverts to asynchronous function, termed noise mode operation (Fig. 7.13). Finally, functional undersensing results from the normal operation of pacemaker features designed to eliminate other problems, such as during ventricular safety pacing or after a post-premature ventricular contraction (PVC) extension of the PVARP. Mode switching, appropriate or not, is a relatively common cause of atrial undersensing.

Pacing stimuli absent

To place a malfunction in this group, one must be certain that this is not an artifact of a diminutive bipolar pacing stimulus further obscured by being isoelectric in a given lead. As previously discussed, one should record multiple leads simultaneously or sequentially. There are a number of causes that can be associated with this type of pacing system malfunction (Table 7.4). An accurate assessment is critical, since the consequences in a pacemaker-dependent patient can be catastrophic.

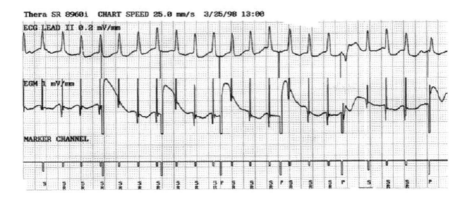

Thera SR 8960i CHART SPEED 25.0 mm/s 3/25/98 13:00

Fig. 7.13 Noise reversion. A patient with a VVI pacemaker developed sustained monomorphic ventricular tachycardia. Due to the rapid ventricular rate, each ventricular tachycardia event is falling into the ventricular sensed refractory period (SR). Continuous refractory sensing triggers a noise reversion mode, in which asynchronous pacing (P) is delivered at the lower pacing rate.

An important cause for this condition is oversensing of either a non-physiological or a physiologically inappropriate signal. When oversensing is suspected, it is important to exclude the possibility that ectopic activity is present but being missed since it is isoelectric to the lead being monitored. Once again, review of multiple leads, if possible, is helpful.

Skeletal muscle potentials (myopotentials) can inhibit output if detected on the ventricular channel (resulting in long pauses or "skipped beats") or trigger a ventricular output when sensed on the atrial channel of a DDD system. Myopotentials are a frequent cause for oversensing and can result from oversensing of the pectoralis, rectus abdominis or diaphragmatic muscles. Bipolar leads are much less susceptible to this phenomenon than unipolar leads; the latter are especially susceptible since the pacemaker case (the system's anode) remains in close proximity to these muscle structures.

Oversensing can also be related to normal intracardiac signals. For example, detection of a far-field R wave often causes oversensing on the atrial lead, and detection of the T wave can cause oversensing on the ventricular lead. In these cases, it is helpful to reduce the sensitivity on the affected lead to eliminate oversensing, assuming that the native signal for which sensing is desired is sufficiently large to allow it to continue to be appropriately sensed. Prolonging the cross-chamber blanking period or refractory periods may be needed, especially for oversensing pacing output.

Another cause for oversensing is exposure to EMI, which can be related to environmental sources, such as electrical current leaks from appliances, electric motors and electronic surveillance systems, or to medical devices, such as electrocautery equipment, magnetic resonance imaging machines, and radiotherapy equipment.[16,17] However, in many cases, the exact source of the EMI

Table 7.4 Differential diagnosis of pauses—pacing stimuli absent

Etiology	Diagnostic evaluation	Management
Oversensing • T wave, P wave, R wave • Myopotential/diaphragm • Pacing afterpotential • EMI • Crosstalk • Make–break potentials	Magnet application (pauses eliminated), reduce sensitivity	Reduce sensitivity or program to bipolar sensing configuration, replace with bipolar sensing lead
Open circuit • Conductor fracture • Loose set-screw • Air in pocket (unipolar system) • Lead pin/header mismatch	Lead impedance—high Magnet—pauses persist Chest radiograph—terminal pin not seated properly, lateral may visualize air in pocket, conductor coil discontinuity	Apply pressure dressing (air in pocket), reprogram to unipolar, replace lead, reoperate to tighten set-screw
Internal insulation failure	Lead impedance low ($< 250\ \Omega$) Magnet—pauses persist Chest radiograph—normal or conductor coil deformity	Program to unipolar until lead can be replaced
Component malfunction	Magnet—pauses persist Telemetry—inconsistencies in measured data	Replace pulse generator, operative reassessment of lead function before pulse generator
Pseudomalfunction • Hysteresis • Mode switching • PMT intervention	Native rate slower than paced rate Pauses follow only sensed beats Interrogation of programmed parameters	Reassurance as normal function

Source: Modified from Levine PA. Pacing system malfunction: evaluation and management. In: Podrid PJ, Kowey PR, eds. Cardiac arrhythmia: mechanisms, diagnosis, and management. Philadelphia, PA: Williams & Wilkins, 1995. By permission of Williams & Wilkins.
PMT, pacemaker-mediated tachycardia.

cannot be identified. That the patient has been exposed to EMI is generally suspected based on retrieval of stored electrograms from the device (Fig. 7.14). Real-time telemetry will reveal no sensing abnormality.

When presented with recurrent pauses in the absence of pacing stimuli, one can usually differentiate oversensing from the other causes of the absence of pacing artifact by applying a magnet to the pacemaker. The magnet will cause most pacemakers to revert to an asynchronous function. In some pacemakers, magnet application can trigger electrogram storage, threshold checks or no response instead of asynchronous pacing. If the pauses are eliminated, the problem is that of oversensing. To determine the source of the oversensing, it is sometimes necessary to record the surface ECG while the patient is in the environment in which the reported symptoms occur. It may also be necessary to have the patient perform provocative maneuvers. For example, one could also have the patient

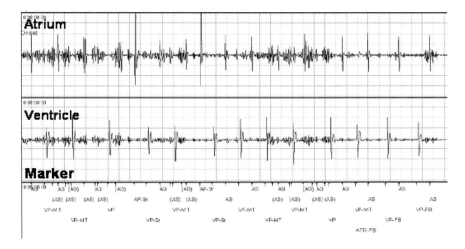

Fig. 7.14 Electromagnetic interference. This electrogram was stored by the device (a Guidant dual-chamber pacemaker) as evidence for an atrial high-rate episode. The electrogram was retrieved during a scheduled pacemaker interrogation; the patient reported no symptoms. Underlying sinus rhythm can be readily appreciated. However, both the atrial and ventricular leads record a high-frequency signal suggestive of electromagnetic interference. The signal is sensed only on the atrial channel (presumably because of the higher sensitivity of the atrial channel compared with the ventricular channel).

do upper extremity isometric exercises, tensing the pectoral muscles, or do sit ups to tighten the abdominal muscles in the case of an abdominal implant. The patient should be asked to take very deep breaths if diaphragmatic oversensing is suspected. These maneuvers should be performed while continuously monitoring the rhythm and, if available, in conjunction with telemetered event markers and electrograms.

Failure to correct the problem with magnet application suggests a complete lead fracture or a pacemaker system malfunction. Although this can be related to a primary component malfunction of the generator, this is quite rare. However, as discussed previously, care should be taken to ensure that the pacemaker generator is not subject to a known product advisory that may explain the observed malfunction. Certainly, a device that has been lost to follow-up and has depleted its battery entirely can present with a failure to output. A transient problem related to the generator occurs when a pacemaker generator change is performed in which a unipolar system is involved. If a large generator is exchanged for a smaller generator, it is possible for air to remain in the pocket; if the air prevents the generator from making contact with the body's tissues, a no-output situation will occur.

The more common possibility is that there is a problem with the lead. This could involve a problem with the connection into the pacemaker generator header block, either because the lead is incompatible with the implanted pacemaker generator's header block or because there is a loose set-screw. Also, programming a generator to bipolar lead configurations when the lead is actually unipolar can result in an open circuit situation. Alternatively, there may be a structural problem with the lead itself (Fig. 7.15). This includes cases in which there are make–break signals (insulation break, partial conductor fracture, lead chatter) or an open circuit (complete conductor fracture). Again, long-term trends of pacing impedance can be useful in trying to differentiate a conductor fracture from an insulation break. In this case, replacement of the lead will be necessary to eliminate the problem.

Finally, absence of expected pacemaker stimuli may simply be related to a misinterpretation of normal device function. Hysteresis or enabling of a sleep or rest rate algorithm should be expected when device markers demonstrate neither evidence for ineffective pacing output nor inappropriate sensing. Other examples include the device being programmed to a lower rate than recalled by the physician, the output being intentionally programmed to zero volts, the mode being programmed to "off" (OAO, OVO, ODO), or the activation of a specific "therapeutic" algorithm within the device, such as automatic mode switching or pacemaker-mediated tachycardia termination. In each case, the device itself would be functioning properly even though the initial rhythms may be misinterpreted as a malfunction. All of these causes can be readily identified by interrogating the pacemaker as to its programmed parameters.

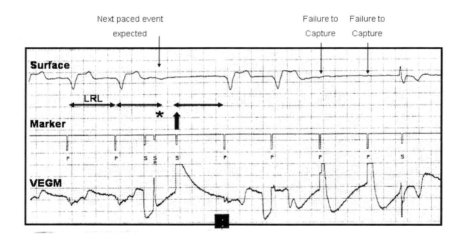

Fig. 7.15 Oversensing. A patient with a previously implanted VVI pacemaker for management of complete heart block presented with symptoms of intermittent light-headedness. During threshold testing at maximal output, two problems were observed: oversensing and failure to capture. The horizontal arrows demarcate the lower pacing rate of the pacemaker. The (*) depicts the time when the next pacing stimulus should have been delivered. However, the device was inhibited due to oversensing of noise evident on the marker channel (S, sensed event; SR, sense in refractory period) and on the ventricular electrogram (VEGM). The vertical arrow depicts another oversensed event, which resets the pacemaker. The surface ECG shows no cardiac activity to account for the sensed events. The combination of problems is consistent with a defect in the pacemaker lead.

Pacemaker malfunctions specific to dual-chamber systems
Crosstalk

Crosstalk is the sensing of the far-field signal originating in the opposite cardiac chamber, causing the pacemaker to either inhibit or trigger an output, depending on its design. Far-field sensing can occur in single-chamber atrial pacing systems in which the far-field QRS is sensed, inhibiting and resetting the basic pacing interval, but crosstalk most commonly refers to ventricular sensing of the far-field atrial stimulus in a DVI, DDI or DDD pacing system. Sensing this stimulus will result in inhibition of the ventricular output and resetting of the atrial escape interval. In the presence of concomitant AV block, crosstalk can be catastrophic and result in ventricular asystole (Fig. 7.16).

Crosstalk inhibition of ventricular output is most likely to occur in the setting of unipolar pacing leads (atrial and ventricular), high atrial output voltage, high ventricular sensitivity, and short post-atrial ventricular blanking/ refractory periods. Crosstalk is suggested by the failure of ventricular pacing following atrial-paced but not atrial-sensed events. Crosstalk is confirmed by telemetered marker channels showing ventricular sensing in the absence of a QRS complex, and is corrected by asynchronous pacing (with magnet application or reprogramming), reducing atrial pacing output or by extending the post-atrial ventricular blanking period initiated by the atrial output pulse (Fig. 7.16). As an added insurance against crosstalk-mediated ventricular output inhibition, a special detection or sensing window was added on the ventricular channel. Following the post-atrial blanking period, this window varies in duration from 51 to 150 ms depending on the manufacturer. A signal sensed during this interval will be treated by the pacemaker as if it were crosstalk, so that rather than inhibiting the ventricular output, a ventricular output will be triggered at an abbreviated AV interval (safety pacing, Fig. 7.16).

Another form of crosstalk is far-field R-wave (FFRW) oversensing. This has become a significant challenge for mode-switching algorithms that allow the pacemaker to detect rapid atrial rhythms and revert to a non-tracking mode (DDI, VVI) from a tracking mode (DDD, VDD). To detect rapid atrial rhythm, these devices can sense atrial events in the PVARP and, in some cases, within the AV delay. If the far-field paced or native R wave is detected in this period in addition to the native P wave, the system may recognize a falsely high atrial rate and initiate the mode switching (Fig. 7.17). Management requires programming of the absolute refractory portion of the PVARP, which is termed the post-ventricular atrial blanking (PVAB) period.[18]

Pacemaker-mediated tachycardia

A pacemaker-mediated tachycardia (PMT) is a tachycardia that is sustained by the continued active participation of the pacemaker in the rhythm. There are several forms of PMT encountered in clinical practice. In the DDD mode, the normally functioning pacemaker should sense atrial activity and trigger a ventricular output in response to the detected P wave. The DDD pacemaker in a patient in whom atrial fibrillation or flutter develops may track the pathological

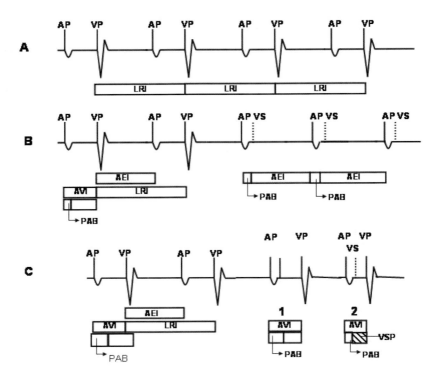

Fig. 7.16 Schematic illustrating the phenomenon of crosstalk. (A) At baseline, 100% atrial and ventricular pacing is present. The lower rate interval (LRI) is the sum of the AV interval (AVI), which includes the post-atrial ventricular blanking period, and the atrial escape interval (AEI). (B) Crosstalk is suggested by the inhibition of ventricular output following an atrial paced event. No actual ventricular event is present. Telemetry demonstrates ventricular sensing in the AVI outside the post-atrial ventricular blanking period (PAB). In addition, crosstalk can be recognized by an acceleration of the atrial paced rate in a dual-chamber pacemaker using ventricular-based timing and programmed to a non-rate-responsive mode. Since ventricular sensing occurs simultaneously with atrial pacing, the AVI is eliminated. Therefore, atrial pacing occurs at an interval equal to the sum of the AEI and blanking periods. (C) Extension of the post-atrial ventricular blanking period will militate against crosstalk, since nothing can be sensed on the ventricular channel during this period (Inset 1). Alternatively, delivery of a ventricular safety pulse can prevent the potential adverse sequelae of crosstalk (Inset 2). After the blanking period, there is a brief crosstalk sensing window. An electrical event sensed during this safety pacing window triggers a ventricular paced event at a shortened (typically 100–120 ms) AV interval rather than inhibiting output.

atrial signals (e.g. flutter or fibrillatory waves). This will drive the ventricular channel of the pacemaker at or near its maximum tracking rate (MTR). Another form of PMT may be driven by undesired rate-responsive sensor behavior. An example would be the activation of respiratory sensors in intubated patients.

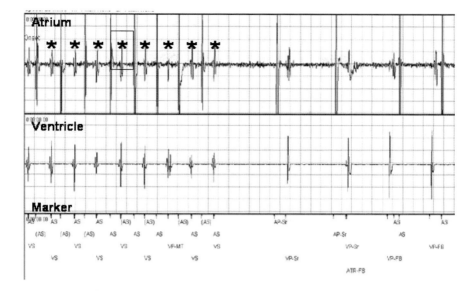

Fig. 7.17 Inappropriate mode switching due to far-field R-wave oversensing. This electrogram was stored by the device (a Guidant dual-chamber pacemaker) as evidence for an atrial high-rate episode. The left-hand portion of the tracing shows an atrial tachycardia at a cycle length of ~500 ms. The automatic mode switching algorithm was triggered by far-field R-wave oversensing (*), which "doubled" the sensed atrial rate.

The term PMT is applied most commonly to sensing retrograde atrial activity arising from ventricular pacing. This sets up a repetitive sequence of the sensed retrograde P wave, triggering a ventricular output at the end of the maximum tracking rate interval (MTRI). The delay created by waiting for the MTRI to complete before the ventricular stimulus is released allows the atrium and AV node to physiologically recover. The depolarization resulting from a ventricular paced beat is again able to conduct in a retrograde direction. This next retrograde P wave would be sensed, triggering another ventricular output and resulting in a sustained PMT (Fig. 7.18A). The onset of such a tachycardia requires at least transient AV dissociation to allow retrograde conduction to occur. Thus, the appearance of PMT should initiate a search for causes of AV dissociation such as atrial undersensing, atrial oversensing, loss of atrial capture, or magnet application to the pacemaker.

Once initiated, PMT will continue unless there is spontaneous ventriculoatrial block or loss of atrial sensing. The latter can be "forced" by application of a magnet. Alternatively, pacemaker algorithms have been developed to prevent PMT by extending the PVARP after a sensed ventricular event that is not preceded by an atrial event (a PVC as defined by the pacemaker). This ensures that any retrograde P wave will fall in the refractory period and not be tracked. Additionally, PMT may be automatically terminated by specialized

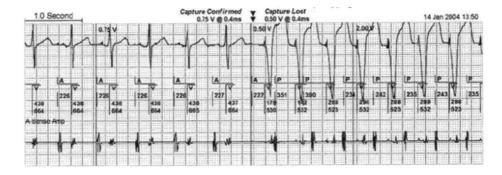

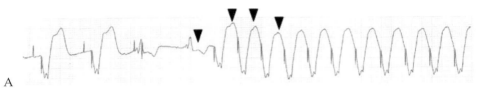

A

Fig. 7.18 This figure shows both a pacemaker-mediated tachycardia (PMT) and a repetitive non-re-entrant ventriculoatrial synchronous (RNRVAS) rhythm. These were recorded from the same patient at the time of a follow-up evaluation. Both rhythms were induced by careful programming of the pacemaker. The base rate was increased to 90 bpm during the atrial capture threshold test. (A) Top panel: To allow PMT to occur in this patient with known retrograde conduction, the postventricular atrial refractory period (PVARP) was reduced to 125 ms. Upon loss of atrial capture, there was full ventricular capture at the end of the AV delay followed by retrograde conduction. The retrograde P wave was detected by the atrial sensing circuit and triggered the next ventricular output after the sensed AV delay was extended so as not to violate the programmed maximum tracking rate. This rhythm would persist until the pacemaker was reprogrammed or an automatic termination algorithm intervened. Bottom panel: spontaneous PMT initiated by premature ventricular contractions (PVCs). AV pacing is interrupted by two PVCs, the second resulting in a retrograde P wave (arrowhead). This is sensed and tracked resulting in pacing at the upper tracking rate. (B) Top panel: To demonstrate the RNRVAS rhythm, atrial threshold testing is performed with the AV delay increased to 300 ms and the PVARP increased to preclude detection of the retrograde P wave. Loss of atrial capture initiates the tachycardia. The paced ventricular event is associated with a retrograde P wave (noted by the arrows), which falls within the PVARP (functional undersensing). With continued atrial pacing, each atrial paced event fails to capture the atrial myocardium since it is refractory from the prior retrograde atrial event (functional non-capture). However, the atrial paced event is "tracked" and results in ventricular pacing. This pattern occurs repetitively. Bottom panel: Spontaneous onset of non-re-entrant AV dyssynchrony initiated by a PVC. The PVC produces a retrograde P wave (arrowhead) that is not sensed in the PVARP. AV pacing ensues with atrial pacing during atrial refractoriness and perpetuation of retrograde conduction by ventricular pacing.

algorithms. These algorithms typically extend the PVARP or withhold a ventricular output for one cycle after tracking at the upper rate limit for a number of cycles and intermittently thereafter. If the tachycardia is due to PMT, it is terminated by the failure to track the retrograde P wave. If tachycardia is due to sinus rhythm, the tracking will continue after a single missed beat.

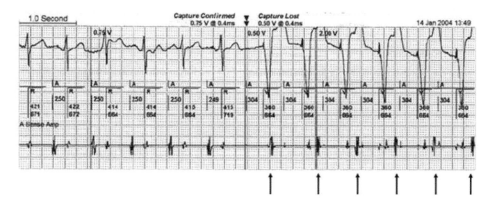

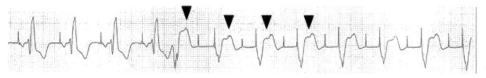

Fig. 7.18 (*Continued.*)

Repetitive non-re-entrant ventriculoatrial synchronous rhythm

This rhythm represents a mismatch between the alert and refractory periods of the pacemaker and the heart. It is functionally equivalent to VVI pacing with intact retrograde conduction, but it occurs in the setting of AV pacing. The trigger for this rhythm is identical to the initiating factors for pacemaker-mediated tachycardia (i.e. AV dissociation) that allow retrograde conduction to develop. In this rhythm, the PVARP is programmed to a sufficiently long interval to preclude the retrograde P wave from being detected; hence, a PMT does not begin. If the AV paced rate is sufficiently rapid, typically due to a high programmed base rate or sensor drive, the P wave occurring within the PVARP is not detected (functional undersensing), thus allowing the atrial escape interval to complete, resulting in the delivery of an atrial output pulse (Fig. 7.18B). At the high rates or long AV delays, the atrial escape interval is relatively short and may result in the delivery of an atrial output pulse at a time when the atrial myocardium is still refractory on a physiological basis. This pattern may then be repetitive (AS–AP–VP). A new algorithm, called non-competitive atrial pacing, has been introduced in an attempt to preclude such a rhythm by extending atrial output to at least 300 ms after an atrial sensed event.

Pacemaker eccentricities and pseudomalfunction

Pacemaker eccentricity is a unique behavior of the pacemaker that would be unexpected based on knowledge of the pacing mode, but that is normal for that model of pacemaker. A pseudomalfunction is a misdiagnosed problem with pacemaker function that in fact results from normal operation of a pacemaker algorithm or function. The eccentricities of pacemaker function are often not popularized in the literature or the physician's manual for the device. They are frequently brought to the attention of the physician only after consulting with technical support for the manufacturer regarding unexplained pacemaker behavior. Examples are shown in Fig. 7.19. Pseudomalfunctions are a challenge for even the seasoned pacemaker physician given the increasing complexity of the newer devices with less than obvious interactions between available algorithms. A list of common features causing pseudomalfunctions in current pacemaker systems is shown in Table 7.5.

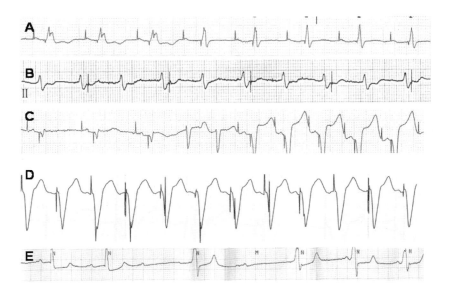

Fig. 7.19 Five examples of pseudomalfunctions. (A) Intrinsic AV search function. After the first three cardiac cycles with atrial pace (Ap)-ventricular pace (Vp) with full ventricular capture, the AV delay is extended to allow for intrinsic conduction. The narrow QRS complexes are pseudofusion complexes that may be mistaken for loss of capture. (B) Safety pacing during a junctional rhythm simulating ventricular undersensing. With every other cycle the atrial pacing is occurring at the start of the QRS. The QRS is sensed early in the AV delay to trigger safety pacing. (C) Rate smoothing causing sudden pacing above the lower rate limit. The two premature ventricular contractions (PVCs) after the third AV pacing cycle initiate AV pacing to decrement incrementally from the faster rate established by the ectopy. (D) St Jude Medical ventricular autocapture algorithm performing threshold determination. After the third QRS complex several complexes occur with two pacing artifacts. The second artifact is the backup pulse that ensures capture, whereas the first pulse is decremented in output. This function can be mistaken for displacement of an atrial lead into the ventricle in a dual-chamber pacemaker or pacemaker malfunction. (E) Medtronic Minimal Ventricular Pacing algorithm. Essentially, AAI pacing occurs until AV block produces an AA interval without an interposed ventricular sensed event. This causes ventricular pacing at the end of the AA interval. If two of four consecutive intervals result in ventricular pacing, the device switches to DDD mode, as in this example.

Table 7.5 Pacemaker functions associated with pseudomalfunctions

	Diagnostic clue
Pacing when not expected	
Rate smoothing	Graded rate slowing toward lower rate limit
Rate drop response	Abrupt pacing 90–110 bpm after sudden slowing
Dynamic atrial overdrive	Atrial pacing after atrial ectopy
Ventricular rate regularization	Pacing after shorter VV intervals in atrial fibrillation
Ventricular based timing	Faster ventricular rate during $A_PV_S–A_PV_P$ cycle
Safety pacing	Ventricular pacing with shortened AV delay
Separate mode switch rate or post-mode switch overdrive rate	Pacing during or after atrial tachyarrhythmia or oversensing
Atrial pace for AV resynchronization	Pacing simultaneous with PVC or delayed after atrial ectopy
Atrial pacing preference	Atrial pacing after atrial sensed events
Automated capture determinations	Closely coupled stimuli for P wave or QRS, sudden increase in paced rates
No pacing when expected	
Hysteresis	Pause after sensed events
Rate smoothing	Graded rate acceleration toward upper rate limit
PMT intervention	Ventricular output absent after A_SV_P near upper rate limit
Mode switching	Failure to track atrial activity
Separate mode switch rate	Lower pacing rate during mode switch
Intrinsic AV conduction search	Periodic extension of AV delay
Non-competitive atrial pacing	Delay in atrial output following atrial sense in PVARP
Separate sleep rate	Reduced lower rate limit at rest
Atrial based timing	Prolongation of VV interval during $A_PV_S–A_PV_P$ cycle
Automatic sensing check	Periodic delay in pacing after prolonged pacing
Minimal ventricular pacing algorithms	AAI pacing behavior until AA interval without interposed ventricular event is followed by ventricular pacing
Apparent undersensing	
Mode switching	Failure to track atrial activity
PMT intervention	Failure to track single P wave during prolonged A_SV_P at upper rate limit
Rate-adaptive AV delay	Evidence of shorter AV delays at faster rates
Non-tracking modes (DDI, DVI, etc.)	Typical non-tracking behavior
Blanked flutter search	Failure to track P wave when atrial tracking at rate < 2 times TARP
Noise mode	Evidence of EMI
PVARP extension post-PVC	Failure to sense P wave after PVC
Minimal ventricular pacing algorithms	Single ventricular events in AA interval do not reset atrial pacing

AV, atrioventricular, PVC, premature ventricular contraction; PMT, pacemaker-mediated tachycardia; PVARP, postventricular atrial refractory period; TARP, total atrial refractory period; EMI, electromagnetic interference.

Pacemaker diagnostics

Given the multiplicity of confusing pacemaker rhythms, most manufacturers include various aids within the pacemaker to assist the physician in evaluating the system. These include both real-time diagnostic aids as well as system overview capabilities. Many real-time diagnostic capabilities have been discussed in this chapter. The pacemaker physician should make full use of these features to assist in troubleshooting the pacing system.[19–21]

Measured data

Measured data is the ability of the pacemaker to provide data regarding battery status, with specific measurements such as battery voltage, current drain and internal impedance. A decrease in the battery voltage is an appropriate marker to identify the point at which there is an increase in the frequency of pacemaker surveillance for signs of battery depletion. Today, several devices provide a gauge that serves as a graphic display of estimated device longevity (Fig. 7.20).

Measured data also include measurements of sense amplitude, pulse voltage, charge, current, energy, and stimulation impedance. The atrial and ventricular sensed amplitude may be particularly useful in the evaluation of issues related to over- or undersensing. Similarly, lead impedance measurements may be particularly helpful in identifying an open circuit, which will be associated with very high impedance or a breach of the internal insulation of a bipolar coaxial lead, in which case the impedance will be very low. Again, the ability of devices to plot long-term trends (Fig. 7.8) allows one to make a better assessment of lead integrity than episodic evaluations at the time of a scheduled device interrogation.

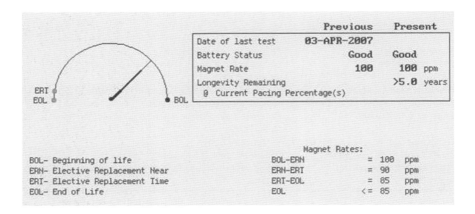

Fig. 7.20 Assessment of battery longevity. The "diagnostic evaluation" window of a Guidant Insignia I Ultra dual-chamber pacemaker. For convenience at follow-up, the current battery status is depicted as a "gas gauge" and an estimate of remaining longevity is provided.

Event markers

Event markers have been shown in multiple figures in this chapter. These comprise timing information telemetered from the pacemaker to the programmer and are displayed on a screen or printed. Basically, these markers are a report of what the pacemaker is doing. Unique notations or marks are generated for paced and sensed events; in some cases, marks are generated for events occurring during the refractory period as well as an indication of refractory period duration. For proper interpretation, the clinician should be familiar with the markers used by a specific manufacturer (Fig. 7.21).

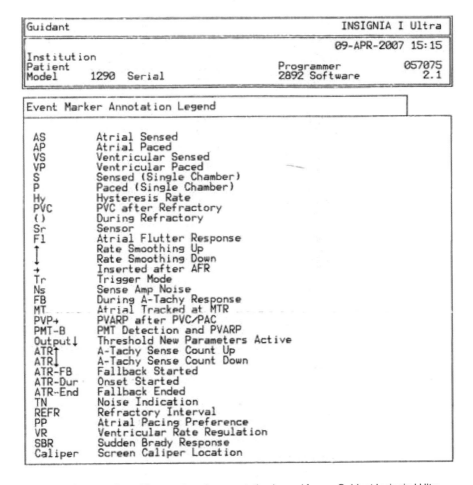

Fig. 7.21 Event markers. The event marker annotation legend from a Guidant Insignia I Ultra dual-chamber pacemaker.

Event markers are an extremely powerful tool, especially when combined with the simultaneously recorded electrocardiogram. Pauses can be identified as due to oversensing or an open circuit. With diminutive bipolar output pulses that may not be visible on the standard electrocardiogram, telemetered event markers will identify whether the P wave or QRS complex is paced or sensed. The ECG also confirms the response to a pacing stimulus.

Event counters

Event counters provide information about the function of the pacing system over time. This feature may provide an overview of the behavior of the pacing system with respect to specific events or activation of various algorithms, an overview of the general behavior of the system, or a report of the pacing system with respect to time. Each manufacturer has its own set of unique labels for the specific counters in its various products, but, generically, there are several separate capabilities.

Total system performance counters

Total system performance counters report the total number of events within each pacing state (atrial sense–ventricular sense, atrial pace–ventricular sense, etc.), sometimes with a further separation as to rate distribution within each pacing state. Many systems will also report the number of premature ventricular sensed events. The potential value to the medical staff caring for the patient is that these counters provide an overview of the behavior of the pacing system since the last evaluation. The interpretation of these counters requires knowledge of the patient's clinical status and the integrity of capture and sensing within the pacing system (Fig. 7.22). For example, if the system reports that all the complexes were paced in the ventricle, either AV or PV, it is a report of the pacemaker's behavior. Loss of atrial or ventricular capture cannot be ascertained from these counters, and a true pacing system problem might go unrecognized if one relied only on the counters.

If the pacing system is functioning properly with respect to capture and sensing, the total system performance counters provide insight into the chronotropic function based on the distribution of sensed atrial activity, the response of the sensor, the percentage of time the sensor is controlling the pacemaker, and the status of AV nodal conduction based on the percentage of paced and sensed complexes. Frequent "PVCs" at a low rate may be a marker for intermittent atrial undersensing with intact AV nodal conduction or for accelerated junctional rhythms; a large number of PVCs at a high rate may reflect true ventricular ectopic beats. The data provided by all the event counters need to be correlated with the clinician's knowledge of the patient.

Subsystem performance counters

Subsystem performance counters track and report the behavior of specific algorithms or features of the pacing system. These include, but are not lim-

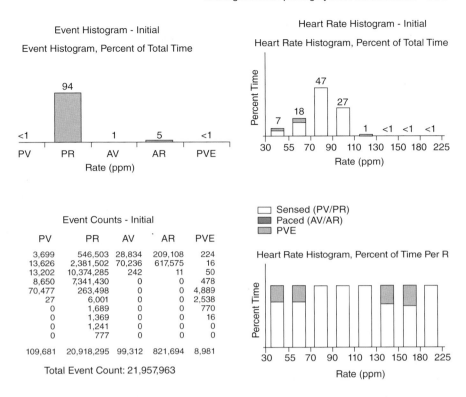

Fig. 7.22 Total system performance counter (event histogram) from a St Jude Medical Integrity 5342 pulse generator demonstrating the relative distribution of pacing states, the heart rate based on atrial events (paced or sensed), and the absolute number of events in each pacing state at each rate bin over the preceding 192 days, 7 h, 23 min, and 20 s. The PVE in this counter reflects events that the pacemaker will treat as premature ventricular contractions (PVCs). As these may also be junctional beats, episodes of atrial undersensing with intact conduction, or noise on the ventricular channel, and not a true PVC as would be implied to the clinical staff, these are labeled PVEs. Key programmed parameters and system statistics are displayed toward the top of the printout (not shown).

ited to, sensor-indicated rates, number of times the PMT algorithm was activated, the amount of time spent at the programmed maximal tracking rate, the number of automatic mode-switch episodes, the peak atrial rates that triggered the mode-switch episodes or occurred above a predefined rate, atrial or ventricular high-rate episodes, and a long-term threshold record for those systems with automatic capture assessment algorithms. The value of these counters is that they separate specific events from the overall total system performance counter and provide information with respect to the frequency with which that algorithm or feature was used. These event counters may also provide data that are not obtainable from a standard ECG or Holter monitor. These counters may be displayed as a summary total, a table of events, a histogram, or a more detailed presentation of each event, depending on the design of the specific counter and the information that is stored. Commonly, these counters also incorporate a time-stamp.

Stored electrograms
Evaluation of device diagnostics clearly assists with the care of the patient with an implanted pacemaker. However, an important component of this capability is the recent ability to review stored intracardiac electrograms, which are stored whether automatically in response to a programmed trigger or in response to patient-activated application of a magnet over the device. It has previously been discussed how these electrograms can be used to evaluate intermittent problems of sensing, which may allow for the diagnosis of unrecognized problems with the integrity of the pacing system.

An additional important value to the stored electrogram is to be able to identify asymptomatic and symptomatic arrhythmias in a given patient, which may be paroxysmal and otherwise difficult to diagnose. The most important arrhythmia in a pacemaker patient is atrial fibrillation; however, on occasion, ventricular tachycardia can also be diagnosed (Fig. 7.23). However, it is important to review the electrogram carefully, as misclassifications are frequently observed (Figs 7.6 and 7.16).

Summary

As mentioned at the beginning of this chapter, it is important to maintain appropriate records containing all the baseline data and results of the periodic detailed evaluations of the pacing system. These records provide the substrate on which to assess a new observation or information. For biventricular systems, it is helpful to have 12-lead ECGs showing the native depolarization, RV pacing, LV pacing and biventricular pacing. Depending on the capabilities of the implanted system, it may need to be recorded during the implant procedure. One should also take advantage of the diagnostic capabilities incorporated into many present-generation pacemakers. These features include programmed parameter interrogation, lead and battery function telemetry, event marker and electrogram telemetry, and event counters for native and paced events, including sensor performance and other unique algorithms. Examples of many of these capabilities have been used to illustrate the various conditions described throughout this chapter, and a simplified schematic for pacemaker troubleshooting is shown in Fig. 7.24. Although these features are helpful, there is no substitute for a thorough understanding of the pacing system, the patient, and the fundamental concepts of pacing.

A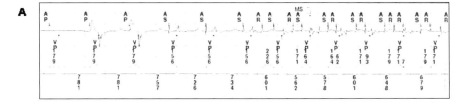

B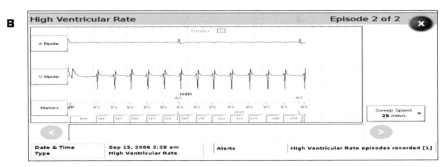

Fig. 7.23 Stored electrograms. (A) A summed electrogram depicting atrial and ventricular activity in a patient with a Medtronic dual-chamber pacemaker. Top: The patient has an episode of paroxysmal atrial fibrillation, which triggers the automatic mode switching (MS) algorithm. Bottom: A stored electrogram of a high ventricular rate episode retrieved from a patient with a St Jude Medical dual-chamber pacemaker. The device stores the atrial and ventricular electrogram, which shows a rapid ventricular rhythm (cycle length ~400 ms) with clear VA dissociation. This is consistent with ventricular tachycardia.

When a true pacing system malfunction is encountered, the full differential diagnosis should be considered. This includes primary problems arising with the pulse generator, the lead(s), and the patient, as well as the interaction between these three components. It is embarrassing, expensive, and potentially dangerous to subject the patient to an operative procedure to replace a normally functioning pacemaker when the observed "problem" could have been easily corrected by programming the pacemaker, or reflected a system eccentricity and was normal. Thus, any prior data that are available should be reviewed, the programmed parameters of the pacing system should be obtained, and all available diagnostic features of the given device should be used before arriving at a final decision and plan. If there are still concerns, each manufacturer provides 24/7 technical support before deciding on an operative intervention. To do less than this may result in an incorrect diagnosis—to the detriment of the patient, the physician, and the overall healthcare economy.

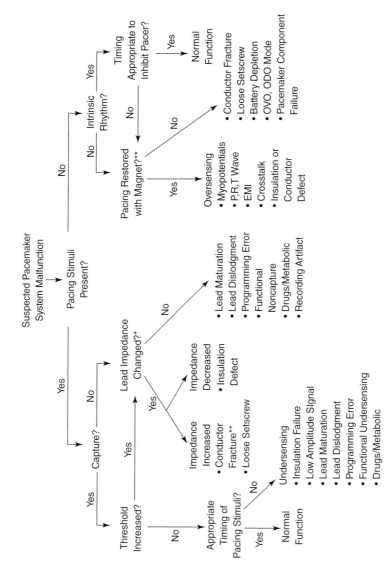

Fig. 7.24 Simplified schematic for pacemaker troubleshooting. EMI, electromagnetic interference. *> 300-Ω change in impedance as measured at the time of malfunction; **or programmed to asynchronous mode; can have no change in impedance with concomitant insulation failure.

References

1 Levine PA. Evaluation and management of pacing system malfunctions. In: Ellenbogen KA, Wood MA, eds. Cardiac pacing and ICDs. Boston: Blackwell Publishing, 2005:322–75.

2 Hayes DL. Effect of drugs and devices on permanent pacemakers. Cardiology 1991; 8:70–75.

3 Kahloon MU, Aslam AK, Aslam AF, Wilbur SL, Vasavada BC, Khan IA. Hyperkalemia induced failure of atrial and ventricular capture. Int J Cardiol 2005; 105:224–6.

4 Maisel WH, Moynahan M, Zuckerman BD et al. Pacemaker and ICD generator malfunctions: analysis of Food and Drug Administration annual reports. JAMA 2006; 295:1901–6.

5 Santini M, Brachmann J, Cappato R et al. Recommendations of the European cardiac arrhythmia society committee on device failures and complications. PACE 2006; 29:653–69.

6 Ribeiro ALP, Rincon LG, Oliveira BG et al. Automatic adjustment of pacing output in the clinical setting. Am Heart J 2004; 147:127–31.

7 Sperzel J, Milasinovic G, Smith TW et al. for the worldwide EnPulse™ study investigators. Automatic measurement of atrial pacing thresholds in dual-chamber pacemakers: Clinical experience with atrial capture management. Heart Rhythm 2005; 2:1203–10.

8 Boriani G, Rusconi L, Biffi M et al. on behalf of the Autocapture study group. Role of ventricular autocapture function in increasing longevity of DDDR pacemakers: a prospective study. Europace 2006; 8:216–20.

9 Park HW, Kim KH, Sohn IS et al. Acute massive rise in the capture threshold: successful management with long-term oral prednisolone. Int J Cardiol 2006; 111:453–4.

10 Castillo R, Cavusoglu E. Twiddler's syndrome: an interesting cause of pacemaker failure. Cardiology 2006; 105:119–21.

11 Hughes JC Jr, Tyers GFO, Torman HA. Effects of acid–base imbalance on myocardial pacing thresholds. J Thorac Cardiovasc Surg 1975; 69:743–6.

12 Magney JE, Flynn DM, Parsons JA et al. Anatomical mechanisms explaining damage to pacemaker leads, defibrillator leads and failure of central venous catheters adjacent to the sternoclavicular joint. Pacing Clin Electrophysiol 1993; 16:445–57.

13 Jacobs DM, Fink AS, Miller RP et al. Anatomical and morphologic evaluation of pacemaker lead compression. Pacing Clin Electrophysiol 1993; 16:434–44.

14 Magney JE, Staplin DH, Flynn DM et al. A new approach to percutaneous subclavian venipuncture to avoid lead fracture or central venous catheter occlusion. Pacing Clin Electrophysiol 1993; 16:2133–42.

15 Ong LS, Barold SS, Lederman M et al. Cephalic vein guidewire technique for implantation of permanent pacemakers. Am Heart J 1987; 114:753–6.

16 Niehaus M, Tebbenjohanns J. Electromagnetic interference in patients with implanted pacemakers or cardioverter-defibrillators. Heart 2001; 86:246–8.

17 Sweesy MW. Understanding electromagnetic interference. Heart Rhythm 2004; 1:523–4.

18 Kolb C, Willie B, Maurer D et al. on behalf of the FFS-test study group. Management of far-field R wave sensing for the avoidance of inappropriate mode switch in dual chamber pacemakers: results of the FFS-test study. J Cardiovasc Electrophysiol 2006; 17:992–7.

19 Pollak WM, Simmons JD, Interian A, Castellanos A, Myerburg RJ, Mitrani RD. Pacemaker diagnostics: a critical appraisal of current technology. Pacing Clin Electrophysiol 2003; 26:76–98.

20 Scher DL. Troubleshooting pacemakers and implantable cardioverter-defibrillators. Curr Opin Cardiol 2004; 19:36–46.

21 Roberts PR. Follow up and optimization of cardiac pacing. Heart 2005; 91:1229–34.

22 Nowak B, Sperzel J, Rauscha F et al. Diagnostic value of onset-recordings and marker annotations in dual chamber pacemaker stored electrograms. Europace 2003; 5:103–9.

## CHAPTER 8

The implantable cardioverter defibrillator

Frank A Cuoco, Michael R Gold

The implantable cardioverter defibrillator (ICD) has undergone a remarkable transformation over the past 25 years. The early pulse generators were large, requiring thoracotomy for epicardial patch placement, and were implanted in the abdomen. This complex surgery resulted in postoperative hospitalization averaging approximately 1 week. The pulse generators had a longevity of < 2 years, had almost no diagnostic capabilities, and had pacing capabilities that were limited to only backup ventricular pacing. Modern devices provide detailed information about the morphology and rates of arrhythmias, and store electrocardiographic signals before, during and after therapy. Heart rate variability, activity level, transthoracic impedance and atrial and ventricular rates are catalogued independent of arrhythmias, and lead impedances and sensed electrogram amplitudes (i.e. R waves and P waves) are measured automatically and stored in memory. The downsizing of pulse generators, in combination with improvements of lead design and shock waveforms, allows the simplicity of defibrillator implantation to approach that of pacemakers, with outpatient placement now feasible. Subcutaneous systems are in development that may further simplify implants by obviating the need for transvenous leads altogether. Despite the marked reduction in size and increase in diagnostic capabilities, device longevity is now > 6 years. Devices have the capabilities to treat multiple problems, not only life-threatening ventricular arrhythmias but also bradyarrhythmias with dual-chamber devices, atrial arrhythmias, and congestive heart failure (CHF) with biventricular pacing.

Indications

The indications for ICD implantation remained unchanged for many years. Initially, the devices were only implanted in patients who survived an aborted cardiac arrest or an episode of sustained ventricular tachycardia (VT) that was refractory to antiarrhythmic drug therapy. The use of ICDs for the secondary prevention of sudden cardiac death (SCD) was the standard for more than a

Cardiac Pacing and ICDs, 5th edition. Edited by Kenneth A. Ellenbogen and Mark A. Wood.
© 2008 Blackwell Publishing, ISBN: 978-1-4051-6350-7

decade. However, several landmark studies established the role of ICD therapy for primary prevention of sudden death in high-risk subjects, and today the vast majority of new implants in the USA are performed for this indication. A summary of the current indications for ICD therapy is shown in Table 8.1.[1]

The AVID study has compared ICD implantation with antiarrhythmic drug use (primarily amiodarone) among patients with aborted cardiac arrest or poorly tolerated VT.[2] Patients were randomized to initial therapy with an ICD or to class III antiarrhythmic drugs. There was a significant reduction in mortality in the group randomized to ICD implantation. The benefit of the ICD was most marked among patients with a reduced left ventricular ejection fraction (LVEF) (≤ 0.35). In the Canadian Implantable Defibrillator Study (CIDS), 659 patients with VT, ventricular fibrillation (VF) or syncope were randomized to antiarrhythmic therapy with amiodarone or ICD implantation. A 20% reduction in mortality was observed in the ICD group, although this did not reach statistical significance. However, subsequent analyses have shown that an LVEF < 0.35, age > 70 years, and advanced CHF were characteristics of the patients who were most likely to benefit from ICD im-

---

Table 8.1 Summary of indications for implantable cardioverter defibrillator (ICD) therapy

Secondary prevention
Class I
Patients with a history of sudden cardiac arrest (SCA), VF, hemodynamically unstable VT, or unexplained syncope with LV dysfunction and inducible VT

Primary prevention
Class I
Patients with ischemic cardiomyopathy who are at least 40 days post-MI with an LVEF $\leq$ 30–40%, NYHA functional class II or III, receiving optimal medical therapy, and have reasonable expectation of survival with a good functional status at > 1 year
Patients with non-ischemic cardiomyopathy, NYHA class II–III, LVEF $\leq$ 30–35%, receiving optimal medical therapy, and have reasonable expectation of survival with a good functional status at > 1 year
Class IIa
Ischemic cardiomyopathy patients with NYHA functional class I, LVEF $\leq$ 30–35%, receiving optimal medical therapy, and have reasonable expectation of survival with a good functional status at > 1 year
ICD in combination with biventricular pacing in patients with NYHA functional class III or IV, receiving optimal medical therapy, in sinus rhythm with a QRS > 120 ms, and a reasonable survival expectation of > 1 year
Patients who are at high risk of SCA due to genetic disorders, such as long QT syndrome, Brugada syndrome, hypertrophic cardiomyopathy and arrhythmogenic right ventricular cardiomyopathy (ARVC), and have reasonable expectation of survival with a good functional status at > 1 year
Class IIb
Non-ischemic cardiomyopathy patients with NYHA functional class I, LVEF $\leq$ 30–35%, receiving optimal medical therapy, and have a reasonable expectation of survival with a good functional status at > 1 year

---

VF, ventricular fibrillation; VT, ventricular tachycardia; LV, left ventricular; MI, myocardial infarction; LVEF, left ventricular ejection fraction; NYHA, New York Heart Association.

plantation.[3] In the CASH study, 288 patients with a history of cardiac arrest were randomized to receive metoprolol, amiodarone, propafenone, or to undergo ICD implantation. There was increased mortality in the group treated with propafenone, and a 28% decreased mortality among the patients who received ICDs.[4] These studies established the benefit of ICD therapy as first-line treatment among patients with a history of life-threatening arrhythmias (i.e. secondary prevention), particularly in individuals with left ventricular dysfunction; thus, antiarrhythmic drugs have been relegated to adjunctive therapy to reduce arrhythmia recurrence rates.

Once the relative safety of ICD implantation became apparent, the use of this therapy for primary prevention of sudden death was studied. The MADIT and MUSTT trials have evaluated patients with coronary artery disease, left ventricular systolic dysfunction, non-sustained VT and inducible sustained monomorphic VT. In the MADIT study, patients were randomized to receive either an ICD or "conventional" medical therapy, which was most commonly amiodarone.[5] In the MUSTT study, patients were randomized to either no antiarrhythmic therapy or electrophysiologically guided drug therapy. In 46% of the latter group, ICD implantation was performed because of the failure of antiarrhythmic drugs to suppress inducible arrhythmias.[6] Despite these differences in study design, the results of the two trials were remarkably similar; ICD use decreased mortality > 50% in these cohorts with ischemic cardiomyopathy.

It is interesting that the magnitude of mortality reduction in these primary prevention trials appears even larger than in the studies of patients with a history of aborted cardiac arrest or sustained VT. One likely explanation for this apparent paradox is that the groups who were evaluated in primary prevention studies had lower mean LVEFs and a higher incidence of CHF, two potent predictors of mortality.

Expanding the indications for ICD use has been an area of intense investigation. The analysis of the MUSTT registry of patients with coronary artery disease, reduced ejection fraction, and no inducible sustained VT demonstrated a disturbingly high mortality rate, even though it was significantly lower than that among patients with inducible VT.[7] This indicates that methods of risk stratification, other than by electrophysiology testing, are necessary. The MADIT II study was a prospective randomized trial of 1232 subjects with previous myocardial infarction (MI) and ejection fraction of ≤ 0.30.[8] Spontaneous non-sustained VT or electrophysiology testing were not required for enrollment in this trial. The ICD and control groups had similar clinical characteristics with a mean age of approximately 65 years, 67% with CHF [New York Heart Association (NYHA) II–IV] and mean LVEF of 0.23. In addition, β-blocker and angiotensin-converting enzyme inhibitor use was approximately 70% among each group. During a mean follow-up of 20 months, the mortality rates were 14.2% in the ICD group and 19.8% in the control group [hazard ratio (HR) 0.69, 95% confidence interval, 0.51, 0.93; $P = 0.016$].

Several other primary prevention studies have evaluated patients with a reduced LVEF without requiring the presence of coronary artery disease. The

SCD HeFT study evaluated 2521 subjects with CHF (NYHA II and III) and left ventricular systolic dysfunction (ejection fraction ≤ 35%), irrespective of etiology (i.e. ischemic or non-ischemic cardiomyopathies).[9] ICD implantation, but not amiodarone, was shown to reduce all-cause mortality. Similar mortality reductions were observed among the subgroups with ischemic and non-ischemic cardiomyopathies. The DEFINITE study randomized 458 subjects with dilated, non-ischemic cardiomyopathy and frequent ventricular ectopy to receive an ICD or optimal medical therapy. There was a strong trend toward a mortality reduction in the ICD cohort, and a significant reduction in the incidence of SCD ($P = 0.006$).[10]

Not all high-risk groups benefit from ICD implantation, as shown by the CABG Patch and DINAMIT trials. In CABG Patch, patients with ischemic cardiomyopathy and an abnormal signal-averaged electrocardiogram (SAECG) were randomized to receive an ICD or no antiarrhythmic treatment at the time of coronary artery bypass surgery. No effect on mortality was observed with ICD use in this cohort.[11] The DINAMIT study evaluated patients with acute MI, left ventricular systolic dysfunction and reduced heart rate variability (HRV). No mortality benefit was observed with ICD implantation. The reasons for the failure of these studies to show a benefit of ICD therapy are unclear. The use of non-invasive risk modifiers, such as signal-averaged ECG or heart rate variability, may be insufficient to identify a high-risk cohort. Also, the competing mortality risks early post-MI or post-bypass surgery may offset any benefit of ICD therapy. However, these studies have clearly demonstrated that clinical trials and not "common sense" need to guide the decision to implant devices. Table 8.2 summarizes the major ICD trials for primary prevention of SCD.

One cohort that is particularly difficult to manage is those patients with structural heart disease and a history of syncope. These patients have been excluded from most prospective, randomized studies because, on one hand, they do not have documented arrhythmias to be included in secondary prevention studies, and, on the other hand, they cannot be classified as asymptomatic to be included in primary prevention trials. Present guidelines recommend ICD implantation in patients with inducible VT and syncope. However, initial treatment with an ICD in patients with syncope and dilated cardiomyopathy, regardless of the results of electrophysiology testing, is rapidly becoming standard clinical practice, despite the lack of randomized studies to support this strategy. Many of these patients now meet other indications for ICD implantation (e.g. MADIT II or SCD HeFT), so their management is less controversial.

Another group of patients in whom ICD implantation may be indicated are those with hypertrophic cardiomyopathy who have one or more risk factors for SCD. These risk factors include a history of VT (sustained or non-sustained detected by Holter monitor), recurrent syncope, high-risk genetic mutations, a family history of sudden death, exercise-induced hypotension, and marked septal thickness (> 30 mm).[12] ICD use is also becoming more common among patients with primary electrical disease, such as the Brugada syndrome and

Table 8.2 Selected implantable cardioverter defibrillator (ICD) trials for primary prevention of sudden cardiac death (SCD)[5-11]

Trial	No. of patients	Etiology	Major inclusion criteria	Hazard ratio for overall mortality (ICD)	P value
MADIT	196	ICM	EF ≤ 35%, NSVT, inducible VT	0.46	0.009
MUSTT	704	ICM	EF ≤ 40%, NSVT, inducible VT	0.45*	< 0.001
MADIT II	1232	ICM	EF ≤ 30%, prior MI	0.69	0.016
SCD-HeFT	2521	ICM & NICM	EF ≤ 35%, CHF NYHA Class II or III	0.77	0.007
DEFINITE	458	NICM	EF ≤ 35%, PVCs or NSVT	0.65	0.08
COMPANION	1520	ICM & NICM	EF ≤ 35%, CHF NYHA Class II or III, QRS > 120	0.64†	0.003
DINAMIT	676	ICM	EF ≤ 35%, ¯HRV, recent MI (< 40 days)	1.08	0.66
CABG-PATCH	900	ICM	EF ≤ 35%, CABG, abnormal SAECG	1.07	0.64

MADIT, Multicenter Automatic Defibrillator Implantation Trial; MUSTT, Multicenter Unsustained Tachycardia Trial; SCD-HeFT, Sudden Cardiac Death in Heart Failure Trial; DEFINITE, Defibrillators in Non-Ischemic Cardiomyopathy Treatment Evaluation; COMPANION, Comparison of Medical Therapy, Pacing, and Defibrillation in Heart Failure Trial; DINAMIT, Defibrillator in Acute Myocardial Infarction Trial; CABG-PATCH, Coronary Artery Bypass Graft Patch.
*MUSTT results listed are the adjusted relative risk for overall mortality for patients receiving electrophysiologically guided therapy with an ICD compared with no antiarrhythmic therapy.
†COMPANION results listed are for CRT+ICD vs. medical therapy alone. The hazard ratio for overall mortality for CRT alone vs. medical therapy was 0.76 (P = 0.059).
ICM, ischemic cardiomyopathy; EF, ejection fraction; NSVT, nonsustained VT; VT, ventricular tachycardia; MI, myocardial infarction; NICM, nonischemic cardiomyopathy; CHF, congestive heart failure; NYHA, New York Heart Association; PVC, premature ventricular contraction; HRV, heart rate variability; SAECG, signal-averaged ECG.

long QT syndrome, particularly among patients with a history of syncope or a family history of sudden death.[13]

One major challenge today is to develop better methods to risk stratify patients for SCD, allowing clinicians to implant devices only in those patients who will be likely to use them appropriately. The major trials for primary prevention mentioned above have shown that only approximately one-third of patients who receive ICDs for primary prevention will receive an appropriate shock for a ventricular tachyarrhythmia over 4–5 years. The results of retrospective analyses of clinical predictors of ICD shocks or mortality generally show that the incidence of shocks or mortality increases with the severity of heart failure, the lower the ejection fraction, QRS prolongation, atrial fibrillation, renal failure and age.

Many non-invasive tools for SCD risk stratification, including signal-averaged ECG and measures of autonomic dysfunction, have been evaluated, but their value is limited by low sensitivity and positive predictive values. One such tool that is gaining popularity is microvolt T-wave alternans (TWA), which measures beat-to-beat changes in repolarization. TWA has a very high negative predictive value, especially in patients with a history of MI (> 99%), and hence it has been given a Class IIa recommendation in the American College of Cardiology/American Heart Association/European Society of Cardiology Guidelines for use in risk stratification for life-threatening ventricular arrhythmias.[1] However, like the aforementioned risk stratifiers, TWA has a low positive predictive value, and its negative predictive value drops in patients with non-ischemic cardiomyopathy and those with heart failure. Additionally, its use is also limited by the fact that many results are indeterminate (30–40%) for a variety of technical and clinical factors. Unfortunately, more recently, a large prospective substudy of SCD HeFT has failed to confirm the utility of TWA in the first evaluation of this technology in a randomized ICD trial.[14]

Finally, perhaps the most important dilemma with regard to prevention of SCD and prophylactic use of ICDs is the fact that most of the SCD victims do not meet current indications for ICD implantation. Population-based studies from both Maastricht, the Netherlands and Oregon have shown that about one-half of SCD victims had an LVEF > 50% prior to their event, and only 20–30% of these patients had severe left ventricular dysfunction that warranted ICD implantation according to current guidelines.[15,16] In order to make an impact on the absolute number of sudden deaths per year, further studies are needed to identify those patients who are at high risk for SCD, but do not have advanced structural heart disease.

Pulse generators and lead systems

Early ICD pulse generators were large and bulky. The size (115–145 cm^3) and weight (195–235 g) of these devices mandated abdominal implantation, typically in the left upper quadrant either subcutaneously or most often under the rectus muscle. The surgical procedure for abdominal ICD implantation is more extensive than for endocardial pacemakers, in part because it requires tunneling leads from the chest. The abdominal location of the pulse generator and the surgical procedure required were probably responsible for the higher complication rates observed with early ICD implantation, particularly infection and lead fractures.

Modern pulse generator size has decreased significantly. With downsizing of these devices (30–39 cm^3, 70–84 g), routine subcutaneous pectoral implantation is possible, although these pulse generators are still significantly larger than pacemakers. This implantation approach is not associated with any increased risk of complications.[17] Despite the large size of the early pulse generators, their battery life was only approximately 2 years. With improvement in battery design and reduction of monitoring current drain, the expected life span of many ICD pulse generators is now > 6 years. This has obvious and important implications for the cost effectiveness of this therapy.

ICDs, unlike pacemakers, are designed to deliver high-energy shocks within seconds of detection of tachycardia. This has implications in the design of power systems for ICDs. ICD batteries are constructed in thin layers, with anode and cathode layers separated by a porous film and bathed in a highly conductive electrolyte solution. Nearly all modern ICDs are powered by lithium–silver vanadium oxide batteries, whose charge times have been optimized by varying the ratios of anode and cathode material in the battery. Unlike pacemakers, ICDs also require multiple high-voltage capacitors to store and deliver the energy required for defibrillation. These capacitors are mainly responsible for the larger size of ICDs compared with pacemakers. ICD capacitors are usually made with aluminum or tantalum, and can be manufactured in stacked-plate or cylindrical construction. An important concept for efficient ICD capacitor function is reformation. Over time, if a capacitor is not used, the anode surfaces develop imperfections which "deform" the oxide film. These imperfections can result in increased charge times as these defects are "reformed" as the capacitor is charged to high voltage. Thus, ICD capacitors need to be periodically reformed (every 1–6 months) to maintain optimal charge times.

ICD pulse generators have very sophisticated programmability and internal circuitry. All pulse generators have non-invasive pacing induction, with the capabilities for programmed ventricular stimulation. With real-time telemetry of intracardiac electrograms, pacing and shocking impedances, and pacing thresholds of the ICD lead systems can be monitored non-invasively as well, to aid in the assessment of lead function. Sudden changes in impedances or electrogram amplitudes, or the sensing of non-physiological short RR intervals, are indicators of lead dislodgement or malfunction. Detailed data logging is present, including precise measurements of arrhythmia rates, time of occurrence, and response to therapy. ICDs can store both near-field and far-field electrograms, as well as marker channels, which can be useful for arrhythmia discrimination (Fig. 8.1). These stored electrograms provide a recording of the arrhythmia at the time of device activity. This is most useful in assessing the appropriateness of therapy (i.e. shocks for atrial fibrillation vs. VT) and any malfunction of the system. Finally, the capacitors in the pulse generator need to be charged periodically to avoid very prolonged charging during spontaneous arrhythmia; such capacitor reformation would mandate office visits every 2–3 months for patients, but now capacitor reformation is performed automatically by the pulse generator.

The lead systems for sensing, pacing, and the delivery of shocks have also changed significantly over the past decade. Although transvenous defibrillation was developed by Mirowski in his pioneering studies of the ICD,[18] the initial commercial systems used epicardial sensing leads and patches placed on the heart. Subsequently, the development of integrated leads incorporating both rate-sensing electrodes and defibrillation coils led to the routine use of non-thoracotomy lead systems. The pectoral placement of pulse generators allowed further improvement in lead technology, because the pulse generator shell can serve as an extrathoracic electrode (e.g. "hot or active can") and actually become part of the lead system. These active pulse generator systems

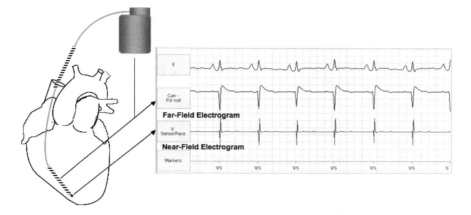

Fig. 8.1 Implantable cardioverter defibrillator (ICD) electrograms. Near-field electrograms (bottom) are true-bipolar recordings between the tip and ring electrodes of the right ventricular (RV) lead. The far-field electrograms (top) are recorded between the RV coil and the ICD can, which gives a more global representation of ventricular activity, not dissimilar to a precordial ECG lead. A surface ECG lead (top) and a marker channel are also printed on this output, illustrating how the ICD interprets these signals (VS indicates sensed ventricular activity).

further simplify the implantation procedure while enhancing defibrillation efficacy.[19]

ICD leads can be coaxial or multilumen, with insulation of silicone, polyurethane or fluoropolymers. Both single-coil and dual-coil defibrillation leads are available, with active or passive fixation. Coaxial lead design was dominant until the mid-1990s. This is characterized by a coiled conductor with an outside insulation layer, both surrounded by another conductor. Typically, the tip conductor would be central with the ring conductor and then the defibrillation conductor more peripheral. Multilumen leads are preferred today, with conductors running in parallel through a single insulating lead body. The advantages of this design include greater space efficiency resulting in smaller leads, and greater resistance to compressive forces by including extra lumens within the lead body. Figure 8.2 illustrates a schematic and diagram of a modern ICD lead design. A radiograph of a single-lead system, including a dual-coil integrated defibrillation lead and an active left pectoral pulse generator, is shown in Fig. 8.3.

Lead insulation can have an important impact on long-term stability and function. Silicone is inert, biostable, and biocompatible, but has a high coefficient of friction. It is soft, making it prone to damage during implantation, and can swell over time. Polyurethane is biocompatible, has a high tensile strength, making small lead diameters possible, and a low coefficient of friction, but is prone to environmental stress cracking and metal ion oxidation. Recent reports have highlighted the high failure rate of polyurethane leads,[20] so they should be avoided given the superiority of alternative insulators. Fluoropoly-

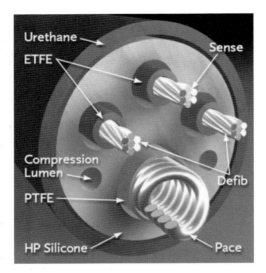

A

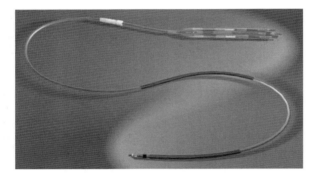

B

Fig. 8.2 (A) A schematic cross-section of a modern dual-coil implantable cardioverter defibrillator (ICD) lead. (B) An illustration of a dual-coil ICD lead. (Reproduced with permission from Medtronic, Inc., Minneapolis, MN, USA.)

mers [e.g. polytetrafluoroethylene (PTFE) and ethylene-tetrafluoroethylene] are the most biocompatible, have high tensile strength allowing small lead size, but are stiff, susceptible to damage from traction when the lead migrates, and they are prone to insulation micro defects and have a difficult manufacturing process. Today's lead systems have an insulating body made of silicone, in some instances supplemented by an outside polyurethane layer (not used for insulation) to reduce friction, abrasion and scar formation. Metal ion oxidation is avoided as polyurethane is not in direct contact with the conductors. The conductors are often insulated with an extra thin layer of fluoropolymer. Coating of leads with expanded PTFE or backfilling shocking coils with medi-

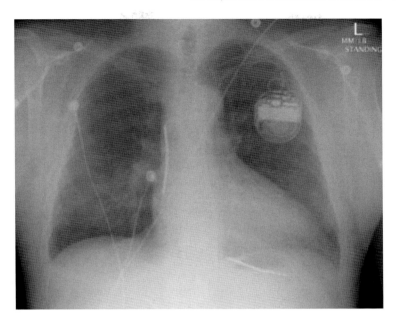

Fig. 8.3 A radiograph of a single-chamber implantable cardioverter defibrillator system. Note the left pectoral pulse generator and the integrated, dual-coil lead with the tip in the right ventricular apex.

cal adhesive have been shown to reduce tissue ingrowth into the lead coils and thereby make future extraction easier, if necessary.[21]

Dual-chamber ICDs are now used more frequently than single-chamber devices. For dual-chamber systems, a separate atrial lead is used. These are typically simple bipolar pacemaker leads, with no unique design for being part of an ICD. Despite the rapid acceptance of this technology, all of the early large studies establishing ICD indications evaluated only single-chamber systems. The first large study to evaluate directly the impact of dual-chamber pacing among ICD patients was DAVID.[22] This was a single-blind, randomized trial of 506 subjects with standard indications for ICDs. Patients underwent implantation with a dual-chamber ICD and were randomized to ventricular backup pacing (VVI at 40 bpm) or dual-chamber rate-responsive pacing (DDDR at 70 bpm). Surprisingly, dual-chamber pacing was associated with worse clinical outcomes. The 1-year survival free of the primary end-point of mortality or CHF hospitalization was 83.9% for patients randomized to VVI pacing and 73.3% for those patients randomized to DDDR pacing (HR 1.61, $P \leq 0.03$). The results of this study have challenged the approach of indiscriminate use of dual-chamber pacing among ICD patients. Recently, the INTRINSIC RV study has shown that the deleterious effects of dual-chamber pacing could be avoided by using advanced algorithms to minimize ventricular pacing by automatically prolonging the atrioventricular (AV) delay.[23] The David II study has shown that AAIR pacing is safe and prevents the adverse effects of DDDR pacing among patients with no standard pacing indications.

Implantable cardioverter defibrillator implantation

ICD systems are implanted by electrophysiologists in nearly 90% of patients, often without the use of an operating room or general anesthesia. The downsizing of ICD pulse generators allows for implantation techniques that approach that of a permanent pacemaker; however, the acute testing and management of these devices still require electrophysiology expertise. It is for this reason that current guidelines require the presence of an electrophysiologist for the implantation procedure.[24]

Whether implanted in an operating room, a multipurpose procedure room, or an electrophysiology laboratory, and whether general anesthesia or conscious sedation is employed, the basic concepts of ICD surgery are the same. Meticulous sterile technique must be used and patients should receive perioperative intravenous antibiotics. The antibiotics chosen should provide adequate activity against staphylococcal species, as these are the most common bacteria associated with early device infections. Typically, vancomycin or a cephalosporin is used. Local irrigation of the pulse generator pocket with antibiotic solution is often performed, although controlled data establishing the efficacy of this additional step are lacking. A physiological recorder is useful for recording and evaluating electrophysiological signals, and heart rhythm, blood pressure and respiration must be monitored. This can be performed either invasively with an arterial line and endotracheal intubation or, more commonly, with electrocardiographic monitoring, a brachial cuff, and pulse oximetry. Finally, the patient should be connected to a transthoracic defibrillator with skin pads for backup defibrillation therapy if needed during defibrillation testing. Two functional external defibrillators (preferably with a biphasic waveform) should always be available during defibrillation testing.

The sites of venous access and methods of obtaining access are similar to those for permanent pacemakers. Unless contraindicated by an AV fistula, venous anomaly, previous chest surgery (i.e. mastectomy), severe dermatological conditions, or scarring, a left-sided approach is preferred. Cutdown to the cephalic vein or percutaneous axillary vein access may be preferable to subclavian puncture to reduce the incidence of subclavian crush observed with these large leads. Leads need to be well secured to the pectoral fascia, because dislodgment of defibrillation leads remains the most common perioperative complication.[25] The transvenous defibrillator leads are implanted in the same fashion as pacemaker leads. The preferred location is the right ventricular apex, with the distal coil entirely within the right ventricular cavity. Adequate sensing (R waves > 5 mV) and pacing (threshold < 1.0 V) of the right ventricular lead need to be established. If a dual-chamber ICD is implanted, then a separate atrial lead is placed, again with adequate sensing and pacing parameters required. Only bipolar atrial leads are used in ICD systems. Such leads should have closely spaced electrodes to reduce the risk of far-field sensing of ventricular electrograms. For biventricular pacing ICDs (CRT-D), a third lead is implanted, typically in a posterior or lateral branch of the coronary sinus venous system. These leads are passive fixation and may be unipolar or bipolar. Novel active fixation methods are being developed for left ventricular leads, which may be very useful given the high incidence of dislodgement compared with right-sided pacing leads.

Acute defibrillation testing is performed to ensure an adequate safety margin for the treatment of spontaneous arrhythmias. In common usage, the defibrillation threshold (DFT) is defined as the lowest energy that successfully terminates VF. Unlike the pacing threshold, however, the DFT is not an absolute value above which defibrillation will always be successful and below which it will always fail. Instead, the likelihood of defibrillation at any energy level is a probability of success. The relationship between probability of successful defibrillation vs. the energy delivered yields a sigmoidal shaped curve (Fig. 8.4). The goal of defibrillation testing is to ensure that the maximal energy output of the device has an extremely high (> 99%) probability of terminating VF in a given patient. There are different methods to determine the DFT, and each method provides a value with different significance.

The DFT value derived from each testing method establishes different positions on the defibrillation success curve for a given patient. For example, a single termination of fibrillation with a given energy level (DFT, Table 8.3) identifies an energy that may terminate fibrillation in as few as 25% of repeated attempts due to the probabilistic nature of defibrillation. However, by demonstrating that this same shock energy terminates VF three times without failure, it is established that energy level is high on the probability curve for success and in fact has at least a 75% chance of terminating fibrillation on further attempts.

Understanding precisely what a given DFT value represents allows the physician to program an appropriate safety margin of energy output above the DFT to ensure termination of all VF episodes. In practice, the simple convention of programming output to 10 J greater than the DFT is widely accepted and usually provides reliable defibrillation. This method is expedient at implant, but lesser energy margins may be satisfactory as well if more thorough testing is performed[26] (Table 8.3).

There are many testing algorithms to assess defibrillation efficacy and to determine a value for DFT (Fig. 8.5), but two methods predominate: the single-energy success and step-down protocols. For both methods, the first shock is typically set at least 10 J less than the maximal output of the device. VF is induced by pacing through the right ventricular electrode or with a low-energy shock on the T wave. The pulse generator will then automatically sense the arrhythmia, charge, and deliver a shock. If the first shock is successful, then this energy level can be repeated once or twice more (single-energy success method). This technique allows for minimal testing to establish adequate

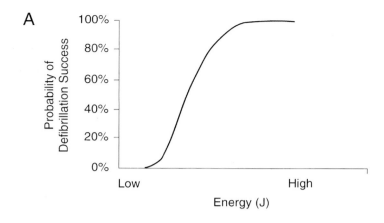

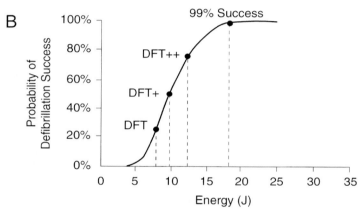

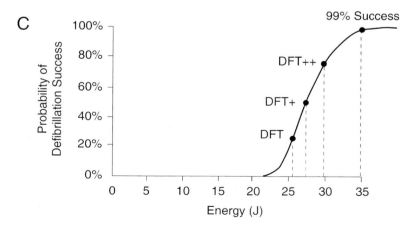

Table 8.3 Safety margins for implantable cardioverter defibrillators based on defibrillation threshold (DFT) method

Method	Technique	Definition	Estimated minimal energy for 99% success
DFT	Step-down to failure	Lowest energy level yielding a single successful defibrillation	$2 \times$ DFT
DFT+	Step-down to failure and repeat last successful energy	Lowest energy level yielding two successful defibrillations without a failure	$1.5 \times$ DFT
DFT++	Step-down to failure and repeat last successful energy twice	Lowest energy level yielding three successful defibrillations without a failure	$1.2 \times$ DFT or $+ 5$ J
Bayesian	Testing in up or down increments based on response to previous attempt	Completion of a four-shock algorithm	Bayesian DFT $+100$V
Single energy, two successes	Single energy level tested twice	Two successful defibrillations without failure at the same energy level	$2 \times$ DFT
Single energy, three successes	Single energy level tested three times	Three successful defibrillations without failure at the same energy level	$1.7 \times$ DFT

Recommendations are based on extensive animal studies and mathematical modeling; appropriate testing in each patient is mandatory. (See Singer I, Lang D. The defibrillation threshold. In: Kroll MW, Lehmann MH, eds. Implantable cardioverter defibrillator therapy. The Engineering Clinical Interface. Norwell: Kluwer Academic, 1996:89–129.)

Fig. 8.4 Graphical representation of the relationship between probability of successful defibrillation vs. energy level of shock. (A) The generalized defibrillation success curve is sigmoidal in shape. (B) Defibrillation success curve for a hypothetical patient. If the defibrillation threshold (DFT) is measured as a single successful defibrillation at a given energy level (DFT), the confidence for repeated success is lower than if an energy level is tested that defibrillates two (DFT) or three times (DFT) without failure. The safety margin for programming is the difference between the measured value of DFT and the energy needed for > 99% successful defibrillation. In this case the safety margins are approximately 10, 8 and 6 J for DFT, DFT+ and DFT++, respectively (see Table 8.3). The energy level for 99% success is never really known for any patient, however. The safety margins for any measure of DFT are estimated empirically based on the assumption that the shape of the DFT curve is relatively consistent between patients. (C) In this hypothetical patient, all measures of DFT are high. Using a safety margin of 10 J added to the DFT+ or DFT++ would require a device with at least 37 J output to ensure > 99% successful defibrillation. This patient would require revision of the lead system to reduce the DFTs or the implantation of a high-output device.

Step Down Protocols

Binary Search

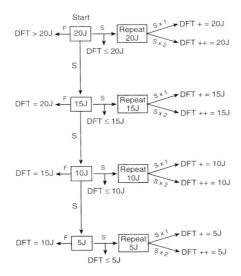

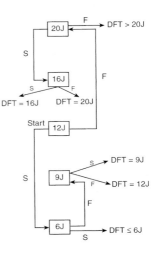

Bayesian Search

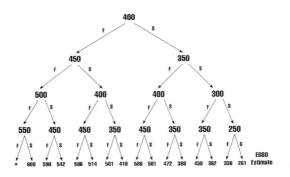

Fig. 8.5 Defibrillation threshold (DFT) testing algorithms. The step-down protocol is most commonly used clinically. Starting at 10 J less than the maximal output of the device (20 J in this example), successful defibrillation may either be repeated at this energy (single-energy success protocol) or stepped down incrementally until failure. The lowest energy level to defibrillate successfully is the DFT. By repeating this energy once or twice without failure, the DFT+ and DFT− are defined. J, joules; S, successful defibrillation; F, failed defibrillation. The binary search protocol starts at intermediate energy levels and again the lowest energy level to defibrillate is the DFT. This energy may be repeated for verification. The Bayesian search protocol shown here was developed for use with St Jude Medical defibrillators. The numerical values represent the voltage output for defibrillation testing using Ventritex devices. The algorithm was constructed mathematically and verified in clinical testing. The voltage output specified by the algorithm after completing the series of four inductions of ventricular fibrillation identifies the ED80 or energy that terminates 80% of fibrillation episodes (*DFT > 550 V). (Bayesian protocol reproduced with permission from Malkin RA, Herre JM, McGowen L *et al.* A four-shock Bayesian up-down estimator of the 80% effective defibrillation dose. J Cardiovasc Electrophysiol 1999; 10:973–80.)

acute defibrillation efficacy. Alternatively, in the "step-down method" the shock energy is decreased on each trial until a shock energy is reached that fails to defibrillate. The lowest energy level to defibrillate successfully is the DFT. This energy level may be tested an additional one or two times if desired to ensure further the likelihood of success. Other algorithms that can be used to determine DFT are the binary search method, in which shock energy is decreased or increased depending on the results of the preceding defibrillation trial, or the Bayesian search method (Fig. 8.5). When ICD shocks fail, a high-output internal or transthoracic shock should be given immediately for arrhythmia termination. There is increasing interest in minimizing defibrillation testing. Consequently, the practice of testing only one episode of VF and then programming devices to maximum output is gaining in popularity. Typically, this is performed at an energy 15–20 J below the maximum output of the device. This strategy probably works because of the very high efficacy of modern lead systems and shock waveforms.[27] There is even a growing practice of performing no defibrillation testing at the time of implantation, although the prospective data to support this strategy are lacking.

Alternatively, determination of the upper limit of vulnerability (ULV) has been used to estimate the DFT while minimizing or even eliminating the need for VF inductions.[28] By delivering shocks of decreasing energy synchronized to the T wave, a minimal energy level is found that does not induce VF while lower energies induce fibrillation. The lowest energy value that does not induce fibrillation is the ULV. The ULV is probabilistic, as is the actual DFT. The ULV is highly correlated with the DFT, and may obviate inductions of VF although multiple shocks in sinus rhythm are required.[28]

At least 2 min, and more typically 3–5 min, should be allowed between defibrillation episodes to ensure full hemodynamic recovery and minimize any cumulative effects of multiple shocks. The appropriate sensing of each episode of induced arrhythmia should be confirmed after each induction. The sensitivity is typically decreased at implant testing (e.g. from 0.3 to 1.2 mV) as an additional safety measure to ensure that there will be adequate sensing of spontaneous ventricular arrhythmias. Although acute defibrillation testing is typically performed using the implanted pulse generator, an external defibrillator that delivers identical shocks to the pulse generator was often used in earlier generations of ICDs and can also be used.

The postoperative management of the patient includes monitoring of vital signs and heart rhythm during the recovery from anesthesia or conscious sedation, as well as the completion of a course of perioperative antibiotics. A chest radiograph is performed to document lead position and to rule out complications from the implantation such as a pneumothorax. Typically, the lead function is assessed non-invasively before the patient is discharged from the hospital. Repeat predischarge defibrillation testing is no longer recommended. The duration of postoperative hospitalization has decreased remarkably with modern ICD technology. Often patients are discharged < 24 h after surgery, and some implants can be performed on an outpatient basis for primary prevention indications.

The follow-up of patients after ICD implantation usually consists of an early evaluation of wound healing and lead integrity. This is often performed approximately 2–4 weeks after implantation. At that visit, chronic pacing outputs can be programmed and lead function can be assessed non-invasively. Traditionally, ICD patients are evaluated with device interrogation and threshold testing every 3 months. However, given the reliability of modern pulse generators and leads, follow-up every 6 months among clinically stable patients is rapidly becoming the norm. Transtelephonic monitoring of ICDs is growing in popularity, and this approach can further reduce the frequency of office visits.

Rate sensing

Sensing of ventricular tachyarrhythmias is a critically important function of an ICD system. The ability to sense small-amplitude signals rapidly during VF, while not oversensing T waves or noise in the absence of tachyarrhythmias, is mandatory for proper ICD function. This goal was difficult to achieve with fixed gain sensing, as is used in pacemaker systems. All ICD pulse generators use automatic adjustment of amplifier gain or sensing threshold to ensure appropriate detection of ventricular arrhythmias. These algorithms effectively increase the amplifier sensitivity over time between sensed or paced ventricular events to search for low-amplitude fibrillatory electrograms that may be missed at lower sensitivities. One such algorithm is shown in Fig. 8.6. In addition to these sophisticated sensing algorithms, the need for stable lead performance is mandatory to ensure normal detection of tachyarrhythmias.

Undersensing of VF was rarely noted with early epicardial or bipolar transvenous leads after automatic gain or sensitivity was employed. Data from large clinical trials of integrated transvenous leads have demonstrated excellent detection of VT and VF, indicating that clinically important undersensing is very rare.[29] At present, both true bipolar sensing, with a dedicated tip and ring, and integrated sensing, where the distal coil is used for both sensing and shocks, are available.

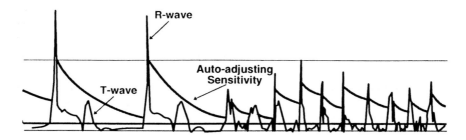

Fig. 8.6 A schematic representation of automatic sensitivity during sinus rhythm and ventricular fibrillation. In sinus rhythm, sensitivity increases slowly to avoid oversensing T waves. However, with the onset of ventricular fibrillation, high sensitivity is maintained to minimize undersensing. (Reproduced with permission from Medtronic Inc., Minneapolis, MN, USA.)

Another area of potential difficulty with sensing occurs when ICDs are used in conjunction with separate pacemakers. The proximity of the endocardial pacemaker and ICD leads within the ventricle can lead to several problems, including double-counting during pacing, which can cause inappropriate shocks, and sensing of pacemaker pulses during VF, which can inhibit detection of VF and thus therapy. The problems of pacemaker–ICD interactions are largely of historical interest with the development of dual-chamber, rate-responsive ICD systems. Such systems provide all of the basic capabilities of permanent pacemakers, obviating implanting or retaining separate devices.

Although undersensing of ventricular tachyarrhythmias is very unusual with modern lead systems and pulse generators, oversensing of other biological signals is now more common. The maximum sensitivity of pulse generators is increased (up to 0.15 mV) with contemporary low-noise amplifiers. At maximal sensitivity, myopotentials arising from the diaphragm or pectoral muscles can cause inappropriate ICD discharges. This problem is more likely to occur during periods of ventricular pacing, when the amplifier sensitivity is maximized, and with integrated bipolar ICD leads. Often a history of coughing or straining preceding ICD discharges can be elicited from the patient, suggesting that myopotential oversensing is present. Such oversensing can be confirmed by monitoring ventricular electrograms during provocative maneuvers such as handgrip, Valsalva, or deep inspiration. Several strategies have been used to prevent further ICD oversensing, including decreasing the maximum sensitivity of the pulse generator, decreasing the bradycardic pacing rate or increasing the AV delay to minimize ventricular pacing, prolonging the detection intervals to prevent shocks from transient oversensing, and implanting a separate rate-sensing lead in the right ventricular outflow tract more distant from the diaphragmatic surface. Oversensing of T waves with double-counting is another problem observed more frequently with modern pulse generators because of increased maximum sensitivity and aggressive sensing algorithms. Again, this can often be avoided with device reprogramming including reducing the maximum sensitivity, prolonging the refractory period or reducing the aggressiveness of the autosensitivity algorithm.

Extensive data logging capabilities are present in pulse generators. All systems provide beat-to-beat interval data for detected tachyarrhythmias. This is helpful for identifying the arrhythmias associated with shocks. For example, very irregular intervals are suggestive of atrial fibrillation, whereas the sudden onset of a regular tachycardia is indicative of either monomorphic VT or paroxysmal supraventricular tachycardia (SVT). A very rapid rhythm with non-physiological intervals (< 130 ms) is indicative of a sensing malfunction, typically due to either a lead defect or a loose set-screw in the pulse generator header.

Stored electrograms can be used as a further diagnostic tool (see Fig. 8.1). This significantly improves the physician's ability to interpret the appropriateness of defibrillation shocks.[30] The electrodes used to record the electrogram may or may not be the same electrodes used for the detection of arrhythmias.

"Near-field" electrograms are recordings of the local bipolar ventricular electrogram, which is also used for arrhythmia detection. This can either be a true bipolar sensing, with recording from the electrode tip to a more proximal ring, or extended bipolar sensing from the tip to a right ventricular shocking coil. For "far-field" electrograms, recordings are made between shocking electrodes, which for a typical transvenous lead system includes a right ventricular coil, a left pectoral active pulse generator, and often a more proximal coil in the right atrium or superior vena cava. Far-field recordings potentially allow for the identification of atrial activity to aid in arrhythmia classification. In addition, the change in morphology of ventricular arrhythmias is often more obvious in the far-field electrograms. The source of stored electrograms is important for interpreting arrhythmia episodes, particularly inappropriate therapy. For example, if the far-field electrogram recorded from the shocking electrodes is being monitored, then this is not the same signal that is being sensed by the amplifier for the determination of tachyarrhythmias. Thus, if no tachycardia is noted at the time of therapy for a rapid rate, then oversensing of the rate-sensing lead can be deduced, but extraneous "noise" may not be demonstrated. Examples of stored electrograms with a lead malfunction are shown in Fig. 8.7. With dual-chamber ICDs, direct atrial recordings further simplify the interpretation of arrhythmias (Fig. 8.8).

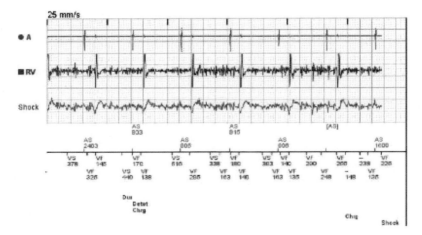

Fig. 8.7 Stored electrograms from a dual-chamber implantable cardioverter defibrillator (ICD) with a fracture of the pace–sense component of the right ventricular ICD lead. Note the oversensing of non-physiological electrical activity, seen on both the near-field (RV tip-coil) and far-field (Shock, RV coil-can). This was interpreted by the device as ventricular fibrillation, as highlighted on the marker channel, and a shock was delivered. The patient received multiple inappropriate shocks for this noise, necessitating a lead revision procedure. A, near-field atrial channel; RV, near-field RV tip-coil (integrated bipolar configuration); Shock, far-field RV coil-can; AS, atrial sensed event; VS, ventricular sensed event; VF, ventricular sensed event in VF rate zone.

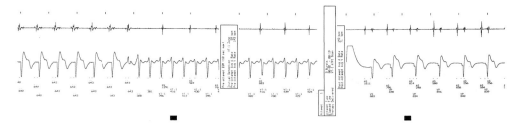

Fig. 8.8 Stored electrogram from a dual-chamber implantable cardioverter defibrillator. The bipolar atrial electrogram is shown in the top panel. Below is the far-field electrogram in the triad configuration (sensing from right ventricle to right atrium and left pectoral pulse generator). Initially the patient is in sinus rhythm, but ventricular tachycardia with clear AV dissociation develops. Following a burst of antitachycardia pacing (not shown), sinus rhythm is restored on the far right panel of the electrogram. Note how the atrial electrogram simplifies the interpretation of rhythms.

Arrhythmia detection

Arrhythmia detection requires effective sensing of the intrinsic cardiac activity and the fulfillment of the programmed detection algorithm. For VT, most ICDs require that a certain number of consecutive R–R intervals be shorter than the tachycardia detection interval for the VT zone (Fig. 8.9). Because the VF electrograms may transiently be very low in amplitude and undersensed, the VF detection algorithms require that a certain percentage (typically 75%) of R–R intervals in a rolling window of cardiac cycles be shorter than the VF detection interval (see Fig. 8.9). After each delivered therapy, the ICD must determine whether the tachycardia was terminated. The redetection criteria after therapies are usually somewhat less demanding than the initial detection criteria for each zone. The detection criteria in the VT zone may be modified by algorithms to prevent inappropriate therapy for SVTs.

Supraventricular tachycardia discrimination

Multiple algorithms have been employed to allow ICDs to discriminate between ventricular and supraventricular tachycardias, which is critical to minimize inappropriate therapies. There are several basic interval-based discrimination algorithms that vary slightly in their programming amongst device manufacturers. These can be programmed to be used in isolation or together, depending on physician preference. Once criteria for SVT are met, the device will withhold therapy, sometimes for a predefined period of time, after which if tachycardia continues in the VT zone, therapy will be delivered. Interval stability is useful in discriminating irregular SVTs (e.g. atrial fibrillation) from VTs, which are usually regular. There are, however, exceptions in which VTs may be irregular and interval stability algorithms may inappropriately withhold therapy (i.e. VT with concomitant antiarrhythmic therapy or polymorphic VT). Onset algorithms help discriminate sinus

VT DETECTION

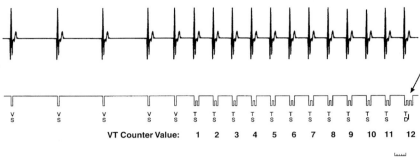

VT Counter Value: 1 2 3 4 5 6 7 8 9 10 11 12

200 ms

VF DETECTION

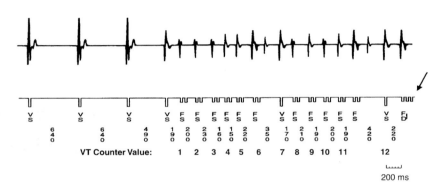

VT Counter Value: 1 2 3 4 5 6 7 8 9 10 11 12

200 ms

Fig. 8.9 Basic ventricular tachycardia (VT) and fibrillation (VF) detection algorithms. In both panels, the tracings are from top to bottom: ventricular electrogram, marker channel, and counter value (labeled) for detection. VS, ventricular sensing below tachycardia detection rate; TS, sensing in the VT zone; TDI, tachycardia detection completed (arrow); FS, sensing in the VF zone; FDI, fibrillation detection completed (arrow). Top: For ventricular tachycardia detection in this example, the criteria are 12 consecutive intervals shorter than the tachycardia detection interval of 400 ms. If an interval > 400 ms had occurred in this episode, the counter would have been reset to zero at that point. Bottom: For VF detection, occasional undersensing is anticipated. The detection criteria in this example are 12 out of 16 consecutive intervals shorter than the fibrillation detection interval of 320 ms. Here two long intervals of 350 and 420 ms are recorded due to signal drop out; however, fibrillation is still detected. (Courtesy of Medtronic, Inc., Minneapolis, MN, USA.)

tachycardia, which usually gradually increases its rate into the detection zone, from tachycardias which rapidly "jump" into the VT zone. The rate of onset for discrimination is a programmable feature on most devices. This algorithm is limited by the fact that paroxysmal SVT and atrial flutter also rapidly change rates and are classified as VT by the device, leading to the delivery of therapy inappropriately.

More complex algorithms compare AV relationships, and withhold therapy if the atrial rate is greater than the ventricular rate (e.g. atrial fibrillation or flutter). Finally, ICDs can also employ morphology algorithms, which allow the device to compare stored baseline electrograms (i.e. in sinus rhythm) with those during tachycardia and withhold therapy if morphologies "match." Like the other algorithms, morphology discriminators have their limitations; for example, aberrant conduction during SVT can cause major changes in electrogram morphology that will result in low match scores. Figure 8.10 illustrates an example of how morphology algorithms work and are used in the discrimination of SVT and VT.[31] Additionally, many modern devices can use combinations of these algorithms to discriminate between VT and SVT.

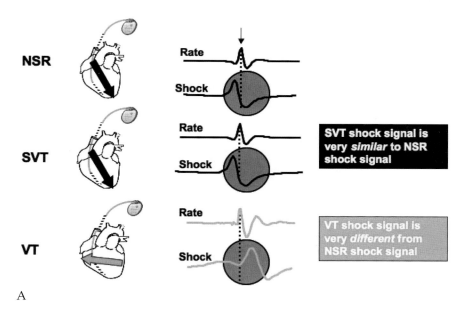

A

Fig. 8.10 An example of a morphology discrimination algorithm (Rhythm ID, Boston Scientific, Inc.).[31] (A) The algorithm works by comparing shock electrogram morphology during tachycardia with that obtained and stored during normal sinus rhythm (NSR), under the premise that the morphology and timing relationships between the two electrograms during supraventricular tachycardia (SVT) will be similar to that during NSR (barring any aberrant conduction), whereas the shock electrogram will be markedly different during ventricular tachycardia (VT) compared with NSR. (B) The correlation between the shock channel morphologies during NSR and the unknown rhythm is calculated from amplitudes for eight time-prescribed comparison points. (C) If the correlation between the shock channel morphologies during NSR and the unknown rhythm is > 94%, the algorithm identifies the rhythm as an SVT, otherwise it indicates that it is VT. (*Continued.*)

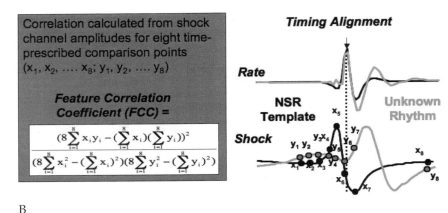

B

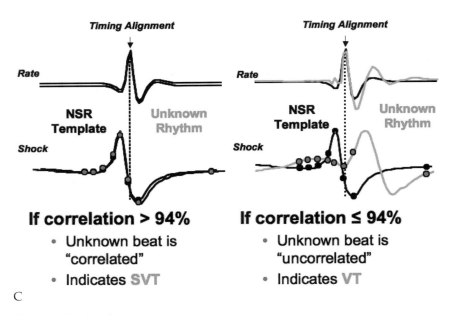

Fig. 8.10 (*Continued.*)

Implantable cardioverter defibrillator therapies

Pacing

All ICD pulse generators have pacing capabilities. This can be simple back-up bradycardia support (VVI mode), more physiological pacing modes with or without rate responsiveness (e.g. DDDR), or high-rate pacing for the termination of VT or supraventricular tachyarrhythmias (SVT or atrial flutter). Ventricular pacing prevents long pauses that occur spontaneously or following shocks for ventricular tachyarrhythmias. Such post-shock pauses can contribute to the hemodynamic compromise associated with these arrhythmias. In fact, in some patients, syncopal episodes associated with appropriate ICD therapy are due to the post-shock pause and not to the primary tachyarrhythmia.

The use of dual-chamber ICD systems has increased dramatically since they were first approved in 1997. It is estimated that approximately 70% of new ICD systems (not including biventricular pacing devices) implanted in the USA were dual-chamber devices in 2005. This is a much greater percentage than the 5–10% of patients who received both pacemakers and ICDs previously, suggesting that this usage is not due solely to the need for atrial pacing for standard indications. Many factors are probably responsible for this discrepancy. Dual-chamber ICDs are likely to be being implanted in an "anticipatory" manner, such as in patients who may receive negative chronotropic drugs or those with conduction system abnormalities (e.g. first-degree AV block or QRS prolongation), when permanent pacemakers would not have been used. Also, dual-chamber ICDs are being implanted for reasons other than to provide atrial-based bradycardia pacing, such as to improve arrhythmia discrimination or to provide therapy for atrial tachyarrhythmias. However, the DAVID study has demonstrated the potential adverse effects of dual-chamber pacing.[22] Moreover, the results of dual-chamber discrimination algorithms to prevent inappropriate shocks have been disappointing.[32] For these reasons and because of regulatory restriction on dual-chamber ICDs, their usage has decreased somewhat. Multiple studies have demonstrated the long-term deleterious effects of frequent right ventricular pacing. Such pacing can be minimized in single-chamber systems by programming a low rate (e.g. VVI 35–40 bpm). For dual-chamber ICD systems, prolonging the AV delay, or activating features such as AV search hysteresis or mode switching from AAI mode to DDD mode during heart block, can serve to reduce the percentage of ventricular pacing. In contrast to avoiding ventricular pacing with single- and dual-chamber devices, biventricular ICDs (CRT-D) are designed specifically to pace the right and left ventricles. These systems are indicated for patients with severe CHF (NYHA III–IV), left ventricular systolic dysfunction and QRS prolongation, typically left bundle branch block.

Antitachycardia pacing

High-rate, overdrive pacing is very effective for terminating VT. Adaptive algorithms are used, in which the pacing rate is programmed based upon the tachycardia cycle length of each episode of tachycardia (Fig. 8.11). Randomized studies have shown similar efficacy of burst (constant cycle length in the train) and ramp (decremental cycle lengths in the train) pacing in this setting (Fig. 8.12). Interestingly, the success rates for pace termination of spontaneous episodes of VT are higher than for induced episodes, typically approximately 90%, whereas arrhythmia acceleration rates are low (1–3%).[33] Presumably, the high efficacy of terminating spontaneous VTs is due to the

BURST

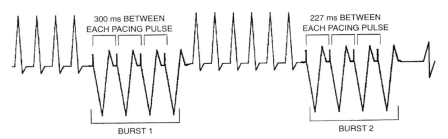

RAMP

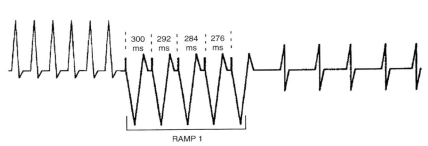

Fig. 8.11 Schematic representation of burst and ramp antitachycardia pacing (ATP). Top: Four beats of ventricular tachycardia are followed by the first burst of ATP at 300 ms for four beats. The rate for this burst is determined as a programmable percentage of the tachycardia cycle length. Tachycardia continues after burst 1, so after redetection burst 2 is delivered at a programmable rate faster than burst 1 (227 ms in this example). The pacing interval for subsequent bursts will decrement further until a minimum pacing cycle length is reached, all ATP attempts are delivered, or the tachycardia terminates. Bottom: In ramp ATP there is a decrement in the pacing interval between consecutive stimuli. The initial pacing rate starts as a percentage of the tachycardia cycle length. Multiple ramp attempts can be programmed with shorter intervals in each subsequent attempt. (Courtesy of Guidant Corp.)

slower rates of these episodes compared with induced tachycardias. These observations support a strategy of empiric programming of antitachycardia pacing in patients with the underlying substrate for monomorphic VT (Table 8.4).[34] There is a relative paucity of data concerning the clinical predictors of unsuccessful pace termination of VT, other than rapid tachycardia rates (> 200 bpm) and very poor left ventricular function.[34] However, even very rapid tachycardias can be pace terminated in a sufficient proportion of episodes to justify programming empiric pacing at rates above 200 bpm to reduce the number of shocks.[34]

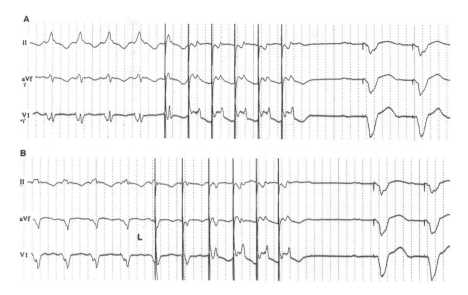

Fig. 8.12 Antitachycardia pacing termination of ventricular tachycardia. Examples of (A) burst and (B) ramp pacing to terminate tachycardia in a patient are shown. Note that the morphology and rate of ventricular tachycardia differ in two episodes in the same patient, illustrating the utility of adaptive rate pacing from the implantable cardioverter defibrillator. Bradycardia pacing is present at the termination of ventricular tachycardia.

Table 8.4 Guidelines for ICD programming

Programming should take into account:
Use of β-blockers
Heart rate during exercise
Rate of prior documented VT
Rate of prior documented non-sustained VTs
Rate of prior documented SVTs
Device programming

VF Zone: 18 out of 24 last R–R intervals CL < 320 ms (> 188 bpm): if last eight R–R intervals were < 240 ms (> 250 bpm), episode detected as VF and treated as shock at DFT + 10 J shock. If all the last eight R–R intervals were ≥ 240 ms (≤ 250 bpm), episode detected as FVT: single ATP sequence (eight pulse burst pacing train at 88% ventricular tachycardia CL, failed ATP followed by shock at DFT + 10 J).
VT zone with a CL of 320 to ≥ 360 ms (≤ 167 to 188 bpm): three sequences of ATP at 88% of VT cycle length with 20-ms decrement between sequences.
SVT discrimination programmed on in the VT zone of all dual-chamber ICDs with the SVT limit of 320 ms.
All devices programmed to store far-field electrogram before the onset of detected episodes.
ATP, antitachycardia pacing; CL, cycle length; SVT, supraventricular tachycardia; VF, ventricular fibrillation; VT, ventricular tachycardia.

Defibrillation

Defibrillation is achieved when a critical mass of myocardium is depolarized by establishing a critical voltage gradient throughout the ventricular tissue. The dispersion of the voltage gradient and current flow depends on the positioning of the high-voltage lead electrodes in and/or around the heart. Failure to defibrillate may be due to a residual mass of fibrillating tissue or immediate reinduction of fibrillation in areas of low electrical gradient. All ICD pulse generators achieve defibrillation by applying voltage to a capacitor, which is then discharged through the lead system. The resulting waveform is an exponentially declining voltage, which is prematurely terminated or truncated before full capacitor discharge. Thus, the maximal delivered energy for an ICD is always less than the stored energy necessary to charge the capacitor fully. In the early ICD systems, monophasic waveforms were used that were truncated at about 35% of the leading edge voltage; this is referred to as a 65% tilt monophasic shock (Fig. 8.13). This waveform was chosen because animal studies have shown a lower defibrillation efficacy with shorter or longer duration pulses. However, more recent human studies have demonstrated that DFTs are not affected by pulse duration over a wide range of pulse widths, including tilts up to 95%.[35] Accordingly, adjusting pulse width is unlikely to have significant effects on defibrillation efficacy. The truncation of shocks from ICD pulse generators allowed the development of more complex waveforms, because the undelivered voltage remaining on the capacitors at the end of the pulse is still available. Biphasic waveforms were shown consistently to reduce defibrillation energy requirements compared with monophasic shocks.[36] For biphasic shocks, the polarity of the voltage pulse is reversed after the termination of the initial positive phase and a second negative phase is delivered. Biphasic waveforms are now the standard waveform for all ICD pulse generators. More complicated ascending ramp waveforms can reduce defibrillation energy requirements further, but it is unlikely that there will be a sufficient reduction of DFTs to merit changing waveforms in implantable devices.

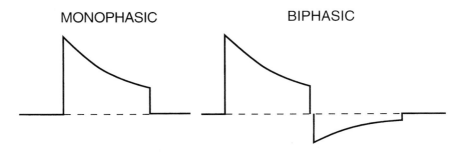

MONOPHASIC   BIPHASIC

Fig. 8.13 Schematic representation of defibrillation waveforms. The time course of the delivered voltage for monophasic and biphasic shocks is shown. Note that shock waveforms are truncated exponentially declining pulses.

Another factor that can affect DFTs is the polarity of the defibrillation shock. Initially, studies of transvenous lead systems used the right ventricular coil as the cathode for shocks. However, reverse polarity, or anodal shocks, result in significantly lower DFTs.[37] Shock polarity has a smaller effect on biphasic DFTs, but anodal first phase shocks are still preferred.[37,38] The polarity of the shock is programmable, but to minimize defibrillation testing the initial configuration to evaluate should be the right ventricular coil as the anode. In some devices different high-voltage electrodes may be reprogrammed in or out of the circuit as well.

Capacitance is another factor that may affect defibrillation efficacy. Capacitors are important components of pulse generator size, so if DFTs are decreased with lower capacitance, then pulse generator size could be reduced. Decreasing capacitance to 60 or 90 μF has reduced DFTs modestly in some studies,[39] but has had no effect on stored energy requirements and increased peak voltage in other studies. The defibrillation safety margin is reduced with lower capacitance because of the higher peak voltages required, so the strategy of marked reductions of pulse generator capacitance is unlikely to be pursued in the future.

Once biphasic waveforms became ubiquitous, the most important advance for lowering DFTs was the development of active pulse generators. With the downsizing of pulse generator size to allow for pectoral placement, the pulse generator shell can become part of the lead system. Such active pulse generators are also known as "hot cans" or "active cans." The active can was first evaluated in humans using a shocking configuration from a right ventricular coil to a left pectoral pulse generator. This lead system was termed the unipolar configuration because only a single endocardial electrode is used, analogous to unipolar pacing where the pacemaker pulse generator serves as the return pathway for current from the right ventricular electrode. These investigators showed that adequate DFTs (< 20 J) could be achieved in approximately 90% of patients with this simple single-coil lead system. Subsequently, it was confirmed that DFTs were lower in the unipolar configuration than in a dual-coil, transvenous configuration (where current is delivered between two coils, one in the right ventricle and the other in the superior vena cava). DFTs are relatively insensitive to pulse generator size, indicating that defibrillation efficacy will not be affected adversely as pulse generators get progressively smaller.

The effect of combining an active pectoral pulse generator with a dual-coil lead was evaluated independent of the development of the unipolar lead configuration. This was called the "triad" configuration because of the presence of three shocking electrodes, the active can and two transvenous coils. In the initial study of this lead system, it was shown that the mean DFT decreased by 36% compared with a dual-coil shocking vector.[40] This benefit was due more to the lowering of impedance with the active can than to an improvement in the shocking vector. Subsequent studies have compared the defibrillation efficacy of multiple lead configurations. DFTs in the triad lead configuration were again much lower than in the dual-coil transvenous lead configuration, as well as 23% lower than in the single-coil unipolar configuration. In the largest study comparing active can defibrillation configurations, the unipolar and triad configurations were measured in 50 patients.[41] Both the mean and the variability of DFTs were lower in the triad configuration. In this study, 98% of patients had a threshold < 15 J. Of particular clinical relevance is the reduction of the number of patients with high thresholds, because such patients have an inadequate safety margin and often require complicated implantation procedures to test multiple lead positions or shocking vectors. The uniformly low thresholds with dual-coil, active can lead systems have simplified implantation testing of these systems.

The effect of proximal coil position has also been evaluated. When shocking between two coils and no active can, positioning a second lead in the left subclavian vein is optimal because it directs current more toward the left side of the heart compared with a more proximal position in the superior vena cava. However, no such benefit of the proximal coil position is observed when an active can is part of the shocking circuit,[42] indicating that single-pass dual-coil leads with fixed intercoil spacing should minimize DFTs without the need for additional leads. The intercoil spacing should be sufficient to ensure that the proximal coil is in the innominate vein and not in the right atrium. This has become the standard lead system for implants. Single-coil leads are still used in pediatric patients and in some other situations where complications from the proximal coil are more likely. Single-coil leads are easier to extract, so they are chosen at times in patients at higher risk for infections (e.g. hemodialysis, immunocompromised, severe dermatological disease, etc) or younger patients with a long life expectancy.

The anatomical position of an active pulse generator is important for determining its effect on DFTs. In the right pectoral region, there is no significant change in thresholds with the use of an active can compared with a dual-coil transvenous lead.[43] This is because an active can increases defibrillation current requirements due to a worsened shock vector, which is directed away from the left ventricle and toward the right shoulder. The reduction in impedance with the active can offsets the increased current, resulting in no net effect on threshold. Active can DFTs are lower with left-sided systems than right-sided systems. Moreover, long-term mortality is much higher among patients with right-sided ICDs, probably due to the comorbidities mandating such an anatomical approach (e.g. AV fistula, previous mastectomy, etc.).

Despite the marked reduction of defibrillation thresholds with active pectoral pulse generators, there are still some patients with unacceptably high thresholds. Unfortunately, identifying these patients prospectively is difficult. Raitt and colleagues have evaluated the clinical predictors of defibrillation efficacy in 101 patients with a unipolar defibrillation system.[44] The only independent predictors of the biphasic DFT were left ventricular mass and resting heart rate. However, all correlations with DFTs were weak. Similarly, no routine clinical factors reliably predict high thresholds in the triad configuration.[45] The possible causes of high DFTs at implant and potential corrective measures are listed in Table 8.5.

Fortunately, the proportion of patients with high DFTs is small with left pectoral active can lead systems. If an adequate safety margin cannot be demonstrated at implantation, then further testing is necessary. The simplest change is to reverse the polarity of the shocks. Other changes that can be made include repositioning leads, placing a second coil, implanting a subcutaneous patch or array,[46] or adding a type III antiarrhythmic drug such as dofetilide or sotalol that can reduce thresholds. Although most popular ICDs have maximal energy outputs of about 30–35 J, most manufacturers also produce high-energy units with delivered energy up to 41 J. These high-output devices are useful in patients with elevated DFTs despite testing different lead configurations. However, pulse generator longevity is reduced and charge times are prolonged with high-output devices, so they are not used routinely. Figure 8.14 illustrates an algorithm to guide the approach to managing the patient with high DFTs.

Table 8.5 Causes and corrections for high defibrillation thresholds (DFTs) at implant

Cause of elevated DFT	Diagnosis	Correction
Poor lead position	On fluoroscopy distal coil out of RV, proximal coil low in atrium	Reposition lead
Increased high-voltage impedance	Data from defibrillation attempt, commanded determination of impedance	Check header connections, reposition lead and/or coils, add SVC to single-coil system, add SQ array, relieve pneumothorax
Pneumothorax	High shock impedance, fluoroscopy, dyspnea	Relieve pneumothorax
Hypoxia	Low oxygen saturation	Lighten sedation, assist ventilation
Ischemia	Chest pain, ECG changes, hypotension	Anti-ischemic therapy
Multiple defibrillations	Numerous previous defibrillation attempts	Implant device in best configuration and retest
Antiarrhythmic drugs or anesthetics	Exclude other etiologies	Retest after stopping drugs, stop inhaled anesthetics
Poor current distributions	High or low shocking impedance, poor lead positions	Reposition coil, add SVC coil to single-coil system, add SQ array
Shunting current through guidewires or retained leads	Retained guidewires, temporary or permanent pacing leads	Retest after removing wires or leads
Poor myocardial substrate	Exclusion of other causes, failure of multiple lead configurations and polarity	Add coils, SQ array, epicardial patches to circuit, use high-output device, add class III antiarrhythmic drugs that reduce DFTs

RV, right ventricle; SVC, superior vena cava; SQ, subcutaneous.

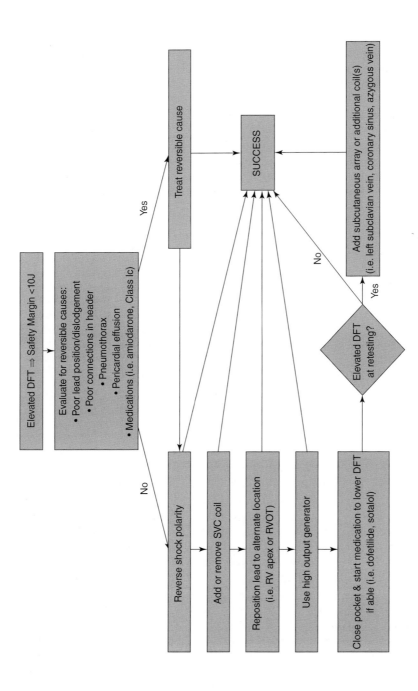

Fig. 8.14 Suggested algorithm for management of the patient with elevated defibrillation threshold (DFT), defined as a safety margin < 10 J below maximal device output. The implanter should first rule out and treat reversible causes of elevated DFTs, and then attempt further modifications to configurations and/or treatment regimen as illustrated. RV, right ventricular; RVOT, right ventricular outflow tract; SVC, superior vena cava.

Historically, an implantation safety margin of at least 10 J between the measured DFTs and the maximal output of the pulse generator is considered adequate. This is because such safety margins are associated with very low arrhythmic death rates in patients with first-generation devices and epicardial patch lead systems.[47] This has led to the common practice of programming shock strengths to at least 10 J greater than the DFTs measured at implantation. Results from the Low Energy Safety Study (LESS) suggest that a safety margin of approximately 5 J may be adequate with modern ICD systems employing biphasic waveforms, transvenous leads, and active pectoral pulse generators when rigorous DFT testing (DFT++) is used.[26]

Traditionally, DFTs were measured only at implantation. This strategy was supported by studies showing no significant change of DFTs chronically with epicardial lead systems. However, mean DFTs with transvenous leads and monophasic waveforms increase over time, and this can lead to an inadequate safety margin that may require operative revision of the lead system. However, more recent studies indicate that DFTs are stable with biphasic waveforms. In a study evaluating chronic changes of monophasic and biphasic DFTs in the same patients, monophasic thresholds increased 23% during a mean follow-up time of 8 months, whereas biphasic thresholds were essentially unchanged.[48] More long-term follow-up evaluations have confirmed the overall stability of biphasic DFTs, although a small minority of patients may show an increase.[26] Thus, routine re-evaluation of defibrillation function is no longer commonly performed. Such testing is still necessary among patients treated with antiarrhythmic drugs, particularly amiodarone, those patients with marginal defibrillation efficacy at implantation and among patients in whom the initial shock has failed to terminate a spontaneous episode of VT or fibrillation.

Summary

ICD therapy has undergone a remarkable transformation in the 25 years since the devices were first approved for human use. The early devices were "shock boxes" with almost no diagnostic capabilities, and they required median sternotomy or thoracotomy for epicardial patch implantation, with typical postoperative hospitalizations of approximately 1 week. Pulse generator longevity was < 2 years. Modern devices provide detailed information about the rate and morphology of electrocardiographic signals before, during and after therapy. The simplicity of defibrillator implantation now approaches that of pacemakers, because of the downsizing of pulse generators and improvements of lead design and shock waveforms. Despite the increase in diagnostic capabilities and the marked reduction in size, device longevity is now > 6 years. Routine outpatient ICD implantation is feasible and will certainly increase. Further advances in lead technology and arrhythmia discrimination algorithms should increase the efficacy and reliability of therapy. Finally, devices have the capabilities to treat multiple problems in addition to life-threatening ventricular arrhythmias, such as atrial arrhythmias and CHF.

References

1 Zipes DP, Camm AJ, Borggrefe M *et al.* ACC/AHA/ESC 2006 guidelines for management of patients with ventricular arrhythmias and the prevention of sudden cardiac death. Circulation 2006; 114:385–484.

2 The Antiarrhythmic Versus Implantable Defibrillator (AVID) Investigators. A comparison of antiarrhythmic-drug therapy with implantable defibrillators in patients resuscitated from near-fatal ventricular arrhythmias. N Engl J Med 1997; 337:1576–83.

3 Sheldon R, Connolly S, Krahn A *et al.* Identification of patients most likely to benefit from implantable cardioverter-defibrillator therapy: the Canadian Implantable Defibrillator Study. Circulation 2000; 101:1660–4.

4 Kuck K-H, Cappato R, Siebels J *et al.* Randomized comparison of antiarrhythmic drug therapy with implantable defibrillators in patients resuscitated from cardiac arrest: the Cardiac Arrest Study Hamburg (CASH). Circulation 2000; 102:748–54.

5 Moss A, Hall J, Cannom D *et al.* Improved survival with an implanted defibrillator in patients with coronary disease at high risk of ventricular arrhythmias. N Engl J Med 1997; 335:1933–40.

6 Buxton AE, Lee DL, Fisher JD *et al.* A randomized study of the prevention of sudden death in patients with coronary artery disease. N Engl J Med 1999; 341:1882–90.

7 Bigger JT. Prophylactic use of implanted cardiac defibrillators in patients at high risk for ventricular arrhythmias after coronary-artery bypass graft surgery. Coronary Artery Bypass Graft (CABG) Patch Trial Investigators. N Engl J Med 1997; 337:1569–75.

8 Buxton AE, Lee KL, DiCarlo L *et al.* Electrophysiologic testing to identify patients with coronary artery disease who are at risk for sudden death. N Engl J Med 2000; 342:1937–45.

9 Bardy GH, Lee KL, Mark DB *et al.* Amiodarone or an implantable cardioverter-defibrillator for congestive heart failure. N Engl J Med 2005; 352:225–37.

10 Kadish A, Dyer A, Daubert JP *et al.* Prophylactic defibrillator implantation in patients with nonischemic dilated cardiomyopathy. N Engl J Med 2004; 350:2151–8.

11 Moss AJ, Zareba W, Hall WJ *et al.* Prophylactic implantation of a defibrillator in patients with myocardial infarction and reduced ejection fraction. N Engl J Med 2002; 346:877–83.

12 Spirito P, Seidman CE, McKenna WJ, Maron BJ. The management of hypertrophic cardiomyopathy. N Engl J Med 1997; 366:775–85.

13 Nademanee K, Veerakul G, Mower M *et al.* Defibrillator versus β-blockers for unexplained death in Thailand (DEBUT): A randomized clinical trial. Circulation 2003; 107:2221–6.

14 Gold MR, Ensley D, Chilson D *et al.* T-wave alternans SCD HeFT study: primary endpoint analysis. Circulation 2006; 114:18:2113.

15 de Vreede-Swagemakers JJ, Gorgels AP, Dubois-Arbouw WI *et al.* Out-of-hospital cardiac arrest in the 1990's: a population-based study in the Maastricht area on incidence, characteristics and survival. J Am Coll Cardiol 1997; 30:1500–5.

16 Stecker EC, Vickers C, Waltz J *et al.* Population-based analysis of sudden cardiac death with and without left ventricular systolic dysfunction: two-year findings from the Oregon Sudden Unexpected Death Study. J Am Coll Cardiol 2006; 47:1161–6.

17 Gold MR, Peters RW, Johnson JW *et al.* Complications associated with pectoral cardioverter-defibrillator implantation: comparison of subcutaneous and submuscular approaches. J Am Coll Cardiol 1996; 28:1278–82.

18 Mirowski M, Mower MM, Gott VL *et al.* Feasibility and effectiveness of low-energy catheter defibrillation in man. Circulation 1973; 47:79–85.

19 Bardy GH, Johnson G, Poole JE *et al.* A simplified, single-lead unipolar transvenous cardioversion-defibrillation system. Circulation 1993; 88:543–7.

20 Ellenbogen KA, Wook MA, Shepard RK *et al.* Detection and management of an implantable cardioverter defibrillator lead failure: incidence and clinical implications. J Am Coll Cardiol 2003; 41:73–80.

21 Wilkoff BL, Belott PH, Love CJ *et al.* Improved extraction of ePTFE and medical adhesive modified defibrillation leads from the coronary sinus and great cardiac vein. PACE 2005; 28:205–11.

22 The DAVID Investigators. Dual-chamber pacing or ventricular backup pacing in patients with an implantable defibrillator: the dual chamber and VVI implantable defibrillator (DAVID) trial. JAMA 2002; 288:3115–23.

23 Olshansky B, Day JD, Moore S *et al.* Is dual-chamber programming inferior to single-chamber programming in an implantable cardioverter defibrillator? Result of the INTRINSIC RV (Inhibition of Innecessary RV Pacing With AVSH in ICDs) study. Circulation 2007; 115:9–16.

24 Hayes DL, Naccarelli GV, Furman S *et al.* NASPE training requirements for cardiac implantable electronic devices: selection, implantation, and follow-up. PACE 2003; 26:1556–62.

25 Gold MR, Peters RW, Johnson JW, Shorofsky SR. Complications associated with pectoral implantation of cardioverter-defibrillators. Pacing Clin Electrophysiol 1997; 20:208–11.

26 Gold MR, Higgins S, Klein R *et al.* Efficacy and temporal stability of reduced safety margins for ventricular defibrillation. Primary results from the Low Energy Safety Study (LESS). Circulation 2002; 105:2043–8.

27 Gold MR, Breiter D, Leman R *et al.* Safety of a single successful conversion of ventricular fibrillation before the implantation of cardioverter defibrillators. PACE 2003; 26:483–6.

28 Swerdlow CD. Implantation of cardioverter defibrillators without induction of ventricular fibrillation. Circulation 2001; 103:2159–64.

29 Gold MR, Shorofsky SR. Transvenous defibrillation lead systems. J Cardiovasc Electrophysiol 1996; 7:570–80.

30 Marchlinski FE, Callans DJ, Gottlieb CD *et al.* Benefits and lessons learned from stored electrogram information in implantable defibrillators. J Cardiovasc Electrophysiol 1995; 6:832–51.

31 Gold MR, Shorofsky SR, Thompson JA *et al.* Advanced rhythm discrimination for implantable cardioverter defibrillators using electrogram vector timing and correlation. J Cardiovasc Electrophysiol 2002; 13:1092–7.

32 Deisenhofer I, Kolb C, Ndrepepa G *et al.* Do current dual chamber cardioverter defibrillators have advantages over conventional single chamber cardioverter defibrillators in reducing inappropriate therapies? A randomized, prospective study. J Cardiovasc Electrophysiol 2001; 12:134–42.

33 Schaumann A, Muhlen FVZ, Herse B *et al.* Empirical versus tested antitachycardia pacing in implanted cardioverter defibrillators: a prospective study including 200 patients. Circulation 1998; 97:66–74.

34 Wathen MS, Sweeney MO, DeGroot PJ *et al.* Shock reduction using antitachycardia pacing for spontaneous rapid ventricular tachycardia in patients with coronary artery disease. Circulation 2001; 104:796–801.

35 Gold MR, Shorofsky SR. Strength–duration relationship for human transvenous defibrillation. Circulation 1997; 96:3517–20.

36 Saksena S, An H, Mehra R *et al.* Prospective comparison of biphasic and monophasic shocks for implantable cardioverter-defibrillators using endocardial leads. Am J Cardiol 1992; 70:304–10.

37 Shorofsky SR, Gold MR. Effects of waveform and polarity on defibrillation thresholds in humans using a transvenous lead system. Am J Cardiol 1996; 78:313–6.

38 Olsovsky MR, Shorofsky SR, Gold MR. Effect of shock polarity on biphasic defibrillation thresholds using an active pectoral lead system. J Cardiovasc Electrophysiol 1998; 9:350–4.

39 Bardy GH, Poole JE, Kudenchuk PJ *et al.* A prospective randomized comparison in humans of biphasic waveform 60-μF and 120-μF capacitance pulses using a unipolar defibrillation system. Circulation 1995; 91:91–5.

40 Gold MR, Foster AH, Shorofsky SR. Effects of an active pectoral-pulse generator shell on defibrillation efficacy with a transvenous lead system. Am J Cardiol 1996; 78:540–3.

41 Gold MR, Olsovsky MR, Pelini MA *et al.* Comparison of single- and dual-coil active pectoral defibrillation lead systems. J Am Coll Cardiol 1998; 31:1391–4.

42 Gold MR, Olsovsky MR, DeGroot PJ *et al.* Optimization of transvenous coil position for active can defibrillation thresholds. J Cardiovasc Electrophysiol 2000; 11:25–9.

43 Kirk MM, Shorofsky SR, Gold MR. Right sided active pectoral pulse generators do not reduce defibrillation thresholds. Pacing Clin Electrophysiol 1999; 22:747.

44 Raitt MH, Johnson G, Dolack GL *et al.* Clinical predictors of the defibrillation threshold with the unipolar implantable defibrillation system. J Am Coll Cardiol 1995; 25:1576–83.

45 Hodgson DM, Olsovsky MR, Shorofsky SR *et al.* Clinical predictors of defibrillation thresholds with an active pectoral pulse generator lead system. PACE 2002; 25:408–13.

46 Higgins SL, Alexander DC, Kuypers CJ *et al.* The subcutaneous array: a new lead adjunct for the transvenous ICD to lower defibrillation thresholds. Pacing Clin Electrophysiol 1995; 18:1540–8.

47 Epstein AE, Ellenbogen KA, Kirk KA *et al.* Clinical characteristics and outcome of patients with high defibrillation thresholds: a multicenter study. Circulation 1992; 86:1206–16.

48 Gold MR, Kavesh NG, Peters RW *et al.* Biphasic waveforms prevent the chronic rise of defibrillation thresholds with a transvenous lead system. J Am Coll Cardiol 1997; 30:233–6.

## CHAPTER 9

Cardiac resynchronization therapy

Michael O Sweeney

A heart failure epidemic

There are 4–5 million people living with chronic heart failure and an additional 400 000 newly diagnosed yearly.[1] Chronic heart failure is a cardiogeriatric condition. The incidence of heart failure is 10 per 1000 for individuals who are > 65 years of age, and increasing, due primarily to the advancing age of the population with coronary artery disease, which is now the principal cause of heart failure associated with reduced ventricular function [dilated cardiomyopathy (DCM)].[2] Almost all heart failure patients will have at least one acute episode with symptoms requiring hospitalization and treatment with intravenous medications to stabilize their condition. Hospital discharges with a primary diagnosis of heart failure totaled ~1000 000 in 2001 and have increased over 150% from 1979. Approximately 800 000 of these patients have advanced heart failure [New York Heart Association (NYHA) class III–IV]. An additional ~2000 000 hospitalizations with heart failure as a secondary diagnosis are recorded annually. Furthermore, the typical patient has ~10 medical contacts during the first 3 months after a heart failure hospitalization. Hospitalization for management of heart failure imposes the highest cost by diagnosis-related grouping to the healthcare system.

Mortality due to progressive heart failure associated with DCM has declined. In the Framingham study total mortality was 24% and 55% within 4 years of developing symptomatic heart failure for women and men, respectively.[2] These statistics approximate well to the natural history of heart failure, as the subject population was untreated by contemporary standards. β-Blockers and afterload reduction (angiotensin-converting enzyme inhibitors, angiotensin receptor blockers) have yielded substantial reductions in mortality due to progressive pump failure. However, despite these improvements in medical therapy, symptomatic heart failure still confers a 20–25% risk of premature death in the first 2.5 years after diagnosis.

Cardiac Pacing and ICDs, 5th edition. Edited by Kenneth A. Ellenbogen and Mark A. Wood. © 2008 Blackwell Publishing, ISBN: 978-1-4051-6350-7

Disordered electromechanical events in dilated cardiomyopathy

Disordered electrical timing frequently accompanies heart failure associated with DCM. Disordered electrical timing disrupts critical mechanical relationships that further impair left ventricular (LV) performance. There are five major disruptions to normal electromechanical events: (i) atrial de-coupling (interatrial conduction delay), (ii) atrioventricular (AV) de-coupling (AV conduction delay), (iii) ventricular de-coupling (interventricular synchrony), (iv) intraventricular conduction delay (LV dyssynchrony), and (v) LV transmural (endocardial to epicardial) delay. These disruptions may occur in isolation or in combinations and serve as potential electrical targets for mechanical reconstitution.

Atrial decoupling

The right atrium and left atrium are activated nearly simultaneously (within 50–80 ms) during sinus rhythm. Preferential sites of interatrial conduction exist at the posterior-superior interatrial septum (Bachman's bundle region), fossa ovalis, and coronary sinus (CS) ostium. Significant interatrial conduction delays (up to ≥ 200 ms) can occur in myopathic atria. These conduction delays can also be induced, or exacerbated, by right atrial pacing. Delayed left atrial contraction can disrupt optimal left-sided AV coupling. In the most severe form of atrial decoupling, delayed left atrial contraction occurs simultaneously or after LV contraction, resulting in atrial transport block. This causes increased left atrial pressures, retrograde flow in the pulmonary veins, and counter-physiological neurohormonal responses termed "pseudo-pacemaker syndrome."

AV decoupling

Optimal AV coupling contributes to ventricular pump function. The normal AV interval results in atrial contraction just before the pre-ejection (isovolumic) period of ventricular contraction. This timing maximizes ventricular filling (LV end-diastolic pressure, or preload) and cardiac output by the Starling mechanism. This optimal timing relationship also results in diastolic filling throughout the entire diastolic filling period, prevents diastolic mitral regurgitation (MR) and maintains mean left atrial pressure at low levels (Fig. 9.1).

Disruptions to AV coupling can be understood by analysis of Doppler mitral inflow patterns (Fig. 9.2A). Prolonged AV conduction disrupts these relationships and may degrade ventricular performance. Significantly prolonged AV conduction results in displacement of atrial contraction earlier in diastole, so that atrial contraction may occur immediately after or even within the preceding ventricular contraction. This may result in atrial contraction before venous return is completed. The result is a reduced atrial contribution to preload that may diminish ventricular volume and contractile force. It may also initiate early mitral valve closure, limiting diastolic filling time. Diastolic MR may also occur with prolonged AV conduction because, once closed, valve cusps may separate again before ventricular contraction as a result

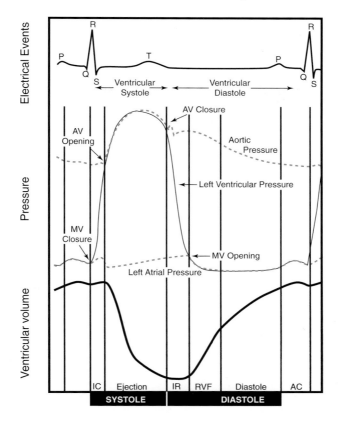

Fig. 9.1 Events of the cardiac electrical cycle. Atrial contraction followed by relaxation produces a negative pressure gradient, causing a surge of blood in the left ventricle (LV) at end diastole. Reversal of the atrioventricular (AV) pressure gradient initiates mitral valve (MV) closure because of a rapid decrease in pressure between the MV cusps pulling them into apposition. A brief period of isovolumetric contraction exists after MV closure and before AV opening, during which the maximum rate of pressure change (peak + dP/dt) occurs. Rapid ejection occurs during ventricular systole and is terminated when ventricular pressure falls below aortic pressure, closing the AV. A brief period of isovolumic relaxation follows, during which the maximum rate of pressure decline (peak − dP/dt) occurs. As the LV pressure continues to decline and fall below atrial pressure, the MV opens and diastolic ventricular filling begins. Normal diastolic filling is characterized by an initial rapid increase in ventricular filling during early diastole followed by a slow phase of filling during mid-diastole. A second rapid increase in ventricular filling occurs in late diastole as a result of atrial contraction.

of the development of a left ventricular–left atrial gradient in late diastole induced by atrial contraction with premature and incomplete mitral valve closure (Fig. 9.2B).

Interventricular and intraventricular conduction delay

Normal ventricular electrical activation is rapid and homogeneous with minimal time delay throughout the ventricular myocardial wall. This elicits synchro-

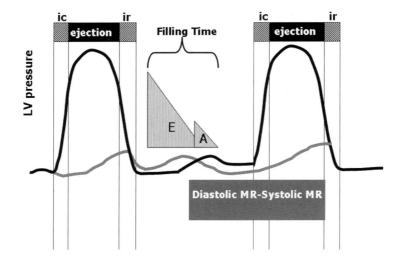

A

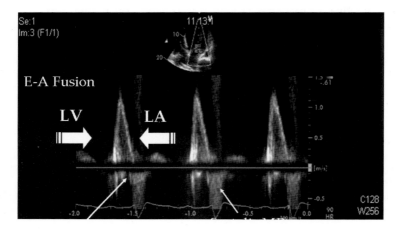

B

Fig. 9.2 (A) Intracardiac pressures and mitral inflow during atrioventricular (AV) decoupling (prolonged AV interval). ic, isovolumic contraction; ir, isovolumic relaxation. The mitral inflow pattern has two constituents. The initial component (E wave) is due to ventricular filling. The subsequent A wave is due to atrial contraction. The sum of these two constituents comprises the diastolic filling period, which is the interval from the onset of the E velocity to the cessation of the A velocity. (B) Effect of left ventricular (LV) conduction delay and prolonged AV conduction on diastolic filling patterns. LV filling is displaced rightward in time, whereas atrial contraction is displaced leftward in time. The result is fusion of filling and atrial contraction (E–A fusion).

nous mechanical activation and ventricular contraction. The resulting coordinated myocardial segment activation maximizes ventricular pump function.

Optimal inter- and intraventricular coupling is more important than AV coupling for maximum ventricular pumping function. Interventricular coupling refers to coordinated contraction of the right ventricle (RV) and LV. Interventricular delay refers to a delay in mechanical activation of one ventricle in relation to the other, most commonly left bundle branch block (LBBB) in which the RV begins its contraction before the LV. The delay in onset of LV activation results in reversal of the normal sequence between RV and LV mechanical events, which persists throughout the cardiac cycle and reduces the regional contribution to global ejection fraction.[3]

However, physiological evidence indicates that conduction delay within the LV (intraLV delay) is primarily responsible for reduced pump function. Delayed LV conduction causes a dyssynchronous contraction, which is mechanically inefficient, with diminished ejection at an increased metabolic cost. Chronic asynchronous ventricular activation redistributes the mechanical load within the ventricular wall and leads to reduction of blood flow and myocardial wall thickness over the site of early activation.[4] This ventricular remodeling contributes to progression of heart failure. In addition to these effects, delayed, sequential activation of papillary muscles may aggravate MR.[5]

LV mural delay

Studies of activation maps have shown different activation timing and sequence between endocardial and transmural activation. This suggests the possibility of intramural activation delay between the endocardial and myocardial layer.[6] The negative effects, if any, of intramural delay on ventricular pumping function are uncertain. However, reversal of the intramural activation sequence during LV epicardial pacing is an important constituent in the mechanism of potentially lethal ventricular proarrhythmia.[7]

Cardiac resynchronization therapy

Recognition that disordered electromechanical coupling at multiple levels contributes to reduced ventricular pump function suggested the possibility that novel pacing techniques could favorably modulate contractile dyssynchrony and AV coupling. The fundamental premise of this therapeutic strategy is stimulation of the LV earlier than would have occurred because of prolonged ventricular conduction. The first-order effect of this intervention is correction of ventricular conduction delay, which is necessary for ventricular resynchronization. The second-order effect is modulation of left-sided AV coupling, which may improve diastolic performance and, indirectly, LV pumping function.

Mechanisms of cardiac resynchronization therapy
Improved pumping function: AV optimization and ventricular resynchronization

Correction of physiologically disadvantageous prolonged AV conduction (AV optimization) can be achieved with left ventricular pre-excitation. Optimization of the AV interval during cardiac resynchronization therapy (CRT) can be conceptualized by examining mitral flow velocity curves using 2-D echocardiography.

When LV pre-excitation is inadequate, the result is similar to a prolonged AV interval, as shown in Fig. 9.2B. Note atrial contraction occurs too early in relation to LV activation and does not contribute to increased LV end diastolic pressure (LVEDP), as evident by the absence of an A wave on the mitral inflow velocity. Atrial contraction occurs before venous return is completed, causing reduced ventricular volume and contractile force. It may also initiate early mitral valve closure, thereby limiting diastolic filling time. Diastolic MR may also occur because, once closed, the mitral valve may drift open again before ventricular contraction.

When the programmed AV interval is too short, LV pre-excitation occurs too early relative to atrial systole (Fig. 9.3). Note that diastolic filling occurs throughout all of diastole. Atrial contraction now occurs simultaneously with LV contraction, resulting in increased left atrial pressure and loss of atrial contribution to ventricular systole, reducing cardiac output. A shorter AV interval lengthens the diastolic filling period by abolishing premature mitral valve closure due to the LV–left atrial pressure gradient seen with long AV delays. This also eliminates diastolic MR. However, the diastolic filling period should not be used as the only guideline to optimize the AV interval. Despite optimization of the diastolic filling period, hemodynamic deterioration will occur at too short an AV interval if atrial contraction occurs against a closed mitral valve (atrial transport block). This could result in a decrease in cardiac output and increase in mean left atrial pressure despite optimization of the diastolic filling period.

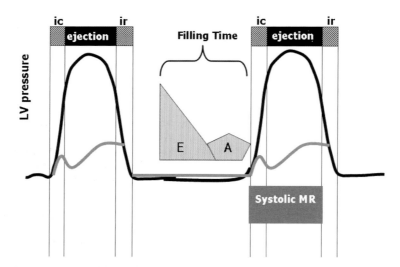

Fig. 9.3 Intracardiac pressures and mitral inflow at short atrioventricular interval. ic, isovolumic contraction; ir, isovolumic relaxation.

LV pre-excitation at the optimal AV interval is shown in Fig. 9.4. The relation of atrial contraction to the onset of ventricular contraction is now optimal, resulting in diastolic filling throughout the entire diastolic filling period. An appropriate relation now exists between mechanical left atrial and left ventricular contraction so that mean left atrial pressure is maintained at a low level with left atrial contraction occurring just before left ventricular contraction. This causes an increase in LVEDP (preload) and cardiac output. Note diastolic MR is eliminated and systolic MR is reduced. Acute hemodynamic studies have shown that AV delay is a significant determinant of changes in all LV systolic parameters (+ dP/dt, aortic systolic pressure, aortic pulse pressure).[8] For CRT "responders" (see below), LV + dP/dt and aortic pulse pressure AV delay functions are positive and unimodal, with a peak effect at approximately 50% of the native PR interval. The optimal AV delays for the same pacing chamber and parameter vary widely among patients and often differ for pulse pressure and LV + dP/dt within an individual.[8] The acute increase in LV + dP/dt with optimal AV delay may be in the range of 15–45%.[8] Whereas optimal AV delay maximizes preload, a diastolic performance metric, the primary effect on pump function relates to ventricular resynchronization that can be modulated by varying the AV delay. This reflects the interactive relationship between AV interval and interventricular interval during LBBB (reviewed[9]).

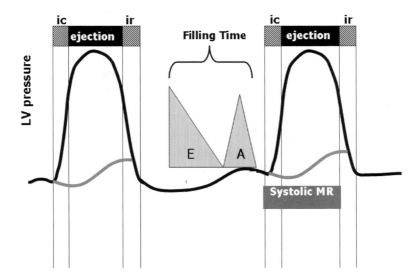

Fig. 9.4 Intracardiac pressures and mitral inflow at optimal atrioventricular interval. ic, isovolumic contraction; ir, isovolumic relaxation.

Reverse LV remodeling

In addition to improvement in acute hemodynamic performance, it has now been clearly demonstrated that CRT can improve chronic LV pumping function. This improvement is accompanied by Doppler echocardiographic (conventional 2-D and tissue imaging) evidence of reverse LV remodeling.[10–12] These remodeling effects include reduction in LV volumes, redistribution of cardiac mass, and improvement in ejection fraction.

Other effects of CRT: reduction in functional MR

Functional MR frequently accompanies DCM and results from an imbalance between the closing and tethering forces that act on the mitral leaflets.[13] This is strongly dependent on alterations in ventricular shape as the tethering forces that act on the mitral leaflets are higher in dilated, more spherical ventricles. These geometrical changes alter the balance between tethering and closing forces and impede effective mitral closure. Ventricular dilation and increased chamber sphericity increase the distance between the papillary muscles to the enlarged mitral annulus as well as to each other, restricting leaflet motion and increasing the force needed for effective mitral valve closure. This mitral valve closing force is determined by the systolic LV pressure–left atrial pressure difference, which is called the transmitral pressure gradient. Under these conditions, the mitral regurgitant orifice area will be largely determined by the phasic changes in transmitral pressure. Increasing the transmitral pressure can reduce the effective regurgitant orifice area. CRT acutely reduces the severity of functional MR and this reduction is quantitatively related to an increase in LV + dP/dt_{max} and transmitral pressure.[13] This is distinct from the reduction in MR due to reduced LV dimensions from remodeling associated with chronic CRT. Functional MR may also occur due to delayed sequential activation of the papillary muscles due to intraventricular delay.[5]

Implementation of CRT

There are currently three approaches to achieving LV pacing. The transvenous approach utilizes specially designed delivery sheaths and tools for cannulating the CS in order to permit delivery of pacing leads into the epicardial venous circulation serving the LV free wall. LV pacing lead placement can also be achieved under direct visualization using a cardiac surgical approach. Finally, transvenous LV endocardial pacing via trans-septal puncture has been described in the rare circumstance in which neither the transvenous epicardial nor surgical options are viable.[14,15]

Approach to transvenous LV lead placement

Early attempts at epicardial LV pacing via the coronary veins utilized standard endocardial pacing leads designed for RV pacing or CS leads designed for left atrial pacing.[16] This approach was met with predictable difficulties, including lead dislodgement, high pacing thresholds and inability to reach the target coronary venous branch. Currently available tools and techniques achieve a > 90% transvenous LV lead placement success rate.

Typically, the CS is cannulated with a specially designed sheath that serves as a workstation for LV lead placement. These preformed sheaths are available in a variety of diameters and shapes and are intended to overcome unpredictable anatomical variation in right heart anatomy. These sheaths are intended to engage the CS os during withdrawal from the RV. This approach overcomes the obstruction to the os commonly produced by the eustacian valve. Deflectable sheaths are also available and some implanters cannulate the CS with a deflectable electrophysiology catheter or a coronary angiography catheter. The sheath is then advanced into the CS body using a guidewire or catheter as a railing system (Fig. 9.5).

Once the CS is successfully cannulated, retrograde venography is performed to delineate the coronary venous anatomy. This is done with a standard balloon occlusion catheter and hand injections of contrast. Care must be taken to achieve a good seal within the main body of the CS in order to obtain maximal opacification of the distal vasculature. Underfilling the coronary venous system is a common mistake that may result in failure to identify potentially suitable targets for LV pacing lead placement. Occasionally, the inflated balloon will occlude the ostium of a suitable branch vessel for LV lead placement; therefore occlusive venography at multiple levels within the main CS may be needed (Figs 9.6 and 9.7). Most operators use both a right anterior oblique and left anterior oblique view to image the CS and its branches.

Transvenous LV pacing leads may be either stylet driven or use an over-the-wire (OTW) delivery system similar to percutaneous coronary intervention (PCI). The necessary reduction in lead diameter for coronary venous

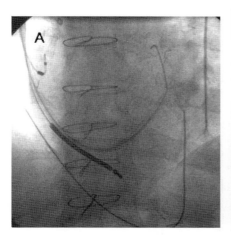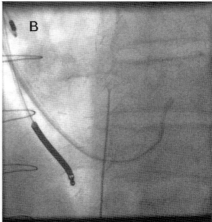

Fig. 9.5 Cannulation of the coronary sinus using a coronary guide catheter and an over-the-wire technique. Note left ventricle lead delivery sheath within main body of coronary sinus.

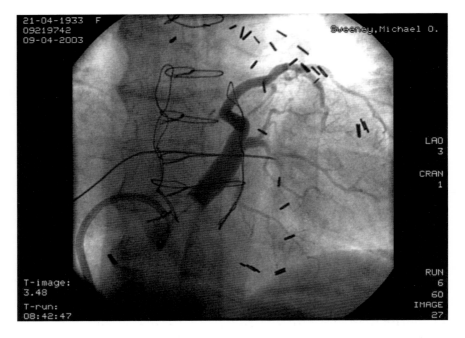

Fig. 9.6 Retrograde coronary venogram via femoral approach. Note large lateral vein with three second-order branches, and a smaller posterolateral vein.

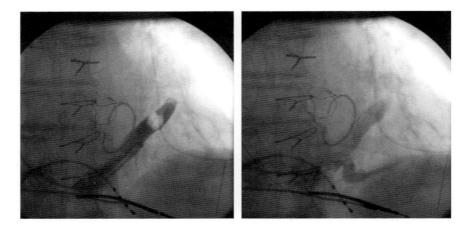

Fig. 9.7 Retrograde coronary venogram via left superior approach. Left: Balloon is inflated in mid-coronary sinus (CS). No target veins are visualized. Right: Sheath and balloon are withdrawn to proximal CS. Venography now reveals a large posterolateral vein. The ostium of this vein was occluded by the sheath on the first injection.

postioning can be reduced in only three ways: reducing lumen size, eliminating a conductor (unipolar) or reducing insulation (undesirable). In general the smallest diameter leads are unipolar and are delivered exclusively over a PCI guidewire. Larger diameter leads may accommodate a conventional stylet or a PCI guidewire ("hybrids"). In some cases, fixation relies primarily on "wedging" the lead tip into a distal site within the target vein so that the outer diameter of the lead closely approximates the inner luminal diameter of the vein. Other LV lead designs incorporate one or more tines, which may assist with fixation by catching on a valve or promoting thrombosis, but are probably otherwise irrelevant. Finally, some other LV leads have a self-retaining cant at the tip that has two intended purposes (see Chapter 2). The cant unfolds within the target vein, simultaneously compressing the distal segment of the lead against the outer wall of the vein, improving fixation, and forcing the tip electrode against the epicardium, thus improving electrical contact for pacing. More recently, enhancements to lead design have been directed at combining the maneuverability of smaller diameter leads with the mechanical stability of large leads. This is achieved by incorporating reversible, self-retaining S- or pigtail-shaped curves at the lead tip, which increase the "effective" diameter of smaller leads for mechanical stability without degrading maneuverability.

Factors limiting successful transvenous LV lead placement

Complex and unpredictable anatomical and technical considerations may preclude successful delivery of the LV lead to an optimal pacing site.

Inability to cannulate the coronary sinus

It is difficult to estimate the true percentage of cases in which the CS cannot be cannulated because this is clearly influenced by operator experience. It is probably in the range of 1–5% and may be commonly due to marked right atrial enlargement, very posterior origin of the CS os or obstruction by the eustacian valve. When the CS cannot be located by the superior approach, an adaptation of the inferior approach described for complex electrophysiology procedures is often successful in localizing the CS ostium (Fig. 9.6). Rarely, left coronary arteriography is needed to define the CS os in levophase. The angiography may be performed at the time of implant or review of previous angiography may provide the needed information. Intracardiac ultrasound may also locate the CS os at implant.

Coronary venous anatomy: absent or inaccessible target veins

The coronary venous circulation demonstrates considerably more variability than the parallel arterial circulation (Fig. 9.8). Careful studies of retrograde coronary venography have revealed that the anterior interventricular vein is present in 99% of patients and the middle cardiac vein is present in 100%. These veins are generally undesirable for LV pre-excitation because they do

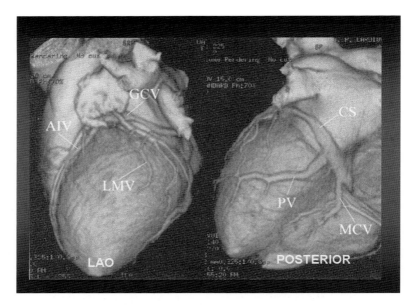

Fig. 9.8 Three-dimensional reconstruction of epicardial coronary venous anatomy using computed tomography. AIV, anterior interventricular vein; GCV, great cardiac vein; LMV, lateral marginal vein; PV, posterior vein; MCV, middle cardiac vein; CS, coronary sinus. Adapted from reference 41 with permission.

not reach the late activated portion of the LV free wall. Unfortunately, approximately 50% of patients have only a single vein serving the LV free wall. Anatomically, this is a lateral marginal vein in slightly more than 75% and a true posterior vein that ascends the free wall in approximately 50% of patients.[17] Thus, as many as 20% of patients may not have a vein that reaches the optimal LV free wall site for delivery of CRT. In some instances, target veins are present but too small for cannulation with existing lead systems, or paradoxically too large to achieve mechanical fixation (Fig. 9.9).

Coronary venous tortuosity
Another commonly encountered difficulty in transvenous LV lead placement is tortuosity of the target vessel take-off or main segment. These anatomical constraints can be extremely difficult to overcome and often require the use of multiple LV lead designs and delivery systems (Figs 9.10 and 9.11). Tortuous take-offs may be overcome with the use of firm guidewires to straighten out the vessel or by subselecting the target branch with the guide sheath. Use of a "buddy wire" may also straighten the vessel while the lead is placed in parallel over a separate wire. Small-diameter unipolar leads may navigate tortuosities impassable to larger leads.

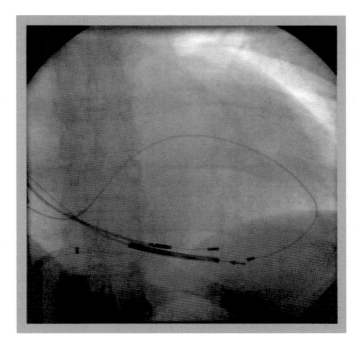

Fig. 9.9 Massive lateral coronary vein extending around the apex of the left ventricle (LV). All available LV leads descended to terminus of lateral marginal vein and into middle cardiac vein, circumnavigating the LV. Despite attempts with multiple leads, mechanical stability could not be achieved more proximally within the vein.

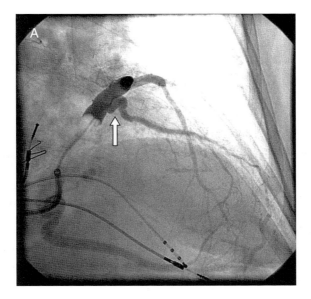

Fig. 9.10 "Shepherd's Crook" take-off of lateral marginal vein, with kink just beyond second bend (arrow). A 4-French over-the-wire left ventricular lead cannot navigate venous kinking.

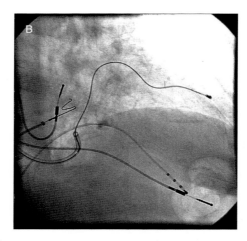

Fig. 9.11 Same patient as shown in Fig. 9.10. Alternate 4-F over-the-wire lead successfully navigated kinked portion of vein.

High LV stimulation thresholds and phrenic nerve stimulation

The principal limitation of the transvenous approach is that the selection of sites for pacing is entirely dictated by navigable coronary venous anatomy. A commonly encountered problem is that an apparently suitable target vein delivers the lead to a site where ventricular capture can be achieved at only very high output voltages or not at all. This presumably relates to the presence of scar on the epicardial surface of the heart underlying the target vein and cannot be anticipated by fluoroscopic examination *a priori* (Fig. 9.12). If this is not successful,

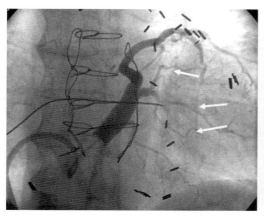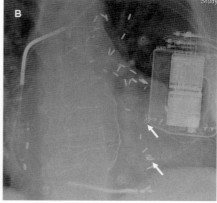

Fig. 9.12 (A) Multiple diminutive lateral marginal veins. Left ventricular (LV) pacing threshold exceeded 6 V in all locations due to epicardial scar due to prior infarct (note surgical clips associated with prior coronary revascularization). (B) Chest radiographs of surgically placed epicardial LV pacing leads in same patient. Note LV free wall position of leads approximates obtuse marginal artery location in circumflex territory, where epicardial mapping identified viable sites for LV pacing.

surgical placement of LV leads permits more detailed mapping of viable sites in the anatomical region of interest (Fig. 9.12).

A second common problem is that the target vein delivers the lead to a site that results in phrenic nerve stimulation and diaphragmatic pacing. This can be difficult to demonstrate during implantation when the patient is supine and sedated, but may be immediately evident when the patient is later active and changes body positions, even in the absence of lead dislodgement. Occasionally, if there is a significant differential in the capture thresholds for phrenic nerve stimulation vs. LV capture, this can be overcome by manipulation of LV voltage output. However, many experienced implanters recognize that once phrenic nerve stimulation is observed during implantation, it is almost invariably encountered during follow-up despite manipulation of output voltages, and therefore alternative site LV pacing is sought (Fig. 9.13). As with high LV capture thresholds, occasionally phrenic nerve stimulation can be overcome by repositioning the LV lead more proximally within the target vein (Fig. 9.14). Use of bipolar leads and pulse generators with programmable LV pacing lead configurations may allow for "electronic repositioning" after implant.

Approach to surgical LV lead placement

The first clinical trial of CRT utilized a hybrid epicardial LV, endocardial RV pacing lead configuration for multisite ventricular stimulation simply because the technique for transvenous epicardial LV pacing had not been developed.[18]

There are several current approaches to surgical placement of LV pacing leads. Many surgeons still use a full left lateral thoracotomy, which permits full visualization of the LV free wall, but results in significant postoperative pain and an extended recovery period. More recently, a minimally invasive approach has been developed. In this approach, the patient is prepared lying on their right side with left arm suspended over their head. Two or three "porthole" incisions are made in the left axillary space for access to the LV free wall (Fig. 9.15). Two

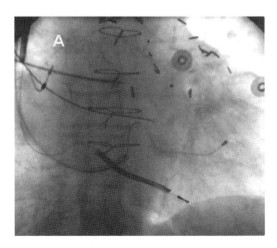

Fig. 9.13 Left ventricular lead is positioned in a lateral marginal vein, but this site was rejected due to insuperable phrenic nerve stimulation.

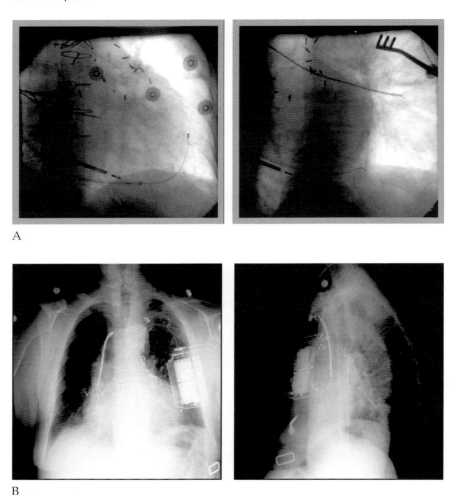

A

B

Fig. 9.14 Same patient as in Fig. 9.13. (A) Repositioning of the left ventricular (LV) lead in a large posterior vein which ascending the LV free wall eliminated phrenic nerve stimulation. (B) Chest radiographs of LV lead in posterior vein.

epicardial LV leads are typically placed using the obtuse marginal branches of the circumflex coronary artery as regional landmarks, approximately 1 cm apical to the mitral annulus. A common pitfall with less experienced implanters is to place the lead too anteriorly. After the leads are placed, the capped terminal pins are tunneled to a provisional pocket on the chest wall. The patient is then reprepared and draped on their back; the provisional pocket is opened and terminal pins are tunneled to the pectoral pocket. One critical difference in patient preparation for surgical vs. transvenous LV lead placement is that it is

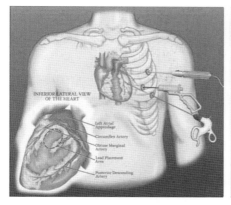
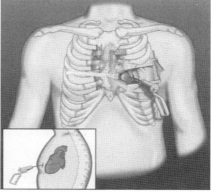

Fig. 9.15 Surgical approach to minimally invasive placement of epicardial left ventricular pacing leads via "port hole" approach (left) or limited left lateral thoracotomy (right).

better to have the patient a little "dry" (well diuresed) in the former and a little "wet" (diuretics withheld) in the latter. In the case of the transvenous approach, adequate hydration may minimize the risk of contrast-induced renal failure. In contrast, during the surgical approach, volume overload may increase lung volume. This increases the hemodynamic consequences of single lung ventilation, particularly on right heart function, and may limit LV visualization if complete left lung deflation cannot be achieved.

Optimal LV lead placement

At present there is no compelling evidence that the position of the RV lead greatly influences the response to CRT. In contrast, the optimal site for LV pacing is an unsettled and complex consideration. It is probably true that the optimal site varies between patients and is likely to be modified by venous anatomy, regional and global LV mechanical function, myocardial substrate, characterization of electrical delay and other factors. The success of resynchronization is dependent on pacing from a site that causes a change in the sequence of ventricular activation that translates to an improvement in cardiac performance. Presumably, this site corresponds to the site of maximal mechanical delay. Such systolic improvement and mechanical resynchronization does not require electrical synchrony[19] and explains the lack of correlation between change in QRS duration and clinical response to CRT. Ideally, the pacing site or sites that produce the greatest hemodynamic effect would be selected.

However, current clinical evidence permits some generalizations regarding LV pacing site selection for optimal acute hemodynamic response. Generally, free wall sites yield greater hemodynamic improvement than anterior wall sites or any other LV region[18,20,21] (Figs 9.16 and 9.17). This may be interpreted as evidence that stimulating a later activated LV region produces a larger response because it more effectively restores regional activation and synchrony. Recent

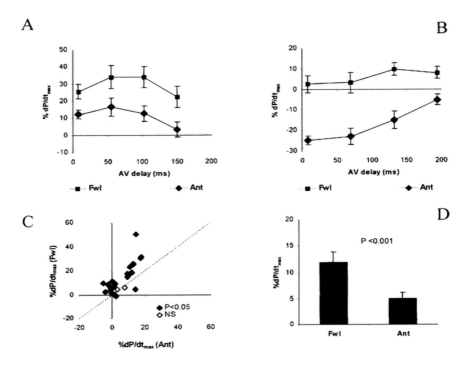

Fig. 9.16 Effect of cardiac resynchronization therapy stimulation site on acute hemodynamic response. Thirty patients enrolled in PATCH-CHF-II trial. Left ventricular (LV) stimulation was delivered at free wall (FWL) or anterior wall (ANT) sites. FWL sites yielded significantly larger LV + dP/dT and pulse pressure than ANT sites. In 1/3 of patients stimulation at ANT sites worsened hemodynamic function, whereas FWL stimulation improved it. The opposite pattern was never observed. See text for details.

animal studies have suggested that the optimal pacing site may include a fairly broad area of the LV lateral wall, and that small deviations in the anterior or posterior direction may still provide substantial hemodynamic benefit.

Methods for identifying the best site during implantation are not yet of proven clinical benefit. Furthermore, even if optimal LV pacing sites could be identified *a priori*, access to such sites is potentially constrained by variations in coronary venous anatomy. Despite rapid evolution of implantation techniques, including guiding sheaths and catheters and over-the-wire delivery systems, a suitable pacing site on the LV free wall cannot be achieved in 5–10% of patients. Even when the coronary venous anatomy is suitable and navigable, some free wall sites are rejected due to unacceptably high pacing thresholds or unavoidable phrenic nerve stimulation. Surgical placement of epicardial LV pacing leads or endocardial LV stimulation[14] are options when the coronary venous approach fails.

A

B

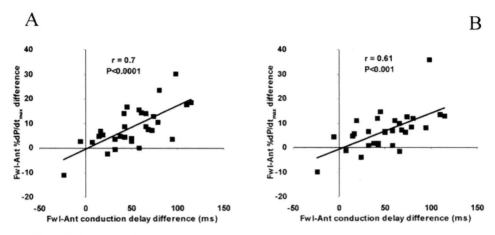

Fig. 9.17 Correlation between free wall (FWL) and anterior wall (ANT) intrinsic conduction delay differences and the LV + dP/dt$_{max}$ response differences during FWL and ANT stimulation for LV cardiac resynchronization therapy (CRT) (A) and BV CRT (B). Positive conduction delay differences correspond to more delayed FWL activation. Positive LV + dP/dt$_{max}$ differences correspond to a larger FWL stimulation response (percentage change from baseline).

CRT pacing systems
Leads and electrodes
Non-independently programmable ventricular polarity configurations
Transvenous and epicardial LV pacing leads may be either unipolar or bipolar. Multiple ventricular pacing polarity configurations are therefore possible. Since programmed polarity settings are common to both ventricular leads and since the type (bipolar or unipolar) of these leads may not be the same, the following considerations apply.

In a dual bipolar polarity configuration, both lead tips are the active electrodes (cathodes) and the ring(s) are the common (non-stimulating) anode. However, the types of ventricular leads implanted define the pacing/sensing vector (Fig. 9.18). With two unipolar leads, the bipolar setting results in no pacing or sensing. If both leads are bipolar, both rings act as the common electrode. If one lead is bipolar (RV) and the other lead is unipolar (typically LV), the ring on the bipolar lead acts as the common electrode (non-stimulating anode). This configuration results in "shared-ring" bipolar pacing and sensing. This hybrid bipolar/unipolar stimulation configuration has until recently been employed in most contemporary CRT pacing systems.

In a dual unipolar polarity configuration, the lead tips are the active electrodes; the non-insulated device case is the common electrode (Fig. 9.18). This configuration is uncommonly used in CRT pacing systems and is not feasible in CRT with defibrillation capability (CRTD) systems due to the concerns regarding ventricular oversensing.

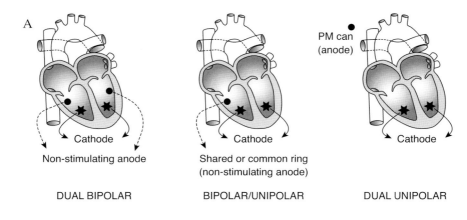

A

PM can
(anode)

Cathode

Non-stimulating anode

Cathode

Shared or common ring
(non-stimulating anode)

Cathode

DUAL BIPOLAR

BIPOLAR/UNIPOLAR

DUAL UNIPOLAR

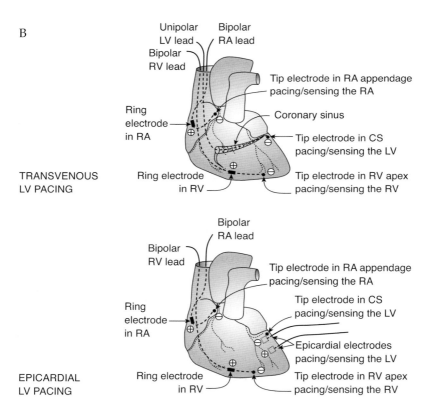

B

Unipolar
LV lead

Bipolar
RA lead

Bipolar
RV lead

Tip electrode in RA appendage
pacing/sensing the RA

Ring
electrode
in RA

Coronary sinus

Tip electrode in CS
pacing/sensing the LV

TRANSVENOUS
LV PACING

Ring electrode
in RV

Tip electrode in RV apex
pacing/sensing the RV

Bipolar
RA lead

Bipolar
RV lead

Tip electrode in RA appendage
pacing/sensing the RA

Tip electrode in CS
pacing/sensing the LV

Ring
electrode
in RA

Epicardial electrodes
pacing/sensing the LV

EPICARDIAL
LV PACING

Ring electrode
in RV

Tip electrode in RV apex
pacing/sensing the RV

Fig. 9.18 (A) Various combinations of lead polarities for biventricular pacing. (B) Lead polarities and configurations for transvenous and epicardial biventricular pacing. Adapted from reference 42 with permission. (Artist: A.F. Sinnaeve.)

Pulse generators

Conventional dual-chamber pulse generators or specially designed multisite pacing pulse generators may be used for CRT applications (Fig. 9.19). A con-

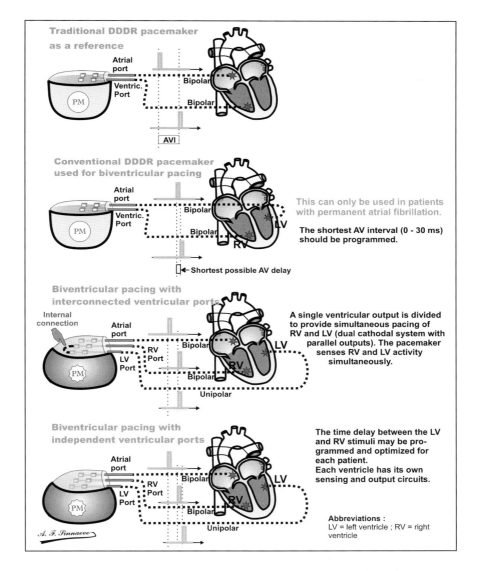

Fig. 9.19 Various pulse generator configurations for biventricular pacing. Adapted from reference 42 with permission. (Artist: A.F. Sinnaeve.)

ventional dual-chamber pulse generator is well suited for CRT in patients with permanent atrial fibrillation (AF). In this situation, the ventricular port is used for the RV lead and the atrial port is used for the LV lead. This permits programming of independent outputs and ventricular–ventricular timing by manipulation of the AV delay. The programming mode can be either DDD/R or DVI/R (see below). A conventional dual-chamber pulse generator can also be used for atrial-synchronous biventricular pacing. The single ventricular output must be divided to provide simultaneous stimulation of the RV and LV (dual cathodal system with parallel outputs). This is achieved with a Y-adaptor and results in simultaneous RV and LV sensing, which may result in ventricular double-counting and loss of CRT (see later) or pacemaker inhibition in the case of LV lead dislodgement into the CS with sensing of atrial activity.

First-generation multisite pacing pulse generators similarly provide a single ventricular output for simultaneous RV and LV stimulation; however, two separate ventricular channels internally connect in parallel. This connection is made for both the lead tip and ring connections and eliminates the need for a Y-adaptor. However, this configuration still provides simultaneous RV and LV sensing with associated limitations.

Second-generation multisite pacing pulse generators have independent ventricular ports. Each ventricular lead therefore has separate sensing and output circuits. This arrangement permits optimal programming of outputs and time delay between RV and LV stimulation for each patient. It also eliminates the potential complications of biventricular sensing.

Biventricular or univentricular stimulation for CRT

It is important to note that uncertainty about the requirement of RV stimulation during CRT, uneasiness about long-term LV lead performance, and unavailability of pacing systems with separately programmable ventricular outputs have influenced the use of biventricular pacing, as opposed to LV pacing alone, in large-scale randomized clinical trials. A particular concern is LV lead dislodgement, which carries a risk for potentially lethal bradycardia and has a reported incidence of 5–10% in larger studies.[22–24] However, there is some scientific evidence that RV stimulation might not be necessary for optimal CRT response. LV pacing alone has acute hemodynamic effects that are similar or superior to those achieved with biventricular pacing in some patients.[25–27]

At present it is not possible to identify patients who will respond better to LV alone compared with biventricular pacing, or neither; and it is not clear how to identify the optimal pacing site. Other factors will warrant RV lead placement in many patients. Patients with reduced LV ejection fraction and at least moderately symptomatic heart failure are at risk for sudden cardiac death due to ventricular arrhythmias, and this risk can be reduced by ICD therapy. Current ICD systems require an RV lead for tachyarrhythmia sensing and high-voltage therapies and have a long record of safety and reliability in this regard. The site of RV pacing does not appear to be a critical determinant of the response to CRT.

Programming considerations in CRT
Pacing modes
It is axiomatic that, for maximal delivery of CRT, ventricular pacing must be continuous, i.e. > 90% of heart beats should be paced. DDD mode guarantees AV synchrony and ventricular pacing with all atrial events in the physiological heart rate range. However, DDD mode increases the probability of atrial pacing (depending upon programmed lower rate limit) that may alter the left-sided AV timing relationship due to interatrial conduction time and atrial pacing latency.

VDD mode guarantees the absence of atrial pacing and synchronizes all atrial events to ventricular pacing at the programmed AV delay. However, if the sinus rate is below the lower programmed rate limit, AV synchrony is lost because the VDD mode is operationally VVI.

Although conventional dual-chamber pacemakers are not designed for bi-ventricular pacing and generally do not allow programming of an AV delay of zero, or near zero, they are being increasingly used with their shortest AV delay (0–30 ms) for CRT in patients with permanent AF. The advantages include programming flexibility, elimination of the Y-adaptor (required for conventional VVIR devices), protection against far-field sensing of atrial activity (an inherent risk of dual cathodal devices with simultaneous sensing from both ventricles) and cost. The DVIR mode is ideally suited for this application. The DVIR mode behaves like the VVIR mode, except that there are always two closely coupled independent ventricular stimuli, thereby facilitating comprehensive evaluation of RV and LV pacing and sensing performance. The DVIR mode also provides absolute protection against far-field sensing of atrial activity in case of LV lead dislodgement, since no sensing occurs on the "atrial" (LV) lead in the DVIR mode.

Ventricular double-counting causing loss of CRT and spurious ventricular therapies
In first-generation CRT and CRTD systems, pacing and sensing occur from RV and LV simultaneously. Double-counting involves the spontaneous wide QRS complex of LBBB (Fig. 9.20). This produces temporal separation of RV and LV electrograms (EGM). The degree of separation depends on the severity of the interventricular conduction delay and the location of the electrodes. The LV EGM may be sensed some time after detection of the RV EGM if the LV signal extends beyond the relatively short ventricular blanking period initiated by RV sensing. This is more likely to occur when a long postventricular atrial refractory period (PVARP) is programmed. In this circumstance, sinus P waves, particularly during sinus tachycardia and first-degree AV block (which are common in heart failure patients), displace the P wave into the PVARP, where it cannot be tracked. This results in loss of ventricular pacing and CRT. This situation is commonly triggered by PVARP extensions after a premature ventricular contraction (PVC). Spontaneous AV conduction occurs in the form of a pre-empted upper rate Wenckebach response with loss of ventricular pacing

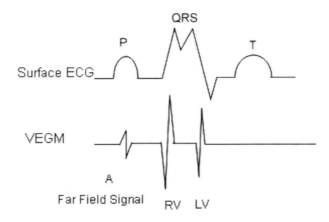

Fig. 9.20 Origin of temporally dispersed right ventricular and left ventricular electrograms during biventricular sensing.

and CRT (Fig. 9.21). In CRTD systems, this may result in ventricular double-counting and misclassification of sinus tachycardia or rapidly conducted AF as ventricular tachycardia, resulting in spurious therapies. During true ventricular episodes, such as ventricular tachycardia, the LV EGM may precede the RV EGM and may result in spurious shocks because the rate is misclassified as VF.

Failure to deliver CRT at high sinus rates can be minimized by shortening the PVARP, increasing the upper tracking limit and deactivating the PVC response in the DDD/R mode. Additionally, AF should be aggressively treated to prevent rapid ventricular response and emergence of spontaneous QRS complexes. New CRT systems prevent ventricular double-counting by sensing only the RV or by employing an interventricular ventricular refractory period (IVRP). Ventricular sensed events (i.e. LV sensing) during the IVRP do not restart PVARP (Fig. 9.22).

AV optimization

AV optimization is important for maximal hemodynamic response to CRT, but not essential, since CRT even in the presence of permanent AF can improve ventricular pumping function. Nonetheless, acute hemodynamic studies have consistently demonstrated that AV optimization "re-times" the left atrial–left ventricular relationship and can result in 15–40% improvement in indices of LV systolic performance acutely. Furthermore, small changes in AV delay may nullify the hemodynamic benefit of CRT. As noted previously, it is now generally understood that the effect of AV delay on pump function relates to ventricular resynchronization, not modification of preload.

At present, two methods of AV optimization are commonly applied. One method uses an echo-guided Doppler analysis of transmitral blood flow ve-

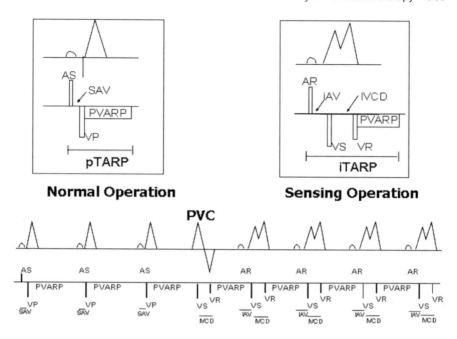

Fig. 9.21 Onset of ventricular double-counting and failure to deliver cardiac resynchronization therapy (CRT) due to loss of atrial tracking during CRT. See text for details. AS, atrial sensed event; SAV, sensed atrioventricular (AV) delay; VP, ventricular paced event; PVARP, postventricular atrial refractory period; AR, atrial refractory event (sinus event within iTARP); iAV, intrinsic AV interval (pacing inhibited); VS, ventricular sensed event (pacing inhibited); IVCD, interventricular conduction delay (interventricular interval, pacing inhibited); VR, ventricular refractory event; pTARP, programmed total atrial refractory period; iTARP, implied total atrial refractory period during pacing inhibition; PVC, premature ventricular contraction.

locities to approximate an optimal timing relationship between atrial systole and ventricular filling. This is a rather tedious process and may be physiologically unsound, since the basis for the technique was derived from studies of patients with permanent AV block and conventional dual-chamber pacing with RV apical stimulation. Nonetheless, this was the technique for AV optimization used in the MIRACLE study.[22] Empirical observation suggested that most optimized AV delays derived using this technique were in the range of 80–100 ms regardless of other considerations. The process of AV optimization using this technique is shown in Figs 9.23–9.25.

A second approach to AV optimization for maximal positive change in LV + dP/dt is derived from the intrinsic AV interval measured from the local right atrial and RV endocardial EGMs using two linear equations.[28] If the native QRSd is > 150 ms, then estimated optimal AV delay EOAVD = A × iAVI + B (ms) and EOAVD = C × iAVI + D (ms), where iAVI = intrinsic AV interval, and A, B, C and D are constant coefficients determined from an empirical dataset.

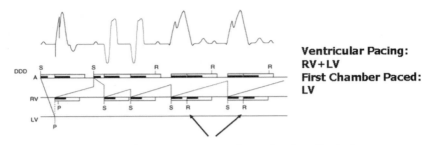

Ventricular Pacing:
RV+LV
First Chamber Paced:
LV

Double Senses without Interventricular Refractory Period

Double Senses
with
Interventricular
Refractory Period

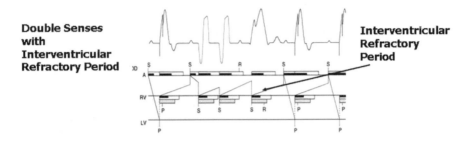

Interventricular
Refractory
Period

Fig. 9.22 Prevention of ventricular double-counting with an interventricular refractory period. See text for details.

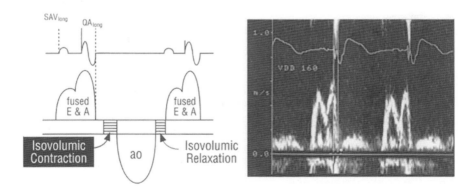

Fig. 9.23 Doppler echo of transmitral blood flow with long atrioventricular (AV) delay. When the AV delay is too long, mitral valve closure may not be complete, since atrial contraction is not followed by a properly timed ventricular systole. Left ventricular pressure increases above the LA pressure at the end of the diastolic filling period and results in diastolic, or "pre-systolic" mitral regurgitation.

These regression formulae can be very closely approximated by the following simple rules: the estimated optimal programmed AV delay for patients with QRSd > 150 ms is 50% of the intrinsic AV interval, and 75% for QRSd

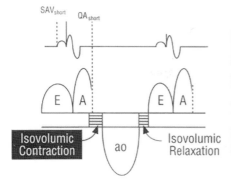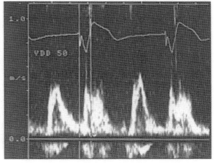

Fig. 9.24 Doppler echo of transmitral blood flow with short atrioventricular delay. Note truncation of diastolic filling period due to premature closure of mitral valve (atrial and ventricular contraction occur simultaneously).

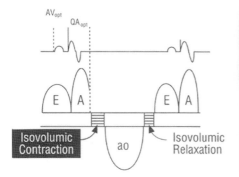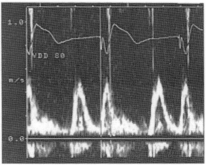

Fig. 9.25 Doppler echo transmitral blood flow at optimal atrioventricular (AV) delay. The relation of atrial contraction to the onset of ventricular contraction is now optimal, resulting in diastolic filling throughout the entire diastolic filling period. An appropriate relation now exists between mechanical left atrial and left ventricular (LV) contraction so that mean left atrial pressure is maintained at a low level with left atrial contraction occurring just before LV contraction. AV optimization is noted by return of the normal E–A separation. Transmitral flood and LV diastolic filling time are increased, which leads to increased stroke volume. If a large amount of diastolic mitral regurgitation can be abolished, a beneficial effect is obtained because of lower left atrial and higher LV preload at the onset of ventricular contraction.

of 120–150 ms (Fig. 9.26). This strategy was used in the study design of the Comparison of Medical Therapy, Pacing, and Defibrillation in Heart Failure (COMPANION) trial,[23] which showed significant reductions in mortality and heart failure hospitalizations with CRT at 1 year.

It is almost certainly true that the optimal AV delay will be likely to differ as heart rate and cardiac loading conditions change, so that the optimal AV delay at one point in time may not predict optimal AV timing under other

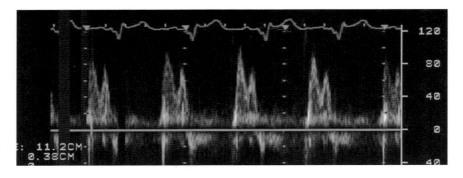

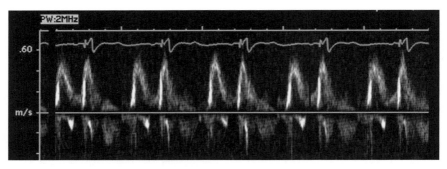

Fig. 9.26 Top: Note E–A fusion due to left ventricular conduction delay and atrioventricular (AV) conduction delay. QRS duration is 160 ms, intrinsic AV interval is 200 ms (not shown). Bottom: Estimated optimal delay is 100 ms (see text). Note correction of E–A relationship at this AV delay.

conditions. Furthermore, the importance of AV delay optimization at rest for chronic clinical and hemodynamic effect remains to be shown.

Pacing outputs

It is critically important that voltage output be adjusted to exceed ventricular capture threshold for LV and RV in common cathodal devices. For devices with common RV and LV voltage outputs, this output must exceed capture threshold in the chamber with the highest threshold (usually the LV) (Fig. 9.27). Newer pulse generators that permit independent programming of ventricular outputs provide greater flexibility in this regard. Similarly, RV and LV voltage outputs may be separately programmable in the situation where a standard DDD device is used to provide RV and LV stimulation in the DVI mode for CRT in permanent AF (see above).

Sequential ventricular pacing

Implantation of a biventricular pacing system with programmable LV and RV stimulation timing would allow correction of interventricular conduction delay. It is presently unclear what benefit, if any, manipulation of interventricular timing would provide during biventricular pacing.[11]

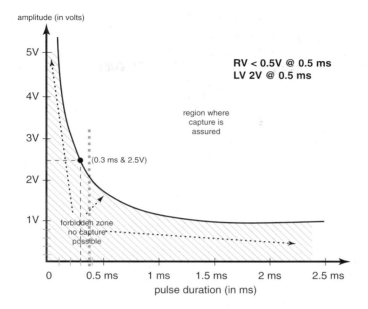

Fig. 9.27 Strength–duration curve considerations for biventricular pacing. The ventricular output must exceed the capture threshold for the chamber with the highest threshold, typically the left ventricle, in common cathodal systems. Adapted from reference 42 with permission.

CRT pacemaker electrocardiography/determining LV and RV capture

The 12-lead ECG is essential to ascertain RV and LV capture during follow-up of CRT systems without separately programmable ventricular outputs. It is recognized that five distinct 12-lead ventricular activation patterns may be seen during threshold determination. These are: (i) intrinsic rhythm during loss of RV and LV capture or pacing inhibition (native QRS), (ii) isolated RV stimulation, (iii) isolated LV stimulation, (iv) biventricular stimulation, and (v) biventricular stimulation with anodal capture (Figs 9.28–9.32).

Ventricular pacing thresholds should ideally be performed independently and in the VVI mode at a rate faster than the underlying ventricular rate to obtain continuous ventricular capture without fusion. Alternatively, thresholds can be performed in the VDD or DDD mode at very short AV delays to ensure full ventricular capture without fusion. In general it is advisable to initiate threshold determinations at maximum output (voltage and pulse duration), since there is often a significant differential in capture thresholds between RV and LV.

In devices without separately programmable ventricular outputs, RV and LV capture can be determined only by ECG analysis during common ventricular voltage decrement. This requires inspection of a 12-lead ECG to demonstrate a change in electrical axis that confirms independent LV and RV capture.

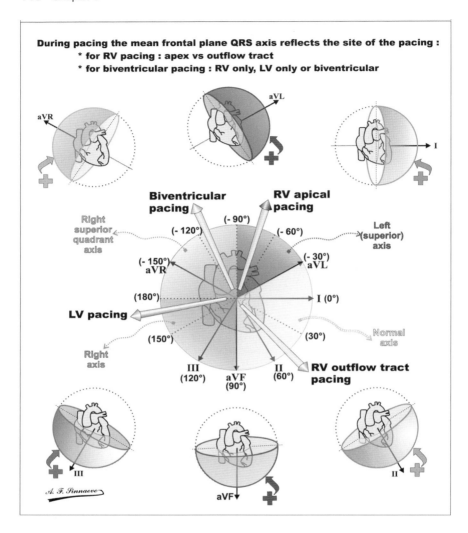

During pacing the mean frontal plane QRS axis reflects the site of the pacing :
* for RV pacing : apex vs outflow tract
* for biventricular pacing : RV only, LV only or biventricular

Fig. 9.28 Mean QRS axis in the frontal plane during ventricular pacing. Adapted from reference 42 with permission. (Artist: A.F. Sinnaeve.)

Pacing from the RV apex produces a negative paced QRS complex in the inferior leads simply because the activation starts in the inferior part of the heart and travels superiorly away from the inferior leads. The mean QRS frontal plane axis is superior either in the left or right superior quadrant. Pacing from the right ventricular outflow tract produces a frontal plane axis that is "normal," meaning inferiorly directed (positive QRS in inferior leads). Isolated LV pacing produces a rightward axis, similar to maximal ventricular pre-excitation over a left-sided accessory pathway. Biventricular pacing (RVapex + LV)

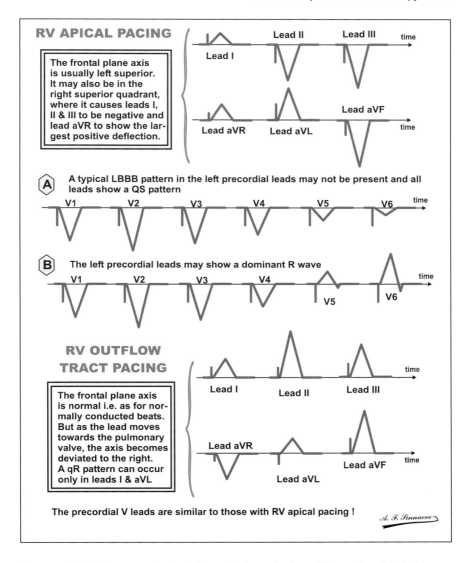

Fig. 9.29 EKG QRS patterns during right ventricular pacing from different sites. Adapted from reference 42 with permission. (Artist: A.F. Sinnaeve.)

produces a right superior axis as a result of fusion of RV and LV electrical axes. A qR or Qr complex in lead I is rare in uncomplicated RV apical pacing, but is present in 90% of cases of biventricular pacing. In biventricular pacing, loss of the q or Q wave in lead I is 100% predictive of loss of LV capture. Another algorithm that is 93% specific and 94% sensitive for detection of LV capture with biventricular pacing is an R/S $\geq$ 1 in lead V1 and a R/S $\leq$ 1 in I.

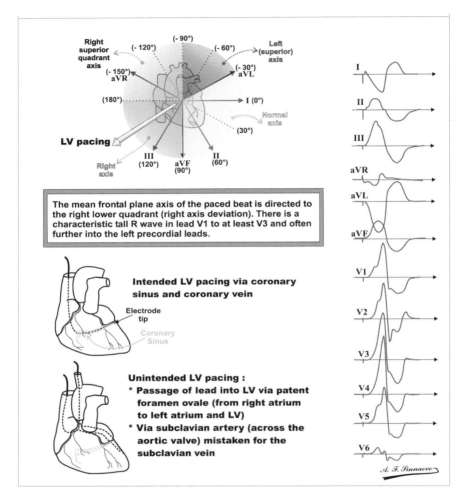

Fig. 9.30 ECG QRS patterns during left ventricular free wall pacing. Adapted from reference 42 with permission. (Artist: A.F. Sinnaeve.)

CRT responders and non-responders

Despite the technical limitations for achieving reliable, long-term transvenous LV stimulation, the majority of appropriately selected patients respond to CRT. Nonetheless, approximately 18–30% of patients fail to respond clinically to CRT.[22,29] In some cases, failure to respond may simply indicate that, despite delayed ventricular activation, mechanical activation is not dyssynchronous.[30] It is likely, however, that technical limitations are a major factor. In the MIRACLE study, a lateral marginal vein site serving the LV free wall was obtained in only 43% of patients. This number is probably an overestimate, since the

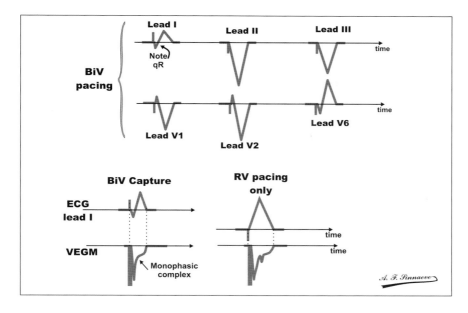

Fig. 9.31 Analysis of ECG QRS patterns to ascertain right ventricular and left ventricular capture in cardiac resynchronization therapy systems without separately programmable ventricular outputs. Adapted from reference 42 with permission. (Artist: A.F. Sinnaeve.)

larger diameter stylet-driven leads used during MIRACLE typically traverse the "Shepherd's Crook" curve of the anterior interventricular vein before they descend the LV. Many of the "lateral" sites were probably really anterolateral rather than true lateral marginal vein sites. Thus, at least 57% of patients in MIRACLE may have had suboptimal LV lead positions. It is conceivable that some of these patients were actually made worse by CRT due to LV pacing at suboptimal sites, particularly among the patients with relatively narrow QRSd (< 150 ms).[21] As reviewed previously, CRT with stimulation at an LV free wall site consistently improves short-term systolic function more than stimulation at an anterior site does (Figs 9.33, 9.34). These differences may account for the varied results and large individual differences observed among clinical studies.

Patient selection for CRT

Ventricular dyssynchrony is the pathophysiological target of CRT. Techniques for selecting patients with significant ventricular dyssynchrony likely to benefit from CRT are rapidly evolving. The optimal criteria would identify all patients with a high probability of response and reject all patients with a low probability of response. To date, QRSd determined from the surface ECG has been most extensively evaluated as a selection criterion for CRT on the premise that electrical delay is a reliable marker for spatially dispersed

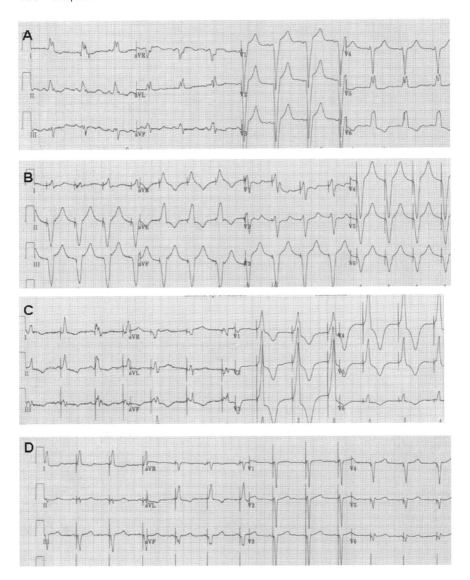

Fig. 9.32 Twelve lead ECGs showing: (A) intrinsic ventricular activation (LBBB); (B) right ventricular only pacing; (C) left ventricular only pacing; (D) biventricular pacing.

mechanical activation (Table 9.1). Numerous studies have reproducibly demonstrated that baseline QRSd > 150 ms is predictive of acute hemodynamic improvement with CRT, whereas patients with QRSd < 150 ms are less likely to respond.[8]

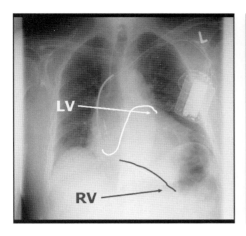
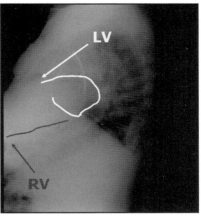

Fig. 9.33 Cardiac resynchronization therapy (CRT) non-responder. Note position of left ventricular (LV) lead in anterior interventricular vein. Note lack of spatial separation of right ventricular and LV leads in lateral view. This patient required an LV assist device within days of CRT implantation, followed by cardiac transplantation.

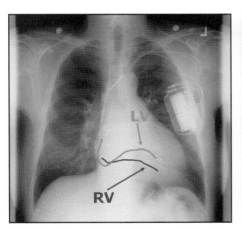
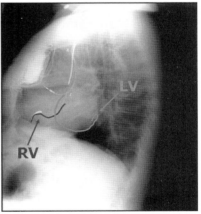

Fig. 9.34 Cardiac resynchronization therapy responder. Note position of left ventricular (LV) lead in lateral marginal vein on LV free wall. Note spatial separation of right ventricular and LV leads in lateral view. This patient had a two-step improvement in New York Heart Association class (IV to II), reduction in mitral regurgitation from severe to trace, and improvement in left ventricular ejection fraction from 20% to 35%.

Prediction curves for contractile function response using baseline QRSd derived from the PATH-CHF and PATH-CHF-II studies are shown in Fig. 9.35.[31] The specificity curve indicates that 80% of CRT non-responders had a QRSd < 150 ms. The sensitivity curve indicates that 80% of CRT responders had

Table 9.1 Guidelines for cardiac resynchronization therapy in patients with congestive heart failure and cardiomyopathy

Advanced symptomatic heart failure, NYHA class III and IV, despite optimal medical therapy
LVEF ≤ 35%
QRS duration ≥ 120 ms

NYHA, New York Heart Association; LVEF, left ventricular ejection fraction.

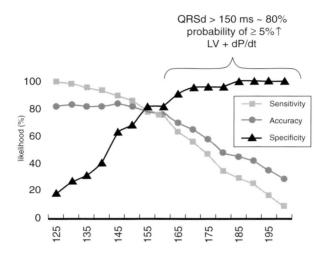

Fig. 9.35 Sensitivity, specificity and accuracy likelihoods are plotted for different QRS thresholds between 120 and 200 ms using acute hemodynamic data from PATH-CHF and PATH-CHF-II. Specificity curve indicates that 80% of non-responders have QRSd < 150 ms. Sensitivity curve indicates that 80% of responders have QRSd > 150 ms. Cardiac resynchronization therapy response is defined as > 5% acute increase in LV + dP/dt.

a QRSd > 150 ms. The overlap between these QRSd ranges was populated with CRT responders and non-responders. The predictive accuracy of QRSd to separate responders from non-responders is fairly constant around 80%, with a threshold cut-off between 120 and 150 ms. If the QRSd is > 150 ms, the likelihood of CRT response is greater. An important qualification is that this analysis is based on acute hemodynamic response to CRT. It is possible that acute hemodynamic response does not correlate precisely with chronic clinical improvement. However, these observations appear to be corroborated by the COMPANION Trial, where little or no benefit of CRT or CRTD on death or heart failure hospitalization was observed among patients with baseline QRSd < 150 ms. An approach to the CRT non-responder is summarized in Fig. 9.36. Clinical characteristics of patients who are CRT responders and non-responders are summarized in Table 9.2.

QRSd may not reliably predict CRT response, for several reasons. It is important to remember that QRSd reflects both RV and LV activation. In many

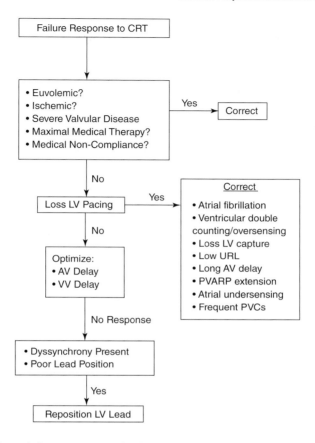

Fig. 9.36 Schematic for management of patients who are cardiac resynchronization therapy non-responders.

Table 9.2 Clinical characteristics of cardiac resynchronization therapy responders and non-responders

	Response more likely	*Response less likely*
QRS duration	> 150 ms	< 150 ms
Heart disease	Non-ischemic	Ischemic
Dyssynchrony	Present	Absent
Bundle branch block	Left	Right
Scar burden (MRI)	Low burden	High burden
	Non-transmural	Transmural
	Posterolateral segments spared	Posterolateral segments involved
Severity of mitral regurgitation	Mild–moderate	Severe
Lead position	Posterior–lateral	Anterior or inferior

patients with LBBB, the delay in ventricular activation resides entirely within the left ventricle, as anticipated. However, in some patients with LBBB, delayed RV activation accounts for a significant proportion of electrical delay manifest on the surface ECG. There are scant data on CRT in right bundle branch block, which suggests that meaningful clinical improvements are unlikely.[23,32] Another reason is the intriguing observation that a prolonged QRSd may not be accompanied by dyssynchronous, mechanical activation. In this situation, despite electrically delayed ventricular activation, CRT would not be anticipated to modify mechanical performance.

Recognition of the potential limitations of QRSd for predicting CRT response has stimulated interest in techniques for directly measuring baseline ventricular dyssynchrony. Intraventricular synchrony can be assessed echocardiographically from the delay between the maximal posterior displacement of the septum and the maximal displacement of the LV posterior wall measured from an M-mode short-axis view of the LV. A septal–posterior wall delay > 130 ms predicted LV volumetric remodeling in one study.[33] Another promising echocardiographic technique to identify dyssynchrony and target patients for CRT is tissue Doppler imaging. Ventricular dyssynchrony detected by tissue Doppler imaging has been shown to predict acute and chronic response (including remodeling) to CRT in several studies.[29–34]

In addition, patients with extensive scar burden in the LV, especially posterior–lateral scar, as demonstrated by magnetic resonance imaging or echo perfusion studies, may respond poorly to CRT. Patients with inotrope-dependent class IV heart failure are also generally felt to be poor candidates for CRT. Although patients with narrow QRS complexes can demonstrate echocardiographic evidence of dyssynchrony, the utility of CRT in these patients is not settled. Similarly, the benefits of CRT for Class II heart failure patients in alleviating symptoms or slowing the progression of heart failure are unknown.

Clinical trials of cardiac resynchronization therapy

CRT is an effective adjunctive treatment for moderately to severely symptomatic heart failure associated with DCM and ventricular dyssynchrony.[22,35–37] The aggregate experience with CRT among clinical trials involving > 5000 patients demonstrates a consistent clinical benefit (Fig. 9.37; Tables 9.3–9.6). The magnitude of the benefit is modest and concordant, although the effects are heterogeneously distributed among different patient subtypes. These include about a one-step improvement in NYHA class, a 10-point improvement in quality of life measures, a 1–2 ml/kg per min improvement in peak VO_2, a 50–70 m improvement in 6-min hall walk, and reduced heart failure hospitalizations. A meta-analysis of randomized trials of CRT using these first-generation pacing systems in 1634 patients has found that heart failure deaths were reduced by 51% (from 3.5% to 1.7%) and heart failure hospitalizations were reduced by 29%.[38]

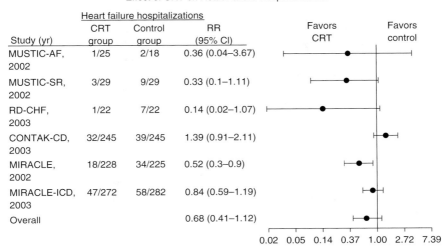

Effect of CRT on Heart Failure Hospitalizations

Study (yr)	Heart failure hospitalizations		RR (95% CI)
	CRT group	Control group	
MUSTIC-AF, 2002	1/25	2/18	0.36 (0.04–3.67)
MUSTIC-SR, 2002	3/29	9/29	0.33 (0.1–1.11)
RD-CHF, 2003	1/22	7/22	0.14 (0.02–1.07)
CONTAK-CD, 2003	32/245	39/245	1.39 (0.91–2.11)
MIRACLE, 2002	18/228	34/225	0.52 (0.3–0.9)
MIRACLE-ICD, 2003	47/272	58/282	0.84 (0.59–1.19)
Overall			0.68 (0.41–1.12)

Fig. 9.37 Effect of cardiac resynchronization therapy on heart failure hospitalizations. Adapted from reference 40 with permission.

Table 9.3 Clinical trials of cardiac resynchronization pacing therapy (CRTP)

Study	Design	N	NYHA class	QRSd	EF
PATH-CHF	Randomized, single blind, controlled	42	II–IV	> 120	< 35
VIGOR-CHF	Randomized, controlled	53	II–IV	> 120	< 30
PATH-CHF II	Acute hemodynamic	43	II–IV	> 120	< 30
InSync OUS	Uncontrolled	81	III–IV	> 150	< 35
MUSTIC	Uncontrolled	67	III–IV	> 150	< 35
MIRACLE	Randomized, double blind, controlled	266	III–IV	> 130	< 35
CARE-HF	Randomized, single blind, controlled	813	III–IV	> 120*	< 35

*Echocardiographic evidence of dyssynchrony required if QRSd 120–150 ms only

Cardiac resynchronization pacing therapy (CRTP, Table 9.3) induces significant volumetric remodeling of the failing LV in some patients, which may reasonably reduce the risk of death by several potential cardiac mechanisms, most importantly favorable substrate modification. Nonetheless, the prevalence of sudden death in this patient population has led to an accelerated

Table 9.4 Clinical trials of cardiac resynchronization defibrillation therapy (CRTD)

	MIRACLE ICD	*CONTAK CD*	*COMPANION*
Target population	CHF + QRSd prolongation + ICD	CHF + QRSd prolongation + ICD	CHF + QRSd prolongation + ICD
Treatment	ICD vs. CRTD	ICD vs. CRTD	CRT vs. CRTD vs. OFT
Patients enrolled	364	581	1602
Arrhythmia qualifier	ICD indication	ICD indication	ICD indication
LVEF (%) qualifier	< 35	< 35	< 35 + LVEDD > 60
CHF qualifier (NYHA class)	II–IV	II–IV	III–IV
QRS duration qualifier (ms)	> 120	> 130	> 120
Death or CHF hospitalization	Not reported	Not reported	40% ↓ CRTD 35% ↓ CRT
Death	Not reported	Not reported	36% ↓ CRTD 24% ↓ CRT

effort to hybridize CRT with defibrillation capabilities (CRTD). Three studies of CRTD involving > 2500 patients have been reported (Table 9.4). The study populations were similar to trials of CRTP except that there was a conventional indication for ICD therapy. CONTAK CD has shown a significant improvement in NYHA class, 6-min hall walk, peak VO_2 and standardized quality of life.[39] *Post-hoc* analysis has shown that the greatest benefit was observed in patients with the most advanced heart failure. However, the primary goal of a 25% reduction in heart failure, as measured by a composite outcome of death, heart failure hospitalization, worsening heart failure requiring other interventions, and ventricular arrhythmias, was not met. Patients receiving CRTD had a 21% reduction in this composite end-point ($P = 0.17$). However, the study was probably underpowered to detect significant differences in this composite end-point, particularly because 80% of the patients were NYHA I or II after 6 months of CRTD. MIRACLE ICD showed a reduction in NYHA class and improvement in quality of life, but not 6-min hall walk.[24] Importantly, neither of these studies has provided data on the effect of CRTD on mortality, or whether the clinical benefits of CRTP or CRTD are sustainable for > 12 months.

The COMPANION trial compared CRTP, CRTD and optimal medical therapy among 1520 patients with DCM (ischemic and non-ischemic), LV ejection fraction < 35%, QRSd > 120 ms and PR interval > 150 ms (Table 9.5). Mortality was reduced by CRTD (36%) and CRTP (24%) compared with medical therapy alone, although only the reduction associated with CRTD was statisti-

Table 9.5 Mortality and heart failure 12-month outcomes in COMPANION

	OPT event rate (%)	CRT rate reduction (%)	P, CRT vs. OPT	CRT-D rate reduction (%)	P, CRT-D vs. OPT
Combined all-cause mortality and all-cause hospitalization*	67.7	18.6	0.015	19.3	0.005
Combined all-cause mortality and heart failure hospitalization	46.1	35.8	< 0.001	39.5	< 0.001
All-cause mortality**	19.0	23.9	0.12	43.4	0.002

*Primary endpoint
**Secondary endpoint

cally significant.[23] Although a mortality reduction with CRTD was expected, the observation that CRTP alone might reduce mortality in the same patient population was particularly intriguing. However, the study was stopped once a mortality advantage was observed in either active therapy, which occurred sooner in the CRTD arm. Had follow-up been extended it is quite likely that a statistically significant reduction in mortality with CRTP would have been recorded.

The mortality benefit of CRTP in systolic heart failure has been definitively demonstrated in the CARE-HF Trial[37] (Table 9.6). A total of 813 patients with DCM, ejection fraction < 35%, NYHA class III–IV heart failure, QRSd > 150 ms (or QRSd 120–150 ms plus echocardiographic evidence of dyssynchrony) were randomized to optimal medical therapy or CRTP. Treatment with CRTP unaccompanied by backup defibrillation was associated with a 36% reduction in relative risk of death compared with optimal medical therapy. The magnitude of this effect virtually overlaps with the mortality benefit of CRTD in COMPANION.

Important future questions that remain unanswered include the use of dyssynchrony measurements to better predict which patients will be CRT responders, and the role of CRT in patients with class I and II heart failure and in patients with narrow QRS with dyssynchrony.

Non-excitatory cardiac contractility modulation

Cardiac contractility modulation is an evolving device-based therapy for heart failure that does not rely upon the presence of ventricular dyssynchrony for a therapeutic effect. Using standard pacing leads and an implantable pulse

Table 9.6 Mortality and heart failure outcomes in CARE-HF

Outcome	Medical therapy alone n = 404		Medical therapy plus cardiac resynchronization n = 409		Hazard ratio (96% CI)	P
	No.	%	No.	%		
Primary outcome						
Death or unplanned hospitalization for a cardiovascular event	224	55	159	39	0.63 (0.61–0.77)	< 0.001
Unplanned hospitalization for a cardiovascular event	184	46	125	31	0.61 (0.49–0.77)	< 0.001
Secondary outcome						
Death from any cause	120	30	82	20	0.64 (0.48–0.85)	0.002
Death from any cause or unplanned hospitalization with worsening HF	191	47	118	29	0.54 (0.43–0.68)	< 0.001
Unplanned hospitalization with worsening HF	133	33	72	18	0.48 (0.36–0.64)	< 0.001

generator, non-excitatory electrical stimuli are delivered to the RV myocardium 30–60 ms after the sensed local electrogram. The pulse is biphasic with a duration of 20–40 ms and amplitude up to 10 V. Because this stimulus is delivered during ventricular refractoriness, it does not participate in the electrical activation of the ventricle (Fig. 9.38). Instead, this stimulus prolongs the local action potential duration, thereby enhancing the sarcolemmal calcium transient. This in turn increases cardiac contractility. A significant inotropic effect has been demonstrated in animal and human studies.[43] In patients enrolled in a multicenter study, improvements in ejection fraction, symptoms and functional status have been demonstrated.[44] At the time of writing, this therapy is in clinical trials in the USA, but is available in Europe. The benefits of this therapy as an alternative or adjunct to CRT are unknown.

Summary: CRTP and CRTD

The field of electrical device therapy has benefited from two basically independent lines of investigation demonstrating improved survival from either CRT or ICD therapy in patients with heart failure. Current clinical evidence data are insufficient to conclude that CRTD offers an advantage over CRTP

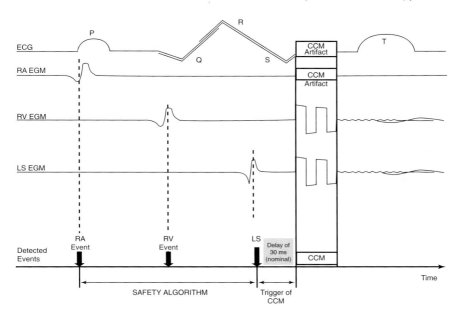

Fig. 9.38 Schematic timing of electrical events in a device for cardiac contractility modulation (CCM). Surface ECG, right atrial electrogram (RA EGM), right ventricular (RV) EGM, and local sensed (LS) ventricular EGM are represented. The CCM pulse is delivered 30–60 ms after the sensed local ventricular EGM to correspond to the plateau of the local action potential. The pulse is visible on surface ECG as a stimulus artifact in the terminal portion of the QRS complex. (Reproduced by permission from Pappone C *et al.* First human chronic experience with cardiac contractility modulation by nonexcitatory electrical currents for treating systolic heart failure: mid-term safety and efficacy results from a multicenter study. J Cardiovasc Electrophysiol 2004; 15:418–27.)

alone. The cost of adding a defibrillator to the CRTP device is substantial and will act as a barrier to wide-scale penetration. Annualized sudden death rates are very low in certain primary prevention populations. Consequently, the potential for overtreatment is very large and the negative costs of ICD therapy are distributed equally among those patients who will have a life-saving benefit and those who were "destined" never to require the therapy. Clinical trials comparing conventional ICDs, CRTP and CRTD are necessary to rationalize the use of expensive hardware resources among different patient populations. Additionally, the importance of patient preference regarding end-of-life care should receive greater emphasis. While CRTP may be considered palliative in terminal heart failure, the decision to offer CRTD must include a discussion with the patient regarding mode of death and the potential for the defibrillator to replace a sudden and peaceful death with prolonged death from progressive pump failure.

References

1 Massie BM, Shah NB. Evolving trends in the epidemiologic factors of heart failure. Am Heart J 1997; 133:703–12.
2 Kannel WB, Plehn JF, Cupples A. Cardiac failure and sudden death in the Framingham Study. Am Heart J 1988; 115:869–75.
3 Grines CL, Boshore TW, Boudoulas H, Olson S, Shafer P, Wooley CF. Functional abnormalities in isolated left bundle branch block: the effect of interventricular asynchrony. Circulation 1989; 79:845–53.
4 Prinzen FW, Cheriex EC, Delhaas T et al. Asymmetric thickness of the left ventricular wall resulting from asynchronous electric activation: a study in dogs with ventricular pacing and in patients with left bundle branch block. Am Heart J 1995; 130:1045–53.
5 Kanzaki H, Bazaz R, Schwartzman D, Dohi K, Sade LE, Gorscan J 3rd. A mechanism for immediate reduction in mitral regurgitation after cardiac resynchronization therapy: insights from mechanical activation strain mapping. J Am Coll Cardiol 2004; 44:1619–25.
6 Auricchio A, Fantoni C, Regoli F et al. Characterization of left ventricular activation in patients with heart failure and left bundle branch block. Circulation 2004; 109:1133–9.
7 Fish JM, Di Diego JM, Nesterenko V, Antzelevitch C. Epicardial activation of left ventricular wall prolongs QT interval and transmural dispersion of repolarization: implications for biventricular pacing. Circulation 2004; 109:2136–42.
8 Auricchio A, Stellbrink C, Block M et al. Effect of pacing chamber and atrioventricular delay on acute systolic function of paced patients with congestive heart failure. The Pacing Therapies for Congestive Heart Failure Study Group. The Guidant Congestive Heart Failure Research Group. Circulation 1999; 99:2993–3001.
9 Vernooy K, Verbeek XAAM, Cornelussen RNM et al. Calculation of effective VV-interval facilitates optimization of AV-delay and VV-interval in cardiac resynchronization therapy. Heart Rhythm 2006; 4:75–82.
10 St John Sutton MG, Plappert T, Abraham WT et al. for the MIRACLE Study Group. Effect of cardiac resynchronization therapy on left ventricular size and function in chronic heart failure. Circulation 2003; 105:1985–90.
11 Sogaard P, Egeblad H, Pedersen AK et al. Sequential versus simultaneous biventricular resynchronization for severe heart failure: evaluation by tissue Doppler imaging. Circulation 2002; 106:2078–84.
12 Lau CP, Yu CM, Chau E et al. Reversal of left ventricular remodeling by synchronous biventricular pacing in heart failure. Pacing Clin Electrophysiol 2000; 23:1722–5.
13 Breithardt OA, Sinha AM, Schwammenthal E et al. Acute effects of cardiac resynchronization therapy on functional mitral regurgitation in advanced systolic heart failure. J Am Coll Cardiol 2003; 203:765–70.
14 Garrigue S, Jais P, Espil G et al. Comparison of chronic biventricular pacing between epicardial and endocardial left ventricular stimulation using Doppler tissue imaging in patients with heart failure. Am J Cardiol 2001; 88:858–62.
15 Jais P, Takahashi A, Garrigue S et al. Mid-term follow-up of endocardial biventricular pacing. Pacing Clin Electrophysiol 2000; 23:1744–7.
16 Daubert CJ, Ritter P, LeBreton H et al. Permanent left ventricular pacing with transvenous leads inserted into the coronary veins. Pacing Clin Electrophysiol 1998; 21:239–345.
17 Meisel E, Pfeiffer D, Engelmann L et al. Investigation of coronary venous anatomy by retrograde venography in patients with malignant ventricular tachycardia. Circulation 2001; 104:442–7.

18 Auricchio A, Stellbrink C, Sack S *et al.* The Pacing Therapies for Congestive Heart Failure (PATH-CHF) study: rationale, design, and endpoints of a prospective randomized multicenter study. Am J Cardiol 1999; 83:130D–135D.

19 Leclercq C, Faris O, Runin R *et al.* Systolic improvement and mechanical resynchronization does not require electrical synchrony in the dilated failing heart with left bundle-branch block. Circulation 2002; 106:1760–3.

20 Auricchio A, Klein H, Tockman B *et al.* Transvenous biventricular pacing for heart failure: can the obstacles be overcome? Am J Cardiol 1999; 83:136D–142D.

21 Butter C, Auricchio A, Stellbrink C *et al.* for the Pacing Therapy for Chronic Heart Failure II Study Group. Effect of resynchronization therapy stimulation site on the systolic function of heart failure patients. Circulation 2001; 104:3026–9.

22 Abraham WT, Fisher WG, Smith AL *et al.* for the MIRACLE Study Group. Cardiac resynchronization in chronic heart failure. N Engl J Med 2002; 346:1845–53.

23 Bristow MR, Saxon LA, Boehmer J *et al.* the Comparison of Medical Therapy, Pacing, and Defibrillation in Heart Failure (COMPANION) Investigators. Cardiac-resynchronization therapy with or without an implantable defibrillator in advanced chronic heart failure. N Engl J Med 2004; 350:2140–50.

24 Young JB, Abraham WT, Smith AL *et al.*, Multicenter InSync ICD Randomized Clinical Evaluation (MIRACLE ICD) Trial Investigators. Combined cardiac resynchronization and implantable cardioversion defibrillation in advanced chronic heart failure: the MIRACLE ICD Trial. JAMA 2003; 289:2685–94.

25 Kass DA, Chen CH, Curry C *et al.* Improved left ventricular mechanics from acute VDD pacing in patients with dilated cardiomyopathy and ventricular conduction delay. Circulation 1999; 99:1567–73.

26 Blanc JJ, Etienne Y, Gilard M *et al.* Evaluation of different ventricular pacing sites in patients with severe heart failure: results of an acute hemodynamic study. Circulation 1997; 96:3273–7.

27 Blanc JJ, Bertault-Valls V, Fatemi M, Gilard M, Pennec PY, Ym E. Midterm benefits of left univentricular pacing in patients with congestive heart failure. Circulation 2004; 109:1741–4.

28 Auricchio A, Kramer A, Spinelli J *et al.* Can the optimum dosage of resynchronization therapy be derived from the intracardiac electrogram? J Am Coll Cardiol 2002; 39:124 (Abstract).

29 Bax JJ, Mohoek SG, Marwick TJ *et al.* Left ventricular dyssynchrony predicts benefit of cardiac resynchronization therapy in patients with end-stage heart failure before pacemaker implantation. Am J Cardiol 2003; 92:1238–40.

30 Kerckhoffs RC, Bovendeerd PH, Kotte JC *et al.* Homogeneity of cardiac contraction despite physiological asynchrony of depolarization: a model study. Ann Biomed Eng 2003; 31:536–47.

31 Kadhiresan V, Vogt J, Auricchio A *et al.* Sensitivity and specificity of QRS duration to predict acute benefit in heart failure patients with cardiac resynchronization. Pacing Clin Electrophysiol 2000; 23:555 (Abstract).

32 Egoavil CA, Ho RT, Greenspon AJ, Pavri BB. Cardiac resynchronization therapy in patients with right bundle branch block: analysis of pooled data from MIRACLE and ContakCD trials. Heart Rhythm 2005; 2:611–5.

33 Pitzalis MD, Iacoviello M, Romito R *et al.* Cardiac resynchronization therapy tailored by echocardiographic evaluation of ventricular asynchrony. J Am Coll Cardiol 2002; 40:1615–22.

34 Yu C-M, Fung W-H, Lin H *et al.* Predictors of left ventricular reverse remodeling after cardiac resynchronization therapy for heart failure secondary to idiopathic dilated or ischemic cardiomyopathy. Am J Cardiol 2003; 91:684–8.

35 Cazeau S, Leclerlq C, Lavergne T *et al.* Effects of multisite biventricular pacing in patients with heart failure and intraventricular conduction delay. N Engl J Med 2001; 344:873–80.

36 Auricchio A, Stellbrink C, Sack S *et al.*, Pacing Therapies in Congestive Heart Failure (PATH-CHF) Study Group. Long-term clinical effect of hemodynamically optimized cardiac resynchronization therapy in patients with heart failure and ventricular conduction delay. J Am Coll Cardiol 2002; 39:2026–33.

37 Cleland JGF, Daubert JC, Erdmann E *et al.*, the Cardiac Resynchronization—Heart Failure (CARE-HF) Study Investigators. The effect of cardiac resynchronization on morbidity and mortality in heart failure. N Engl J Med 2005; 352:1539–49.

38 Bradley DJ, Bradley EA, Baughman KL *et al.* Cardiac resynchronization and death from progressive heart failure: a meta-analysis of randomized controlled trials. JAMA 2003; 289:730–40.

39 Higgins SL, Hummel JD, Niazi IK *et al.* Cardiac resynchronization therapy for the treatment of heart failure and intraventricular conduction delay and malignant ventricular tachyarrhythmia. J Am Coll Cardiol 2003; 42:1454–9.

40 McAlister FA, Ezekowitz JA, Wiebe N *et al.* Systematic review: cardiac resynchronization in patients with symptomatic heart failure. Ann Intern Med 2004; 141:381–90.

41 Tada H, Naito S, Koyama K, Taniguchi K. Three-dimensional computed tomography of the coronary venous system. J Cardiovasc Electrophysiol 2003; 14:1385.

42 Barold SS, Stroobandt RX, Sinnaeve AF. Cardiac pacemakers step by step: an illustrated guide. Malden, MA: Blackwell, 2004.

43 Pappone C, Augello G, Rosanio S *et al.* First human experience with cardiac contractility modulation by nonexcitatory electrical current for treating systolic heart failure: midterm safety and efficacy results from a multicenter trial. J Cardiovasc Electrophysiol 2004; 15:418–27.

44 Neelagaru SB, Sanchez JE, Lau SK *et al.* Nonexcitatory, cardiac contractility modulation electrical impulses: feasibility study for advanced heart failure in patients with normal QRS duration. Heart Rhythm 2006; 3:1140–7.

## CHAPTER 10

ICD follow-up and troubleshooting

Sumeet S Chugh, Mark A Wood

The implantable cardioverter defibrillator (ICD) is the treatment of choice for prevention of sudden cardiac death. The expansion of indications for ICDs to include prophylactic implantation based on the presence of severe left ventricular dysfunction without arrhythmic events has resulted in a large and growing population of ICD recipients. As a consequence, the need for regular follow-up by physicians and allied health personnel, equipped with the knowledge to ensure appropriate functioning and also troubleshoot any problems, has grown significantly.

Follow-up after implantable cardioverter-defibrillator placement

After implanting the device and before discharging the patient from the hospital, the implanting physician should observe the following procedures:

1 Inspect the ICD site for evidence of hematoma or infection.

2 Counsel the patient about keeping the ICD site clean and dry for 1–2 weeks, as well as to avoid raising the arm ipsilateral to the ICD above the shoulder for 2–4 weeks.

3 Interrogate the ICD and perform a non-invasive check of lead resistances as well as lead sensing and pacing thresholds.

4 Obtain chest radiographs in the anteroposterior and lateral views to ascertain appropriate lead positions.

5 Discuss driving, activity and occupational restrictions appropriate for the patient's condition. The recommendations for the period immediately following a primary prevention ICD implant are to avoid driving for at least 1 week; for a secondary prevention implant this period is 6 months.[1] In the USA, most states have mandatory driving restrictions for 6 or 12 months following an episode of syncope.

In addition, some devices emit audible alert tones or vibrate to indicate battery depletion, high lead impedances or prolonged charge times. These tones should be demonstrated to the patient and their importance emphasized.

The ICD patient should be seen again 1–2 weeks after the implantation surgery to ascertain whether the wound is healing appropriately. The ICD

Cardiac Pacing and ICDs, 5th edition. Edited by Kenneth A. Ellenbogen and Mark A. Wood.
© 2008 Blackwell Publishing, ISBN: 978-1-4051-6350-7

pocket should be carefully examined for evidence of infection. The ICD system should be checked as outlined below to ensure that the lead is stable and the device is functioning. Patients should be seen every 3–6 months thereafter until the device approaches elective replacement indicators, at which time more frequent follow-up assessments are warranted.

Routine follow-up

The purpose of subsequent follow-up visits is to assess the patient's condition, check the stability and performance of the ICD system and the adequacy of programmed therapies, provide patient education, and investigate potential device malfunctions.

History and physical examination

The history and physical examination is the essential first step toward evaluating the performance of a patient's ICD. The patient should be asked about the occurrence of shock therapies, palpitations or syncope. In particular, conditions such as congestive heart failure and cardiac ischemia, which may precipitate ventricular tachyarrhythmias, should be evaluated. Conditions such as chronic obstructive pulmonary disease, infection, anemia and dehydration, that can precipitate supraventricular tachyarrhythmias and inappropriate shocks, should be investigated. The patient should be asked whether particular body positions tend to trigger ICD therapy or skeletal muscle stimulation from resynchronization devices. The latter suggests phrenic nerve stimulation from the left ventricular lead. Since antiarrhythmic drugs are often used in ICD recipients to prevent arrhythmia recurrence, a drug history should be obtained at each visit. Some medications could change pacing, sensing and defibrillation thresholds; others could cause electrolyte imbalances that may interfere with appropriate ICD function.[2] Furthermore, patients who have congestive heart failure or recurrent cardiac ischemia should be placed on effective doses of β-blockers, angiotensin-converting enzyme inhibitors and "statins," all of which are likely to reduce the incidence of sudden cardiac death, atrial fibrillation (AF) and possibly the frequency of delivered ICD therapy.[3–5] Device safety alerts are more common with ICDs than with pacemakers. The response to a safety alert should be individualized for each patient. Factors influencing the decision to replace a device at risk for malfunction include the degree of patient dependency for bradycardia pacing, the risk of death from malfunction, the likelihood of device failure and the risk of complications (primarily device infection) from device replacement (see Chapter 11). The patient should also be examined for ICD infection or erosion. Early detection of impending device erosion can prevent the possibility of catastrophic ICD system infection.

Device interrogation

At each visit, information retrieved from the device using an ICD programmer should be examined carefully in a systematic fashion.

Programmed parameters

These include detection and treatment algorithms for ventricular tachyarrhythmias, therapies for bradyarrhythmias, and various alert settings. Review of these parameters may reveal erroneous programming that can potentially result in inappropriate or suppressed ICD therapy. For example, failure to program a ventricular tachycardia (VT) zone could prevent delivery of effective therapy for undetected VT. On the other hand, failure to use supraventricular tachyarrhythmia (SVT) discrimination schemes could allow SVTs such as AF to trigger inappropriate ICD therapy. Occasionally, patients who have ICD therapies suspended when they undergo surgery are left unprotected when these therapies are not reactivated after completion of their procedures.

System data

These include lead impedances, battery voltage, capacitor charge time and defibrillation circuit resistance. Initial examination of these data can rapidly reveal potential problems with the ICD system, including battery depletion (low battery voltage or prolonged charge time), faulty capacitor function (prolonged charge time), lead insulation failure (low impedance), or lead conductor fracture (high impedance). These values should be compared with information recorded from previous visits and with the guidelines for the specific ICD model. In particular, lithium–silver–vanadium oxide batteries are used in ICDs. These batteries have unusual voltage discharge characteristics and approach end-of-life voltage in a less predictable fashion than pacemaker batteries.

Elective replacement indicators for ICDs are based on battery voltage, in some cases combined with charge time criteria specific for each model of ICD. The charge times reflect the time required to charge the capacitor to high voltages. Prolonged charge times may indicate battery depletion, capacitor or component malfunction, or excessive times between capacitor reformation. The reformation process restores the insulating dielectric between the capacitor plates, and is required for optimal capacitor function. This process is usually performed automatically by the device at 3–6-month intervals. When the ICD battery voltage is approaching elective replacement status, the patient should be observed on a more frequent basis (i.e. monthly or bimonthly) to allow for timely ICD generator replacement.

Event logs

Event logs include ventricular and supraventricular tachyarrhythmia episodes/ electrograms and therapies, bradyarrhythmia information, and system component alerts. Each episode of VT, ventricular fibrillation (VF) and SVT should be reviewed carefully to ensure that detection was appropriate and that the therapy was effective.

Remote monitoring of implantable cardioverter-defibrillators

All manufacturers have either initiated or are in the process of initiating remote monitoring of ICDs using monitoring stations based in the patient's home. The retrieved data from the ICD are transmitted by telephone line to a secure server that may be accessed by authorized healthcare providers over the Internet (Fig. 10.1). This information may allow physicians to assess the device programming, activity and performance without the patient leaving home. Some initial evaluations of these monitoring systems have been conducted and these would suggest that remote ICD interrogation is likely to be convenient and safe. The decreased frequency of clinic visits may also contribute to satisfaction expressed by patients in such surveys.[6]

System component testing

The system components that require intermittent testing include the sensing and pacing thresholds. These should be determined at each visit. Occasionally, defibrillation threshold testing may need to be done.

Sensing

Sensing of intrinsic intracardiac signals by atrial and ventricular leads must be determined, as an indication that atrial and ventricular tachyarrhythmias will be reliably detected. Current ICDs include a semiautomated check of sensing, whereas older devices require that bradycardia pacing be temporarily inhibited while a telemetered, calibrated intracardiac electrogram strip is printed. Myocardial infarction, congestive heart failure, cardiac surgery, lead dislodgment, and lead maturation, fracture or perforation can all cause significant decreases in sensed intracardiac electrogram amplitude.

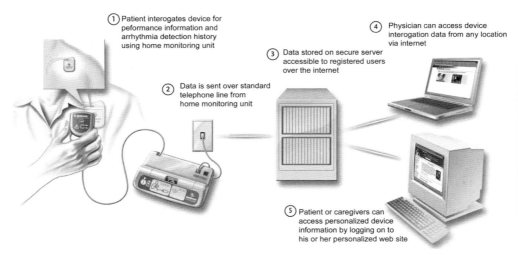

① Patient interogates device for peformance information and arrhythmia detection history using home monitoring unit

② Data is sent over standard telephone line from home monitoring unit

③ Data stored on secure server accessible to registered users over the internet

④ Physician can access device interogation data from any location via internet

⑤ Patient or caregivers can access personalized device information by logging on to his or her personalized web site

Fig. 10.1 Schematic of home-based remote implantable cardioverter defibrillator monitoring system. (Figure courtesy of Medtronic, Inc.)

For suspected noise on the sensing lead, the intracardiac electrogram should be observed while the patient is performing arm movements, deep breathing, coughing, and other maneuvers. If high-frequency signals are seen or there is a failure to sense surface electrocardiographic events, lead conductor fracture, insulation failure or lead/header problems are likely. The intracardiac electrogram should also be examined for diaphragmatic myopotentials, T-wave sensing or far-field sensing.

In biventricular devices, sensing of both left and right ventricular leads should be ascertained. Potential double-counting of sensed ventricular events should be checked in older devices that sense between right and left ventricular tip electrodes to right ventricular ring or defibrillation electrodes.

Pacing thresholds
Pacing thresholds for atrial and ventricular leads should be checked to ensure reliable pacing for bradyarrhythmias. Significant changes in pacing thresholds could be caused by lead fracture, perforation, or dislodgment; congestive heart failure or ischemia; and medications or serum electrolyte abnormalities. Since bradycardia pacing can shorten the longevity of the ICD battery by months or even years, every attempt should be made to optimize pacing outputs and to minimize unnecessary pacing [e.g. preventing ventricular fusion, optimizing the lower rate limit, inactivating rate-responsive and rate-adaptive atrioventricular (AV) delays, etc.].

In biventricular ICDs, both right and left ventricular pacing thresholds should be checked to ensure that biventricular pacing is effective. Additionally, diaphragmatic and chest wall pacing should be checked at maximal left ventricular voltage and pulse duration.

Defibrillation threshold testing
Defibrillation threshold (DFT) testing may have to be repeated using the non-invasive electrophysiology study capability of the ICD. This is mostly warranted for the evaluation of failed therapies, especially if a new DFT-raising drug is initiated or the patient has an event such as myocardial infarction or cardiac surgery. Both DFT as well as sensing during VT or ventricular fibrillation can be re-evaluated. The practice of routine yearly defibrillation testing is controversial.

Implantable cardioverter-defibrillator programming
The successful programming of an ICD depends on a good understanding of a particular patient's arrhythmias and the symptoms from those arrhythmias, as well as the underlying cardiac pathophysiology and the patient's medications. In addition, a thorough knowledge of the capabilities of the patient's ICD is essential. The various parameters that may be programmed are shown in Table 10.1.

Table 10.1 Basic parameters for ICD programming

Parameter	Function	Programming*	Comments	Cautions
VF zone	Detection rate for fastest VF zone: rate of VF zone must be on at all VT/VF in multizone hemodynamically programming or rate for single zone	VF zone: rate of hemodynamically unstable VT; single zone: 10 bpm; spontaneous VT	VF zone must be on at all times, only shock RX available	Programmed rate, spontaneous VT rate causes failure to detect
VT zone	Detection rate for slower VTs in multizone programming	On or off; usually 10 bpm; spontaneous VT	ATP and cardioversion RX available	Programmed rate; spontaneous VT rate causes detection failure
Initial detection (no. of intervals and/or duration)	Number of intervals or time above rate limit to diagnose VT/VF	VF zone: 75% intervals; VF rate; VT zones: number of consecutive intervals or time (seconds) above rate limit	VF typically 12 of 16, or 18 of 24 beats; VF rate of 1–2 s; VT typically 8–20 beats; VT rate of 2–5 s	Short criteria may treat criteria delay; RX
Redetection	Number of intervals or time after RX to assess RX success or failure	Similar to initial detection but shorter criteria	Similar to initial detection but shorter criteria	Same as initial detection
Ventricular sensitivity	Amplitude of EGM that can be detected	Usually 0.18–0.3 mV	High sensitivity needed to detect small EGM in VF	Failure to detect VF if not sensitive enough; oversensing if too sensitive
SVT discriminators	Differentiates SVT from VTs	See Table 10.2. On or off	See Table.10.2. Often initial RX for VTs < 240 bpm	See Table 9.2. May prolong time to shock RX; may accelerate VT to shock RX
ATP	Painless pace termination of VT			
Type of sequence (burst or ramp)	Burst: all paced intervals the same Ramp: decrements between paced intervals in sequence	Burst or ramp	Ramp therapy considered more aggressive but equal efficacy for spontaneous VTs	May prolong time to shock RX; may accelerate VT to shock RX
Coupling interval	Interval from VT beat fulfilling detection to first beat of ATP	Typically 80–90% of VT cycle length	May be same as R-R%	Too long or short an interval prevents capture
R-R%	Sets rate for first sequence of ATP	Typically 80–90% of VT cycle length	Consider number of sequences to deliver	Values ≥ 80% VT cycle length likely to accelerate VT
No. of pulses	Number of paced beats delivered within each ATP sequence	Typically 5–15 beats	Some algorithms add 1 pulse to each sequence	Short trains may fail to penetrate VT circuit; long trains may reinitiate VT

Parameter	Description	Typical value		
Decrement	Amount the intervals shorten between (burst) and/or within sequence (ramp)	Typically 10–30 ms	Value should consider number of sequences to be delivered	Large decrements may rapidly reach minimal ATP interval value
No. of sequences	Maximal number of ATP sequences attempted	Typically 3–6 sequences	Most VT terminated with 3 sequences	Large number of sequences prolongs time to shock RX
Sustained high rate	Overrides SVT discriminators to initiate RX after programmed duration	Highly individualized for each patient, typically 1–5 min	Only requires programming when discriminator algorithms active	Excessively long duration will delay therapy for misdiagnosed VT
Minimum ATP interval	Limits maximal rate of ATP pacing	Typically 240–300 ms	VT ≥ 200 bpm less likely to terminate with ATP	Short intervals may accelerate VT
Cardioversion/defibrillation	Shock therapy	Always on in all zones (rarely is disabled in a very slow VT zone)	Only RX in VF or single zone; initial RX or follows ATP in VT zones	Painful at all energy levels
Energy	Magnitude of shock in joules or as voltage	VF: DFT 5–10 J; VT: at or above smallest successful energy	VT often terminated with 2–10 J	Failed first shocks prolong time to effective RX and are painful
Pathway/polarity	Path of current flow between electrodes	Typically RV coil negative (cathodal) and can proximal coil positive (anodal)	Most devices can reprogram polarity; new devices can program coils in or out of circuit	Reprogramming may significantly alter DFT
Tilt	Voltage drop on capacitor during shock	Usually 40–65%	Programmable in some devices; programming based on shock impedance	Reprogramming may significantly alter DFT
Pulse width	Duration of each phase of shock	For biphasic shock, typically 8–16 ms total	Based on shock impedance	Reprogramming may significantly alter DFT
Capacitor reformation interval	Restores capacitor dielectric	Usually every 3 months	Requires capacitor charge	Too frequent drains battery, too infrequent delays charging
Patient alert	Activates audible or vibratory alert for malfunction	Alert at scheduled time of day		Demonstrate to patient post implant

*All programming must be individualized for each patient.
ATP, antitachycardia pacing; DFT, defibrillation threshold; EGM, electrogram; RX, ICD therapy; SVT, supraventricular tachycardia; VF, ventricular fibrillation; VT, ventricular tachycardia.

Ventricular tachyarrhythmia detection

Most devices allow for multiple zones of ventricular tachyarrhythmia detection based on heart rate (Fig. 10.2). Whereas a "shock box" programmed to detect and treat VF in a single zone works to reduce sudden death in large clinical trials, the use of VT zones allows for the use of antitachycardia pacing therapies (ATP) and SVT discrimination algorithms in most patients The performance of SVT–VT discriminators is linked to boundaries between detection zones. Therefore, it is common practice to have a zone programmed for slower, relatively well-tolerated VT (VT zone), and another zone programmed for faster, hemodynamically unstable ventricular tachycardia or fibrillation (VF zone). The rate limits for these zones are usually set 10 bpm slower than the documented ventricular arrhythmia rate to ensure reliable detection. VT induced by electrophysiological testing is often much faster than the patient's spontaneous arrhythmia and is not usually an accurate guide to setting the rate limits.

The ventricular sensitivity must allow for the detection of very low-amplitude VF signals and is typically set to 0.3 mV, or more sensitive settings. Criteria for the number of beats or the time duration above the tachycardia rate in each zone must also be programmed to complete the detection algorithm. In the VT zone, various enhancements are available to decrease the risk of supraventricular tachyarrhythmias, triggering therapy. In single-chamber ICDs, stability, suddenness of onset, as well as duration of arrhythmia may be used to increase the specificity for ventricular arrhythmias. These features are described further in Table 10.2. In addition, algorithms derived from analysis of ventricular electrogram morphology have proven useful in differentiation of VT from SVT.[7] All of these algorithms are derived from a series of steps that compare the recording of a baseline rhythm electrogram template with tachycardia electrogram recordings. Depending on the fraction of electrograms that have morphological similarity to the baseline template, the tachycardia is classified as SVT or VT. In some ICDs, the number of electrograms that need to have a required degree of morphology matching can be programmed, e.g. the recommended programming for Medtronic ICDs is a requirement of at least three out of eight electrograms having at least a 70% match with baseline sinus rhythm, in order for the ICD to call it SVT. There are situations in which morphology algorithms fail, particularly when the baseline template changes (e.g. narrow QRS changing to bundle branch block) or there is electrogram truncation due to an increase in the amplitude of the recorded electrogram signal, or if alignment of compared electrograms does not occur perfectly. The utility of using changing QRS morphology to differentiate between supraventricular tachycardias and VT is shown in Fig. 10.3.

With the incorporation of atrial sensing and bradycardia pacing in ICDs, information recorded from the atrial lead allows for further discrimination based on the relationship of atrial to ventricular activity. As demonstrated in Figs 10.3 and 10.4, the addition of an atrial electrogram is invaluable in proving ventriculoatrial dissociation, thus confirming the diagnosis of VT.

ICD **Model**: Gem DR 7271
Serial **Number**:

Nov 17, 2000 09:44:38
9960 Software Version 3.0
Copyright (c) Medtronic, Inc. 1997

Detection Report   Page 1

Detection

	Enable	Interval (Rate)
VF	On	290 ms (207 bpm)
FVT	Off	320 ms (188 bpm)
VT	On	400 ms (150 bpm)

Number of Intervals to Detect

	Initial NID	Redetect NID
VF	18/24	12/16
VT	16	8

Sensitivity

| Atrial | 0.45 mV |
| Ventricular | 0.3 mV |

Dual Chamber SVT Criteria

AFib/AFlutter	On
Sinus Tach	On
Other 1:1 SVTs	On
SVT Limit	320 ms

Ventricular SVT Criteria

| VT Stability | 40 ms |

A

ICD **Model**: Gem DR 7271
Serial **Number**:

Nov 17, 2000 09:41:33
9960 **Software Version 3.0**
Copyright (c) **Medtronic, Inc. 1997**

VT Therapies Report   Page 1

VT Therapies	Rx1	Rx2	Rx3	Rx4	Rx5	Rx6
VT Therapy Status	On	On	On	On	On	On
Therapy Type	Burst	Ramp	CV	CV	CV	CV
Initial # Pulses	8	10				
R-S1 Interval=(%RR)	91 %	84 %				
S1S2(Ramp+)=(%RR)						
S2SN(Ramp+)=(%RR)						
Interval Dec	10 ms	20 ms				
# Sequences	5	3				
Smart Mode	On	On				
Energy			5 J	15 J	35 J	35 J
Pathway			AX>B	AX>B	AX>B	AX>B
Anti-Tachy Pacing Minimum Interval		280 ms				

B

Fig. 10.2 (A) Ventricular arrhythmia detection parameter report for the Medtronic model 7271 dual-chamber implantable cardioverter defibrillator (ICD). Up to three tachyarrhythmia detection zones are programmable based on ventricular rate. In this example, two zones are programmed: a ventricular tachycardia (VT) zone is from 150 to 206 bpm, and a ventricular fibrillation (VF) zone is over 207 bpm. An intermediate zone [fast VT (FVT)] can also be programmed. This example shows the number of intervals to detection (NID) for the VT and VF zones. After initial detection, a redetect NID must also be satisfied before therapy delivery. Also shown are atrial and ventricular sensitivities and discriminator algorithms for supraventricular tachyarrhythmia. (B) Therapies for the VT zone programmed for a Medtronic 7271 dual-chamber ICD. Up to six progressively more aggressive therapies (Rx) may be programmed. The initial therapy (Rx1) is a burst-type antitachycardia pacing (ATP) with eight pulses being delivered in five sequences; each successive sequence pacing cycle length is decremented by 10 ms. The second therapy (Rx2) is a more aggressive ramp ATP scheme. Therapies three to six (Rx3 to Rx6) are progressively higher energy shocks, up to the maximal output for the device (35 J). For all ICD therapy, each successive therapy should be more aggressive than the last.

Table 10.2 Detection enhancements in implantable cardioverter defibrillators (ICDs) for differentiation of SVT from VT

Parameter	What it does	Potentially useful for	Potential problems
Stability	Suppresses therapy for tachyarrhythmias with variable ventricular rate	Atrial fibrillation	Underdetection of VT with irregular rate; failure to suppress therapy for SVTs with regular ventricular response
Onset	Suppresses therapy for tachyarrhythmias that slowly accelerate	Sinus tachycardia	Underdetection of gradually accelerating VT or VT onset during sinus tachycardia; failure to suppress therapy for sudden onset SVTs
Ventricular electrogram morphology	Suppresses therapy for tachyarrhythmias with ventricular EGM morphology similar to that in sinus rhythm	Potentially useful for differentiation of SVT from VT	Limited specificity with bundle branch block
Sustained rate duration	Therapy for tachyarrhythmias finally delivered after this period of time, even if enhancements still met	Prevents indefinite inhibition of therapy for VT misdiagnosed as SVT	Therapy will eventually be delivered if the SVT continues after sustained rate duration expires
Atrial to ventricular ratio	Compares atrial to ventricular rate	Atrial fibrillation	Atrial undersensing can result in false diagnosis of VT
Atrial to ventricular timing	Evaluates the temporal relation of atrial electrogram to ventricular electrograms	Atrial fibrillation, 1 : 1 SVTs retrograde conduction	Variable AV timing, long antegrade or retrograde AV conduction times

Some detection enhancements are available only in certain models of ICD.
EGM, electrogram; SVT, supraventricular tachycardia; VT, ventricular tachycardia.

In some dual-chamber ICDs, discrimination between supraventricular tach-yarrhythmia and VT is based on stability of the atrial rate and whether the atrial rate is faster than the ventricular rate. Often, supraventricular tach-yarrhythmia discrimination algorithms are subject to a sustained rate-dura-tion limit that, once exceeded, triggers therapy. In Medtronic dual-chamber ICDs, the algorithm involves determining timing of atrial activity in relation to ventricular activity (PR Logic, Medtronic, Inc., Minneapolis, MN, USA). Certain patterns are associated with supraventricular tachyarrhythmias, AF, sinus tachycardia as well as far-field R-wave sensing, and will inhibit therapy. Other patterns showing AV dissociation or retrograde conduction consistent with VT will allow therapy. Generalized algorithms for arrhyth-mia detection using these discriminators in single- and dual-chamber ICDs are shown in Fig. 10.5.

Despite the introduction of dual-chamber ICDs, the rate of inappropriate ICD discharges, mostly due to supraventricular arrhythmias, still ranges be-

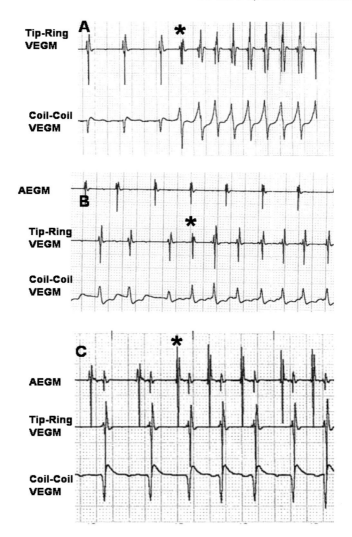

Fig. 10.3 Electrogram morphology changes during ventricular tachycardia (VT) and supraventricular tachyarrhythmia. (A) Ventricular tachycardia. Ventricular electrograms (VEGM) from the closed spaced tip-ring configuration and coil–coil configuration of a single-chamber implantable cardioverter defibrillator (ICD). With the onset of ventricular tachyarrhythmia (*) there is a marked change in the morphology of the electrograms recorded from both electrode pairs. (B) VT from a patient with a dual-chamber ICD. AEGM, atrial electrogram. At the onset of VT (*), there is AV dissociation; however, there is minimal change in the ventricular electrogram morphologies. Similar electrogram morphologies may be seen with VT and sinus rhythm in 10–15% of patients. (C) Atrial tachycardia triggering ICD detection. The onset of atrial tachycardia (*) is evident by the change in the AEGM morphology and the atrial rate change precedes the ventricular rate change. Note that the VEGM morphologies do not change. (D) VT in the same patient as panel C. There is AV dissociation. In this case the ventricular rate change (*) precedes the atrial rate change. With VT there is a subtle change in the tip-ring VEGM, but a more marked change in the coil–coil VEGM. (*Continued.*)

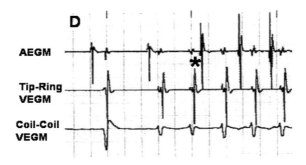

Fig. 10.3 (*Continued.*)

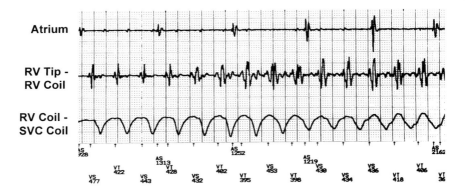

Fig. 10.4 Ventricular tachycardia, as recorded by a dual-chamber implantable cardioverter defibrillator. AV dissociation is clearly demonstrated when comparing the atrial electrogram (Atrium, top tracing) with the ventricular electrogram (RV Tip–RV Coil, middle tracing), which is recorded from the distal tip electrode to the right ventricular defibrillation coil. The bottom tracing (RV Coil–SVC Coil) is a ventricular electrogram recorded from a coil on the portion of the ventricular lead that is in the superior vena cava to the distal coil located on the portion of the lead which is in the right ventricle. The marker channel annotations below the electrograms are: AS, atrial sensed event; VS, ventricular sensed event; VT, ventricular sensed event meeting VT rate criteria. The numbers are the intervals in milliseconds between consecutive events.

tween 20 and 40%.[8] Clinical predictors of inappropriate therapy in ICD patients include New York Heart Association heart failure score (class I patients have a higher incidence of inappropriate shock) and history of AF.[9] Supraventricular tachyarrhythmias with sudden onset and a regular ventricular response (i.e. atrial flutter where P waves fall in atrial channel-blanking periods) or 1 : 1 SVTs are especially problematic for present generation ICDs. Although further programming to discriminate these arrhythmias could be done, it comes at the expense of decreased sensitivity of the algorithm with the increased potential for failure to sense VT.

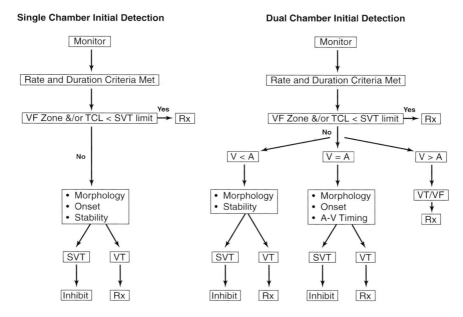

Fig. 10.5 Generalized detection algorithms for single- and dual-chamber implantable cardioverter defibrillators (ICDs) incorporating discrimination enhancement features. For the dual-chamber algorithm, a primary "decision point" is the difference between the atrial and ventricular rates. VF, ventricular fibrillation; TCL, tachycardia cycle length; Rx, ICD therapy; SVT, supraventricular tachycardia; VT, ventricular tachycardia; V, ventricular; A, atrial.

Ventricular tachyarrhythmia therapies

ATP is the preferred mode of initial therapy because it has a > 90% success rate in terminating VT, particularly at rates < 200 bpm.[10,11] The benefits of ATP are that it is painless to the patient and contributes to preservation of battery life when compared with cardioversion. Even in patients who received an ICD for ventricular fibrillation, a VT detection zone with ATP as initial therapy should be empirically programmed because > 50% of these patients will subsequently have VT amenable to successful treatment with ATP.[12]

The traditional practice of programming ATP only for VT rates < 200 bpm has been challenged by the publication of two recent trials.[13,14] These studies have suggested that programming ATP therapies for VTs in the 188–250 bpm range (fast VT zone) can terminate such VTs in 70–85% of these cases. As a result, some devices will allow programming in three separate zones: VT, fast VT and VF. One manufacturer allows for the delivery of ATP during device charging for shock therapy. On the other hand, if a review of the stored episodes of VT shows that ATP does not reliably terminate or possibly accelerates VT, this therapy should be disabled and low-energy cardioversion (5–10 J) should be the initial therapy. Cardioversion energies < 5 J should be avoided since they could precipitate AF.[15] Usually, up to six therapies are available for a VT zone, progressing from ATP and/or low-energy shocks to high-energy shocks. An example of programming multiple VT therapies is shown in Fig. 10.2.

Because defibrillation of VF at any given shock energy is a probability function, the initial defibrillation energy for the VF zone should include an appropriate safety margin. What this margin should be is somewhat controversial, but programming a 10-J safety margin above the DFT energy is traditionally practised. A randomized study has demonstrated that safety margins of 4–6 J above carefully defined DFT at implant (DFT++) have the same efficacy in follow-up as full-output shocks.[16] More recently, an alternative has been suggested to this traditional approach of DFT testing. In current generation devices with a dual-coil lead and active pulse generator, it is equally safe and efficacious to limit DFT testing to the first successful 14-J shock, as long as all shocks are programmed to 31 J.[17] If testing demonstrates that the DFT has increased over time, possible remedies include discontinuation of any drugs that could increase DFT (Table 10.3); addition of pure class III agents, such as sotalol, which can decrease the DFT; or revision of the ICD system, which may include repositioning or replacing the defibrillation lead, addition of a subcutaneous electrode array, or substituting another ICD with higher defibrillation energy output.

Some new devices allow for programmable energy pathways, waveforms, tilt, pulse width, and polarity to non-invasively optimize the DFT. Up to six

Table 10.3 Drugs that may elevate the defibrillation threshold

Class IA
  Quinidine*
  Procainamide*
Class IB
  Lidocaine
  Mexiletine*
  Tocainide
Class IC
  Flecainide*
  Moricizine
  Propafenone*
Class II
  Propranolol
  Carvedilol
Class III
  Amiodarone*
Class IV
  Verapamil
  Diltiazem
Other
  Sildenafil
  Enflurane inhaled anesthetic
  Fentanyl

*Data in the literature regarding effects on DFT are mixed.

progressively higher shock energies are usually available for VF zones, with maximal output mandatory for the final shocks.

Atrial antitachycardia therapies

Some devices incorporate ATP and shock therapies for atrial arrhythmias that are analogous to ventricular therapies in most respects (Fig. 10.6). Different arrhythmia zones, usually defined as atrial tachycardia and atrial fibrillation zones, are programmable based on atrial rate and duration criteria. Because

Patient Activated Therapy (AT/AF)					
Status	Off				
Therapy Type					
Energy					
Pathway					

AF Therapy	Rx1	Rx2	Rx3		
Status	On	On	On		
Therapy Type	A-50Hz	A-CV	A-CV		
Burst Duration	1 sec				
# Sequences	10				
Energy		5 J	30 J		
Pathway		AX>B	AX>B		

AT Therapy	Rx1	Rx2	Rx3	Rx4	Rx5
Status	On	On	Off	On	On
Therapy Type	A-Ramp	A-Burst+		A-CV	A-CV
Burst Duration					
# Sequences	6	6			
Energy				1 J	5 J
Pathway				AX>B	AX>B
Initial #S1 Pulses	8	15			
A-S1 Interval (%AA)	91 %	91 %			
S1S2 (%AA)		69 %			
S2S3 Decrement		10 ms			
Interval Dec	10 ms	10 ms			

Parameters shared by all A-CV therapies

Episode Duration Before Delivery		Automatic A-CV Limits	
Pacing	10 min	Start Time	03:00 for 1 hr
A-CV	6 hr	Maximum shocks per day	2
		Device Time	15:56
Time To Stop Therapy	48 hr		

Fig. 10.6 Atrial antitachycardia therapies programmed for a Medtronic dual-chamber implantable cardioverter defibrillator with combined ventricular and atrial therapies. AT, atrial tachycardia; AF, atrial fibrillation; Rx, therapy; A, atrial; CV, cardioversion; AX>B, current path for high-energy delivery with ventricular coil negative and proximal coil and can positive. Three AF therapies are programmed: first high-frequency (50 Hz) atrial burst pacing for 1 s and 10 sequences if needed. Low-energy (5 J), then high-energy (30 J) cardioversions follow failed pacing therapies. Note that the shocks will be delivered only within a 1-h window starting at 03.00 h to minimize patient discomfort (Automatic A-CV Limits). AT therapies include two ATP schemes, followed by two attempts at low-energy cardioversion.

there is rarely time urgency to terminate atrial arrhythmias, extensive, tiered ATP therapies may be programmed as initial therapies. Efficacy for pace termination of atrial arrhythmias in the atrial tachycardia zone is usually around 50%. Some devices provide high-frequency (50 Hz) burst pacing in the AF zone, although the efficacy of ATP for AF is limited (approximately 25%). Nevertheless, there is usually little disadvantage to attempts at ATP for atrial arrhythmias, and every effort should be made to avoid shock therapy for atrial arrhythmias. Because even very low-energy shock therapy at 1–2 J is poorly tolerated, shock therapy for AF is rarely programmed on. Again, because of the lack of urgency to terminate AF, shock therapies may be delayed for extended periods (hours) and warning of impending shock may be issued by some device in the form of a very low-energy shock. In some devices, shock therapy for AF may be programmed to be delivered only at a scheduled time of day or at night to reduce the level of discomfort. Some devices allow for the patient to divert therapy or command a shock using an external activator if all other detection criteria are met. The number of shocks delivered in 24–48 h is typically programmable.

Management of implantable cardioverter defibrillators in the operating room, endoscopy suite and radiofrequency ablation procedures

It is logical for the increase in the population of ICD recipients to also manifest as increased encounters with hospital-based sources of electromagnetic interference (EMI). Both electrocautery and radiofrequency ablation have the potential for EMI. Sensing of cautery output by the ICD may trigger therapy for presumed ventricular arrhythmias and/or inhibit pacing output. Transmission of cautery current down the pacing/defibrillation leads may increase the pacing threshold. There is a possibility that the ICD may potentially be damaged or reprogrammed.

To prevent these problems, tachyarrhythmia detection as well as therapies should be disabled for the duration of the procedure. Ideally, this is done with the ICD programmer. However, it is likely that operating rooms and endoscopy suites may not have people with the necessary knowledge or expertise to re-program the ICD. Alternatively, therapies can be disabled by placing a magnet over the device during surgery and removed at the conclusion of the procedure. For most devices, this effect is reversible and the ICD therapies become available when the magnet is removed. Some innovations have been introduced in specific magnets, e.g. the Medtronic Smart Magnet™ contains an indicator light that confirms correct placement of the magnet over the device. There are also some notable make-specific features related to the magnet response. In Guidant ICDs, response of the ICD to a magnet is a programmable parameter. Therefore, if therapies are unaffected by a magnet (indicated by absence of audible tones when a magnet is placed on the device), the Guidant ICD has this programmable feature turned off. If there are intermittent tones, the feature is turned on and the therapies have been disabled. Once the magnet is removed for 30 s, the therapies are resumed and this is indicated by a continuous tone. There are specific Guidant CRT-D devices that will have the Enable Magnet Use feature turned off due to a field advisory (communication to physicians June 23, 2005). As a result, for these devices, suspension of tachyarrhythmia therapy can only be performed using a programmer. In general, while tachyarrhythmia detections and therapies are turned off, the patient's electrocardiogram should be continuously monitored and external defibrillation should be readily available. Other procedures that have the potential to trigger therapies, inhibit therapies or otherwise damage the device include transcutaneous electrical neurological stimulation units, lithotripsy, magnetic resonance imaging and radiation therapy.

ICD patients with separate pacemaker systems

Since the use of separate temporary or permanent bradycardia pacing systems in the ICD patient may cause a multitude of problems, these merit special mention. The main reason is that the ICD cannot "blank" pacing stimuli from separate pacing units. Therefore these stimuli and subsequent R waves may be double-counted, thereby triggering inappropriate therapies. An example of inappropriate double-counting in a patient with a single-chamber ICD and a separate dual-chamber pacing system is demonstrated in Fig. 10.7A. In some situations, if the pacing unit is not sensing ventricular tachycardia or fibrillation in an appropriate manner, it may continue to deliver pacing stimuli during these arrhythmias. Due to the sensing characteristics of automatic gain and automatic threshold sensing algorithms, ICDs may only count the pacing stimuli; this could lead to underdetection of the ventricular arrhythmia and failure to deliver therapy, as shown in Fig. 10.7B.

Elective cardioversion and external defibrillation in ICD recipients

The procedure for elective cardioversion and external defibrillation in the ICD patient is similar to that for pacemaker patients described elsewhere in this text. Most ICDs are implanted in the left pectoral region, but older ICD systems may have been implanted in the left upper abdomen. For the ICD patient presenting with cardiac arrest, standard advanced cardiac life-saving protocols for cardiopulmonary resuscitation and external defibrillation should be followed as for any other patient. One should not wait for the ICD to deliver therapy, as malfunctions or ineffective therapies may already have occurred.

Troubleshooting implantable cardioverter defibrillators

Troubleshooting ICD problems encompasses all aspects of bradycardia pacemaker malfunctions as well as evaluation of the appropriateness of therapies for VT. Several scenarios with ICD patients demand sleuth work on the part of the follow-up physician. These scenarios include patients presenting with (i) pacing malfunction, (ii) single ICD discharge, (iii) multiple ICD discharges,

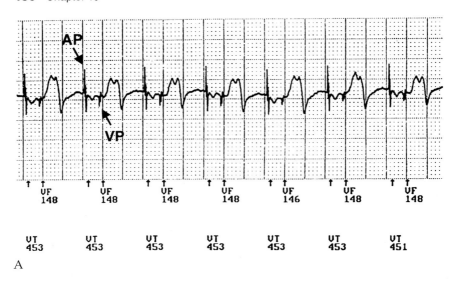

A

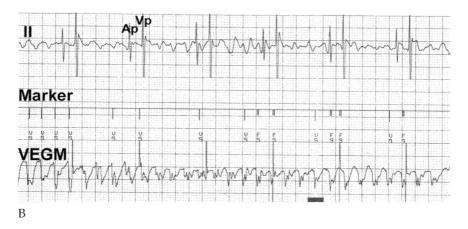

B

Fig. 10.7 Problems with separate bradycardia pacing systems in patients with implantable cardioverter defibrillators (ICDs). (A) Double-counting of atrial and ventricular pacing artifacts from a dual-chamber pacemaker by a Guidant PRx single-chamber ICD. The ICD detects alternating ventricular cycle lengths of 148 and 453 ms, which meet the rate criteria for ventricular tachycardia (VT) and ventricular fibrillation (VF) detection annotated on the marker channel. (B) Undersensing of VF by a single-chamber ICD due to interaction with a separate dual-chamber pacemaker. II, surface lead II; VEGM, ventricular electrogram; VS, ventricular sensed event; FS, ventricular fibrillation sensed event. At ICD testing the pacemaker is programmed to DOO mode at maximal outputs (bipolar pacing). After induction of VF the atrial (Ap) and ventricular (Vp) outputs are sensed by the ICD, which decreases the automatic sensitivity setting so that the ventricular electrograms are not sensed following the pacing artifacts.

(iv) syncope with no perceived ICD therapy, and (v) documented sustained VT without ICD therapy.[18,19] A careful history and physical examination, and inspection of the comprehensive data logs and stored electrograms will often provide answers to all of these scenarios. Further information can be obtained from the programmed device parameters, the device battery and capacitor status, and the lead performance. It is also important to remember that the companies keep a record of individual implanted patients. In the event that a patient is not able to provide basic information, such as the make of the device, physicians can contact individual companies to obtain this vital information.

Bradycardia pacing by the implantable cardioverter defibrillator

Although most of the bradycardia pacing functions of the ICD are identical to a simple pacemaker, some features are different. Because of the high ventricular sensitivity and limited blanking periods needed to optimally detect VF, oversensing by the ICD may be more difficult to avoid or correct. Different parameters may be programmed for post-shock pacing and standard bradycardia pacing; unipolar pacing modes are not available in the ICD. As described previously, application of a magnet to an ICD inhibits tachycardia therapies, but does not trigger the asynchronous bradycardia pacing mode. Asynchronous and triggered modes are not available in ICDs. In addition, there are sometimes limitations on the pacing intervals that can be programmed due to overlap and interference with tachycardia detection algorithms.

Biventricular ICDs incorporate simultaneous left and right ventricular pacing for treatment of congestive heart failure caused by left ventricular dyssynchrony. Failure of either right or left ventricular pacing because of elevated pacing thresholds or lead dislodgment may change QRS morphology on the electrocardiogram. Double-counting of conducted ventricular events could inhibit pacing.

Single implantable cardioverter defibrillator discharge

Even though ICD therapies form the basis of device utilization, careful evaluation is warranted of patients who receive such therapies. A significant proportion of therapies may be inappropriate, requiring reprogramming of tachycardia detection parameters. Recognition of appropriate shocks, on the other hand, is the critical information needed to proceed with either antiarrhythmic therapy or radiofrequency ablation for prevention of recurrent ventricular arrhythmias. A flow diagram for the evaluation of ICD shocks is shown in Fig. 10.8. Following ICD implantation, patients should be educated about the procedures to follow after an ICD shock, before they are discharged from the hospital. It is advisable to have the patient call the physician's office after the first shock is perceived. It is an opportunity to assess the appropriateness of the therapy as well as to provide reassurance. This allows assessment of the patient's level of anxiety, a part of patient management that could be further strengthened in most practices. We interrogate the device electively within 1–2 days to ensure that the ICD is functioning appropriately. Thereafter, the

Evaluating the ICD Discharge

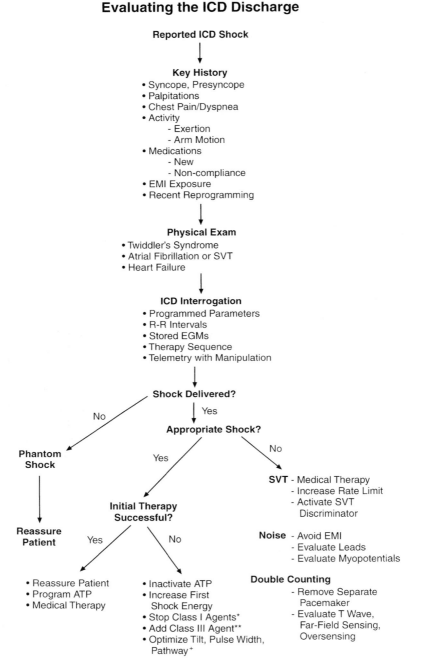

Fig. 10.8 Flow diagram for evaluating implantable cardioverter defibrillator shocks. ATP, antitachycardia pacing; EGM, electrocardiograms; EMI, electromagnetic interference; SVT, supraventricular tachycardia. *See Table 10.3. **Class III drugs include sotalol and dofetilide; not programmable in all devices.

patient may contact us for the infrequent shocks, depending on his or her level of comfort. We advise patients to call immediately when more than two shocks within 24 h are experienced, as this may indicate failed device therapy or inappropriate shocks.

The immediate goal of the physician evaluating a patient who has had an ICD shock is to establish whether the therapy was appropriate. A full account of the events leading up to the shock should be elicited, including activities, medical compliance, use of new medications, syncope, palpitations, exposure to EMI, angina, and heart failure. Shocks preceded by syncope or presyncope are almost always appropriate. Shocks associated with heavy exertion, motion of the arm ipsilateral to the ICD, or exposure to electromagnetic current sources should raise suspicions of sinus tachycardia, lead noise, or EMI interference, respectively. Interrogation of the device therapy log is most useful in determining the cause of the shock. For VT episodes, the stored electrograms will usually confirm the diagnosis by demonstrating AV dissociation or a change in the morphology compared with sinus rhythm. Otherwise, any noise, SVT or sinus tachycardia will be evident.

Regardless of the cause of the shock, hospitalization for an isolated ICD discharge is rarely warranted unless changes in the antiarrhythmic drug therapy are needed. It is important to reassure the patient that the device has functioned properly. However, in an attempt to minimize the chances of recurrent painful therapies, consideration should be given to activating ATP therapies or initiating antiarrhythmic drug therapy. For an inappropriate shock, corrective measures must be taken. To avoid triggering of inappropriate ICD therapies by SVTs, increasing the tachycardia detection rate, activation of SVT discrimination algorithms, or initiation of antiarrhythmic/AV nodal blocking agents may be useful. Myopotential sensing may require reprogramming of device sensitivity and subsequent follow-up electrophysiological testing for appropriate VF detection. The observation of noise on intracardiac recordings should prompt a thorough search for a lead malfunction or any exposure to EMI.

Finally, some patients report ICD discharges but the ICD counters show no therapy being delivered. This phenomenon, called "phantom shocks," often occurs at night and may be due to anxiety, dream states, or hypnagogic contractures. Usually, reassurance is all that is needed, but psychological counseling is occasionally required.

Multiple discharges

Multiple ICD discharges can be either appropriate or inappropriate. A differential diagnosis for multiple ICD discharges is included in Table 10.5. Because multiple ICD discharges often cause significant psychological stress to the patient, they should be considered a medical emergency.

Multiple appropriate discharges

Acute treatment of the patient with multiple appropriate ICD discharges should first focus on treating any underlying causes and/or initiating intravenous antiarrhythmic or β-blockade therapy.[20] When multiple therapies occur within a 24-h period, the event has been referred to as an "electrical storm." Common underlying causes of electrical storm include ischemia, electrolyte abnormalities, decompensated heart failure and drug effects, but many cases have no identifiable etiology. If the patient is receiving multiple appropriate shocks for VT, reprogramming to include ATP for VT may diminish the number of shocks. On occasion, most of the episodes of VT are self-terminating, and in this case the patient may benefit from a longer detection and confirmation time in the VT zone. If multiple shocks are delivered as a result of initial therapies being ineffective (i.e. ATP or a low-energy shock failed to treat VT), more aggressive initial therapy may diminish the total number of discharges the patient receives (Fig. 10.9).

Ineffective therapies may result in multiple shocks for a single arrhythmic episode. If initial therapies fail to terminate VF, the DFT should be re-evaluated, because it may rise over time. An important cause of increased DFT is drug therapy, as outlined in Table 10.3. DFT may also change after myocardial infarction, cardiac surgery and physical movement of the lead or generator. Occasionally, ICD system revision to change the current shock vector, revision of a lead, or installation of a high-output generator may be needed. Finally, catheter-based radiofrequency ablation for VT can be effective in eliminating or decreasing the number of VT episodes in drug-refractory cases.[21]

Although this is rarely used today, some ICDs may still be programmed to "committed" mode, in which therapy will be delivered after initial tachycardia detection criteria are met, even if the arrhythmia spontaneously terminates. This mode of operation may result in frequent or multiple shocks for non-sustained ventricular arrhythmias. Some devices are capable of defibrillation therapy for atrial tachyarrhythmias. Multiple low-energy shocks are

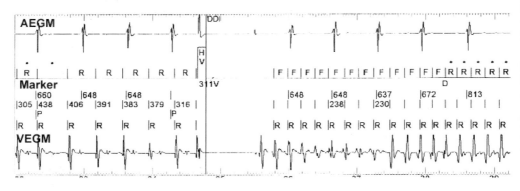

Fig. 10.9 Acceleration of slow ventricular tachycardia (VT) to ventricular fibrillation (VF) by low-energy shock (311 V, approximately 5 J). AEGM, atrial electrogram; VEGM, ventricular electrogram; HV, high-voltage therapy; R, sensed ventricular event; F, ventricular fibrillation sensed event. As initial treatment, this ineffective therapy is counterproductive, leading to more therapies. Antitachycardia pacing or a higher energy shock may be more appropriate to minimize therapy deliveries.

one strategy to terminate AF with these devices as an alternative or prelude to high-energy therapy.

Multiple inappropriate discharges

In the case of repeated inappropriate discharges, the ICD should be promptly inactivated and the patient placed on telemetry with external defibrillation capabilities readily available. Most devices will have therapies inhibited as long as a magnet is in place over the generator. Inappropriate ICD therapies may have many causes, but the most common cause is AF, as shown in Fig. 10.10. Other atrial tachyarrhythmias including atrial flutter and sinus tachycardia may also trigger inappropriate ICD therapy. Examination of stored electrograms from the delivered therapies should always be performed to document the nature of the recorded arrhythmia. Clues to the differentiation of SVT from VT based on stored electrograms are given in Table 10.4. Once the device is inactivated, the atrial arrhythmia can be managed in a conventional manner. If the device cannot be immediately reprogrammed, chemical or electrical conversion of the atrial arrhythmia may be needed if ventricular rate control cannot be achieved. After initial control of the SVT has been achieved, ICD tachyarrhythmia detection features for discrimination of SVT from VT may be useful in preventing further inappropriate therapies. In theory, dual-chamber ICDs should decrease the number of inappropriate ICD therapies for supraventricular tachycardias. A recent evaluation in a randomized study has found that dual-chamber ICDs had a significantly lower rate of inappropriate therapies due to SVT, but this difference was small (30.9% in dual- vs. 39.5% in single-chamber ICDs).[8] Atrial undersensing of AF (resulting in a faster measured ventricular than atrial rate) and rapid ventricular conduction into the VF zone are common causes of therapies for atrial arrhythmias. Additionally, it is unclear whether the use of ventricular electrogram morphology algorithms will decrease inappropriate ICD therapies due to SVTs (Fig. 10.11). Ventricular electrogram morphology discrimination when used in conjunction with other SVT discriminators has a suboptimal sensitivity for atrial tachycardia.[22] SVTs with subtle rate-related changes in the QRS complex can also trigger inappropriate detection of ventricular tachyarrhythmias. Reprogramming of the percent template match to less rigorous criteria may improve SVT detection, without adversely affecting sensitivity for VT detection. Some ICD patients who receive inappropriate shocks repeatedly for AF or atrial flutter require radiofrequency ablation of the AV node for definitive control of the ventricular rate.

Over-counting of ventricular events by the ICD is another important cause of inappropriate ICD discharges. An example of T-wave oversensing in a patient with a ventricular lead with an integrated sensing bipolar lead (right ventricular defibrillation coil and tip electrodes) is shown in Fig. 10.12. This may be corrected by decreasing the ventricular sensitivity and subsequent testing to confirm that VF would be appropriately detected. Some devices allow for change in the slope of the autosensitivity decrement after sensing to better blank T-wave sensing. In other cases, substitution of a lead with a true bipo-

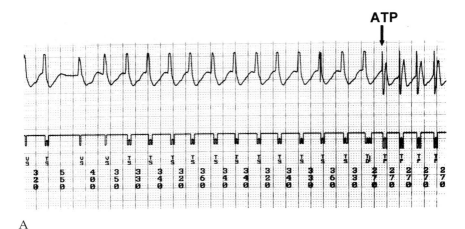

A

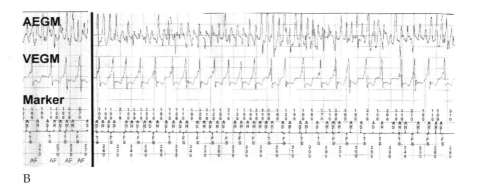

B

Fig. 10.10 Inappropriate therapies due to atrial fibrillation (AF). (A) AF and inappropriate therapy, as recorded by a single-chamber implantable cardioverter defibrillator. Note the marked irregularity of the intracardiac ventricular electrogram (top tracing) and the ventricular cycle length, which varies between 290 and 500 ms (bottom tracing, marker channel). The ventricular rate eventually falls into the ventricular tachycardia (VT) zone (denoted by "TS" marker channel) and is more regular at the rapid rate. Antitachycardia pacing (ATP) therapy is delivered (denoted by "TP" marker channel). (B) AF with very rapid ventricular rate into the ventricular fibrillation zone. Initially, the Medtronic PR Logic algorithm appropriately classifies the tachycardia as AF based on the irregularity and rapid irregular atrial rate (left panel). At rapid ventricular response into the ventricular fibrillation zone, however, the supraventricular tachycardia (SVT) discriminators no longer apply and ventricular therapies are delivered. AEGM, atrial electrogram; VEGM, ventricular electrogram. (C) Inappropriate therapy due to undersensing of AF. The rapid ventricular response to AF is classified as ventricular tachycardia despite 100% match on the morphology algorithm because of "AV dissociation" diagnosed by a faster ventricular rate than atrial rate. The box inserts show the sensed atrial intervals (A–A) longer than the ventricular intervals (V–V) due to atrial electrogram drop out.

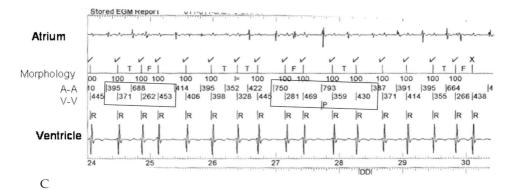

C

Fig. 10.10 (*Continued.*)

Table 10.4 Differentiating SVT and VT by stored electrograms

Finding	Interpretation	Comment
Change VEGM morphology	Suggests VT	Misdiagnosis from aberrancy with SVT, VEGM in VT similar to template
Stable R–R interval	Suggests VT in setting of atrial fibrillation	Misdiagnosis from R–R interval can regularize with rapid response to atrial fibrillation
Gradual onset	Suggests sinus tachycardia	Misdiagnosis from VT onset during sinus tachycardia, slow VT gradually crossing into VT zone, other SVTs usually abrupt onset
VA relationship		
V > A	VT	Misdiagnosis from atrial undersensing,
V = A	Suggests SVT	ventricular oversensing
A > V	Suggests SVT	Misdiagnosis from VT with 1 : 1 retrograde
Change A–A before change V–V	SVT	conduction (uncommon); Misdiagnosis from double tachycardia, atrial oversensing Atrium driving the ventricles
Response to ATP		
Termination	SVT or VT	50% SVTs terminate with ATP
No termination and no change in A–A	AT	Atrial activation not due to retrograde conduction
No termination and VAAV response post pacing	AT	Atria driving ventricles
No termination and VVA response post pacing	VT	Ventricle driving tachycardia
No termination and VAV response post pacing	SVT or VT	AVNRT, AVRT and VT with retrograde conduction give same response

VEGM, ventricular electrogram; VT, ventricular tachycardia; SVT, supraventricular tachycardia; ATP, antitachycardia pacing.

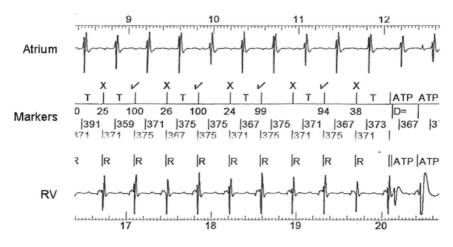

Fig. 10.11 Failure of ventricular electrogram morphology discrimination in a St Jude Medical dual-chamber implantable cardioverter defibrillator. The atrial and right ventricular (RV) channels show 1 : 1 conduction indicative of sinus tachycardia. Checks alternating with "X"s in the marker channel demonstrate an alternating match and mismatch with the stored ventricular electrogram template recorded in sinus rhythm. The poor match with the stored template probably results from misalignment of the electrogram with the template. The patient experienced inappropriate ventricular tachycardia detection and antitachycardia pacing therapy.

lar sensing electrode configuration or repositioning of the ventricular sensing lead may be needed. Double-counting of atrial and/or ventricular pacing spikes on the ventricular lead is a potential problem when the ICD patient has a pacemaker as a separate device. This is remedied by reducing the output of the pacemaker or upgrading the ICD to a dual-chamber device with removal of the pacemaker.

Double-counting of sensed ventricular events may occur in older biventricular ICDs (Guidant Contak, or conventional ICDs with right and left ventricular sensing/pacing electrodes connected via a Y-adaptor), which sense from left and right ventricular tip electrodes to a right ventricular defibrillation coil or ring electrode. Decreasing ventricular sensitivity or increasing the programmed lower rate to ensure continuous pacing may correct this problem. Often, the system must be revised with a biventricular device that senses only in the right ventricle.

In dual-chamber ICDs, far-field R-wave sensing on the atrial lead can be interpreted as AF. In Fig. 10.13, intermittent far-field R-wave sensing during sinus tachycardia caused the ICD to misinterpret a double tachycardia (AF and VT) for which therapy was delivered. In some cases this can be resolved by reprogramming atrial sensitivity. In other cases, the atrial lead must be repositioned to minimize far-field R-wave sensing.

Extracardiac signals may be inappropriately sensed by the ventricular lead and can precipitate inappropriate ICD therapies. Diaphragmatic or chest wall myopotentials may be detected by some ICDs,[23] especially those with auto-

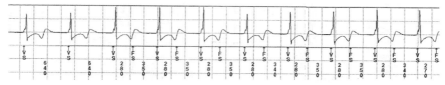

A

#	Date/Time	Type	V. Cycle	Last Rx	Success	Duration
	Aug 03 13:54:12	VF	290 ms	VF Rx 6	No	9.9 min

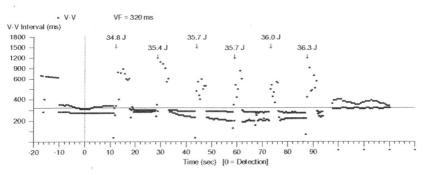

B

Fig. 10.12 T-wave double-counting. (A) The tip-ring ventricular electrogram from this single-chamber implantable cardioverter defibrillator (ICD) is shown. There is sensing of the repolarization artifact ("T wave") causing alternation of the R–R interval between 350 and 280 ms. (B) The R–R interval plot shows the characteristic "railroad track" appearance of the alternating cycle lengths from double-counting. The patient received 84 ICD shocks before reaching the emergency room.

matic gain sensing (Fig. 10.14). Solutions include reprogramming of ventricular sensitivity, repositioning of the ventricular lead, or substitution of a true bipolar ventricular sensing lead. Another important source of inappropriate sensing is a conductor fracture or insulation failure in the ventricular sensing portion of the defibrillation lead. As shown in Fig. 10.15, high-frequency noise secondary to a lead fracture was interpreted by the ICD to be non-sustained VF. In such situations, obtaining a chest radiograph and comparing it with one performed after the initial implant can be helpful. Besides conductor fracture, useful clues may be obtained regarding lead malposition or dislodgment and improper positioning of a pin connector in the header.[24]

External EMI can also trigger ICD therapy. Potential sources include poorly shielded electrical equipment, welding devices, electrocautery, lithotripsy, and electric generators. Figure 10.16 depicts intracardiac electrograms recorded from a patient who was working on an alternator of a running car. The electrograms were interpreted as a "double tachycardia" (simultaneous AF and VF), which triggered therapy. Obviously, treatment is avoidance of the EMI source. EMI from airport metal detectors is rare.[25]

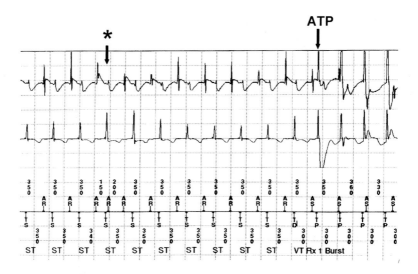

Fig. 10.13 Inappropriate diagnosis of a double tachycardia leading to therapy in a patient with a dual-chamber implantable cardioverter defibrillator (ICD). Far-field R waves are seen in the atrial electrogram (top tracing) during sinus tachycardia ("ST," marker channel, bottom tracing), are intermittently detected by the ICD (*), and are interpreted as atrial fibrillation (AF). In the face of presumed AF being recorded on the atrial electrogram, the ICD assumes that the regular ventricular rhythm as recorded on the ventricular electrogram (middle tracing) is ventricular tachycardia, and it then initiates antitachycardia pacing therapy.

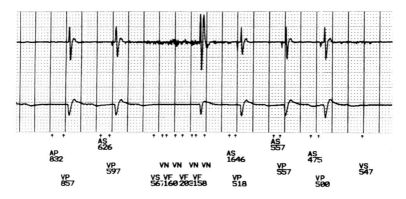

Fig. 10.14 Diaphragmatic myopotential oversensing with an integrated bipolar lead (Guidant ICD). Routine interrogation of the implantable cardioverter defibrillator (ICD) reveals multiple episodes of non-sustained ventricular fibrillation. A stored electrogram for one of the episodes reveals multiple R-wave detections interpreted as ventricular fibrillation (marker channel, bottom tracing), whereas the far-field electrogram (can to coil, bottom tracing) does not show any ventricular activity correlating with these marked ventricular fibrillation events. Examination of the intracardiac ventricular electrogram (distal ventricular lead tip to RV coil, top tracing) reveals low-amplitude, high-frequency myopotentials that are sensed by the ICD and inappropriately interpreted as ventricular fibrillation (VS, ventricular beat sensed; VF, ventricular fibrillation sensed; VN, ventricular noise sensed; bottom marker channel).

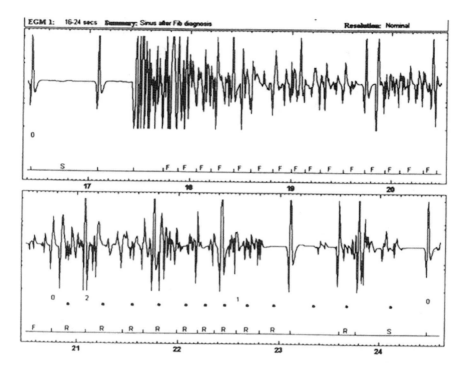

Fig. 10.15 Lead fracture causing noise and inappropriate therapies in a St Jude Medical single-chamber implantable cardioverter defibrillator.

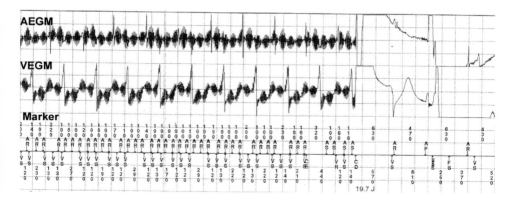

Fig. 10.16 External high-frequency electrical noise causing implantable cardioverter defibrillator therapy. The patient was checking the alternator of his car while it was running. The high-frequency noise simultaneously on both leads is characteristic of external electromagnetic interference. AEGM, atrial electrogram; VEGM, ventricular electrogram; Marker, marker channel.

Sustained ventricular arrhythmias but no delivered implantable cardioverter defibrillator therapy

The most common cause of no ICD therapy despite sustained VT is because the ICD VT rate limit is set above that of the clinical VT. Thus, the ICD does not detect the VT. Slow VT may present *de novo* in the patient who previously only had fast VT or VF, or may result from slowing of VT by antiarrhythmic drugs (Fig. 10.17). Programming errors that may prevent therapy from being delivered for ventricular tachyarrhythmias include:

1 *Failure to reprogram tachyarrhythmia detections/therapies that have been temporarily suspended in patients undergoing surgery.*
2 *Only VF therapies being programmed in the patient who previously has had only VF but subsequently develops a slower VT.*
3 *SVT discrimination schemes that misclassify VT as SVT.*
4 *Intentionally very long initial detection algorithms for hemodynamically stable VT.*
5 *Inadvertent device inactivation due to magnet exposure.*
6 *Low programmed ventricular sensitivity with failure to detect VT/VF.*

System component failure is another important cause of delay or failure in delivery of effective therapy. This may include battery or capacitor failure causing prolonged charge times (Fig. 10.18). Lead problems contributing to failure to detect ventricular tachyarrhythmias or to deliver effective therapy include conductor fracture or insulation failure in either the ventricular rate

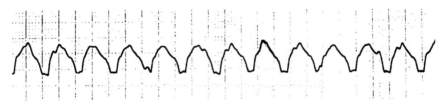

A

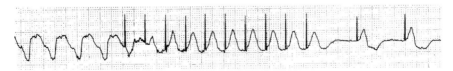

B

Fig. 10.17 (A) Failure to detect sustained ventricular tachycardia (VT) by an implantable cardioverter defibrillator (ICD) due to a tachycardia rate slower than the programmed rate limit. The patient had received amiodarone therapy for 3 years before presenting with sustained ventricular tachycardia at 145 bpm. Because the VT detection rate limit was set at 160 bpm, the ICD did not identify VT as being present. (B) By reducing the rate limit to 130 bpm, the VT was readily detected and terminated with a single burst of antitachycardia pacing.

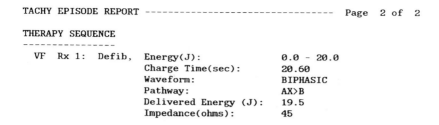

```
THERAPY SEQUENCE
----------------
  VF  Rx 1:  Defib,  Energy(J):              0.0 - 20.0
                     Charge Time(sec):       20.60
                     Waveform:               BIPHASIC
                     Pathway:                AX>B
                     Delivered Energy (J):   19.5
                     Impedance(ohms):        45
```

Fig. 10.18 Prolonged charge time causing a delay in therapy and syncope in a patient with a Medtronic 7221 implantable cardioverter defibrillator. Examination of the therapy sequence report from this patient reveals a charge time of 20.6 s to deliver a 20-J shock for ventricular fibrillation. This could result from capacitor or component failure, or from battery voltage near the end of the battery's life.

sensing or high-voltage circuits. Deterioration of the sensing characteristics of the ventricular lead over time can also result in failure to detect low-amplitude electrograms during VT or VF.

The ICD patient who presents with a sustained ventricular tachyarrhythmia should be promptly treated using accepted advanced cardiac life support protocols. The ICD should be inactivated until possible causes of malfunction have been explored (see Table 10.5).

Table 10.5 Causes for multiple implantable cardioverter defibrillator discharges

Appropriate therapy
1   Electrical storm
2   Ineffective initial therapies
3   Incessant VT
4   Appropriate shocks for AF by atrial defibrillation functions
Inappropriate therapy
1   Supraventricular tachycardias
• Atrial fibrillation
• Atrial flutter
• Sinus tachycardia
• Atrial tachycardia
• Re-entrant SVT
2   Oversensing
• T wave
• Diaphragmatic/chest wall
• Other devices
• Lead dislodgment/double-counting atrium and ventricle
3   Noise
• External electromagnetic noise (alternators/welding/cautery/lithotripsy)
• Loose set-screw/extendable lead screw
• Lead fracture
4   Phantom shocks

VT, ventricular tachycardia; AF, atrial fibrillation; SVT, supraventricular tachycardia.

Syncope with no apparent implantable cardioverter defibrillator discharge

Patients may present with a syncopal episode but no perceived ICD therapy. The patient work-up should focus on whether the likely cause of syncope is due to a ventricular tachyarrhythmia. Table 10.6 lists a differential diagnosis for this scenario. If a ventricular tachyarrhythmia is the presumed cause of the syncope, a full device interrogation and lead testing will provide valuable clues as to whether system failure may have occurred. Often, a system failure has not occurred; rather, the patient has lost consciousness prior to ICD therapy. This may occur because of inappropriately long detection and redetection intervals or very complex tiered therapy schemes for VT that may unnecessarily delay effective treatment. An example of a complex VT therapy scheme that delayed definitive therapy for > 60 s is shown in Fig. 10.19.

The patient may have symptomatic ventricular tachyarrhythmia episodes that are not registered by the ICD. Reasons for this include VT slower than the

Table 10.6 Syncope with delayed or absent implantable cardioverter defibrillator therapy

I   Ventricular tachyarrhythmias present
- Device
  - Battery depletion
  - Capacitor failure
  - Other electronic failure
- Lead related
  - Fracture of defibrillation circuit
  - Fracture of rate-sensing circuit
  - Lead dislodgment
- Programming
  - Device inactivated
  - Detect and redetect intervals too long
  - SVT discrimination inhibits therapy
  - VT rate under rate limit
  - Initial therapies accelerate VT
  - Ineffective initial therapies
  - Undercounting due to signal size
- Underlying substrate
  - Increased defibrillation threshold
  - Drugs
  - Congestive heart failure
  - Ischemia
  - Electrolyte abnormalities

II   Non-arrhythmic causes of syncope: ventricular tachyarrhythmias absent
- Bradyarrhythmia and intolerance of ventricular pacing
- Failure of bradycardia pacing
- Seizure
- Neurocardiogenic syncope
- Orthostasis

#	Date/Time	Type	V. Cycle	Last Rx	Success	Duration
	Nov 21 11:23:30	VT	360 ms	VF Rx 1	Yes	1.1 min

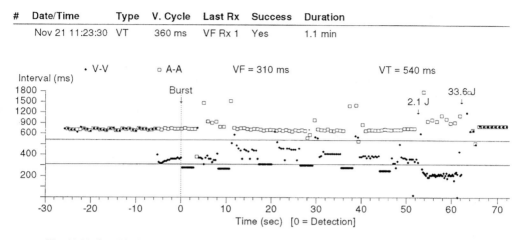

Fig. 10.19 Graphical representation of sequential therapies appropriately delivered by a Medtronic Gem DR implantable cardioverter defibrillator. The time from detection is shown on the horizontal axis. From left to right, ventricular tachycardia (VT) with cycle length of 360 ms is detected at time 0. Six bursts of antitachycardia pacing are delivered that change the VT rate but fail to terminate it. A 2.1-J shock accelerates VT, then a 33.6-J shock terminates the episode. More than 1 min elapsed in VT before successful therapy was delivered (Duration).

programmed rate limits, SVT discrimination algorithms preventing detection of VT, and ventricular undersensing. If this situation is suspected, liberalization of detection criteria or activation of a slow VT zone may help to protect the patient until a definitive diagnosis can be made.

It should be remembered that not all syncope in the ICD patient is due to a ventricular arrhythmia. Bradyarrhythmias are also an important cause. Syncope may result from failure of bradycardia pacing in the pacemaker-dependent ICD patient due to ventricular oversensing, loss of capture, lead malfunction, or ICD battery depletion (Fig. 10.20). Other causes of syncope in the ICD patient include neurocardiogenic syncope, orthostatic hypotension, seizure, hypoglycemia, and psychogenic causes.

Conclusion

Whether in the outpatient setting or facilitated by remote monitoring, follow-up of the ICD by a qualified healthcare professional is central to the appropriate management of the ICD recipient. These follow-up assessments encompass all aspects of pacemaker function, automated tachyarrhythmia detection as well as delivery of therapies. The availability of stored electrograms and built-in non-invasive testing capabilities has simplified the process of troubleshooting these devices in the event of a malfunction. However, there is no substitute for attaining a thorough understanding of device functioning, combined with a step-wise, systematic approach to follow-up of the ICD.

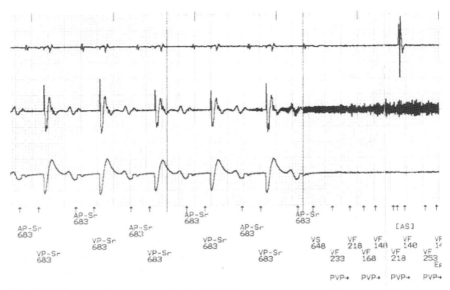

Fig. 10.20 Syncope due to pacemaker inhibition from noise on the ventricular lead of a dual-chamber implantable cardioverter defibrillator. The noise results in ventricular fibrillation detection (VF) based on the short R–R intervals. There is no pacing output during the misdiagnosed ventricular arrhythmia.

References

1 Epstein AE, Baessler CA, Curtis AB *et al.*; American Heart Association; Heart Rhythm Society. Public Safety Issues in Patients with Implanatble Defibrillators A Scientific Statement from the American Heart Association and the Heart Rhythm Society. Circulation 2007; 115:1170–6.

2 Marchlinski FE, Zado ES, Deely MP, Saligan J, Ashar M, Nayak H. Am J Cardiol 1999; 84:69R–75R.

3 Brophy JM, Joseph L, Rouleau JL. Beta-blockers in congestive heart failure. A Bayesian meta-analysis. Ann Intern Med 2001; 134:550–60.

4 Garg R, Yusuf S. Overview of randomized trials of angiotensin-converting enzyme inhibitors on mortality and morbidity in patients with heart failure. Collaborative Group on ACE Inhibitor Trials. JAMA 1995; 273:1450–6.

5 Goldberger JJ, Subacius H, Schaechter A *et al.*; DEFINITE Investigators. Effects of statin therapy on arrhythmic events and survival in patients with nonischemic dilated cardiomyopathy. J Am Coll Cardiol 2006; 48:1228–33.

6 Joseph GK, Wilkoff BL, Dresing T, Burkhardt J, Khaykin Y. Remote interrogation and monitoring of implantable cardioverter defibrillators. J Interv Card Electrophysiol 2004; 11:161–6.

7 Glikson M, Swerdlow CD, Gurevitz OT *et al.* Optimal combination of discriminators for differentiating ventricular from supraventricular tachycardia by dual-chamber defibrillators. J Cardiovasc Electrophysiol 2005; 16:732–9.

8 Friedman PA, McClelland RL, Bamlet WR *et al.* Dual-chamber versus single-chamber detection enhancements for implantable defibrillator rhythm diagnosis: the detect supraventricular tachycardia study. Circulation 2006; 113:2871–9.

9 Nanthakumar K, Dorian P, Paquette M *et al.* Is inappropriate implantable defibrillator shock therapy predictable? J Intervent Card Electrophysiol 2003; 8:215–20.

10 Mont L, Valentino M, Sambola A, Matas M, Aguinaga L, Brugada J. Arrhythmia recurrence in patients with a healed myocardial infarction who received an implantable defibrillator: analysis according to the clinical presentation. J Am Coll Cardiol 1999; 34:351–7.

11 Grosse-Meininghaus D, Siebels J, Wolpert Ch *et al.*; German Ventritex MD-Investigators. Efficacy of antitachycardia pacing confirmed by stored electrograms. A retrospective analysis of 613 stored electrograms in implantable defibrillators. Z Kardiol 2002; 91:396–403.

12 Schaumann A, von zur Muhlen F, Herse B *et al.* Empirical versus tested antitachycardia pacing in implantable cardioverter-defibrillators. Circulation 1998; 97:66–74.

13 Wathen MS, Sweeney MO, DeGroot PJ *et al.*; PainFREE Investigators. Shock reduction using antitachycardia pacing for spontaneous rapid ventricular tachycardia in patients with coronary artery disease. Circulation 2001; 104:796–801.

14 Wathen MS, DeGroot PJ, Sweeney MO *et al.*; PainFREE Rx II Investigators. Prospective randomized multicenter trial of empirical antitachycardia pacing versus shocks for spontaneous rapid ventricular tachycardia in patients with implantable cardioverter-defibrillators: Pacing Fast Ventricular Tachycardia Reduces Shock Therapies (PainFREE Rx II) trial results. Circulation 2004;110:2591–6.

15 Florin TJ, Weiss DN, Peters RW *et al.* Induction of atrial fibrillation with low-energy defibrillator shocks in patients with implantable cardioverter defibrillators. Am J Cardiol 1997; 80:960–2.

16 Gold MR, Higgins S, Klein R *et al.* Efficacy and temporal stability of reduced safety margins for ventricular defibrillation. Circulation 2002; 105:2043–8.

17 Gold MR, Breiter D, Leman R, Rashba EJ, Shorofsky SR, Hahn SJ. Safety of a single successful conversion of ventricular fibrillation before the implantation of cardioverter defibrillators. Pacing Clin Electrophysiol 2003; 26(1 Pt 2):483–6.

18 Swerdlow CD, Friedman PA. Advanced ICD troubleshooting: Part I. Pacing Clin Electrophysiol 2005; 28:1322–46.

19 Swerdlow CD, Friedman PA. Advanced ICD troubleshooting: Part II. Pacing Clin Electrophysiol 2006; 29:70–96.

20 Nademanee K, Taylor R, Bailey WE *et al.* Treating electrical storm: sympathetic blockade versus advanced cardiac life support-guided therapy. Circulation 2000; 102:742–7.

21 O'Donnell D, Bourke JP, Anilkumar R, Simeonidou E, Furniss SS. Radiofrequency ablation for post infarction ventricular tachycardia. Report of a single centre experience of 112 cases. Eur Heart J 2002; 23:1699–705.

22 Boriani G, Biffi M, Dall'Acqua A *et al.* Rhythm discrimination by rate branch and QRS morphology in dual chamber implantable cardioverter defibrillators. Pacing Clin Electrophysiol 2003; 26:466–70.

23 Schulte B, Sperzel J, Carlsson J *et al.* Inappropriate arrhythmia detection in implantable defibrillator therapy due to oversensing of diaphragmatic myopotentials. J Interv Card Electrophysiol 2001; 5:487–93.

24 Gupta A, Zegel HG, Dravid VS, Nierenberg SJ, Freiman DB. Value of radiography in diagnosing complications of cardioverter defibrillators implanted without thoracotomy in 437 patients. Am J Roentgenol 1997; 168:105–8.

25 Kolb C, Schmieder S, Lehmann G *et al.* Do airport metal detectors interfere with implantable pacemakers or cardioverter-defibrillators? J Am Coll Cardiol 2003; 41:2054–9.

## CHAPTER 11

Follow-up assessments of the pacemaker patient

Mark H Schoenfeld, Mark L Blitzer

The goals of pacemaker follow-up assessment

Pacemaker follow-up evaluations entail the repeated assessment of the pacing system and the patient to ensure appropriate and optimal pacer function and to detect and prevent pacemaker-related problems. The follow-up evaluation of a pacemaker patient begins in the immediate postimplantation period and extends throughout the patient's life, rather than throughout the life of the pacemaker system *per se*. The original indications for pacemaker insertion require periodic review, and new indications for modifications of the existing system also warrant continuing evaluation. The pacemaker physician needs to assess those symptoms not satisfactorily treated by the pacemaker as well as those symptoms potentially caused by the pacemaker. Systematic record-keeping is an important part of this process, particularly in following end-of-life parameters and in tracking patients whose systems may be subject to product recall or failure.

It remains a challenge to optimize the functioning and longevity of a pacemaker system in the face of constantly changing patient needs, whether those changes are in lifestyle, medical circumstances, cardiac function, or electrophysiological milieu. The issue of who should perform pacemaker follow-up evaluations remains an ongoing debate—what is clear is that the relevant skills must be continuously and finely maintained.[1] This chapter explores these issues and examines the methodology of the pacemaker follow-up evaluation.[2,3]

The immediate postimplantation period

Following the implantation of a new pacemaker system, the patient is generally observed on a cardiac monitor for 24 h to confirm adequate pacemaker function. The roles of ambulatory pacemaker implantation and shorter hospital stays remain controversial. Most patients receive prophylactic antibiotic coverage for at least 24 h following pacer insertion. This practice is supported by the

Cardiac Pacing and ICDs, 5th edition. Edited by Kenneth A. Ellenbogen and Mark A. Wood. © 2008 Blackwell Publishing, ISBN: 978-1-4051-6350-7

results of a meta-analysis.[4] Posteroanterior (PA) and lateral chest radiographs are obtained within 24 h to confirm satisfactory positioning of the pacer lead(s) and to serve as a baseline for subsequent comparisons. Twelve-lead electrocardiograms both with and without pacing are obtained before discharge.

Most essential in the immediate postimplantation period is education of the patient. The importance of always carrying a pacemaker identification card must be stressed. Medical alert bracelets are often recommended as well. The patient is asked to refrain from vigorous activity involving the ipsilateral arm for a period of approximately 4 weeks to minimize the possibility of lead dislodgment. The patient should also keep the incision completely dry for 5–7 days to minimize the chance of infection. One of the questions most commonly asked by patients prior to discharge is whether microwave ovens need to be avoided; with modern-day generators the answer is "no." Temporary driving restrictions may be appropriate for patients presenting with syncope until the follow-up assessment confirms that the pacemaker is functioning normally. Plans are then made for outpatient wound evaluation and suture or staple removal if needed, generally to occur within 2–4 weeks. Patients are asked to be attentive to any signs of fever or infection such as pain, redness, swelling or drainage at the incision site.

The follow-up clinic and record keeping

The personnel necessary to the pacemaker follow-up assessment include a supervising physician, a pacemaker nurse or technician, and clerical staff for record keeping and outpatient scheduling. Personnel directly involved in the pacemaker follow-up evaluation must be thoroughly familiar with all aspects of pacemaker function. The site of the pacemaker follow-up evaluation should allow history taking and patient examination and should be fully equipped to allow for analysis of pacemaker function (Table 11.1). This includes capabilities for 12-lead electrocardiography (with and without a magnet), radiography (and fluoroscopy, if possible), transtelephonic and ambulatory electrocardiographic monitoring, and availability of the programmer's and physician's manual for every model of pacemaker encountered. The telephone numbers for technical support of all pacemaker manufacturers should be available. Depending on the number of different pacer models employed by the clinic, extensive familiarity with a wide variety of programming devices may be necessary because of the lack of universal programming.[5] A resuscitation cart, defibrillator and transcutaneous pacemaker should be immediately available. The clinic staff should be capable of performing advanced cardiac life support.

Record keeping is an indispensable component of a pacemaker clinic. Its purpose is to record accurately such patient demographics as name and address, to identify specifics of the pacer system used (model and serial numbers, implant values), to track patient symptoms and various parameters of pacemaker function (e.g. sensing and pacing thresholds, identified changes in magnet rate) and to update any changes in programmed parameters. Such records may be computer stored and allow for the generation of comprehen-

Table 11.1 Pacemaker clinic

Clinic personnel
    Pacemaker physician
    Pacemaker nurse or technician
    Clerical staff
Pacemaker and patient data
    Patient's name, age, identification, address, phone number
    Pacemaker generator data: model, serial number
    Pacemaker lead(s): model, serial number
    Operative note from implant with implant data
    Complete follow-up records
    Telephone numbers for pacemaker technical support
Equipment
    Examination room
    Pacemaker programmers
    Pacemaker magnet
    Physician manuals for each model pacer followed
    ECG machine
    External defibrillator and transcutaneous pacemaker
    Code cart
Ancillary requirements
    X-ray and fluoroscopy
    Tilt table
    Blood chemistry laboratory
    Holter/event monitoring

---

sive updated reports. Record keeping also allows for organization and maintenance of strict schedules for patient follow-up assessments. This promotes identification of potential problems with pacer function well before they are actualized, rather than having patients drop in only after the problem has manifested.

The establishment of a federal pacemaker registry was mandated by Medicare guidelines, wherein specifics of pacer data such as patient demographics and model and serial numbers are reported at the time of implantation. This registry, coupled with manufacturer-generated patient lists and accurate record keeping by the pacer physician, should facilitate contacting patients if a systematic problem with a particular type of pacer system is identified or if a product advisory/recall is issued. If the physician has observed such a problem, such as premature battery depletion, the manufacturer can then be consulted to determine whether others may have made similar observations.

Independent of a formal recall, it is the responsibility of the pacer physician to decide whether corrective measures are warranted in a particular case. If a recall or advisory on a particular pacer product has been issued, the nature of the potential malfunction should determine the timing of the pacer system revision, if required at all. If the reported component failure is random and unpredictable, then replacement should be undertaken more rapidly, especially in those patients who are deemed "pacer-dependent." (See sections on

Pacemaker dependence and Device advisories) Unfortunately, as of this writing, there is no manufacturer-independent, large-scale national device/lead database that allows physicians and their patients to be notified in a timely fashion of pacemaker system malfunctions.[6] Thus, the pacer physician must be ever vigilant as to trends of potential pacer malfunction in their practice as well as to reports from others, whether via other physicians or manufacturers' notifications.

The outpatient visit

Even a routine pacemaker follow-up visit is a labor-intensive encounter with much to be accomplished in a timely manner, including a brief history, examination, pacemaker evaluation, troubleshooting, reprogramming and record keeping. By keeping the goals of the visit in focus and maintaining an orderly approach to follow-up, the process can be made efficient (Fig. 11.1).

The first visit, approximately 2–4 weeks subsequent to implantation, is primarily directed toward evaluation of the healing wound. This is particularly important in diabetic patients prone to slower healing and patients requiring anticoagulation (coumadin, aspirin or clopidogrel), in whom pocket hematomas can prove catastrophic. Symptoms are reviewed as with any visit. Chest radiographs (PA and lateral) and electrocardiograms with and without pacing can be repeated at this time. Most problems arising within 2 weeks of implantation relate to either lead dislodgment, exit block, or healing of the incision or pocket. Arrangements for transtelephonic monitoring according to preset guidelines are made, as well as for the 3-month checkup. At that point, the inflammation associated with the tissue–electrode interface has generally resolved, allowing for assessment of chronic pacing and sensing thresholds. After the 3-month checkup, patients are generally seen once or twice yearly, or as otherwise dictated by their clinical needs (Table 11.2). With increasing reliability and automaticity built into modern pacemakers, less frequent in-office checks have become more feasible.

History

Subsequent visits should focus on device maintenance, optimization of function, and evaluation of patient complaints. The elicitation and evaluation of symptomatology require careful sleuthing on the part of the pacemaker physician. Perceptions of pain, well-being, or vigor may vary widely from patient to patient, depending on an individual's "threshold" for discomfort or malaise. These may also be a function of a patient's fears and expectations. If the patient does not feel "100% better" after pacer insertion, does this reflect malfunction, or were the patient's original symptoms multifactorial in etiology and not preventable by pacing alone? As such, it is sometimes difficult to distinguish symptoms that warrant only reassurance from those that may be subtle clues to underlying pacemaker malfunction, malprogramming, or "patient–pacer mismatch."

Pacemaker Follow-up Visit

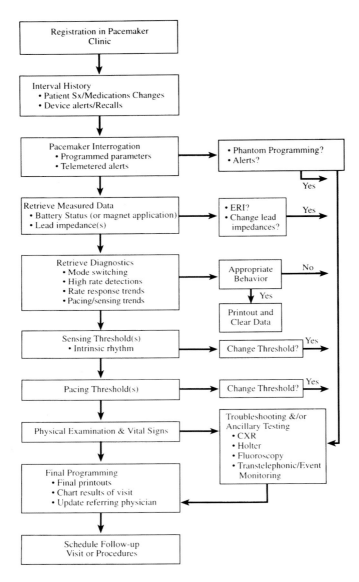

Fig. 11.1 Flow chart for efficient pacemaker follow-up visit. Sx, symptoms; ERI, elective replacement indicators; CXR, chest radiograph.

Table 11.2 Schedules for pacemaker follow-up

	Outpatient office visit		Transtelephonic Monitoring	
	General guidelines	*Medicare Guidelines*	*Medicare Guideline I*	*Medicare Guideline II*
Appropriate patients	All patients	All patients	Pacemakers with proven 5-year longevity > 90% and non-abrupt decline in output over ≥ 3 months	Pacemakers with inability to demonstrate 5-year longevity > 90% and non-abrupt decline in output over ≥ 3 months (applies to most pacemakers)
Schedule	• 2–4 weeks after implant • 3 months after implant, then • Every 6–12 months thereafter until approaching elective replacement indicators.	• Twice in first 6 months after implant, then *Single chamber* • Once every 12 months *Dual chamber* • Once every 6 months	*Single chamber* • First month: every 2 weeks • 2nd to 36th month: every 8 weeks • Thereafter: every 4 weeks *Dual chamber* • First month: every 2 weeks • 2nd to 6th month: every 4 weeks • 7th to 36th month: every 8 weeks • Thereafter: every 4 weeks	*Single chamber* • First month: every 2 weeks • 2nd to 48th month: every 12 weeks • 49th to 72nd month: every 8 weeks *Dual chamber* • First month: every 2 weeks • 2nd to 30th month: every 12 weeks • 31st to 48th month: every 8 weeks • Thereafter: every 4 weeks

In pacer–patient mismatch, the pacer system may be functioning perfectly appropriately, but fails to result in optimal patient functioning and indeed may even produce symptoms. For example, a previously vigorous patient who receives a dual-chamber system for complete heart block may be exertionally limited with an upper tracking rate of only 120 beats per minute (bpm), especially if electrical Wenckebach or 2 : 1 heart block develops at the pacemaker's upper rate limit (Fig. 11.2). Treadmill testing may, on occasion, be useful in assessing exercise tolerance, chronotropic competence and maximal heart rates achievable, either independent of pacing or in the setting of specifically programmed parameters. In rate-adaptive systems it is particularly useful to assess activity-sensing thresholds as well as the rapidity of pacing rate increases and decreases with activity. For example, in an older patient who develops angina it may be important to make the system less sensitive to activity, lower the upper rate limit, and have a relatively quicker decline of pacing rate once activity ceases. Upper rate behavior in dual-chamber systems may also be appreciated with exercise testing (e.g. Wenckebach vs. 2 : 1 block); exercise-induced arrhythmias potentially contributing to pacer-mediated tachycardias may rarely be observed.

Cardiac symptoms of angina or congestive heart failure may arise unrelated to the pacer, or to the arrhythmia that had prompted its original implantation. Pacer adjustments may, however, result in alleviation of these symptoms in some cases. The lower rate limit may be increased in patients with so-called "rate-limited cardiac output" to minimize their congestive heart failure. In contrast, patients with angina requiring increased time for diastolic coronary perfusion may benefit from a reduction in their rate limit or changes to their rate response parameters, as discussed previously.

Symptoms reminiscent of the bradyarrhythmia for which a pacer was inserted may reappear, either because of pacemaker malfunction or, paradoxically, because of appropriate cardiac pacing that is poorly tolerated by the patient. Reported symptoms may include dizziness, presyncope, or syncope, but may extend to more subtle concerns such as weakness, fatigability and dyspnea.

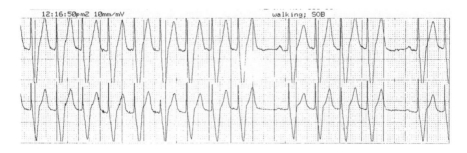

Fig. 11.2 Holter transmission in a dual-chamber system with ventricular tracking at the upper rate of 120 ppm associated with electrical Wenckebach phenomenon. This vigorous patient reported exercise limitation and dyspnea in association with this upper rate limitation.

The appearance of these symptoms in the presence of a well-functioning pacer system may result from "pacemaker syndrome."[8,9] This syndrome reflects the loss of atrioventricular (AV) synchrony during pacing and may produce systemic hypotension, AV valvular regurgitation, reduction in cardiac output, pulmonary congestion, and unpleasant neck pulsations (cannon A waves due to atrial contraction against a closed AV valve). In the worst-case scenario of AV dyssynchrony, retrograde 1 : 1 ventriculoatrial (VA) conduction may occur with ventricular pacing. Retrograde VA conduction is observed in approximately 80% of patients with sick sinus syndrome and even in a small minority of patients (15%) with antegrade high-grade AV block.

A surprising number of patients may experience severe symptoms of presyncope, syncope, malaise, palpitations, or dyspnea from this "pacemaker syndrome." This phenomenon, commonly observed during single-chamber ventricular pacing, results in hemodynamic compromise from retrograde activation of the atria in some cases and from cyclic losses of synchrony between the atria and ventricles in other cases (Fig. 11.3). The presence of retrograde VA conduction should be ascertained with electrocardiography, particularly in the inferior leads (e.g. II, III and aVf), and/or telemetered intracardiac electrograms. Blood pressure determinations should be made in the supine and erect positions with both ventricular pacing and during a non-paced rhythm

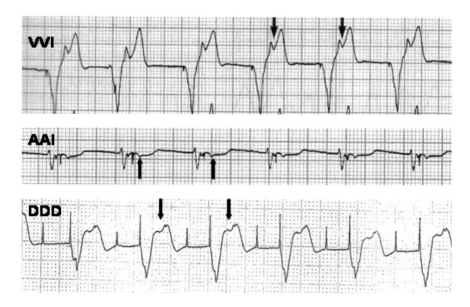

Fig. 11.3 Paced ventriculoatrial activation sequences associated with pacemaker syndrome. The P waves are shown by the arrows. VVI, VVI pacing with retrograde conduction; AAI, atrial pacing at about 80 bpm with very long PR interval; DDD, AV sequential pacing with retrograde conduction due to loss of atrial capture.

if possible. Rarely, cardiac output determinations may also be required to demonstrate hemodynamic compromise associated with ventricular pacing. If pacemaker syndrome is identified, consideration should be given to reprogramming the pacer to reduce pacer dependence (e.g. decrease the lower rate), but ultimately revision to a dual-chamber system may be required. Pacemaker syndrome can occur with AAI pacing secondary to long PR intervals and with DDD pacing in the setting of loss of atrial capture, inappropriate mode switching, pacemaker-mediated tachycardia (PMT), etc.

The patient with a pacer may occasionally report symptoms due to true pacemaker malfunction or inappropriate inhibition. This requires careful evaluation—namely, determination of sensing and pacing thresholds and consideration of the possibility of pacer inhibition by myopotentials or other electromagnetic interference (EMI). Other potentially symptomatic arrhythmias such as ventricular tachycardia (VT), rapid atrial fibrillation, or other supraventricular tachycardias (SVT) need to be investigated as possibilities. Virtually all newer pacing systems have sophisticated diagnostics, often storing the actual electrogram from any such tachycardia. This greatly simplifies evaluation. Many pacemakers allow the clinician to attempt to terminate the SVTs with rapid atrial pacing if the patient were in persistent tachycardia at the time of a follow-up visit. Additionally, certain recent pacemakers even allow for the programming of atrial antitachycardia pacing to be automatically delivered for SVT. PMTs may also arise and generate symptoms. Reprogramming options to "defeat" PMT are addressed later in this chapter. Tilt testing may prove useful in revealing the presence of vasodepressor syncope. Under such circumstances, medical therapy with volume expansion, β-blockers, selective serotonin reuptake inhibitors or vasoconstrictors may prove useful. Pacemaker reprogramming may also be beneficial. Increasing the lower pacing rate or activating certain specialized "rate-drop" algorithms may provide assistance. There is evidence that certain rate-adaptive sensors responsive to cardiac contractility may be particularly efficacious in minimizing recurrent vasovagal spells.[10] The extent that any pacing system can improve on vasovagal syncope remains a source of controversy.[11]

Symptoms that are non-cardiac but pacer-related may include myopectoral stimulation (most common in unipolar systems in which the generator case serves as the anode), concerns related to the pacemaker wound itself (pain, overt erosion) or diaphragmatic stimulation (reflecting pacing either through a thin right ventricular (RV) wall or via a lead in the vicinity of a phrenic nerve). The latter is clearly increasing in frequency with greater use of biventricular pacing systems where the LV lead is often in close apposition to and poorly insulated from the left phrenic nerve. A summary of commonly reported symptoms and their causes is given in Table 11.3.

Physical examination

The physical examination is a critical aspect of pacemaker follow-up evaluations. Most attention will be directed toward the healing incision and pacer

Table 11.3 Common symptoms in pacemaker patients

Symptom	Possible causes
Swelling/pain at pacer site	Infection, hematoma, generator migration, twiddler's syndrome, skin erosion, subclavian thrombosis, pectoral stimulation
Exercise intolerance, dyspnea on exertion	Pacemaker syndrome, low maximal heart rate settings, inadequate rate response settings, failure to capture, chronotropic incompetence
Dyspnea at rest	Pacemaker syndrome, pericardial effusion, failure to capture, pulmonary emboli from pacer leads
Palpitations	Atrial arrhythmias (tracked or conducted), pacemaker-mediated tachycardia, overly aggressive rate-response settings, myopotential tracking, sensor-driven tachycardias, ventricular arrhythmias, pacemaker syndrome
Skeletal muscle/ diaphragmatic stimulation	Pectoral muscle stimulation (unipolar), insulation failure, phrenic nerve stimulation, lead perforation, diaphragm stimulation through ventricle
Chest pain	Pericarditis, lead perforation, angina due to excessive rate response, pacemaker syndrome
Syncope, presyncope	Pacemaker syndrome, failure to capture, oversensing, cross-talk inhibition, electromagnetic interference inhibition, ventricular arrhythmias, neurally mediated vasodepressor syncope
Edema	Loss of capture, pacemaker syndrome, pericardial effusion, superior vena cava or subclavian vein thrombosis (upper extremities)

pocket, looking for erythema, tenderness, incipient or overt erosion, or pocket hematoma. Pocket hematomas occur in approximately 20% of patients who receive subcutaneous or intravenous heparin shortly postprocedure.[12] While a hematoma does not imply an infection exists, the risk of subsequent infection is heightened, and most would advocate prolonging the period of prophylactic antibiotics until the hematoma has resolved. Conservative management is all that is usually required, with temporary cessation of anticoagulants and more frequent follow-up to look for signs of pressure necrosis. Percutaneous aspiration of the pocket may actually be counterproductive, diminishing the tamponading effect and increasing chances of further bleeding and infection.

Patients may note caudal migration of the generator or superficiality of the pacemaker leads, but these phenomena are infrequent and of concern only rarely. In a healthy pocket, the generator is freely mobile beneath the skin. An immobile generator, especially when firmly adherent to the overlying skin, raises the possibility of occult infection or pre-erosion. Erosion of a generator or a lead is potentially quite serious and may result in systemic infection (Fig. 11.4). A variety of approaches to "salvaging" an eroded system have been advocated, although ideally the entire system (including leads) should be explanted and replaced with a new system after an appropriate period of intravenous antibiotics. Swelling over the pulse generator may represent hematoma formation, seroma, or pocket infection. A fluctuant pocket should not be aspirated, as this may introduce infection into a sterile process and will not

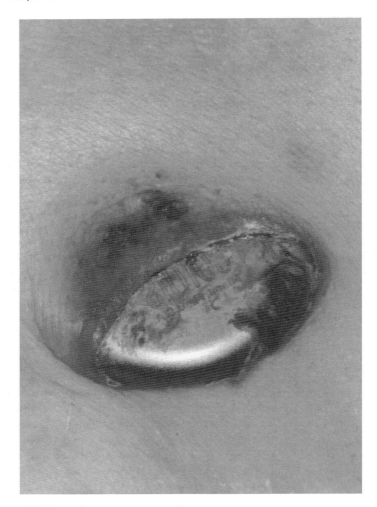

Fig. 11.4 Pacemaker erosion.

treat an infection if present. Suspected pocket infections should be surgically opened to confirm the diagnosis and to remove all hardware from an infected pocket. Pacemaker infections are not adequately treated by prolonged courses of antibiotics alone.

Myopectoral stimulation may be appreciated at the pocket site and is almost exclusively seen in unipolar systems. Certain generators are manufactured with one insulated side meant to be placed against the pectoral muscle. Rarely, myopectoral stimulation may be attributed to placement of such a generator can with the uninsulated side down against the pectoral muscle, leading to anodal stimulation of the underlying muscles; it may thus be corrected by inversion of the generator. It may also indicate lead or insulation fracture close to the muscle layer. Frequently, no problem is identifiable, but the situation may be corrected by reprogramming to a lower output to avoid invasive revision to a bipolar system. Reduction of voltage is often effective in eliminating muscle stimulation—far more so than reduction of pulse width duration.

Diaphragmatic stimulation, if present, is usually apparent on physical examination, but rarely requires fluoroscopy for confirmation. This problem is becoming more frequent with the use of biventricular pacing systems. As mentioned previously, it may indicate direct stimulation of the diaphragm through a thin ventricular wall, or, less commonly, through a perforated ventricle. In the former case, reduction of output may alleviate the problem. Another cause for diaphragmatic stimulation (right-sided) is phrenic nerve stimulation with a misplaced or dislodged atrial or ventricular lead. Depending on which lead is responsible, the corrective approach may entail inactivation of the atrial channel, reduction of atrial output, or repositioning of the displaced lead.

Other important aspects of the physical examination include vital signs, with particular emphasis on pulse and blood pressure. The latter may vary significantly as a function of pacing mode (e.g. VVI vs. DDD) or pacing rate. Neck veins should be evaluated for the presence of cannon A waves; cardiac examination should confirm paradoxical splitting of the second heart sound in most cases of RV pacing, and should exclude the presence of a pericardial friction rub suggestive of cardiac perforation. The arm ipsilateral to the lead insertion site should be examined for edema, perhaps reflecting venous thrombosis, which is usually a spontaneously resolving phenomenon and rarely responsible for thromboembolism. Arm elevation is often helpful while endogenous thrombolysis and recruitment of collateral circulation take place. If symptoms are more marked, short-term anticoagulation with warfarin may speed the process. Edema coupled with inflammation may, less commonly, represent a gouty attack precipitated by the recent surgical implantation of a pacer system.

Physical manipulation of the pacer system should be undertaken to evaluate the integrity of the leads and their connections to the generator can. Rarely, inversion of the generator can lead to myopectoral stimulation and/or loss of capture in unipolar systems. This may result because the generator was implanted with the uninsulated side down or because the patient has reversed the can by "twiddling."

In rate-adaptive systems dependent on sensing vibration, the can may be tapped to demonstrate increases in the pacing rate. Traction applied to the generator may expose a previously unsuspected malconnection or lead fracture and result in loss of capture or myopectoral stimulation. Confirmation of continued capture should be made with the patient in erect as well as supine position in cases where inadequate or insufficient lead "slack" may be present. Myopotential inhibition in single-chamber systems or myopotential triggering of ventricular pacing in dual-chamber systems may be elicited by various movements such as abduction of the arm ipsilateral to the generator. This is ordinarily an issue only for unipolar systems. The ability to observe real-time intracardiac signals as well as the universal adaptation of marker channels has greatly eased this evaluation. If myopotential inhibition is elicited and clinically significant, reprogramming to a reduced sensitivity, to an asynchronous pacing mode, or to a triggered pacing mode may be undertaken to ensure continuous pacing in the pacer-dependent patient. Consideration of changing the unipolar system to a bipolar system is another option. Carotid sinus massage is another physical maneuver that may be employed to induce slowing to the lower rate limit, thereby confirming the ability of the pacemaker to capture. Rarely, carotid massage-induced slowing of the sinus node may be useful in dual-chamber systems to differentiate SVT from physiological sinus tachycardia with ventricular tracking near the upper rate limit.

Radiography

The chest radiograph (PA and lateral using the dorsal spine technique) remains an important feature of the pacemaker follow-up evaluation, conveying a wealth of information. Following implant, it serves to delineate lead positioning and screw-tip advancement in active fixation leads. Lead dislocation is rare beyond the first month after implantation. Subsequent radiographs may be scheduled on a periodic basis or only if specific questions are to be addressed.

In particular, lead conductor fractures may sometimes be identified in cases of lead failure in the setting of elevated lead impedance. These typically occur at sites of acute angulation or at sites of increased external stress such as the first rib–clavicular junction in leads placed via subclavian vein puncture or at anchoring sites if a protective sleeve was not applied at the time of implant. Fluoroscopy, in conjunction with traction on the lead and generator, may be required to delineate the fracture. Previously, a manufacturer's advisory on potential fracture of an inner J-shaped retention wire has recommended periodic cinefluoroscopy to evaluate for fracture in certain active-fixation J-shaped atrial leads (Telectronics Accufix series). The venous insertion site may be apparent on the film; jugular venous cut-down, for example, entails lead entry superior to the clavicle. Anatomical variants (such as persistent left superior vena cava) may also be appreciated. Clues to the polarity of the lead(s) may also be appreciated by analyzing either the distal tip for presence of a ring electrode or the header block, although whether the generator is actually programmed to bipolar or unipolar remains to be determined. Examination of the connector block may disclose retraction of the lead pin.

The generator may also be examined for position and, importantly, to identify the specific model in patients with an unknown system. Various radiographic identification codes exist that are manufacturer-specific and facilitate recognition of the specific device in question (Fig. 11.5). Comprehensive references exist to assist in this process.[13] Older systems not employing such ra-

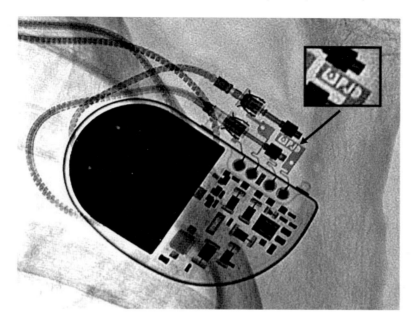

Fig. 11.5 Radiographic identification of a pacer generator has been facilitated by the use of device-specific identification codes. The code appears horizontally in the right upper corner of the device. The code "PJD" following the Medtronic logo identifies the device as a Medtronic Sigma 303 pacemaker (insert).

diographic codes may be identified on the basis of generator shape or battery configuration on the radiograph.

Electrocardiography and magnet application

It is beyond the scope of this chapter to provide a detailed discussion of pacemaker electrocardiography. Rather, a general approach to the use of electrocardiography in assessing pacemaker functioning will be addressed. The 12-lead electrocardiogram, both with and without pacing, is a useful tool in pacemaker follow-up assessments. Aside from confirming the pacer's ability to sense and capture, the electrocardiogram can provide important information on lead integrity and position. For example, the typical morphology of a RV paced complex is that of left bundle branch block, whereas right bundle branch block (RBBB) morphology may suggest LV pacing, whether intentional (e.g. epicardial wires or coronary sinus pacing) or otherwise (e.g. perforation). A superior axis is common in leads in the RV apex, whereas intermediate or inferiorly directed axes are suggestive of leads high on the septum or in the outflow tract.

Although multiprogrammability and telemetered data through the programmer have supplanted magnet application for detailed pacemaker analysis in most cases, magnet application remains an important aspect of pacemaker evaluation. In the absence of a programmer, magnet application with electrocardiographic monitoring confirms the ability to capture a cardiac chamber during asynchronous pacing. This may be otherwise inapparent if the patient's intrinsic rhythm inhibits pacer firing.

Magnet responses vary widely among manufacturers and even among various models of a single manufacturer (Table 11.4). For example, magnet application in single-chamber systems may result in asynchronous pacing at the standard rate or the programmed rate or ventricular demand pacing at a fast rate. Magnet application in dual-chamber systems may result in dual-chamber asynchronous pacing at the programmed rate or at a standard rate, or at the programmed rate plus a fixed percent increment. Elective replacement indicators in some models may be elicited only in the magnet mode. In such instances, routine magnet application may be especially important for determining the need for replacement of a depleting pacer generator.

The application of a magnet over the generator is rarely associated with adverse effects. On occasion, ventricular ectopy may result from asynchronous ventricular pacing, but this is seldom sustained. Caution is warranted if the patient has both a pacer and an implantable cardioverter defibrillator (ICD);

Table 11.4 Pacemaker magnet application

Possible responses to magnet application	Uses of magnet application
1 Asynchronous pacing • SSI to SOO • DDD to DOO with programmed or shortened AV delay • DDD to VOO 2 Triggered mode • SSI to SST 3 Rate change • Programmed rate • Faster rate than programmed 4 Threshold determination • Fixed percentage amplitude reduction over first few paced complexes • Autothreshold search 5 Trigger electrogram storage 6 No change in pacer function • Programmable magnet response (on/off) • ICD	1 Device identification—some manufacturers or models have characteristic response 2 Determination of single-chamber or dual-chamber pacing modes in patient with spontaneous rhythm that inhibits pacer output 3 Elective replacement indicators— characteristic of each model 4 Necessary for programming in some devices— reed switch actuation by magnet in programming head 5 Threshold margin test in some devices 6 Assesses pacing capture capabilities by asynchronous pacing 7 Diagnosis of some problems related to oversensing, such as far-field signals, T-wave sensing, cross-talk inhibition 8 Termination of pacemaker-mediated tachycardias 9 Underdrive pacing to terminate some arrhythmias, such as ventricular tachycardia 10 Ensures pacing when electromagnetic interference may inhibit output, such as electrocautery 11 Triggers electrogram storage 12 Inactivates/activates certain ICDs, audible beep on sensed R wave, asynchronous pacing does *not* occur with ICD magnet application

some implanted defibrillators may have tachycardia therapy inactivated by prolonged magnet exposure.

Because most devices respond to magnet application by asynchronous pacing, magnets may also be employed, both diagnostically and therapeutically, in cases where potential pacer malfunction is attributed to sensing problems (see Table 11.4). Magnet application can be therapeutic to terminate PMT or to restore pacing in cases of oversensing. In cases of pacemaker dependence, rapid magnet conversion to asynchronous pacing may be critical in preventing asystole due to oversensing or crosstalk inhibition (particularly if the appropriate pacemaker programmer is unavailable). In some contemporary pacemakers, however, magnet application may instead trigger specialized pacemaker functions such as threshold search, electrogram storage or no response in programmable devices with the magnet response turned "off".

Pacemaker dependence

Pacemaker dependence refers to a condition in which cessation of pacemaker function may result in symptomatic bradycardia or ventricular asystole that endangers the patient. The term is problematic for a variety of reasons. First, it is often misused in cases when 100% pacing is observed. In this sense any pacer patient may be rendered "pacer dependent" by having the device programmed to a rate greater than their intrinsic heart rate. Second, in patients with conduction abnormalities such as AV block, the degree of impairment may vary from one point in time to another. That is, the ability to conduct 1 : 1 from atrium to ventricle may be somewhat "whimsical" and may also vary with the application of various medications that facilitate or depress conduction (Fig. 11.6). Lastly, with reprogramming of pacers to slower rates, gradual slowing of the pacer rate is more likely to allow the emergence of an escape rhythm than is a sudden cessation of pacing (Fig. 11.7).

In patients in whom gradual reprogramming of the generator to slower rates still results in 100% pacing at the slowest programmable rate, it is still possible to determine the presence (or absence) of an underlying rhythm if the output is temporarily inhibited or programmed to subthreshold values. This practice may result in prolonged asystole during programming and should be attempted only if temporary programming is available that is rapidly reversible. Alternatively, chest wall stimulation may be applied with alligator clip cables from a temporary pacing device via skin electrodes (one situated directly over the generator can) in an effort to produce EMI and thereby inhibit pacer output. This technique is particularly well suited to unipolar systems with limited programming capabilities for rate or output.

Programmers

Pacemaker programmers are complex devices with which the pacemaker physician must be thoroughly familiar.[5] Pacemaker programmers enable both programmability and telemetry of a host of data, including programming com-

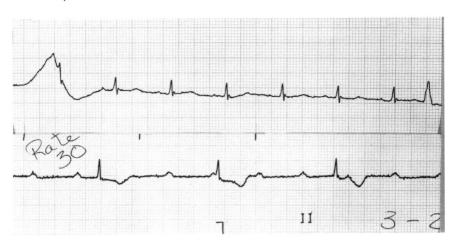

Fig. 11.6 Top: Intact atrioventricular conduction in a pacer patient with resulting inhibition of pacer output. Pacemaker was originally inserted for complete heart block. Bottom: Underlying rhythm in the same patient several months later demonstrating recurrent complete heart block.

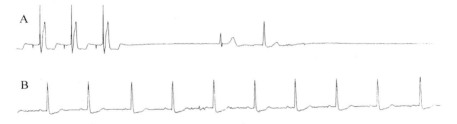

Fig. 11.7 Emergence of escape rhythm in a 56-year-old woman 3 days after mitral valve replacement. (A) The patient has been paced with temporary wires at 90 bpm since her surgery. Abrupt termination of pacing results in asystole lasting a total of 9 s. (B) Hours after gradually decreasing the pacing rate to 50 bpm, sinus rhythm at 70 bpm with normal atrioventricular conduction is noted. The patient was discharged from the hospital 2 days later without permanent pacing.

mands, administrative data, programmed data, measured data and diagnostic data. All programmers, independent of the manufacturer, share certain architectural features. All modern programmers are computer based. There is an input section that allows operator interface with the computer programmer via a keyboard, light pen, and/or touch-sensitive screen. There is a telemetry interface associated with the programmer, usually in the form of a handheld wand that transmits signals to and receives data from the pulse generator. Wireless communication between the programmer and the device is available for some ICDs. The programmer is also associated with a printer for hardcopy printouts of pacemaker data. The printer may be physically integrated with the programmer or a separate component.

The three electromagnetic wave modalities that have enabled coupling between programmer and pacer generator have been magnetic coupling—application of a continuous or pulsed magnetic field that is detected by the generator's reed switch; inductive coupling—detection of pulsed magnetic fields through an antenna coil which then induces current flow that is detected as a coding scheme; and radiofrequency waves.[14] Radiofrequency energy allows for the most rapid transmission of a large amount of information through high-frequency waves emitted by the programmer's antenna and received by the generator's antenna. The carrier frequencies depend upon the manufacturer.

Spurious programming remains a problem that may present in a variety of forms. "Phantom programming" refers to the reprogramming of a device by another physician unbeknown to the original physician programmer. "Dysprogramming" is spurious programming due to an anomalous interference source such as electrocautery. "Misprogramming" is reprogramming of a pacer by a programmer in unanticipated fashion due to faulty program emission counts. Rarely, "cross-programming" may be observed as the unpredictable reprogramming of one manufacturer's pacemaker by another manufacturer's programmer. For this reason, a pacemaker must be interrogated and programmed only with the specific manufacturer's programmer.

Telemetry, stored and real-time data

Pacemaker follow-up assessments can be performed efficiently using a systematic approach to interrogation and threshold testing (see Fig. 11.1). Even before any reprogramming is undertaken or thresholds are determined, the device should be interrogated to document the current programmed settings. All modern devices have such telemetry available. It should be emphasized that independent confirmation of such parameters as mode and rate should be made electrocardiographically after all interventions, because telemetry will not always reflect true programmed settings, although this is rare. This is particularly true in the case of pacer systems that have come into contact with extreme environmental noise (such as electrocautery or defibrillation), causing subsequent resetting of the device or pacer malfunction—in these cases, what you see (via telemetry) is not always what you get. The ability to undertake telemetry, as in the case of programming, is device-specific and requires manufacturer-specific programmers and/or modules. Inability to perform telemetry has several potential explanations, including the wrong programmer has been used, the programmer is correct but lacks software updates to communicate with the present model, the device is an older model incapable of providing telemetry, the device has a circuit malfunction[15] or is at end of life.

The retrieval of stored and real-time data is an important part of each follow-up visit. When obtainable, real-time telemetry of measured data such as battery voltage or lead impedance may prove useful in diagnosing problems with impending battery depletion or lead integrity, respectively (Fig. 11.8). A very low telemetered lead impedance may suggest problems with lead insulation, for example, whereas a very high telemetered impedance may indicate conductor fracture or a loose set-screw, which may not be apparent radiographically. With time, battery voltage declines and battery impedance rises, allowing projections of device longevity. Lead conductor or insulation problems can also be identified by the recording of non-physiologically short intervals between intracardiac events.

Historical information, such as initial implant values, may also be recorded in some systems and be available for recall via telemetry. Some models allow both programmers and generators to have actual times displayed, important in programming certain circadian features, as well as identifying when certain events, such as automatic mode switching, have occurred since the last interrogation.

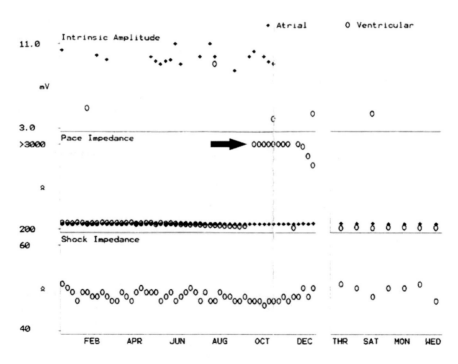

Fig. 11.8 Graphic 6-month trend report of atrial and ventricular electrogram amplitudes, pacing lead and high-voltage lead impedances in a Guidant implantable cardioverter defibrillator. From August to December, high ventricular lead impedances (open circles) were documented (arrow), but returned to normal at the time of the interrogation. The patient was demonstrated to have a fractured ventricular lead.

Aside from identifying programmed settings and measured data, telemetry of event counters is usually possible with current systems. These data may assist in diagnosing certain problems reported by the patient and in optimizing pacer function. Histograms may be obtainable to demonstrate how often different rates occur during rate-adaptive pacing at a particular activity-sensing threshold. The determination of such events (or predicted events) may enable the physician to reprogram the device settings so as to achieve rates thought to be more appropriate or "physiological" for the patient (sensor-indicated rate histogram) (Fig. 11.9).

Histograms of "event records" are available in many models, allowing for precise determination of when some event occurred, symptomatic or otherwise, and at what rate. In this fashion, episodes of tachycardia and other events, such as automatic mode switching or search hysteresis episodes, may be assessed in some models. Pacer generators may thus serve as their own mini-Holter monitors. Storage of these episodes is particularly helpful in patients with atrial tachyarrhythmias. They allow fine tuning of antiarrhythmic and AV nodal blocking medications as well as allowing rational assessment as to the necessity of anticoagulation.

Real-time intracardiac electrograms and marker channels may be available, depending on the system used; they facilitate the physician's ability to diagnose appropriate, or inappropriate, pacer function. The size of the intracardiac electrograms may give the pacer physician a rough idea of the sensing capabilities of the system and may also delineate the amplitude of far-field signals. With some devices, the patient may freeze and store electrograms with external magnet application during symptomatic events, or the device may

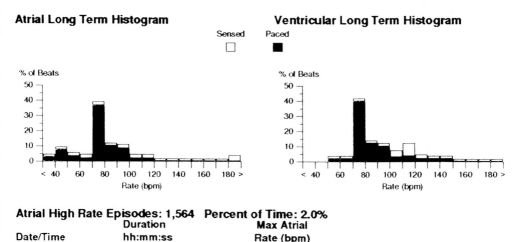

Fig. 11.9 Telemetry of stored rate histogram for a patient with a rate-adaptive dual-chamber pacemaker. The histograms display long-term data for the atrial and ventricular paced and sensed rates.

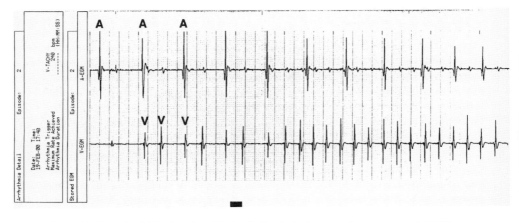

Fig. 11.10 Stored atrial (top) and ventricular (bottom) electrograms from a pacemaker with automated electrogram capture triggered by a high ventricular rate. The patient experienced syncope at the time the electrograms were recorded. The documentation of atrioventricular dissociation is diagnostic of ventricular tachycardia.

automatically store electrograms in response to high heart rates (Fig. 11.10). This corresponds to an event monitor function of the device. The clinical utility of intracardiac electrograms includes identifying retrograde conduction, measuring VA conduction time, assisting rhythm identification, evaluating unusual sensing phenomena, evaluating lead connector integrity, assisting threshold determinations, and evaluating myopotential sensing.

Potentially more useful are marker channels, which denote when a particular channel (atrial or ventricular) is sensing activity or emitting a paced output (Fig. 11.11). By telling the physician what the pacer is "seeing and doing," certain phenomena, such as crosstalk inhibition, may be more easily defined. However, event markers do have their limitations. They describe pacer behavior, but not its appropriateness; a stimulus output report does not necessarily imply capture.

Sensing and pacing thresholds

For manual sensing threshold determination, the device should first be reprogrammed below the intrinsic rate to assess sensing. In single-chamber devices, ventricular sensing thresholds may be determined by then decreasing sensitivity (i.e. increasing the millivolt values) in the VVI mode to determine at what value pacer output is no longer inhibited. The same approach may be applied for establishing atrial-sensing thresholds. The triggered modes may also be used in their respective chambers to determine sensing thresholds. Failure to trigger a pacemaker spike at a given sensitivity value indicates undersensing (Fig. 11.12). Alternatively, triggered pacing by signals other than

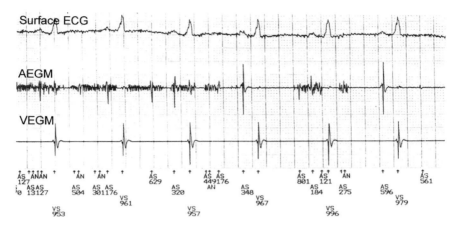

Fig. 11.11 Surface ECG, atrial (AEGM) and ventricular (VEGM) intracardiac electrograms, and marker channel (bottom) demonstrating "noise" and oversensing on the atrial lead of a Guidant implantable cardioverter defibrillator. This resulted from an insulation break from subclavian crush.

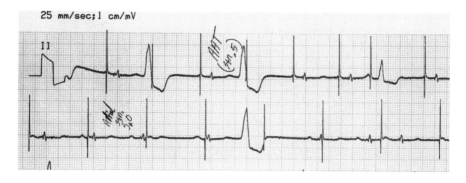

Fig. 11.12 Atrial triggered pacing mode. Top: Maximal sensitivity of 0.5 mV atrial sensing is appropriate. Bottom: With reduction of atrial sensitivity to 5.0 mV, there is a failure of atrial sensing with atrial spikes that do not coincide with native P waves.

the P wave or QRS, such as T waves or myopotentials, indicates oversensing. In dual-chamber systems, atrial sensing can be confirmed by programming to a P-wave synchronous ventricular triggered mode, shortening the AV interval so as to trigger ventricular pacing, and reducing atrial sensitivity progressively until paced ventricular events no longer result. Ventricular sensing can either be checked in a VVI mode with the rate set lower than the intrinsic rate or, alternatively, in the DDD mode as long as the AV delay can be set sufficiently long to inhibit ventricular pacing. Newer devices provide other techniques to check sensing thresholds. Some automatically check atrial and ventricular electrogram amplitudes on a regular basis. The results are available for review upon interrogation. Others require running a sensing protocol that automates the process described above. Finally, in certain devices, the intracardiac signal can be printed on calibrated paper that allows direct reading of the size of the sensed signal. With this technique, small variations may exist compared with the signal measured by the device due to differences in filters between the telemetry circuit and the sensing circuit. In patients with atrial electrical standstill or complete heart block without a viable escape mechanism, sensing thresholds will not be obtainable.

For unipolar systems, particularly in pacemaker-dependent patients, the possibility of myopotential inhibition of ventricular output should be investigated. At increasing ventricular sensitivities, the patient is asked to perform isometric exercise using the arm ipsilateral to the generator, such as pushing the hands together in front of the chest (Fig. 11.13). One should look for "noise" on the surface lead and electrogram with inappropriate sensing of R waves on the marker channel and ventricular pacing inhibition. Likewise, the possibility of myopotential triggering of ventricular pacing from atrial oversensing in a dual-chamber system should be evaluated by having the patient perform deltopectoral isometric exercises at increasing atrial sensitivities. Atrial oversensing of myopotential or far-field R waves is a frequent cause of inappropriate mode switching. In general, the chronic atrial and ventricular sensitivities settings should be set to a twofold to fourfold safety margin unless oversensing occurs (i.e. for an atrial sensing threshold of 2 mV, a sensitivity setting of 0.5–1.0 mV would be appropriate).

The pacing threshold determination is an important feature of pacer follow-up evaluations, because generator longevity may be significantly enhanced if the output can be programmed to the lowest value that will provide an adequate safety margin for pacing. Particular longevity may be obtained if outputs can be programmed to 2.5 V, i.e. less than the lithium–iodine battery voltage of 2.8 V. At this output, the energy inefficient voltage doubling circuit can be avoided. Further decreases in output beyond this point provide dimin-

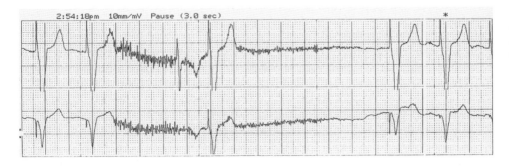

Fig. 11.13 Two-channel Holter (simultaneous V_1 and modified V_5) showing symptomatic inhibition of pacing by myopotentials.

ishing energy savings. In practice, doubling the voltage threshold (at a pulse width of 0.4 or 0.5 ms) or tripling the pulse width threshold (as long as the threshold is < 0.3 ms) will usually provide an adequate safety margin. Energy consumption is directly proportional to the pulse width, but increases with the square of voltage. If tripling the pulse width results in an interval < 0.9 ms, this is usually more energy efficient than doubling the voltage. Programming larger safety margins is typical immediately after implant to allow for the usual post-implant threshold increases. This process is almost always complete by 2–3 months, allowing chronic thresholds to be programmed at that point. Programming larger safety margins should also be considered in the ventricular channel of pacemaker-dependent patients given the possibility of late unexpected threshold rises.[16]

Determination of pacing thresholds should be made for both chambers where applicable. In patients with intact AV conduction, determination of atrial stimulation threshold is easiest measured in the AAI mode with the pacing rate set 10–20 bpm above the intrinsic rate. Atrial output (or pulse width) is progressively lowered until a QRS complex is "dropped" indicating loss of atrial capture. In patients with AV block, atrial capture must be measured in a DDD mode. The threshold may then be determined by noting the loss of a P wave on a surface tracing or the appearance of atrial sensed events on a marker channel or spontaneous atrial signal on an electrogram tracing. The latter two findings indicate return of spontaneous sinus node function after loss of atrial capture. Ventricular stimulation thresholds are most cleanly performed in VVI mode. DDD mode may also be used as an alternative, particularly in patients who feel poorly with the loss of AV synchrony with VVI pacing. The AV delay must be set sufficiently short to "force" ventricular pacing and minimize fusion and pseudo-fusion which can obscure detection of loss of ventricular capture and result in a falsely low perceived stimulation threshold. In pacemaker-dependent patients, loss of ventricular capture may result in asystole. Fortunately, most modern programmers permit rapid restoration of preprogrammed outputs with temporary pacing modes or automated threshold algorithms. It is often helpful to warn the patients what they may feel as threshold is approached during testing. The operator must remain vigilant though to terminate the test immediately after loss of capture is first noted.

Automaticity is a feature that has been applied to a number of pacemaker parameters to allow for device regulation without the need for continual clinician input. This is particularly the case with ventricular capture determinations. To date, auto-capture algorithms have concentrated on the ventricle due to the relative ease of measuring the large evoked response with capture; however, devices capable of automatically measuring atrial capture are also available. In some devices, the generator may be programmed to automatically determine the pacing threshold continuously or at periodic intervals and reset the output so as to ensure an adequate safety margin and simultaneously optimize device longevity. Certain devices which check capture on a beat-to-beat basis allow programming the output to as little as 0.25 V over the stimulation threshold. This option is being used increasingly to facilitate device follow-up.[17]

Programmability of polarity has become increasingly available in current pacemakers and, unfortunately, is not infrequently required. Problems with insulation defects in certain polyurethane leads subject to the "subclavian crush" syndrome, resulting in low impedance values, may be temporarily addressed by reprogramming from bipolar to unipolar mode. Some devices will automatically reprogram the lead configuration to unipolar polarity when bipolar impedances are abnormal. This maneuver generally will increase the lead impedance in these situations and prevent loss of capture and possible undersensing, but will not prevent oversensing from make–break electrical transients arising from contact between the two conductors. Ultimately, lead replacement is required in the pacer-dependent patient. Occasionally, pacing or sensing thresholds will be significantly better in one polarity compared with the other. This may be helpful in the setting of marginal threshold values. General guidelines for chronic programming of common pacemaker parameters are given in Table 11.5.

The atrioventricular interval

Recent data[18] suggesting that RV pacing may worsen symptoms of congestive heart failure in those with underlying cardiomyopathy have refocused attention on appropriate programming of the AV interval. Studies suggest that the risk of heart failure in patients with sinus node dysfunction can be related to the cumulative percent ventricular pacing and the paced QRS duration.[20] The highest risk of heart failure occurs at > 40% cumulative ventricular pacing in the DDD mode.[20] Certainly, in those with diminished LV function and narrow intrinsic QRS duration, one should make attempts to prolong the AV delay sufficiently to minimize RV pacing. This can be accomplished by programming a long fixed AV delay or programming "on" an AV search hysteresis feature which is being increasingly incorporated into new devices. With this feature, a backup AV interval is set as well as a further delay which is added to the programmed value, allowing additional time to encourage native conduction. If no intrinsic R wave has been sensed by the end of the summed interval, the programmed "physiological" AV delay will become active, but with periodic searches for native conduction. Newer algorithms allow programming to a minimal ventricular pacing mode.[19] This provides pacing in an AAI(R) mode with beat-to-beat analysis checking for antegrade conduction. If there is failure of AV conduction block, the device will automatically mode switch to DDD(R) (Fig. 11.14) . Programming the device to DDI(R) mode is sometimes worthwhile as well.

In contrast, patients with normal LV function are rarely able to distinguish between native conduction and P wave synchronous pacing. Nevertheless, the above techniques to minimize ventricular pacing may still be worthwhile, if only to maximize battery duration. However, there is clearly an AV delay sufficiently long that the benefits of inhibiting ventricular pacing are out-

Table 11.5 General guidelines for programming common pacemaker parameters

Parameter	Situation	Chronic setting	Comments
Lower rate limit	General	50–70 bpm	
	Heart failure	70–90 bpm	Benefit of high-rate pacing not proven
Upper rate limit	General	85% maximal predicted heart rate [(220⁻ age) × 0.85] bpm	Based on average levels of activity
	Children/athletes	(220⁻ age) bpm	May require programming short refractory periods
	Coronary artery disease/angina	110–120 bpm	Approximates peak heart rates on maximal β-blockade
Pacing output	Fixed voltage	3× pulse width threshold	Minimizing voltage output is most efficient
	Fixed pulse width	2–3× voltage threshold	Use autothreshold functions
Sensitivity	Atrium	25–50% of threshold value	Need < 1 mV setting for mode switching
	Ventricle	25–50% of threshold value	Evaluate oversensing in unipolar systems
AV delay	AV block	150–180 ms paced AV delay, sensed AV delay 25–40 ms < paced AV delay	Turn on rate-adaptive AV delay in active patients
	Intrinsic AV conduction (no CHF)	Up to 220 ms	Longer AV delays may compromise hemodynamics, use AV interval hysteresis to promote intrinsic conduction
	Hypertrophic cardiomyopathy	Approximately 100 ms	Optimize by Doppler Use negative hysteresis to "force" ventricular pacing Minimize ventricular pacing Lower rate limit 40 bpm
	Risk for CHF	Atrial non-tracking modes (VVI, DDI, DVI)	Hysteresis Long AV delay/AV search algorithm Minimal ventricular pacing algorithm Inactivate rate response Activate sleep rate Inactivate rate-adaptive AV delay Ensure appropriate atrial capture, mode switching, etc.

weighed by the adverse hemodynamic effects which can result with marked first-degree block. Much of this detrimental effect may be linked to atrial contraction occurring during or immediately after ventricular systole, creating "pseudo-pacemaker syndrome." Certain studies have demonstrated that this detrimental effect is seen with PR intervals of > 220 ms.[21] In occasional patients who continue to complain of breathlessness after a pacemaker is implanted,

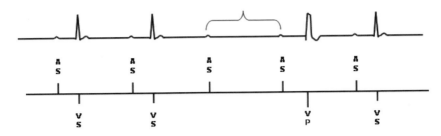

Fig. 11.14 Schematic of Medtronic Inc. minimal ventricular pacing algorithm. AAI(R) pacing is operative until a P–P interval occurs without containing a sensed ventricular event (bracket). AS, atrial sense event; VP, ventricular paced event. Ventricular pacing occurs after the P wave. AAI(R) pacing then resumes until two out of four P–P intervals occur without sensed ventricular events. This triggers a sixth DDD(R) pacing for a preprogrammed number of intervals, then the AAI pacing may again become operative. Because the sensed ventricular event may occur at any time in the P–P interval, minimal ventricular pacing may occur at the cost of atrioventricular dyssynchrony.

an attempt at AV optimization using Doppler echocardiography or impedance cardiography may be warranted. Both AV as well as LV/RV optimization is a subject of particular interest in those with biventricular pacemakers. Traditional mitral inflow and aortic outflow Doppler measurements as well as newer tissue Doppler techniques are being investigated.[22]

In contrast to the previous situations, there are also situations in which ventricular pacing is desired. This is particularly true when dual-chamber pacemakers are placed for symptom relief in those with hypertrophic obstructive cardiomyopathy. Programming a short fixed AV delay is one option, although more sophisticated algorithms such as negative AV interval hysteresis can be effective in allowing for the longest AV interval that still provides 100% ventricular pacing. Patients with biventricular pacemakers represent another group where continuous ventricular pacing is desired. This is often difficult when these patients develop rapid atrial fibrillation. New algorithms are being developed to assist in this situation. One such algorithm automatically increases the ventricular pacing rate after every sensed ventricular event. Another provides a "triggered" mode where each sensed RV beat immediately results in LV pacing resulting in a fused QRS complex which is more synchronized than the intrinsic beat would be alone. Finally, in patients with a "traditional" dual-chamber pacemaker, underlying cardiomyopathy and a baseline RBBB, biventricular pacing can often be simulated. To accomplish this, one carefully programs the AV delay so as to create fusion between the RV paced complex and the native QRS (which, due to the RBBB, is activating the left ventricle first) and thus create some measure of resynchrony.

A differential AV delay is now incorporated into virtually all modern pacemakers. This allows for programming of a shorter AV delay for the sensed AV interval (SAV) compared with the paced AV interval (PAV). This accounts for the fact that the pacemaker does not recognize a sensed atrial event (and start the SAV timer) until atrial depolarization is well under way. The differential AV delay thus keeps the time between atrial and ventricular contraction constant regardless of the presence of atrial pacing. A differential value of 25–40 ms is considered appropriate. Most pacemakers also now have a rate-responsive AV delay feature. This provides for a shortening of the AV interval during exercise, mimicking the normal positive dromotropic effect seen in those with normal AV conduction. This feature provides a hemodynamic benefit as well as allowing for the programming of a higher maximum tracking rate. This feature should ordinarily be programmed "on" in those with AV conduction disturbances.

Special considerations in dual-chamber systems

In dual-chamber systems several problems may require evaluation during follow-up evaluations as the clinical situation arises. The possibility of cross-talk, i.e. inappropriate sensing of the atrial pacing artifact on the ventricular channel resulting in ventricular pacing inhibition, can be assessed by programming the ventricular channel to highest sensitivity and the atrial output to its highest value (Fig. 11.15). The programmed rate should exceed the native rate

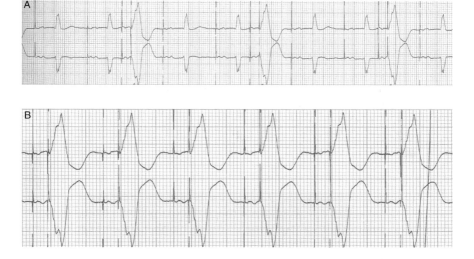

Fig. 11.15 Cross-talk in a unipolar dual-chamber pacemaker. (A) This patient was referred for loss of capture on the ventricular lead. The ECG shows atrial pacing consistently but ventricular output on only the first cardiac cycle. Telemetry showed ventricular sensing within 40–60 ms of the pacing output that inhibits ventricular pacing. (B) After reducing atrial sensitivity from 2.8 to 5.6 mV, inhibition of ventricular output was corrected. This device did not have programmable postatrial pacing, ventricular blanking intervals or safety pacing that would have also resolved the cross-talk.

so as to require continuous atrial pacing, and the programmed AV interval should be shorter than the native PR interval. Cross-talk is most likely to occur with unipolar pacing systems. The absence of cross-talk inhibition at maximal atrial output and maximal ventricular sensitivity suggests that this problem is not likely to be encountered at usual settings. Fortunately, cross-talk is much less of a problem with modern pulse generators that incorporate various techniques to minimize this problem such as ventricular blanking periods and cross-talk sensing windows. Assessment of this phenomenon should be undertaken cautiously in patients with heart block, because ventricular asystole may occur. Identification of cross-talk warrants reprogramming, when possible, to lower atrial output or ventricular sensitivity, prolongation of ventricular blanking period, or consideration of another mode such as VDD.

The propensity for PMT in the DDD mode may be explored by shortening the postventricular atrial refractory period (PVARP) to its minimum and programming atrial output to subthreshold levels. If retrograde ventriculoatrial conduction is present, PMT may be observed if it is triggered by a spontaneous PVC or if loss of atrial capture occurs. In the latter case, the AV sequential paced rhythm fails to capture the atrium, but captures the ventricle, with retrograde conduction leading to activation of the atrium and setting up PMT. PMT may be managed by decreasing the upper ventricular tracking rate, extending the PVARP (which may limit the desired upper tracking limit), changing to a non-atrial tracking mode such as DDI or activating PMT intervention algorithms. These can include an increase in the PVARP after a PVC, which will minimize the chance of initiating a PMT, or periodically "dropping" a ventricular paced beat with any tachycardia near the upper rate limit. This will terminate the tachycardia if it is indeed a PMT, but only create a brief pause if the rhythm were an intrinsic atrial rhythm that the pacemaker was tracking, i.e. sinus tachycardia. Many devices allow programming of a rate-adaptive PVARP that shortens the PVARP at more rapid rates, permitting a long PVARP at rest without unduly imposing limits on the upper rate.

Not infrequently, a patient with a dual-chamber device will present with new-onset atrial fibrillation or flutter. The atrial fibrillation or flutter waves may be sensed and trigger rapid ventricular responses, often irregularly (Fig. 11.16). Automatic mode switching is a very important feature incorporated into many dual-chamber pacemakers for the management of atrial arrhythmias. It allows reversion from dual-chamber pacing to single-chamber ventricular pacing (or to a non-atrial tracking mode such as DDI(R)) when atrial arrhythmias are recognized, and a return to dual-chamber mode when sinus rhythm has been restored. In general, this algorithm works well, but occasional undersensing of fibrillatory waves may result in frequent switches back to DDD mode for several seconds before re-recognizing the atrial dysrhythmia and again mode-switching. This often results in the reporting of hundreds or even thousands of mode-switch events corresponding to a single or just a few more sustained episodes of atrial fibrillation. Separately, one occasionally sees oversensing in the atrial channel during sinus rhythm from

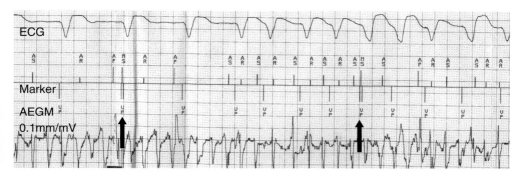

Fig. 11.16 Rhythm strip showing intermittent ventricular tracking of atrial flutter/atrial fibrillation resulting in irregular ventricular pacing near the upper rate limit in the DDD mode. At the start of the tracing, the device is in mode switch non-atrial tracking mode with a slow paced ventricular rate. At the first arrow, the device exits mode switching to DDD mode because of atrial undersensing (MS on marker annotations). The second arrow identifies re-activation of mode switch behavior due to consistent atrial sensing with brief tracking at the upper rate limit. AEGM, atrial electrogram.

far-field R waves. This can result in "double-counting," which can spuriously trigger mode switch. Episodes of mode switching due to far-field R-wave sensing are typically < 5 min in duration. In non-mode-switching devices, the upper tracking rate limit may be reduced to minimize rapid ventricular tracking, but it is often more effective to reprogram the device to a DDIR or VVIR mode. The DDIR mode works particularly well for patients with significant sinus node dysfunction but intact AV conduction, who spend much of their time in sinus rhythm with atrial pacing. In some devices, atrial flutter may be converted to sinus rhythm by temporary burst pacing from the atrial channel manually or as part of automated atrial antitachycardia pacing therapies. Guidelines for chronic programming of basic dual-chamber pacemaker parameters are shown in Table 11.5.

Outpatient monitoring

A variety of electrocardiographic techniques enable ambulatory determinations of pacemaker function between clinic visits. The most important of these is transtelephonic monitoring of the patient's free-running and magnet rates. This technique does not supplant the direct outpatient visit with the pacer physician. It does, however, reduce the frequency of outpatient visits, which may be particularly burdensome for patients who are frail, are unable to travel or live remote from medical facilities. Guidelines for transtelephonic and office follow-up schedules are listed in Table 11.2.

Deviations from the recommended schedules may be needed for pacemaker dependent patients, devices under recall or alert, or for changes in the patient's clinical condition. Despite its limitations, transtelephonic monitoring enables the pacer physician to determine changes in free-running or magnet pacing rates indicative of battery depletion and may indicate problems with pacemaker sensing or capture. Patients experiencing symptoms potentially related to pacer function or malfunction are encouraged to transmit their rhythm when they are symptomatic, independent of the above scheduling guidelines.

As an extension of this approach, 24-h Holter monitoring may be useful for uncovering problems with pacer malfunction that are potentially responsible for a patient's symptoms (Fig. 11.17). The approach is limited by sampling error in patients with infrequent symptoms, as no abnormalities may be identified if the patient is "having a good day." Rather, the technique is more often useful in demonstrating previously unsuspected and asymptomatic malfunctions, such as intermittent undersensing or myopotential triggering. Activity-related rate trends warranting reprogramming, particularly with dual-chamber or rate-adaptive pacing, may be observed with Holter monitoring.

All manufacturers of pacemakers and ICDs have released enhanced outpatient remote monitoring devices. These newer devices vastly increase the amount of data available to the clinician. These systems can "interrogate" the implanted device and provide information equivalent to that when interrogating a device in the office, including stored electrograms from high-rate events in pacemakers as well as printouts from VT/ventricular fibrillation events in defibrillators.[23] This technology is already being expanded to provide additional data on non-arrhythmic variables such as transthoracic impedance measurements from one manufacturer that may provide preclinical information on incipient heart failure and the inclusion of a BP cuff and scale with the system from another manufacturer. These systems are being created to allow specialized datasets so that the general cardiologist or heart failure specialist can access certain data streams while the electrophysiologist can access others.

With the increased automaticity of many devices, pacing and sensing thresholds are often available. Many new ICDs incorporate transmitter/receivers to

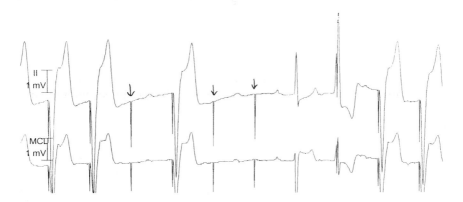

Fig. 11.17 Intermittent loss of ventricular capture documented on ambulatory Holter monitoring.

allow communication with the monitoring device wirelessly. Usually the patient has to be within 15 ft of the receiver, making placement of the device on the nightstand in a patient's bedroom ideal. Once set up, there is often no need for any patient involvement. The monitoring device is plugged into a traditional phone line and the information is then uploaded to a password-protected internet website. The system can be set up to transmit information on a pre-specified schedule, i.e. every 6 months. Certain "alert" situations such as battery at elective replacement indicator (ERI), lead impedances out of range, multiple defibrillator shocks or onset of atrial fibrillation can trigger immediate transmissions. Depending on the system being used, the clinician can be advised of these "alert" transmissions via page, fax, phone or internet review. These systems often allow the patient to "trigger" a transmission if concerned about a possible shock, a symptom such as syncope or an audible alert.

With implanted devices lacking wireless technology, an antenna similar to a programmer head is placed directly on top of the generator.[24] Technical issues such as use with cell phones or with voice over internet telephony are being actively addressed. These monitoring devices are usually portable, i.e. patients can take them when they travel or go to second homes, etc. These enhanced outpatient monitoring devices are presently being utilized for ICDs. The technology is becoming available for PPMs as well and may well supplant traditional transtelephonic monitoring in the future. Updated guidelines for the application of this technology are being developed.[25] Although the technology is already available for the physician to remotely reprogram the device, safety concerns limit access to this feature at present. Similar to stand-alone programmers, manufacturers are using proprietary technology and thus the chance for universal equipment appears remote.

Elective replacement indicators

The behavior of pacemakers approaching battery depletion is highly variable among different manufacturers and even among different models from the same maker. It is important to distinguish end of life (EOL) from ERI. The former connotes gross pacemaker malfunction or lack of function; the latter strives to indicate a time when generator replacement should be considered within a period of a few weeks to months. ERIs should be reached in the absence of patient symptoms or electrocardiographically demonstrated abnormalities in free-running pacer function. Indeed, changes in behavior, such as in magnet rates, may occur years in advance of true end of life. The changes in pacing function at ERI are device-specific and may be found by consulting with the manufacturer or the physician's manual. With all manufacturers, rate response and certain diagnostic and storage features are disabled at ERI. With certain manufacturers, the mode of pacing at ERI is changed as well, i.e. DDD to VVI. These changes may produce symptoms of pacemaker syndrome in some patients. With all devices, the pacing rate in response to magnet application is altered at ERI and provides the primary means of discerning the triggering of ERI, particularly in patients followed transtelephonically. A summary of changes at ERI by manufacturer among more modern pacemakers is illustrated in Table 11.6. When it is available, real-time telemetry of available battery voltage and impedance may be useful in confirming battery depletion, particularly as progressive increases in battery impedance are observed.

As the lithium–iodine battery discharges, the internal impedance of the battery to current flow increases. At or near EOL, transient high-current drain from the battery may further reduce the output voltage. This may result in temporary or persistent loss of device function (Fig. 11.18). True ERI or EOL behavior must be distinguished from "power on reset" (POR) mode that results from loss or corruption of the pacemaker's volatile electronic memory. POR mode is a simple backup pacing mode (typically VVI or VOO) that is stored in non-volatile, read-only memory and allows the device to function after loss of programmable memory. The POR mode and ERI modes and rates of operation may or may not be identical for a given device. If identical, POR may be distinguished from ERI by a satisfactory battery voltage in POR and a low battery voltage in ERI.

A summary of pacemaker behavior throughout the stages of battery life is shown in Table 11.6.

Device advisories and recalls

Recently, there has been increased concern over pacemaker and ICD generator reliability. A meta-analysis of device registries has demonstrated an increase in the rate of ICD malfunctions, whereas pacemaker reliability has substantially improved.[26] Warnings about the potential for device malfunction may be issued by the device manufacturers or by the Food and Drug Administration (FDA) within the USA. Manufacturers are required to submit to the FDA annual performance reports on the reliability of all pacemakers and ICDs. These data are generated from voluntary physician reporting of device failures and post-market surveillance registries. Unfortunately, data on the performance of any device model are never complete due to the voluntary nature of the registries, physician under-reporting of malfunctions and failure to return out of service devices for analysis (especially from deceased patients). Healthcare providers and institutions should also report malfunctions to the manufacturer and also directly to the FDA through the MedWatch program (www.fda.gov/medwatch). Reporting of device-related fatalities is mandatory. All device reports since 1995 are contained in the Manufacturer and User Device Experience (MAUDE) database. This database can be accessed and researched by healthcare providers (www.fda.gov/cdrh/maude.html). When the FDA determines that there exists a significant risk of device failure, a safety alert or "recall" is issued (Fig. 11.19). The term recall is misleading, however, because removal of the device is not mandated, but left to the discretion of the physician who must determine the relative risks and benefits of device replacement. Device manufacturers may directly issue safety alerts as well. Whereas the

Table 11.6 Pacemaker behavior by battery status for lithium–iodine cell

	BOL	ERI	EOL	POR
Cause	No significant battery use	Voltage reduced but still able to support basic or all pacer functions	Voltage unable to support basic or any pacer functions	Loss or corruption of volatile memory controlling pacer function
Voltage	Approx. 2.8 V	Approx. 2.1–2.4 V*	≤ approx. 2.1 V*	> approx. 2.4 V*
Battery impedance	< 1 kΩ	≤ approx. 5–10 kΩ*	≥ approx. 5–10 kΩ*	< approx. 5–10 kΩ*
Behavior	As programmed	• Percent or fixed decrease in free-running rate or magnet rate • Increase in pulse width duration • Change to simpler mode: DDDR to VVI, VVIR to VVI/VOO	• Cessation of all pacer function • Failure to communicate or reprogram • Change to simplest mode: DDDR to VOO, VVI to VOO	• Change to simpler mode: DDDR to VVI, VVIR to VVI • Change to unipolar lead polarity • Percent or fixed change in free-running rate or magnet rate
Diagnosis	High voltage, low battery impedance, BOL magnet/free running rate	Battery voltage reduced, elevated battery impedance, restricted programmability, ERI free running or magnet rate (after 60-s magnet application), telemetered advisory	Failure to communicate or program, failure to pace sense, very low battery voltage, very high battery impedance	Battery voltage > ERI, battery impedance < ERI, telemetered advisory, exposure to EMI, perform battery "stress test"
Correction	None needed	Generator change in weeks to months	Immediate generator change	Reprogram generator

* Specific values will vary from manufacturer to manufacturer.
BOL, beginning of life; EOL, end of life; ERI, elective replacement indicators.

Programmer Application   **1 second**

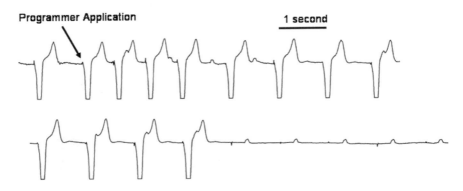

Fig. 11.18 Loss of capture during programmer head (magnet) application in a pacemaker at end of battery life. The pacemaker telemetry was non-functional. Three paced beats at 100 bpm denote magnet application. With continued application of the programming, head capture was lost due to increased current demand on the battery. A temporary pacemaker was in place anticipating such an occurrence.

manufacturer may offer a non-invasive reprogramming strategy to correct or minimize the likelihood of some malfunctions, the physician is otherwise left to make complex outcome decisions for each patient with the affected device. Not surprisingly, the rate of generator replacement in response to a particular advisory varies dramatically among physicians. The mortality and morbidity of generator change is probably underestimated by many physicians, leading to overly aggressive replacement practices.[27] Routine replacement of all devices under advisory (especially in non-pacemaker-dependent patients or low rates of device failure) probably results in more patient deaths than are caused by the device failure.[27] To assist in making rational decisions in response to device advisories, decision analysis models have been created.[28] An example of such an analysis is given in Fig. 11.20. Although many factors weigh in on this decision, the primary determinants identified by decision analysis modeling are (i) the incidence of device malfunction, (ii) estimated risk of device replacement (considering the potential for device infection and extraction) and (iii) the likely effects of device failure, i.e. the degree of patient dependency on the device.[28,29] In general, the lowest threshold for generator change applies to pacemaker-dependent patients. A failure rate approximately 10-fold higher is required to prompt generator change in those with ICDs who are not pacemaker dependent. On the other hand, increased frequency of follow-up (possibly via remote monitoring) or use of magnet-assisted patient monitoring may delay or defer the need for device replacement. Ultimately, decisions will still need to be made on a patient-specific basis. Ongoing efforts at standardizing company reporting of potential device failures and the rapid dissemination of this information will facilitate management of these issues in the future. Physicians and healthcare providers can improve the surveillance of implanted devices by returning all explanted devices to the manufacturer for

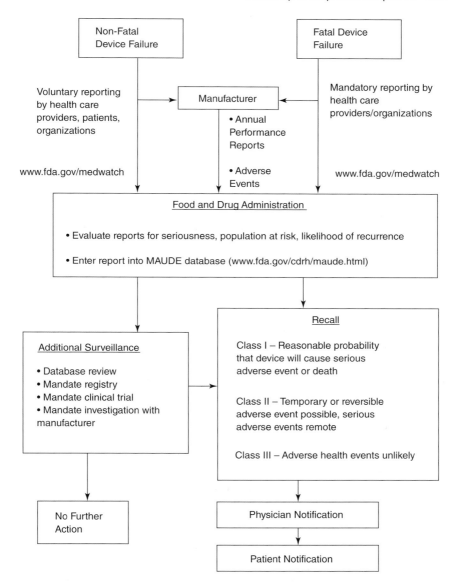

Fig. 11.19 Schematic showing flow of information leading to device recalls or safety alerts. MAUDE, Manufacturer and User Device Experience. After Food and Drug Administration notification, the agency may initiate further surveillance or issue a recall directly.

analysis, reporting all suspected device failures to the manufacturer and the FDA (via Medwatch), and pursuing post mortem interrogation of device and device explant in cases of sudden death in device patients.

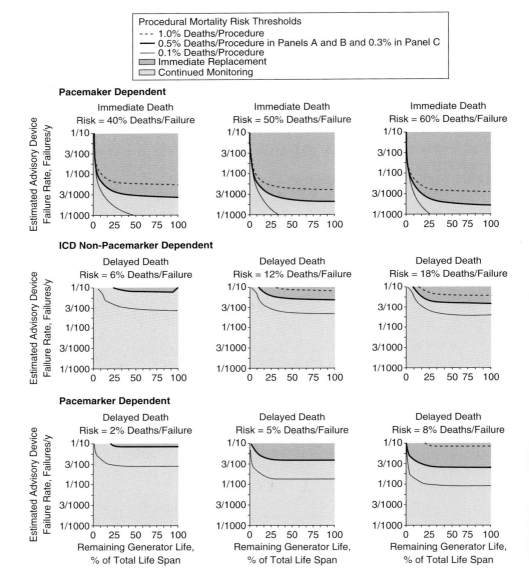

Procedural Mortality Risk Thresholds
- - - 1.0% Deaths/Procedure
── 0.5% Deaths/Procedure in Panels A and B and 0.3% in Panel C
── 0.1% Deaths/Procedure
▨ Immediate Replacement
☐ Continued Monitoring

Pacemaker Dependent

Immediate Death
Risk = 40% Deaths/Failure

Immediate Death
Risk = 50% Deaths/Failure

Immediate Death
Risk = 60% Deaths/Failure

ICD Non-Pacemarker Dependent

Delayed Death
Risk = 6% Deaths/Failure

Delayed Death
Risk = 12% Deaths/Failure

Delayed Death
Risk = 18% Deaths/Failure

Pacemarker Dependent

Delayed Death
Risk = 2% Deaths/Failure

Delayed Death
Risk = 5% Deaths/Failure

Delayed Death
Risk = 8% Deaths/Failure

Estimated Advisory Device Failure Rate, Failures/y

Remaining Generator Life, % of Total Life Span

Special situations encountered by the pacemaker patient

The pacer physician is often asked to evaluate a pacemaker patient before surgery. In addition to obtaining details from the history and physical examination outlined previously, it is essential to establish the degree of pacer dependence and, via telemetry, the current programmed settings. Operating room personnel including the surgeon, nursing staff, and anesthesiologists all need to be aware of the presence of the device, the potential EMI encountered in the operating room, and corrective techniques. An external defibrillator with transcutaneous pacing capabilities should be easily accessible. Electrocautery, often required intraoperatively, may result in a variety of pacemaker phenomena. Electrocautery may cause transient inhibition of pacer output because of oversensing of EMI. If pacer dependence has been demonstrated preoperatively, the device may be programmed to either an asynchronous mode or a triggered mode to pre-empt undue inhibition of pacer output. If such programming is not possible, then a magnet may be taped over the generator during the period of cautery. However, by activating the reed switch, magnet application may make certain older pacemakers vulnerable to spurious re-programming. It is ideal to avoid electrocautery entirely if possible, especially near the pacer generator. The cautery grounding pad should be placed as far as possible from the generator and in a location where the vector from the electrocautery tip to the pad moves directly away from the pacemaker generator. In addition, short bursts of cautery and use of bipolar cautery are recommended. The major issue with an ICD is the risk of oversensing noise resulting in inappropriate defibrillator shocks. The devices should be interrogated after the procedure.

Certain endoscopic procedures require the use of cautery, including treatment of bleeding ulcers and the removal of colonic polyps. Although there is a paucity of reports in the literature regarding interactions during these procedures and implanted devices, a cautious approach still seems rational. With endoscopic procedures where cautery will be used, placing a magnet over the generator in pacemaker-dependent patients and using a magnet or temporarily turning off tachycardia detection with an ICD are reasonable approaches.

Fig. 11.20 Results of decision analysis model for "recalled" device replacement. Each graph shows estimated device failure rate (logarithmic scale ordinate) and the percent remaining device battery longevity (abscissa). The analysis can be used as follows: (1) assign patient to one of three groups: pacemaker dependent [pacemaker or implantable cardioverter defibrillator (ICD)], ICD patients that are not pacemaker dependent and pacemaker patients that are not dependent on the device; (2) within the patient group, select from the three graphs the one which best estimates the mortality rates should the device fail (rates given at top of graph); (3) within each graph, chose among the three lines that which best estimates the mortality rate for elective device replacement in the patient under question (see legend at top of figure); (4) use the estimated device failure rate and device longevity to identify a point in the field of the graph. If this point falls above the line for the patient's replacement mortality rate, device replacement is the preferred strategy. If this point is below the line, continued observation is preferred. (Reproduced with permission from reference 28.)

Capsule endoscopy is an increasingly used novel system for visualizing the small intestine. The labeling of the device reports it is contraindicated in patients with implanted cardiac devices. The contraindication was based more on theoretical concerns rather than hard data. Several publications have reported absolutely no effect of the capsule on pacemaker function. The largest report involved 100 pacemaker patients tested with an external device simulating the capsule transmissions and moved over the generator and along the chest wall. The distances between device and simulator were closer than what would occur *in vivo*. There were no dangerous interactions. In four patients, the device briefly switched to a noise reversion, asynchronous pacing mode.[30] In rare instances, the output of the cardiac device can interfere with the video acquisition from the capsule, i.e. with an abdominal pacemaker generator.

Both electrocautery and defibrillation can produce irreversible damage to the generator. This is more likely in older devices that lack protective mechanisms such as zener diodes, which shunt energy away from the delicate device circuitry. They may also result in resetting of the generator to a backup or noise-reversion mode. Pacemaker interrogation with pacing and sensing thresholds should be performed before and after the surgical procedure. Recommendations for perioperative management in those with implantable devices are discussed in Table 11.7.

Transient undersensing and both acute and chronic rises in pacing threshold have also been observed with defibrillation and cardioversion (Fig. 11.21).[31] Some of this may relate to transmission of current down the lead(s) causing injury at the tissue–electrode interface, resulting in the potential for exit block. The majority of problems seen after electrical cardioversions are encountered

Table 11.7 Intraoperative management of devices

Intraoperative problem	Solution
Cautery-induced pacing inhibition	Program device to asynchronous mode (best) or place and tape magnet over device with pacemaker-dependent patients
	Place grounding pad away from device
	Limit electrocautery to short bursts with pauses between bursts
	Bipolar preferable to monopolar electrocautery
	Coagulation mode preferable to cutting
	Use lowest effective power output
	Monitor telemetry for pacemaker inhibition
	Monitor pulse with second means, i.e. arterial line or oximetry tracing in case of cautery-induced artifact on telemetry
Cautery-induced inappropriate ICD shocks	Turn off tachy detection on device via the programmer (best) or place and tape magnet over the device
Inadvertent device re-programming or device malfunction	Interrogate the device postoperatively to assess for threshold rises, reset modes, or changes in tachy mode
	Have backup transcutaneous pacer and defibrillator readily accessible. Staff should know make and model number of device as well as device settings and pacer dependency

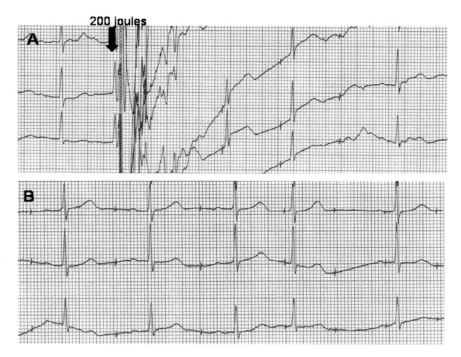

Fig. 11.21 Loss of capture in a VVI pacemaker following DC cardioversion for atrial fibrillation (A). Panel B was obtained 3 min after the shock showing persistent loss of capture at the paced rate of 60 bpm. The threshold increased transiently from 0.6 to 3 V, but returned to baseline within 10 min.

with unipolar pacemakers implanted in the right pectoral fossa. To minimize these types of phenomena, cardioversion or defibrillation should be performed via anteroposterior rather than anteroapical paddles. Minimizing the defibrillating energy by using more efficient biphasic defibrillators is desirable. In addition, pacing and sensing thresholds should be checked following external defibrillation. Finally, equipment for temporary pacing should be nearby, especially for a pacemaker-dependent patient.

Other sources of electromagnetic interference encountered in the hospital setting are magnetic resonance imaging (MRI), extracorporeal shock-wave lithotripsy, radiofrequency ablation, and radiation therapy. MRI presents a particularly noxious environment for cardiac devices. Potential interactions include reed switch closure, pacing inhibition, inappropriate ICD discharges, and rapid pacing, potentially with arrhythmia induction. The latter can be initiated either from the pulse generator or, independently, by the induction of current flow along the lead. Thermal injury at the lead tip–myocardial interface resulting in elevated pacing thresholds is also possible. Lead dislodgment or the induction of torque on the generator itself remain possible, but with diminishing amounts of ferrous material in recently constructed systems there is much less rotational and translational force brought to bear.[32] The presence of a pacemaker or ICD should be considered a relative contraindication to MRI. This caution is encouraged by device labeling, recommendation from MRI manufacturers and by the FDA,[33] who continue to follow this subject with significant interest. Before device placement, the implanter should give careful thought to the potential need for MRI and, when feasible, complete the imaging before implant. It has been estimated that 50–75% of patients with implanted devices will have an MRI exam recommended within the 12 months post implant. There is a growing body of literature reporting on the potential safety of cardiac devices and MRI. All studies require careful monitoring of the patient, including continuous verbal communication, ECG, pulse oximetry, and the presence of emergency resuscitation equipment, radiologist and cardiologist. The pacemaker is interrogated in detail immediately before and then after the exam is completed. The pacemaker is reprogrammed pre-procedure usually to an asynchronous mode in pacer-dependent patients or to a non-sensing or non-tracking mode in patients who require pacing support only rarely. Rate response should be programmed "off. " Recent studies have not had any examples or pacemaker inhibition, arrhythmia induction, lead dislodgement (chronic implants) or generator failure.[34,35] One study has demonstrated an increase in threshold of ≥ 1.0 V in 6/195 (3.1%) leads.[34] In the same study, POR usually to a VVI mode occurred in seven (6.1%) of 115 examinations. The reed switch was activated only in a portion of the exams. This holds out the theoretical possibility of potentially life-threatening pacing inhibition in a pacer-dependent patient whose device is programmed asynchronously but undergoes a POR to VVI. The reed switch may not be activated and the pacemaker may then be subject to inhibition by EMI from the MRI. Although MRIs with PPM are coming closer to acceptance, we continue to advocate referral to a center experienced in these exams until more specific protocols for the correct spin sequences, maximum SAR, acceptable MRI machines and pacemaker models are developed.

Lithotripsy has the potential to cause pacing inhibition,[36] triggered pacing at the URL and activation of rate response. The pacemaker circuitry, particularly piezo-electric crystals, may be damaged if within several inches of the lithotriptor focal point. Great care should be taken with abdominal implants. Lithotripsy synchronized to the R wave is less frequently used nowadays, particularly as it can add to the length of the procedure. This mode should be strongly considered in those with significant ventricular irritability, as the synchronized pulses are less likely to result in ventricular arrhythmias. If the lithotriptor is used in a synchronized mode, care should be taken to ensure that the pulses are synchronized to the R wave and not the P wave or atrial spike, which can result in oversensing and ventricular pacing inhibition. In general, rate response should be turned "off" and consideration given to programming to an asynchronous mode, particularly with pacemaker-dependent patients.

Radiofrequency ablation is often undertaken in the EP lab to effect permanent cure of various atrial and ventricular tachyarrhythmias. This energy can at times result in reprogramming the device to a reset mode, or transiently

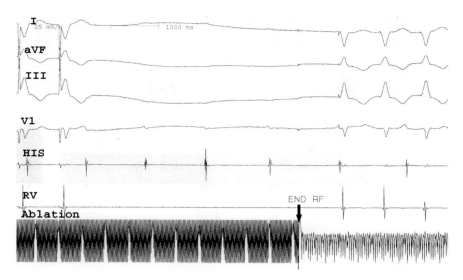

Fig. 11.22 Multichannel recording of a patient with a single-lead implantable cardioverter defibrillator undergoing RF ablation of the atrioventricular node. The ablation is successful, but the RF energy results in ventricular oversensing with resulting inhibition of ventricular pacing and CHB without escape. When the RF delivery is stopped, ventricular pacing resumes.

cause asynchronous pacing due to noise reversion or pacemaker inhibition. The latter can be particularly relevant in the patient undergoing AV node catheter ablation, which results in complete heart block and pacemaker dependency (Fig. 11.22). Reprogramming the device to an asynchronous mode will prevent this issue from arising. RF energy can result in spurious shocks in those with ICDs. Antitachycardia therapies should be programmed "off." Rarely, threshold rises may be observed.

Radiation therapy (e.g. for breast or lung cancer) to the chest may be unavoidable in certain patients with pacemakers. Ionizing radiation can result in random component failure and premature battery depletion. To minimize this risk, appropriate methods of shielding the generator and limiting the field of radiation should be discussed with the radiation therapist. Damage may result in sudden loss of output, alterations in programmed parameters, and rate runaway. Device malfunctions may sometimes become manifest late after radiation exposure. In rare instances, a newly placed contralateral system or generator repositioning using lead extenders should be considered. If included in the radiation field, the device should be interrogated after each treatment; however, delayed malfunctions may still occur.

It has also been recognized increasingly that cellular telephones may interfere with the function of implanted devices. In one study, the potential for any type of interference was 20%, with associated symptoms in 7.2%, when the telephone was placed over the generator.[37] The most common pacemaker interactions include tracking interference on the atrial channel followed by asynchronous pacing and ventricular inhibition. Potential ICD interactions include reed switch activation leading to VT underdetection and erroneous shock therapy, although latter reports have been extraordinarily rare. Interference was more common in older devices without feed-through filters. Interestingly, the incidence of interaction is similar between unipolar and bipolar devices. A reasonable recommendation would be to avoid placing cellular telephones in the breast pocket over the device.[38] Some advocate holding the telephone over the ear contralateral to the device. Particular care should be exercised with high-powered fixed cellular devices such as those in cars and boats.

Anti-theft surveillance systems are becoming ubiquitous in retail centers. Several different technologies are used to detect metal alloy-containing tags on merchandise. These have also been observed to potentially interact with implanted devices, resulting in inappropriate device triggering or, in the case of implanted defibrillators, inappropriate discharge. In these situations, we have observed one patient whose device reverts from dual-chamber pacing to single-chamber ventricular pacing with resultant pacemaker syndrome. These interactions appear to be clinically infrequent, particularly with diminishing use of acousto-magnetic technology. Patients should be told to walk through the store threshold without either lingering or leaning directly against the gates.[39] Similarly, patients may pass through security metal detectors without lingering but will trip the detector. Patients with implanted devices should notify security staff of the presence of the device. The metal-detecting wand may be passed over the device quickly in a single stroke. Repeated back-and-forth motions over the device are to be avoided.

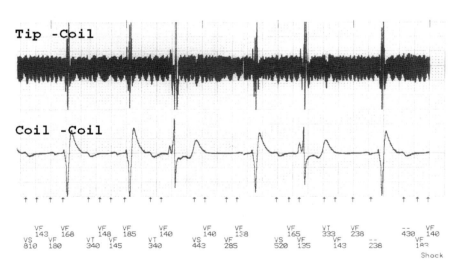

Fig. 11.23 Intracardiac electrogram from a patient with a single-lead implantable cardioverter defibrillator undergoing transcutaneous electronic nerve stimulation. In hopes of achieving better pain relief, the patient independently turned up the output to maximum. This resulted in inappropriate detection of ventricular fibrillation and high-output shock delivery.

Transcutaneous electronic nerve stimulation (TENS) units do not readily interfere with modern bipolar pacemakers. In pacemaker-dependent patients, particularly with unipolar leads, the ECG tracing should be monitored during treatment or reprogrammed to an asynchronous mode. TENS units have clearly resulted in inappropriate defibrillator shocks (Fig. 11.23).[40] Patients with ICDs who absolutely require TENS should have the marker channel observed with the device in a "monitor-only" mode with the first treatment to rule out any interference. Electroconvulsive therapy is safe in the pacemaker patient. Medical diathermy should be avoided in the area of the pulse generator. A summary of EMI–device interactions is shown in Table 11.8.

Table 11.8 Solutions to electromagnetic interference (EMI)/device interactions

Source of EMI	Solutions
Cellular telephones	Keep telephone out of breast pocket over device Use contralateral ear Keep fixed high-output telephones, i.e. car or boat phones, at least 15 cm away from device
Electronic surveillance equipment	Walk through entranceway without pause
MRI	Avoid with pacemaker or ICD unless extreme circumstance
Airport metal detector	Inform security personnel of device; walking through detector will not harm implantable device but may trigger detector; request hand or wand search. Wand should not be held directly over ICD
DC cardioversion	Place pads in anteroposterior position at least 5 cm away from generator. Back-up transcutaneous brady pacing should be available in pacer-dependent patients. Use of biphasic shocks to minimize required energy device should be interrogated post shock
Household appliances (microwave ovens, television, toasters)	No specific concerns, avoid electrical shocks
Transcutaneous electronic nerve stimulation (TENS)	Consider magnet use or reprogramming to an asynchronous mode with unipolar pacemakers or with pacer-dependent patients ICD patients should proceed with caution and consider having the device monitored with the first session to ensure no inappropriate detections
Radiation therapy	Discuss treatment with radiotherapist. Shield device particularly with treatment of thoracic tumors. Continuous ECG monitoring during treatment in pacemaker-dependent patients receiving high-dose treatment. Rarely, the device will need to be moved using lead extenders. Increase frequency of device monitoring
RF ablation	Reprogram to asynchronous mode in pacemaker-dependent patients Turn "off" tachytherapy in ICDs Interrogate the device post procedure
Lithotripsy	Inactivate rate response Synchronize pulses to R wave Avoid submersion of generator if possible

The pacer physician may be called upon to terminate tachyarrhythmias acutely, preferably without the need for cardioversion or defibrillation. Some devices allow for temporary high-rate pacing to > 300 ppm, allowing for the pace termination of atrial flutter. Rarely, application of a magnet with resultant asynchronous pacing may be successful in terminating a tachyarrhythmia. Reprogramming the device to faster rates for overdrive pacing, or using the triggered mode with chest wall stimulation to "program in" extra stimuli, may also prove useful. Some devices allow for programmed stimulation in either chamber using the programmer. In all cases, the intervention should be undertaken cautiously with defibrillator backup.

The diagnosis of myocardial ischemia/infarction in the pacemaker patient is complicated by the left bundle branch block pattern imposed by RV pacing and the classic findings of ischemia are frequently obscured. The presence of an anterior myocardial infarction, age undetermined, may be indicated by the presence of qR complexes in I, aVL, V_5, and V_6, and that of an inferior infarct by a qR, QR or Qr in the inferior leads. The specificity for these signs is quite good, but the sensitivity is poor. Notching of the ascending S wave in mid-precordial leads is another specific finding (Cabrera's sign, Fig. 11.24). An acute infarct can be diagnosed with reasonable specificity during RV apical pacing by the presence of ST elevation ≥ 5 mm in leads with predomi-

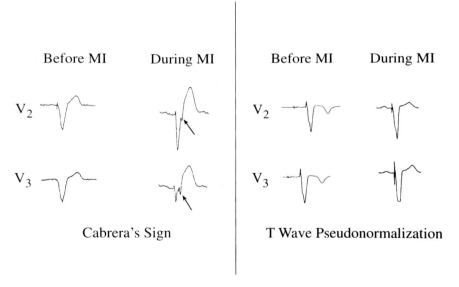

Fig. 11.24 Twelve-lead ECG showing old anteroseptal myocardial infarction during unipolar DDD pacing in a patient with complete atrioventricular (AV) block. The ventricular stimulus does not obscure or contribute to the qR pattern in leads I, aVL and V_6. Leads V_2 to V_4 show Cabrera'a sign and a variant in lead V_5. The lack of an underlying rhythm because of complete AV block excluded the presence of ventricular fusion.

nantly negative QRS complexes.[41] All of these changes are best appreciated by comparing a current ECG with those previously recorded. Inhibition of the pacemaker with a programmer may reveal the patient's intrinsic QRS for a clearer diagnosis of ischemia/infarction. T-wave changes alone should be interpreted with caution in this setting because ventricular pacing may produce T-wave abnormalities, which are persistent after the discontinuation of pacing (T-wave memory). However, these post-pacing repolarization changes do not produce ST segment elevation or depression.

References

1 Schoenfeld MH. Quality assurance in cardiac electrophysiology and pacing: a brief synopsis. Pacing Clin Electrophysiol 1994; 17:267–9.

2 Bernstein AD, Irwin ME, Parsonnet V *et al.* Antibradycardia pacemaker follow-up: effectiveness, needs, and resources. Pacing Clin Electrophysiol 1994; 17:1714–29.

3 Schoenfeld MH. Contemporary pacemaker and defibrillator device therapy: challenges confronting the general cardiologist. Circulation 2007; 115:638–53.

4 DaCosta A, Kirkorian G, Cucherat M *et al.* Antibiotic prophylaxis for permanent pacemaker implantation: a meta-analysis. Circulation 1998; 97:1796–801.

5 Schoenfeld MH. A primer on pacemaker programmers. Pacing Clin Electrophysiol 1993; 16:2044–52.

6 Schoenfeld MH. Recommendations for implementation of a North American multicenter arrhythmia device/lead database. Pacing Clin Electrophysiol 1992; 15:1632–6.

7 Byrd CL, Schwartz SJ, Gonzalez M *et al.* Pacemaker clinic evaluations: key to early identification of surgical problems. Pacing Clin Electrophysiol 1986; 9:1259–64.

8 Ausubel K, Furman S. The pacemaker syndrome. Ann Intern Med 1985; 103:420–9.

9 Ellenbogen KA, Thames MD, Mohanty PK. New insights into pacemaker syndrome gained from hemodynamic, humoral and vascular responses during ventriculoatrial pacing. Am J Cardiol 1990; 65:53–9.

10 Deharo JC, Brunetto AB, Bellocci F *et al.* DDDR pacing driven by contractility versus DDI pacing in vasovagal syncope: a multi-center, randomized study. Pacing Clin Electrophysiol 2003; 26:447–50.

11 Connolly SJ, Sheldon R, Thorpe KE *et al.* Pacemaker therapy for prevention of syncope in patients with recurrent severe vasovagal syncope: Second Vasovagal Pacemaker Study (VPS II): a randomized trial. JAMA 2003; 289:2224–9.

12 Michaud GF, Pelosi F Jr, Noble MD *et al.* A randomized trial comparing heparin initiation 6h or 24h after pacemaker or defibrillator implantation. J Am Coll Cardiol 2000; 35:1915–8.

13 Morse D, Parsonnet V, Gessman L *et al.*, eds. A guide to cardiac pacemakers, defibrillators, and related products. North Carolina: Droege Computing Services, 1991.

14 Schoenfeld MH. Pacemaker programmers: an updated synopsis. Cardiac Electrophysiol Rev 1999; 3:20–3.

15 Blitzer ML, Marieb MA, Schoenfeld MH. Inability to communicate with ICDs: an underreported failure mode. Pacing Clin Electrophysiol 2001; 24:13–5.

16 Danilovic D, Ohm OH. Pacing threshold trends and variability in modern tined leads assessed using high resolution automatic measurements: conversion of pulse width into voltage thresholds. Pacing Clin Electrophysiol 1999; 22:567–87.

17 Schoenfeld MH, Markowitz HT. Device follow-up in the age of automaticity. Pacing Clin Electrophysiol 2000; 23:803–6.

18 Wilkoff BL, Cook JR, Epstein AE *et al*. Dual-chamber pacing or ventricular back-up pacing in patients with an implantable defibrillator: the Dual Chamber and VVI Defibrillator (DAVID) Trial. JAMA 2002; 288:3115–23.

19 Sweeney MO, Shea JB, Fox V *et al*. Randomized pilot study of a new atrial-based minimal ventricular pacing mode in dual-chamber implantable cardioverter-defibrillators. Heart Rhythm 2004; 1:160–7.

20 Sweeney MO. Minimizing right ventricular pacing: a new paradigm for cardiac pacing in sinus node dysfunction. Am Heart J 2007; 153:34–43.

21 Vardas PE, Simantrakis EN, Parthenakis FL *et al*. AAIR versus DDDR pacing in patients with impaired sinus node chronotropy: an echocardiographic and cardiopulmonary study. Pacing Clin Electrophysiol 1997; 20:1762–8.

22 Meluzin J, Novak M, Mullerov AJ *et al*. A fast and simple echocardiographic method of determination of the optimal atrioventricular delay in patients after biventricular stimulation. Pacing Clin Electrophysiol 2004; 27:58–64.

23 Theuns DA, Res JC, Jordaens LJ. Home monitoring in ICD therapy: future perspectives. Europace 2003; 5:139–42.

24 Schoenfeld MH, Compton SJ, Mead RH *et al*. Remote monitoring of implantable cardioverter-defibrillators: a prospective analysis. Pacing Clin Electrophysiol 2004; 27:757–63.

25 Gregoratos G, Abrams J, Epstein AE *et al*. ACC/AHA/NASPE 2002 guideline update for implantation of cardiac pacemakers and antiarrhythmia devices: Summary article: A report of the American College of Cardiology/American Heart Association Task Force on Practice Guidelines (ACC/AHA/NASPE Committee to Update the 1998 Pacemaker Guidelines). Circulation 2002; 106:2145–61.

26 Maisel WH. Pacemaker and ICD generator reliability: meta-analysis of device registries. JAMA 2006; 295:1929–34.

27 Gould PA, Krahn AD. The Canadian Heart Rhythm Society Working Group on Device Advisories: Complications associated with implantable cardioverter defibrillator replacement in response to device advisories. JAMA 2006; 295:1907–11.

28 Amin MS, Matcher DB, Wood MA, Ellenbogen KA. Management of recalled pacemakers and implantable cardioverter-defibrillators: a decision analysis model. JAMA 2006; 296:412–20.

29 Carlson MD, Wilkoff BL, Maisel WH *et al*. Recommendations from the Heart Rhythm Society task force on device performance policies and guidelines. Heart Rhythm 2006; 3:1250–73.

30 Dubner S, Dubner Y, Gallino S *et al*. Electromagnetic interference with implantable cardiac pacemakers by video capsule. Gastrointest Endosc 2005; 61:250–4.

31 Levine PA, Barold SS, Fletcher RD, Talbot P. Adverse acute and chronic effects of electrical defibrillation and cardioversion of implanted unipolar cardiac pacing systems. J Am Coll Cardiol 1983; 1:1413–22.

32 Gimbel JR, Johnson D, Levine PA *et al*. Safe performance of magnetic resonance imaging on five patients with permanent cardiac pacemakers. Pacing Clin Electrophysiol 1996; 19:913–9.

33 Faris OP, Shein M. Food and Drug Administration perspective: magnetic resonance imaging of pacemaker and implantable cardioverter-defibrillator patients. Circulation 2006; 114:1232–3.

34 Sommer T, Naehle CP, Yang A *et al*. Strategy for safe performance of extrathoracic magnetic resonance imaging at 1.5 Tesla in the presence of cardiac pacemakers in non-pace-

maker-dependent patients: a prospective study with 115 examinations. Circulation 2006; 114:1285–92.

35 Nazarian S, Roguin A, Zviman MM *et al.* Clinical utility and safety of a protocol for non-cardiac and cardiac magnetic resonance imaging of patients with permanent pacemakers and implantable cardioverter defibrillators at 1.5 tesla. Circulation 2006; 114:1277–84.

36 Cooper D, Wilkoff B, Masterson M *et al.* Effects of extracorporeal shock wave lithotripsy on cardiac pacemakers and its safety in patients with implanted cardiac pacemakers. Pacing Clin Electrophysiol 1988; 11:1607–16.

37 Hayes DL, Wang PJ, Reynolds DW *et al.* Interference with cardiac pacemakers by cellular telephones. N Engl J Med 1997; 336:1473–9.

38 Blitzer ML, Schoenfeld MH. Effects of electromagnetic interference on implanted cardiac devices. In: Raviele A, ed. Cardiac arrhythmias 2003. Milan: Springer-Verlag Italia, 2004:911–8.

39 McIvor ME, Reddinger J, Floden E, Sheppard RC. Study of pacemaker and implantable cardioverter defibrillator triggering by electronic article surveillance devices (SPICED TEAS). Pacing Clin Electrophysiol 1998; 221:1847–61.

40 Philbin DM, Marieb MA, Aithal KH, Schoenfeld MH. Inappropriate shocks delivered by an ICD as a result of sensed potentials from a transcutaneous electronic nerve stimulation unit. Pacing Clin Electrophysiol 1998; 21:2010–1.

41 Barold SS, Herweg B, Curtis AB. Electrocardiographic diagnosis of myocardial infarction and ischemia during cardiac pacing. Cardiol Clin 2006; 24:387–99.

Index